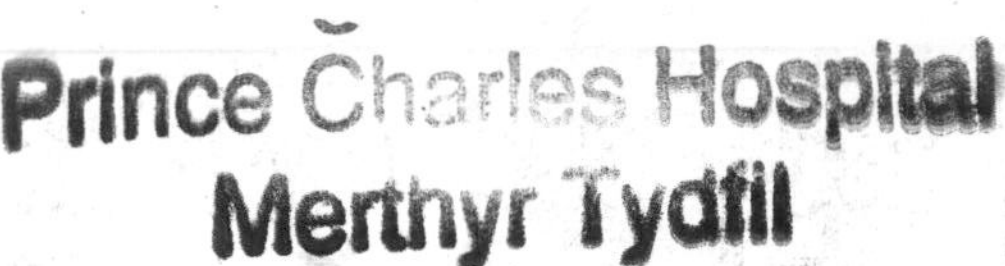

Common Foundation Studies in Nursing

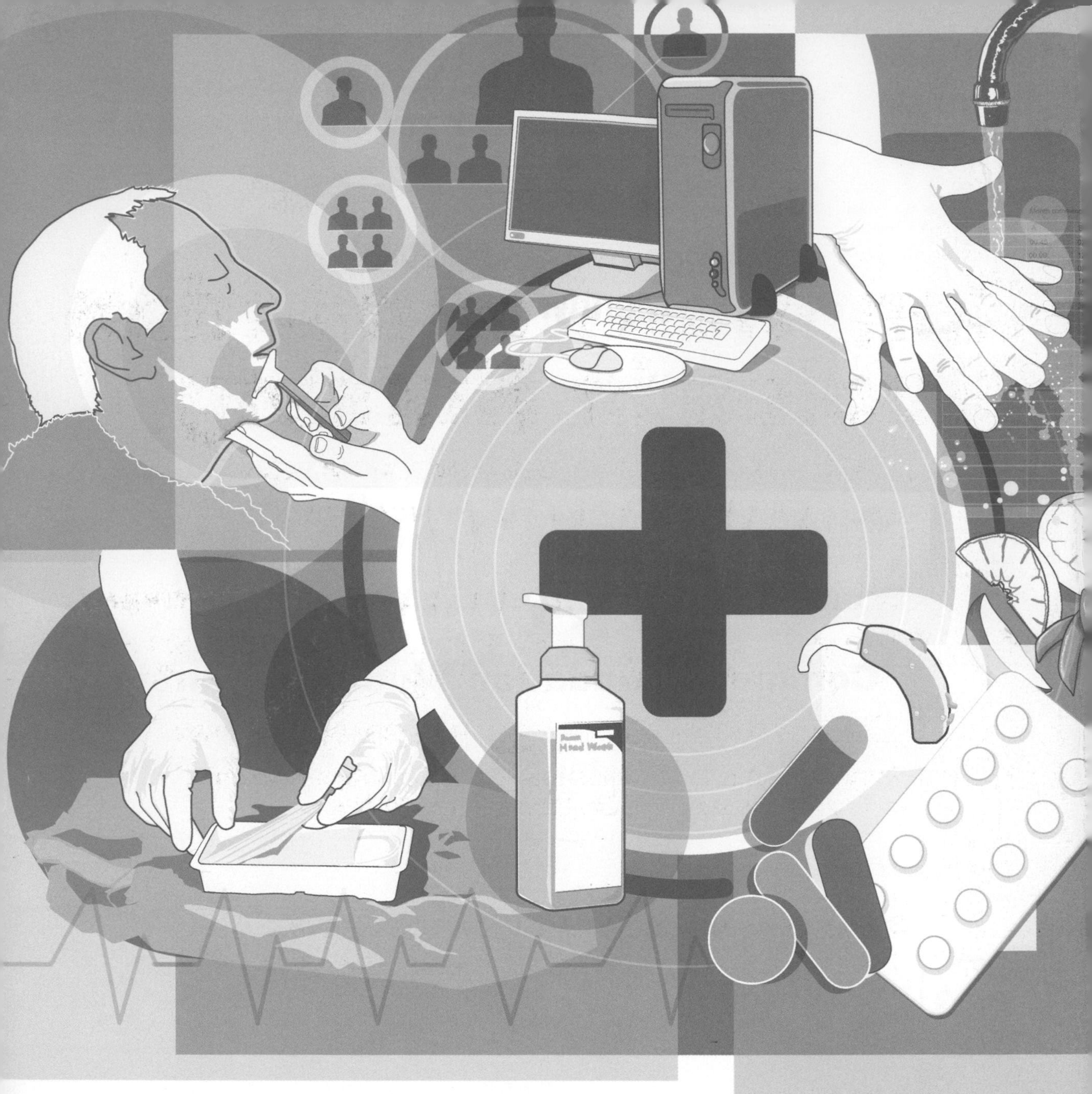

For Elsevier:

Senior Commissioning Editor: *Ninette Premdas*
Development Editor: *Mairi McCubbin*
Project Manager: *Christine Johnston*
Designer: *Stewart Larking*
Illustration Manager: *Merlyn Harvey*
Illustrator: *Graeme Chambers*

Common Foundation Studies in Nursing

Jenny **Spouse** MSc PhD DipN RN SCM RNT RCNT

Associate Dean for Practice Education, St Bartholomew School of Nursing and Midwifery, City University, London, UK

Mike **Cook** MSc(EdMgt) MSc(QuMgt) EdD CertEd DipN(Lond) RN RNT

Deputy Head of Education & Development, East of England Strategic Health Authority, East of England Multi-Professional Deanery, Cambridge, UK

Carol **Cox** BSc(Hons) MSc MAEd PhD PGDipEd CertCHP RN

Professor of Advanced Clinical Practice, St Bartholomew School of Nursing and Midwifery, City University, London, UK

Foreword by

Sir Jonathan Asbridge DSci RGN

Past President, Nursing and Midwifery Council, London, UK

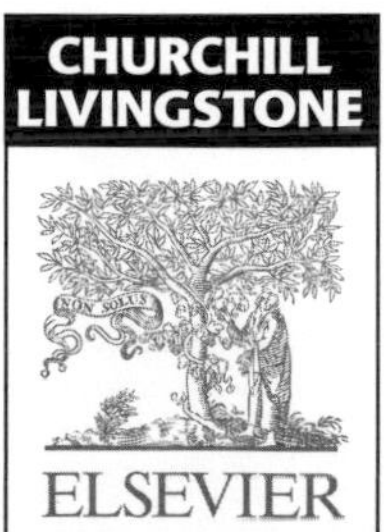

Edinburgh London New York Oxford Philadelphia St Louis Sydney Toronto 2008

CHURCHILL
LIVINGSTONE

First edition 1992
Second edition 1996
Third edition 2002
Fourth edition 2008

ISBN-13: 978 0 443 10154 0

British Library Cataloguing in Publication Data
A catalogue record for this book is available from the British Library

Library of Congress Cataloging in Publication Data
A catalog record for this book is available from the Library of Congress

Notice
Knowledge and best practice in this field are constantly changing. As new research and experience broaden our knowledge, changes in practice, treatment and drug therapy may become necessary or appropriate. Readers are advised to check the most current information provided (i) on procedures featured or (ii) by the manufacturer of each product to be administered, to verify the recommended dose or formula, the method and duration of administration, and contraindications. It is the responsibility of the practitioner, relying on their own experience and knowledge of the patient, to make diagnoses, to determine dosages and the best treatment for each individual patient, and to take all appropriate safety precautions. To the fullest extent of the law, neither the Publisher nor the Editors assumes any liability for any injury and/or damage to persons or property arising out of or related to any use of the material contained in this book.

The Publisher

Printed in China

Contents

Contributors

Jane Akister **MSc(Oxon)**
Senior Lecturer in Social Work, Anglia Polytechnic University, Chelmsford, UK

11 Managing self and setting priorities in placements

William Blows **BSc(Hons) PhD RMN RNT OStJ**
Lecturer in Biological Sciences, St Bartholomew School of Nursing and Midwifery, City University, London, UK

7 Communication between patients, carers and health care professionals

Shuling Breckenridge **MSc RN**
Lecturer, St Bartholomew School of Nursing and Midwifery, City University, London, UK

7 Communication between patients, carers and health care professionals

Mike Cook **MSc(EdMgt) MSc(QuMgt) EdD CertEd DipN(Lond) RN RNT**
Deputy Head of Education & Development, East of England Strategic Health Authority, East of England Multi-Professional Deanery, Cambridge, UK

11 Managing self and setting priorities in placements

13 Promoting safe practice

Alison Coutts **BSc MSc PGCEA RGN**
Lecturer, Applied Biological Sciences, St Bartholomew School of Nursing and Midwifery, London, UK

8 Food and nutrition

Carol Cox **BSc(Hons) MSc MAEd PhD PGDipEd CertCHP RN**
Professor of Advanced Clinical Practice, St Bartholomew School of Nursing and Midwifery, City University, London, UK

9 Hygiene

Maria Dingle **BA MSc RN**
Senior Lecturer in Applied Biological Sciences, St Bartholomew School of Nursing and Midwifery, City University, London, UK

9 Hygiene

Christine Ely **BA MSc RN**
Lecturer, St Bartholomew School of Nursing and Midwifery, City University, London, UK

2 How to study and learn effectively

Ann Jackson Fowler **BSc(Hons) RGN DPSN**
Head of Department, Placement Development and Support, Institute of Health and Social Care, Anglia Ruskin University, East Road, Cambridge, UK

11 Managing self and setting priorities in placements

Alex Grayson **RN**
Freelance writer

9 Hygiene

Anne Harriss **BEd MSc RGN OHNC MIOSH**
Reader in Educational Development and Course Director Occupational Health Nursing, Faculty of Health, London South Bank University, London, UK

13 Promoting safe practice

Margaret Lane **MSc DipNE(Lond) RCNT RSCN**
Associate Dean of Students, St Bartholomew School of Nursing and Midwifery, City University, London, UK

1 Becoming a nurse

Maria Lorentzon **BSc MSc PhD SRN SCM**
Visiting Senior Fellow, European Institute for Health and Medical Sciences, University of Surrey, Guildford, UK

3 The emotional labour of nursing

Scott Reeves **BSc MSc PGCE PhD**
Associate Professor, Faculty of Medicine, University of Toronto, Toronto, Canada

10 Working in a team

Ian Scott **BSc PhD CNAA**
Senior Lecturer, Accreditation of Prior Learning, St Bartholomew School of Nursing and Midwifery, City University, London, UK

2 How to study and learn effectively

Pam Smith **BNurs PhD RGN RNT**
Professor of Nurse Education and Director, Centre for Research in Nursing and Midwifery Education, The European Institute of Health and Medical Sciences, University of Surrey, Guildford, UK

3 The emotional labour of nursing

Alison Spires **BSc(Hons) MSc MA DipNEd RGN RM RCNT**
Principal Lecturer, Adult Nursing, Faculty of Health and Social Care, London South Bank University, London, UK

5 Learning and working as a nursing student in a multicultural world

Jenny Spouse **MSc PhD DipN RN SCM RNT RCNT**
Associate Dean for Practice Education, St Bartholomew School of Nursing and Midwifery, City University, London, UK

1 Becoming a nurse

6 Using a 'toolkit' of activities in your placement

Verina Waights **BSc(Hons) PhD**
Lecturer in Professional Health Care Education, Faculty of Health and Social Care, The Open University, Milton Keynes, UK

12 Decision-making in practice

Hannele Weir **BA(Hons) MSc PGCE RHV RGN**
Lecturer in Applied Sociology, St Bartholomew School of Nursing and Midwifery, City University, London, UK

8 Food and nutrition

Isabelle Whaite **MA CertEd DPSN RGN RM RCNT RNT**
Associate Head of Department of Nursing, University of Central Lancashire, Preston, UK

4 Professional standards and rules: the professional regulatory body and the nursing student

Foreword

I am delighted to recommend this text to people embarking on their studies of nursing and nursing care. Within the past decade, the patient/client has increasingly become the centre of health care provision. Moreover, nursing care has many distinguished practitioners and writers who have long campaigned for holistic patient care and most nursing students embark on their career believing that holistic care is the essence of their practice.

With the rapid changes in health care provision and advances in medical technology, nurses are finding that their contribution is more significant than ever before. Their knowledge, skills and practice have even greater importance for effective patient/client care and the successful provision of health care. As key members of the health and social care team, their skilled contribution is even more vital.

This book introduces the reader to fundamental concepts of nursing that will assist the nursing student in their new role. The vibrancy and energy of nursing is clearly evident within the narrative of this foundation text, which provides an introduction to the professional role within the contemporary health care system, the key biological sciences, concepts of health and illness, the nature of the nurse–patient/client relationship and, most importantly, the essence of care.

This fourth edition builds on the excellent work of its predecessors and reflects the significant changes in nursing education and health care provision. The text recognizes the diversity of knowledge, age and experience that contemporary nursing students bring to the profession, as well as the complexity of modern society and so, inevitably, that of the people who look to good nursing care for their health and recovery from illness.

I welcome you to this first stage of your new profession and commend this text to you.

London, 2007 Jonathan Asbridge

Preface

Welcome to this fourth edition of *Common Foundations Studies in Nursing*. It is a completely new edition, in which every chapter has been totally reviewed; some chapters are completely new and others have been revised and updated. We hope that you will find the chapters and the illustrations informative and supportive of your studies to become a nurse. We have written the text mindful that entering nursing can hold many new experiences and that often these can be quite overwhelming, so much so that for many new nursing students the realization that there is so much to learn and assimilate can be quite shocking. We hope that the various case histories will capture your imagination in a meaningful and memorable manner and that you will be able to draw on the lessons in your reading and relate them to your everyday practice experiences of patient care. Similarly, we hope that you will recognize situations from your own practice when you are reading the text and appreciate the value of studying. With the rapid changes in society, in health care technology and health care provision, the importance of developing your professional knowledge is very great, not only so that you can be successful in your examinations but also so that you can deliver high standards of care to your clients/patients with confidence and expertise.

This book is divided into three sections and the focus is very much on the kinds of knowledge that will take you through the first year of your common foundation programme. The sections reflect the four domains of knowledge identified by the Nursing and Midwifery Council of the United Kingdom for successful completion of the common foundation programme and your branch programme. These domains are concerned with professional and ethical practice, care delivery, care management, and personal and professional development. In each of the sections of the book we have promoted the importance of respecting the rights of the individual and their specific beliefs and values, and this reflects the emphasis on patient-centred care that is communicated in national and professional policies and documents.

The different sections of the book are distinctive. Section 1 is concerned with helping you to become an effective student, both in the academic setting and in your placements, and explores some of the more immediate aspects of learning to become a professional practitioner. Section 2 introduces you to the concepts associated with safe and effective nursing practice, which an American nurse, Barbara Carper, identified as the art and science of essential care. Section 3 is concerned with how you manage your time, your relationships and how to ensure that at all times you act in such a way as to regard the safety of your patients and colleagues, not least yourself.

The contents of this book offer you as a nursing student a broad insight into issues related to practice that are commonly addressed in all common foundation nursing programmes. The book does not claim to be a definitive work, but presents a sample of issues from writers, many of whom have an international reputation in the field of nursing. The difficulty we had as editors was not what to include in the collection, but rather knowing what to leave out, for we truly discovered that there is a vast range of excellent material available for the student to read, much of which we would have loved to have included in this book. The genesis of this book was to provide access to these materials for nursing students studying at foundation level.

Section 1: Personal, professional and ethical aspects of becoming a nurse

In Section 1 we focus on the Nursing and Midwifery Council domains relating to personal, professional and ethical factors of becoming a nurse and being a nursing student. Section 1 is made up of six chapters each dealing with different aspects of being a nursing student. It is concerned with the personal and professional implications and obligations of learning and working in health care settings as a learner. As you start on your professional career and work towards becoming a nursing student, you may find much of the information you receive somewhat overwhelming and even bewildering. Many students start their career with feelings of anticipation and trepidation. Before they start the programme, students rarely anticipate that they will feel confused and perhaps even lonely as they struggle to balance all the different and additional demands on their lives. There is the ambiguity of being a university student, which symbolizes freedom, fun and hours of academic work, whilst also becoming a health care professional, which requires selflessness, discipline and physically hard work when engaging intimately with people who find themselves in distressing circumstances. So for many new entrants to nursing it can feel more like an emotional roller coaster. Experiences are often characterized by times of exhilaration from having achieved a goal or being praised for something done well and the thrill of witnessing a child being born. These experiences may be contrasted with being called upon to support someone in mental anguish or experiencing feelings of personal inadequacy whilst watching a person facing death. Emotions of this nature are natural and are often compounded by the uncertainties of starting a new placement with new people and new challenges whilst also facing piles of texts and studying for assignments. Throughout the first section of this book you will find ideas and strategies for addressing many of these experiences and for developing your inner strength as a person and as a practitioner.

Chapter 1 (Becoming a nurse) introduces you to the idea of joining different communities of practice, an academic community and a professional community of nurses. The case histories illustrate how different people chose to become a nurse and give some of their reasons for choosing a particular branch of nursing. These case histories introduce you to the different kinds of nursing that is practised and the kinds of patients you might meet. The chapter also provides some guidance about the support networks available to students in university: the financial as well as the personal support. It discusses the important contribution that every student can make to their programme, as well as providing some suggestions and activities to help you learn how to learn while working in your practice placements.

Chapter 2 (How to study and learn effectively) provides extensive information about how to become an effective student and offers ideas and strategies for improving your study skills as well as your time management so that you have time to study as well as to enjoy yourself. Developing skills of searching the world wide web to obtain information for assignments and to inform your nursing practice will be an essential part of your studies. This chapter will introduce you to some of these necessary skills, as well as teaching you how to store information and write assignments.

Chapter 3 (The emotional labour of nursing) deals with a significant aspect of learning to become a nurse and is concerned with those frequent situations when you will be supporting ill or distressed people. This chapter draws on several research studies and introduces you to the emotional work that all nurses undertake and, through case histories of everyday situations, provides some guidelines on how to respond effectively and professionally.

Chapter 4 (Professional standards and rules: the professional regulatory body and the nursing student). During your programme you will probably encounter several situations that challenge your thinking and beliefs about life and death, health care practice and even your own values. This chapter introduces you to the 'Nursing and Midwifery Council Code of professional conduct'. Through small case examples it will show you how the 'NMC Code of professional conduct' relates to you as a nursing student whilst introducing some of the ethical dilemmas that you may face. The aim of this chapter is to introduce you to some of the ethical dilemmas you might encounter and to teach you how to develop your own solutions to the different kinds of ethical conundrums you are likely to face as a nurse.

A new version of the Code of professional conduct is published in January 2008. You need to obtain a copy from the NMC website (www.nmc-uk.org) to compare with the 2004 Version in the Appendix.

Chapter 5 (Learning and working as a nursing student in a multicultural world) provides an introduction to the diversity of living and working in a multicultural society. It discusses some of the implications of the global economy on health care provision and working as a nurse in a range of settings. In particular it explores some of the beliefs and values held by people from different cultures about health and illness, and how as a nurse you should be respecting and responding to their needs when they are dependent upon others for their everyday care.

Chapter 6 (Using a 'toolkit' of activities in your placement). In this chapter you will find a sequence of activities designed to help you learn from your practice experiences. It teaches you how to recognize what is happening around you, to understand its significance and to develop the vocabulary needed to function effectively in everyday practice and as a team member. The chapter is made up of a range of different activities for you to do while you are in practice. By undertaking these suggested activities you will also gain in confidence and understanding of your role. If you have clinical placements in more than one practice setting, you will find it helpful to copy the exercises (or download them from the world wide web (http://evolve.elsevier.com/Spouse/commonfoundation) and work your way through them in each new practice placement. You will notice that the exercises are designed to help you meet the outcomes required by the Nursing and Midwifery Council of all common foundation programme students to continue on to their branch programme, so you will find that the exercises will help you prepare for your written and practical assignments.

Section 2: Essentials of care delivery

This section addresses the second major area of study for nursing students: the delivery of patient care that is holistic, patient-focused and evidence-based. Each chapter is concerned with a core element of care delivery: communication between patients, carers and health care professionals; food and nutrition; and personal and oral hygiene. These chapters provide information about relevant anatomy and physiology and some of the frequently encountered disorders of the different aspects of care. We chose these particular areas of care delivery as they have been identified by the Department of Health (in the 'Essence of care' benchmark standards) and by the National Assembly of Wales (in the 'Fundamentals of care' project) as being critical to patient recovery. Other aspects of care delivery, such as documentation, health and safety, are discussed in Section 3.

Each chapter in Section 2 is focused on both the art and the science of nursing practice, and stress the importance of getting the basics right, indicating that this is essential if patient/client/carer care is to improve. The chapters have been written using a patient-focused approach to help you consider your own practice experiences critically by using the knowledge from these chapters.

Chapter 7 (Communication between patients, carers and health care professionals). In this chapter, you will learn about the importance of effective communication that is patient-focused. It stresses that patients and carers should experience effective communication that is sensitive to their individual needs and preferences and how good-quality communication can promote high-quality care for patients. Throughout the chapter there is recognition that for interactions to be effective and therapeutic there must be recognition of the patient as a person who happens to be ill. Some of the factors that can inhibit or affect good communication are discussed in relation to relevant anatomy and physiology and case histories taken from practice. The components of the communication process are described and the style of the interaction required is presented in relation to personality and culture. Throughout the chapter, you are encouraged to think and act in a manner that is sensitive and flexible to the needs and communication style of your patients, their family and your colleagues, in order to strengthen your relationships with them.

Chapter 8 (Food and nutrition). Without adequate food and nutrition, people cannot maintain their health. In many hospitals and care homes, where patients and residents are very dependent on the organization and the carers to ensure that their nutritional needs are met, the quality of food is heavily criticized for not meeting these nutritional needs. This chapter discusses the different policies and strategies being implemented throughout the UK to address this matter. Another important aspect of nutrition discussed in this chapter is the influence of national and international policies on food production and food delivery. It also explores some of the issues and factors that are affecting society and the consequences of so many people having only a poor understanding of the importance of nutrition and the kinds of foods that are essential for a healthy lifestyle. Finally, the chapter explores the importance of nutrition in ill-health where a healthy diet is vital to promote healing and recovery from illness. So this chapter will discuss the nature of a healthy diet, how it contributes to normal cell growth and repair, the processes by which food is assimilated, growth is promoted and tissue repaired in living organisms. In doing so it will consider recent government policies and white papers, practices that shape food availability and selection, and the impact they have on health and illness. The chapter demonstrates the extent to which the production of food has become a globalized and politicized industry and that nutrition is complex and often poorly understood, leading to unhealthy lifestyles and ultimately ill-health.

Chapter 9 (Hygiene). Helping people to maintain their personal hygiene is an essential aspect of mental and physical care. Through such a fundamental activity the knowledgeable nurse can detect a range of factors that might be impacting on their patient's well-being. The chapter provides an opportunity to assess your patient's mental, physical and social state and to begin strategies to address any areas of need. In order to achieve this, nurses need to understand the normal state of the skin (otherwise known as the integumentary system), its supporting structures and the mouth. As you read through this chapter, you will explore how to help maintain personal and oral hygiene and to understand the related anatomy and physiology, including discussion about the hair, glands of the skin and nails and the associated physiological functions of, for example, temperature regulation, infection control and strategies to promote safety, comfort, privacy and dignity.

Section 3: Care management

Section 3 of this book is concerned with the fourth requirement of the professional statutory organization: that nurses should develop management and leadership skills. Thus this section will introduce you to some of the fundamental aspects of working within a multidisciplinary health care team to promote the safety and well-being of your patients and your colleagues.

Chapter 10 (Working in a team) introduces you to the concept of effective teamworking, in particular the role of other health care professionals and the importance of effective communication by the different members of the team. The chapter also discusses the contributions other team members make to enable effective care delivery. It also provides an introduction to working alongside your mentor or practice placement supervisor and how their role is essential to supporting your learning and professional development. Throughout the chapter you will see how you can play an important part in ensuring that high-quality care is delivered.

Chapter 11 (Managing self and setting priorities in placement). In this chapter you will look at some of the processes that you need to consider when working as a member of the clinical team whilst learning in your practice placements. It is well recognized that the pressures of an increasingly technological age and government demands for greater efficiency – measured with throughputs rather than quality – makes compassionate caring more difficult to achieve. What is indisputable is the extent to which good nursing makes a difference to each patient's experience of care. Many practitioners strive to implement their vision of high-quality care that is patient-centred, but they are often frustrated by the pressures under which they are working. As a nursing student learning in and from practice, you will inevitably be exposed to the same kinds of pressures. This chapter will help you to think about how to manage care as it relates to the various aspects of the Nursing and Midwifery Council outcomes for entry to the branch programme. Specifically, you will learn about: managing your time and yourself in relation to other staff and in relation to patients or other service users, whilst learning and working in your practice placement; setting priorities and managing your work and patient care; communication skills and documentation; the importance of confidentiality; and, looking after yourself. Each of these elements examines your role as a developing practitioner and discusses issues that you might encounter through the process. Also explored is the importance of having safeguards to promote ethical practice and to prevent the misuse of power in the caring professions.

Chapter 12 (Decision-making in practice). This chapter focuses on helping you to make clinical decisions associated with care and will help you to understand the importance of effective communication between everyone associated with care delivery and care management. Even though you are just embarking on your nursing career and are a common foundation programme nursing student, you will find that almost every activity that you undertake will require you to make a decision of some kind. In this chapter you will learn some useful strategies that will help you frame a problem, and then to use different approaches to explore how to address it effectively. You will know from reading earlier chapters in this text that nurses are responsible for their decisions at a professional level and the Nursing and Midwifery Council make this clear in their 'Code of professional conduct'. Where possible, these decisions should be made on the basis of sound evidence; but such evidence is not always available, so it then becomes even more important to have a clear framework to help you arrive at a satisfactory decision. In this chapter you will learn about what is evidence-based practice, the importance of decision-making, using the nursing process and the various kinds of models that can be used when assessing a patient for their health and nursing care needs. Using models of assessment, using frameworks for decision-making, some ideas about making decisions on-your-feet, and the importance of documentation and record-keeping are discussed. Understanding these different aspects of decision-making is essential to ensure effective communication between different members of the health care team and to ensure the safety or your patients. By documenting your decisions it means that every other carer will know what and why specific care has been provided to the patient.

Chapter 13 (Promoting safe practice) draws on one of the most publicized of nurses, Florence Nightingale, who in fact was a very able administrator and mathematician. She recognized that 'The very first requirement in a hospital is that it should do the sick no harm'. You will probably have read and heard about health care delivery in the news, and the often cited reports of hospital-acquired infections, as well as incidents that have happened to patients and nursing staff that might have been avoided if the people involved had followed the policies and procedures of their organization. Risk assessment and management, health and safety at work and infection control are all important daily considerations of nurses, and are just a few of the many factors that require close attention if we are to ensure that Nightingale's maxim is observed. In this chapter, you will learn about some of these factors and about some of the strategies designed to promote health and safety at work. You may find that these strategies have relevance to you at home as well as in your daily working life, and we hope that you will consider them thoughtfully to the advantage of you, your colleagues and most of all your patients.

Throughout the book we have emphasized the important contribution you will be making to the health and well-being of your patients and the centrality of patients to all your nursing practice. We very much hope that you will find each of the chapters a useful introduction to the kinds of professional and personal knowledge that will equip you for your common foundation studies in nursing and that you will be successful in your chosen career.

London, 2007

Jenny Spouse
Carol Cox
Mike Cook

Acknowledgements

The editors would like to extend particular thanks to those authors who contributed to the original chapters in the third edition and whose work has provided the foundation for the current volume:

Andrew Betts (7 Communication between patients, carers and health care professionals).

Pat Downer (12 Decision-making in practice).

Tracey Heath (12 Decision-making in practice; 13 Promoting safe practice).

Pam Taylor (12 Decision-making in practice; 13 Promoting safe practice).

They would also like to thank **Rachel Beadle**, City University, who took the photographs specially commissioned for the book.

Section One

Personal, professional and ethical aspects of becoming a nurse

Jenny Spouse

CHAPTERS

This first section of the book is made up of six chapters, each concerned with various aspects of the personal, professional and ethical aspects of being a nursing student. It is concerned with the personal and professional implications and obligations of learning and working in health care settings as a learner. As you start on your professional career towards become a nursing student, you may find much of the information you receive somewhat overwhelming and even bewildering. Many students start their careers with feelings of anticipation and trepidation. What they rarely anticipate is the feeling of confusion and perhaps even loneliness as they struggle to balance all the additional demands on their lives, the ambiguity of being university students (which symbolizes freedom, fun and hours of academic work), while at the same time becoming a health care professional (which insists on selflessness, discipline and physically hard work when engaging intimately with people who find themselves in distressing circumstances). So, for many new entrants to nursing, it can feel more like an emotional roller coaster: times of exhilaration with having achieved a goal or being praised for something done well or the thrill of witnessing a child being born, contrasting with supporting someone in mental anguish or watching a person facing death, and experiencing feelings of inadequacy coupled with anticipation of starting a new placement, with new people and new challenges, facing piles of texts, studying for assignments. In this section, you will find ideas and strategies for addressing many of these experiences and for developing your inner strengths as a person and a practitioner.

Chapter 1 introduces you to the idea of joining different communities of practice: an academic community and a professional community of nurses. It describes the stories of different people who chose to become a nurse and some of their reasons for choosing a particular branch of nursing. The case histories illustrate the different kinds of nursing that is practised and the types of patients you might meet. The chapter also provides some guidance about the support networks that are available to students in university: the financial as well as the personal support. It discusses the important contribution that every student can make to their programme, as well as providing some suggestions and activities to help you work and learn in your practice placement.

Chapter 2 provides extensive information about how to become an effective student, and offers ideas and strategies for improving your study skills as well as your time management so that you have time to study as well as enjoy yourself. Developing skills of searching the world wide web to obtain information for assignments and to inform your nursing practice will be an essential part of your studies. This chapter introduces you to some of these necessary skills, as well as teaching you how to store information and write assignments.

Chapter 3 describes a significant aspect of being a nurse when supporting ill or distressed people. It draws on several research studies and introduces you to the emotional work that all nurses undertake, and provides some guidelines as to how to respond effectively and professionally.

During your programme you will probably encounter several situations that challenge your thinking and beliefs about life and death, health care practice and even your own values. Chapter 4 introduces you to the 'Nursing and Midwifery Council Code of professional conduct'. Through small case examples, you will see how the Code of professional conduct relates to you as a nursing student whilst introducing some of the ethical dilemmas that you may face. It cannot provide any answers but it helps you to develop your own solutions.

Chapter 5 provides an introduction to the diversity of living and working in a multicultural society. It discusses some of the implications of the global economy on health care provision and working as a nurse in a range of settings. In particular, it explores some of the beliefs and values about health and illness that are held by people from different cultures, and their needs when dependent upon other people for their everyday care.

Chapter 6 is rather different as it contains a series of activities for you to do while you are in practice and which are designed to help you recognize what is happening around you and to understand the significance of these happenings. The activities are designed to help you learn how to learn from your practice experiences and to relate what you have learned from your 'classroom sessions' and from your reading to what you are doing in your practice placement.

By undertaking the suggested activities you should gain in confidence and understanding of your role. If you have clinical placements in more than one practice setting, you will find it helpful to copy the exercises (you will find blank copies of the templates at http://evolve.elsevier.com/Spouse/commonfoundation) and work your way through them in each new practice placement. As the exercises are designed to help you meet the learning outcomes required by the Nursing and Midwifery Council of all foundation course students to continue to their branch programme, you will find that the exercises will also help you prepare for your assignments.

Chapter One

1

Becoming a nurse

Jenny Spouse, Margaret Lane

Key topics

- Having a personal vision about being a nurse
- Formalizing the vision
- The professional statutory organization for nursing in the UK
- Careers in nursing
- Learning to become a nurse
- Making the best of learning experiences
- Student services and financial help
- Joining the community of practice in academic settings
- Having a voice in the organization of your programme
- Joining the community of nursing practice
- Learning and working in clinical placement settings

Introduction

This chapter describes some of the experiences you are likely to undergo during your programme to become a nurse. Drawing on various sources of information, including research into how nursing students learn, it introduces you to the idea of becoming a member of several different communities of practice: the global community of the nursing profession and of health care practitioners; the community of your university where you are studying to become a nurse; and the various micro-communities of your peer group and your placement colleagues. As you progress through this chapter, you will be exploring some of the challenges you might face while making the transition from being an outsider to an insider of such communities during your journey to become a nurse. You will be learning strategies for minimizing any difficulties and how to identify and make the most of opportunities; we will also explore some of the factors that have an effect on your experiences of nursing. Guidelines are provided for making successful progress through your programme and in particular why developing strong peer support networks can transform your university and professional experiences and make your success more likely. Also included in the chapter is information about the various university resources that are designed specifically to help students be successful. Resources such as the student services, occupational health department and the students' union could be important to your success or to that of a friend. Being familiar with the university governance structure, designed to promote academic quality, can provide another important resource for students as it is the committee structure of the university that can provide a forum for students to exercise their democratic rights and to contribute to programme development, programme management and policy development. Thus, in this chapter, we also describe how to become a student representative.

What is nursing?

At this point we would like you to think about why you want to be a nurse, what you imagine you will be doing and to introduce some of the factors that regulate the profession and protect the public. Further on, in Section 2, you will read about various definitions of nursing and the specific activities that nurses undertake.

Having a personal vision

Many students enter nursing carrying memories of their own experiences of being nursed, either by a parent or by a professional practitioner. Sometimes such experiences leave a desire to replicate the same kind of care for another person. Many students describe their concept of nursing care along the lines of:

- A professional form of loving.
- Helping someone to feel comfortable and free from physical or emotional pain.
- Helping someone in a quiet and thoughtful manner.
- Recognizing the signs and symptoms of distress as well as knowing what to do to relieve them.
- Being able to put a person at ease.
- Being involved with someone but not in a way that you draw away their energy.
- Being warm and friendly.
- Listening to what a person has to say and trying to be reflective and responsive in a therapeutic manner.

Other students think of nursing more from the technical aspect:

- Being able to give injections.
- Being able to implement a doctor's directions.
- Being able to understand what is happening to someone when they are ill or have injured themselves.
- Understanding why a patient is receiving a particular drug or treatment and how it will help them.
- Giving advice on how to care for someone.

Yet other students see nursing as a means of fulfilling personal ambitions or addressing particular social issues, such as setting up a home for older people, ensuring that a particular group of the community receives better care, as an opportunity to work overseas, and so on (see Activity 1.1).

Activity 1.1

You might find it helpful to jot down your own reasons for wanting to become a nurse.

For many people, nursing entails elements from all of the different aspects listed above. To be successful in your ambition it is important to be clear about what you want to achieve as a nursing practitioner. Many students coming into nursing have seen television programmes in which nursing takes place in emergency or critical-care settings and practice is presented as high drama with close teamwork. This portrayal represents only a tiny fraction of the wide range of opportunities that nursing offers. Rarely represented is what happens to patients in their own homes or the huge contribution nurses make to the general health and welfare of children and their families, to people with mental health problems or to people with long-term illnesses who live successful lives in the community as a result of nurses' work. Case histories 1.1–1.5 describe examples of people who have chosen to work in different areas of nursing. You will see that these nursing students come from a range of backgrounds and experiences and have a clear vision of how they want to be working when they complete their initial programme.

Benjamin's lengthy experience as a teacher inspired him to take the significant step of changing career and to work towards achieving a clear ambition, that of becoming a children's nurse (Case history 1.1, Figures 1.1 and 1.2). He recognized that he would be spending quite a number of years preparing for his new role but felt convinced that this was the right path for him.

Another student, whom we shall call Amina, decided that when she left school she wanted to be a nurse specializing in women's health (Case history 1.2).

Both Benjamin and Amina were influenced by their observations of people around them and were inspired to become nurses as their way of addressing problems they had identified. Mark decided to become a nurse for different reasons, choosing to nurse people with learning disabilities (Case history 1.3).

These students had a strong vision as to why they wanted to be nurses. Other students are less specific but have a clear vision of what they see themselves doing as nurses (see Case histories 1.4 and 1.5).

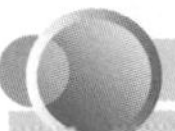

Case history 1.1

Benjamin preparing to be a children's nurse

Benjamin qualified and worked as a teacher in Zimbabwe before coming to teach in the UK. After 5 years he decided that he wanted a change of career and to become a children's nurse. He gave his reasons for the change: "Working in a large city like Leeds I saw many kids who came to school not having had breakfast or who were clearly in a bad shape emotionally. I felt I wanted to learn how to help them from a different perspective. They were not ready to be educated and they needed a different kind of help than what I could give them. I want to train as a children's nurse and then do mental health nursing with the view of helping children and their families in the community as a specialist health practitioner."

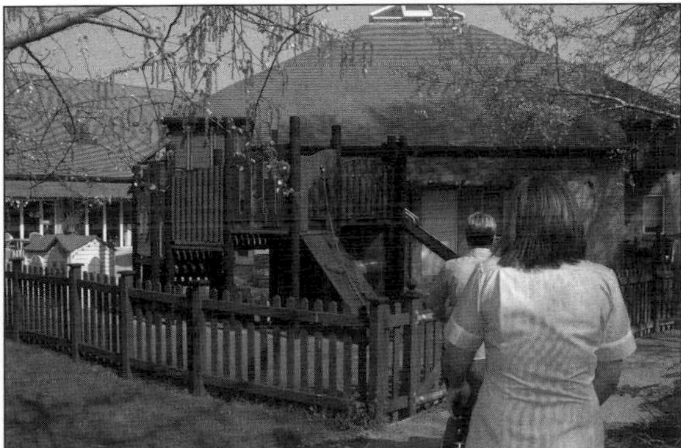

Figure 1.1 • The children's nurse has a role in helping dying children to play.

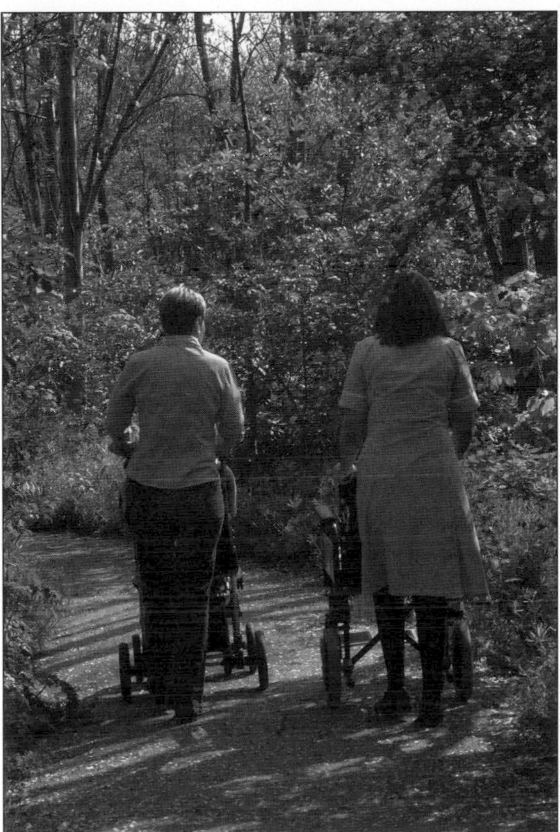

Figure 1.2 • Children's nurses work with the family.

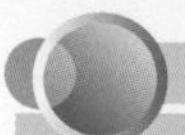

Case history 1.2

Amina's vision of nursing

Growing up in a close Bangladeshi community in the UK, I was aware that many of my mother's friends were suffering from different forms of anaemia and depression caused largely by their life style, which is so different from living in a hot country. I was also aware that, with the rise of HIV and AIDS, Muslim women have very specific needs that they may not be aware of. While I was at school, I saw various adverts for becoming a nurse and decided that perhaps this was something I could do that would improve women's lives. My plan is to train as a nurse and try to concentrate on women's diseases both through placements in hospitals and clinics and in the community. Eventually, I see myself working from a general practice as a specialist advisor for women's health. I expect to take some counselling courses as well as a course in sexual health once I have qualified.

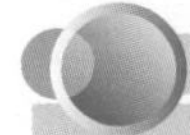

Case history 1.3

Mark, choosing to nurse people with learning disabilities

Being the oldest of four children, I was the one who was responsible for looking after the others. When the youngest one was born I had very mixed feelings about her arrival and I now understand that I was jealous of all the attention she was receiving. It wasn't until some time later, when I noticed that she was not doing the same kinds of things that the others could do, that I began to realize that she was different. In fact, I found out that she had Down's syndrome, a genetic change where someone is born with an extra chromosome. As a result, they often have a number of abnormalities, but the most difficult one is their impaired ability to learn. Hannah was so loving and so much fun, but we had to take special care of her to make sure she was safe as she was always getting into a pickle. I suppose she changed my life, because I realized how difficult it could be for someone with Down's syndrome and for their family if they did not get the right support. My family was very lucky: we had a brilliant community nurse who had trained in learning disabilities. So I decided I would find out more about it as a career. I did some voluntary work in summer camps and worked some shifts in a local community house for a group of four people all with learning disabilities. I found the experience so satisfying that I decided it was what I wanted to do with my life. I was really surprised how much it entailed. It was not just to do with physical and mental health care; education was also a big factor in teaching people to have socially fulfilling lives, as well as knowing about all the state-funded facilities that are available for families and people who have a learning difficulty.

Formalizing nursing practice

All those described in the case histories here chose to become nurses for very personal reasons. However, they also held a strong mental image of how they would be nursing people during their programme and after registration. Quite often the image is a strong incentive to stay on the programme during the times when it feels difficult and even painful. Holding on to a personal vision of what makes good nursing care has been important to good nurses for generations.

Theories of nursing activities and roles

Several notable nurses have recognized that nursing entails a range of special skills and knowledge and have written extensively about how they believe nursing care should be delivered. These writers, known as nursing theorists, have identified approaches to giving care that are based on their specific beliefs about health and illness and the relationship of the nurse to the patient. These approaches, or nursing models, can be used as a guide to providing care. Some models are more appropriate for some specific kinds of nursing and reflect the professional interest of the theorist. Some examples of nursing models and their theorists are:

- Activities of daily living: Roper, Logan and Tierney (1996).
- The nature of nursing: Virginia Henderson (1966).
- A recovery model aimed at specifying the role of the nurse when a patient is in an established recovery stage of their illness: Dorothea Orem (1959).

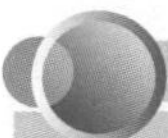

Case history 1.4

Lucy's vision of being a nurse and doing nursing

Both my parents are nurses and I resisted the idea as I felt I wanted to make my own decisions. I got three good 'A' levels at school and decided I should go to university, where I obtained a 2:1 degree in human sciences. However, by the end of the course, having also spent my holidays working as a care assistant, I really felt something was missing from my life and so I began finding out more about nursing. I felt I wanted to care for people and make them feel nice, help them gain their self-esteem and have a fulfilling life. I see myself becoming a 'geriatric nurse'. I know it is a bit of a Cinderella in the nursing profession but I can see myself making a real difference. I am also aware of how complicated the medical condition of older people can be, with so many organs failing and the difficulties of getting medications right for each individual. Doing a postgraduate nursing course means I can qualify more quickly because I get credit for my degree. I am determined to make a career out of this and will go on to do a masters degree and perhaps a doctorate where I can do research into the care of older people.

- The interpersonal relations of nursing (used in some mental health settings): Hildegard Peplau (1952).
- Biophysical aspects of care (often used to support people who are acutely physically ill): Martha Rogers (1970).

Many of the models were developed by American nurses more than 40 years ago and are still used throughout the world. Roper, Logan and Tierney are British nurses, and Henderson's model has been adopted by the International Council of Nurses. If you wish to find out how nursing models are used in practice there are several books that will provide more information (e.g. Pearson et al 2005). Sometimes these models are used at different stages in a patient's illness, going from a high-intervention stage (during the most acute or dependent stage in the illness) to low nurse intervention but high patient autonomy as the person is recovering their independence.

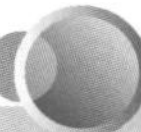

Case history 1.5

Jolene's vision of nursing

Jolene started nursing when she was 35 years old. She has three children between the ages of 7 and 15 years. Before starting her nursing course, Jolene had been a catering manager in her local NHS hospital. As a single parent she had found the hours suited her and was pleased when the Trust introduced a scheme for staff who wanted to take further education courses. Jolene had enrolled and done well, achieving the equivalent of three 'A' levels through national vocational qualifications (NVQs). During her work, she had become aware of what nurses do and she felt that she wanted to improve the quality of her life by becoming a professional. She was accepted at the local university and is now in her third year of the programme. She found the changes difficult to make, especially as many of her mentors were younger than she was. However, what she enjoyed most was the drama of working in the acute surgical wards. She found it very satisfying having people coming in with a lot of discomfort, supporting them through their anxieties of having an anaesthetic and surgery, then making sure they were pain-free afterwards and going home cured. As part of her placement, she had spent three weeks in the intensive care unit (ICU) and had worked alongside some very skilled nurses, caring for patients who were on life-support systems (ventilators, heart monitors and drug infusers). Initially, she had been quite scared of being there, but with her mentor's support she gained in confidence. She then began to see how dependent the patients were on good nursing care and how skilled the nurses were in helping the patients recover both physically and mentally. On a visit to the surgical outpatients department some months later she had been astonished to meet a patient who had recognized her voice from the time she had worked in the ICU. Looking back on the experiences of her course so far, Jolene highlighted these as inspiring her to be a surgical nurse, able to provide total care to people when they are at their most vulnerable. She realizes that she will need to have quite a lot more experience and probably further studies to top-up her diploma to a degree.

Using a nursing model can provide a series of triggers for thinking about how to care for a person when assessing their needs and planning decisions about what care is most appropriate. Normally this process is undertaken collaboratively with the patient and, if permission is given by the patient, in consultation with their carers. Chapter 12 provides detailed help regarding decision-making in nursing practice.

The professional statutory organization for nursing

The Nursing and Midwifery Council of the United Kingdom (NMC) is the current statutory organization charged by the UK parliament to protect the public through regulation of nurses, midwives and health visitors. As part fulfilment of this responsibility, the NMC ensures that every person whose name is on the Professional Register of the Council is fit to practise, fit for purpose and fit for their academic and professional award. To become a registered nurse with the NMC, nursing students must successfully complete a prescribed course of 4600 hours, of which 50% must take place in a practice setting and 50% in the study of theory. The course must also comply with other requirements specified by the European Parliament, which are concerned with the nature of clinical placement experiences. The course may be studied to the level of a diploma in higher education or to a bachelor's degree. England is one of the few nations where nursing students can gain their professional qualification at diploma level and most countries in the UK and Europe require nurses to have studied at degree level in order to register with the NMC.

Throughout the pre-registration nursing course, students' academic and professional knowledge and skills are assessed on a regular basis. These assessments will be undertaken both in the placement setting by registered practitioners and through course work and theory examinations. This means that nursing students are often working in placements while they are studying. This provides an ideal opportunity to learn how theory and practice are interlinked and to use theory in practice and vice versa. Another important factor regulating a student nurse's entry to the Professional Register is assurance that their health and conduct has met the required standards and that they are fit to practise as a professional. You can find out more about the Nursing and Midwifery Council on the NMC website (www.nmc-uk.org).

Careers in nursing

The context of nursing

With changes in demography and patterns of health, many more people are living long and fruitful lives free, for the most part, of acute incidents of illness. However, with improved treatments, many people, including children, are living at home with long-term diseases, whereas several years ago they were either untreatable or required long bouts of treatment in hospitals. As a result, the majority of care is being delivered in the community and many more nurses are training to work as clinical practitioners supporting people in their homes. Health care delivery is also changing to reflect the needs of local communities. The accessibility of walk-in clinics means that many more people can be treated quickly and efficiently without having to visit their general practitioner or go to a hospital. Many general practitioners are offering facilities that were previously only available in hospitals, thereby saving lengthy disruptions to their patients' daily lives. Demographic changes have also had an impact on the health care service needs of the population. In 2003, 23% of the population were more than 60 years of age, many of whom were over 80 years old. For older people, this can mean a full and active life; however, the increasing fragility of their physiological systems predisposes older people to a greater sensitivity to drug therapy and to disease, requiring more skilled care.

The Professional Register

The Professional Register of the NMC has three parts, which distinguish the three categories of practitioners who have specific expertise in health care: midwives, specialist community public health nurses, and nurses. Those wishing to become midwives, specialist community public health nurses or nurses can study on a specific programme designed to prepare them for the role.

The nursing part of the Professional Register has four branches: child health nursing, adult nursing, mental health nursing, and learning disability nursing. Each branch has further specialist areas which registered nurses can study in greater depth. You may be aware that people sometimes first register as, for example, a mental health nurse and then undertake a shorter programme of study to register on another branch of the nursing part of the Professional Register, depending on their career intentions. Others might wish to move their registration to another part of the Register and become a midwife or a specialist community public health nurse.

Specialist community public health nurses practise where they can engage in health promotion work in schools, clinics or in people's homes. Many have previously worked as health visitors, practice nurses, school nurses or community nurses.

Practitioners on all parts of the Professional Register can develop specific expertise and become a consultant (either as a midwife or a nurse). Many practitioners take further courses and study to degree level or to higher degree level (masters or doctoral level) in order to become both practitioner and researcher in their specialist area of nursing care and work as a consultant. Other nurses find that they are more interested in education and want to work as a lecturer or, increasingly, to hold a joint clinical and educational post either within the health care organization or within a university and link across both settings.

Nursing has four specific branches: adult nursing. mental health nursing, children's nursing, and learning disability nursing. Within each branch of nursing there are further clinical specialisms in which practitioners may wish to develop expertise following registration (see, for example, Figure 1.3). For example, a mental health nurse may choose to work with people who suffer from substance abuse (such as alcohol or drugs), or with adolescents, or in forensic psychiatry. Similarly, trained children's nurses can work in a wide range of settings such as caring for children in accident and emergency departments, intensive care units or specialist settings either in hospitals or the community. Others choose to work with families in their homes and have specialist knowledge in

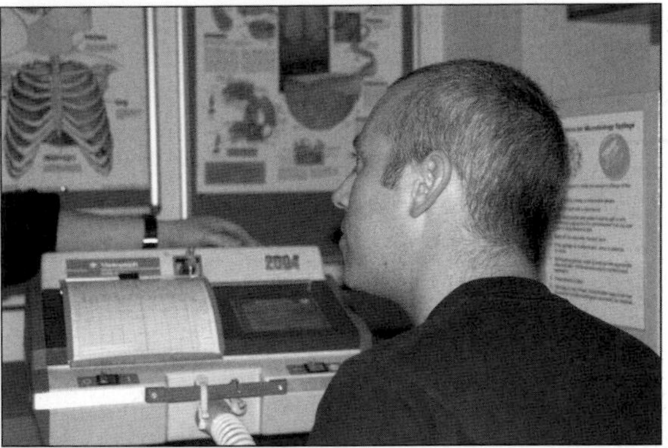

Figure 1.3 • Learning biological sciences.

managing symptoms and diseases such as diabetes or asthma. In adult nursing and learning disability nursing there is a similar range of clinical specialities for which, on registration, a nurse can develop specific expertise and become a consultant nurse.

Learning to become a nurse

Several studies of nursing students (Bradby 1989, Melia 1987, Oleson & Whitaker 1968, Simpson 1967, Spouse 2003) showed that new students find becoming a nurse a considerable challenge. In Spouse's (2003) study, one student described it as having to negotiate his way through the maze of information; another student described the difficulties of juggling all the competing demands on her life (home life, academic life, placements and pleasure). It seemed that the early stages of starting the programme created a state of confusion and disequilibrium for students that only resolved once they realized it wasn't them but the challenge of all the new knowledge they were encountering.

Adjusting to new ways of thinking

A Canadian researching into how adults respond to re-entering learning situations found eight stages in the process (Taylor 1987). She also realized that these stages were cyclical, in that every time adults encountered a radically new approach to thinking, being and working they had to reassess their personal values and beliefs and in essence forgive themselves for not knowing, before they could really absorb the new knowledge! Inevitably, going through each stage is very painful and many people felt confused, perhaps even angry and certainly anxious, which often made them less able to share their sense of inadequacy with their friends and peers. For new students who are used to feeling competent and are respected for their ability to manage tricky situations this is a hard process to go through. Taylor called this stage 'disconfirmation leading to disorientation'. This is a critical stage in learning and some people felt it was too much and decided to leave the course rather than go through the agony of self-doubt, whilst others blamed their teachers for not being good enough in a process called 'projection'. The second major stage Taylor called 'exploration', in which learners came to recognize their difficulties and what was causing them. A useful strategy to get through this stage is talking with friends and peers on the same programme as it is always helpful to gauge personal experiences against those of others in similar situations. Having achieved this stage of exploration, students in Taylor's study began to regain their self-confidence and could then start learning independently. This stage leads onto the stage of 'reorientation', in which learners become more able to make sense of classroom knowledge (or formal knowledge) and to see how all the different elements are related to each other. This is a major step in learning effectively, and some educational researchers describe it as taking a 'deep' approach to learning. With greater familiarity with the language and knowledge, learners could utilize this information in a range of different ways. Having achieved this stage in their learning, Taylor's students were then able to talk and write about their understanding and insights with a certain measure of authority and confidence. Understanding that learning new material is personally challenging and often causes students to feel socially isolated for fear of being 'found out' as being not 'good enough' and the consequent emotional distress this can cause, can help learners to feel more at ease about what they are embarking upon and seek help.

Spouse's (2003) study of nursing students discovered that they progress through similar stages to the students in Taylor's research. However, the differences she identified were related to whether students felt like health care assistants, nursing students or nurses and their progress towards achieving this. Drawing on Taylor's work, Spouse identified four specific stages (see Figure 1.4), each of which seemed to be influenced by the extent to which students felt part of their clinical team and the amount of supported clinical practice they undertook. There also seemed to be significant transition points following long vacation periods. Since most of the students worked as care assistants during their vacations, this meant they could consolidate their clinical learning without having to worry about being formally assessed. When discussing these findings with nursing students of several different nationalities, they all agreed the findings reflected their own experiences and wished they had known that 'this was what it is like'.

Making the most of learning experiences

Financial implications of being a nursing student

Coming into a professional programme either on a grant or a bursary means that for most students their income is going to be considerably less than if they were in full-time, or perhaps even part-time, employment. Consequently, preparation prior to starting the programme is important. Part of this preparation entails developing your own budget for living and studying while on the programme. This may seem sensible, but many students leave their programme because they have not made such calculations and become increasingly distracted by financial difficulties (see Case history 1.6).

Student services: financial and practical help

There are a number of options for financial help available to students undertaking NHS-funded courses.

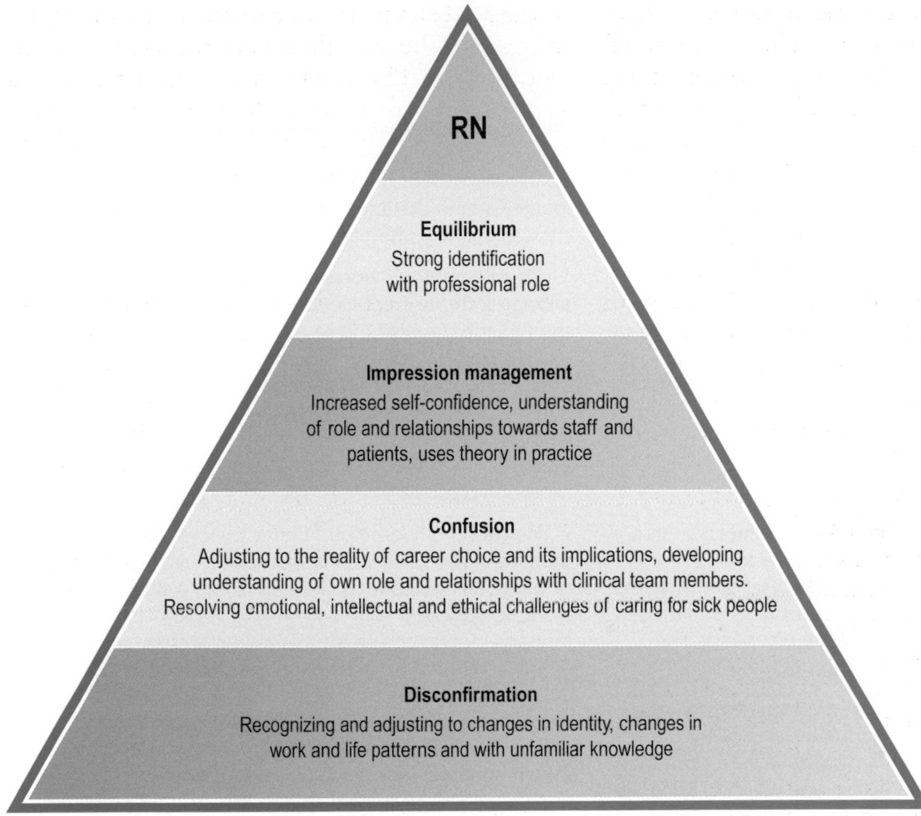

Figure 1.4 • Spouse's four stages in the learning process of becoming a registered nurse (RN). (After Spouse 2003.)

Bursaries for diploma- and degree-course students

Nursing students taking the diploma route receive a non-means-tested bursary, although there is a difference in the amount awarded depending on whether you are studying in an area where the cost of living is identified as being higher than the national average. You can find out what you should be receiving in your bursary by going to the website at www.dh.gov.uk or www.nhsstudentgrants.co.uk (if you live in Wales, Scotland or Northern Ireland, broadly comparable arrangements are in place and you can access the specific details through clicking on the relevant link from this website).

There are also a number of allowances which may be added on to the basic amount. There are some restrictions, so it is advisable to check these out before you start your programme. Students with dependants can apply for a number of allowances which are payable for those who are wholly or mainly financially dependent upon you during your time on the course. The income (net of allowable deductions) of all your dependants, spouse or partner is taken into account in deciding if you are eligible for this extra allowance.

Allowances are reduced for students residing at the parental home. As with diploma students, those enrolling on the BSc may have other allowances added to the means-tested basic award, if you are eligible. You will also have access to the Student Loan to add to your bursary. There are some residency regulations applicable to funding for diploma and degree nursing courses in England and the bursary will be dependent upon your meeting these residency regulations. You should make sure you have checked this out before you start and ask for advice at the university when you apply.

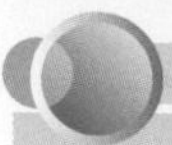

Case history 1.6

Mya

Mya is 28-year-old single parent. Her 6-year-old daughter goes to a local school and when Mya is working an evening shift either a friend or her mother collects her. Mya lives in a council flat and receives income support as well as a rate rebate for being a single parent.

Prior to starting her course to become a mental health nurse, Mya had held several different jobs. None of them had been particularly well paid. Her most recent job had been working as a health care assistant in a home for older people who were mentally frail. Her employers had been so impressed by her ability that they encouraged her to take an access course into nursing at her local college.

Having successfully completed the access course, Mya obtained a place at her local university to undertake the diploma in nursing programme. She was eligible for a bursary and she believed she would be able to continue working during her weekends and holidays after she had started the course.

Once she had started on the course, Mya realized that it was much more intellectually demanding than she had realized and that she would have to do a lot of studying in her spare time if she was going to keep up with the workload and not fall behind with the various course deadlines. Neither had Mya realized that after the first few weeks into the course she would be doing shift work on her clinical placement, which meant she could not work to earn money in the way she had anticipated. Both the hospital and the university were located some distance from her home and so getting there entailed quite a lot of travelling expenses.

To make things worse, her bursary was late in arriving into her bank account and when she went to the finance department to find out what was happening she discovered that her account number had been inaccurate. She had an overdraft limit of £500 which she had now exceeded. Mya also discovered that she was no longer eligible for income support or housing benefit now that she was on the nursing course and receiving a bursary.

Her parents were helping her by looking after her daughter when she was working evening shifts and for one day each weekend. This gave her a chance to work at least one shift a week to supplement her bursary. However, her studying was suffering and, despite Mya trying to study in the mornings when her daughter was at school or when she was asleep at night, her marks for her assignments were not as good as she had got when taking the access course. With mounting debts and an increasing sense of hopelessness, Mya went to see the student services advisor for help and advice.

If you become pregnant during your diploma or degree programme and you are receiving an NHS-funded bursary, you will be able to keep your bursary for a maternity break for up to 45 weeks subject to meeting the Department of Health criteria related to this funding (details can be found on www.nhsstudentgrants.co.uk).

Child Care Allowance

If you have dependent children, you will be eligible to apply for the Child Care Allowance (CCA). This allowance is available to all students with dependent children aged under 15 years, or aged under 17 years if your child has special educational needs. The child care must be provided by a registered or approved child care provider and the allowance pays up to 85% of your actual child care costs with a maximum amount payable for one child and a maximum amount payable for two or more children.

Students with disabilities

You need to let your university know if you have a disability and need extra help or equipment to complete your studies. You will be eligible for the Disabled Students Allowance, which will be assessed on the nature and severity of your disability once you have submitted a claim. All information will be treated as confidential, but it is in your interests to share your personal needs with the designated person at the university so that you can receive both the financial and practical guidance you might need to study and be successful.

Practice placement costs

Normal daily travel between your home and the university is not reimbursed. However, as part of your course will involve practice placements, travel can be reimbursed providing the cost is in excess of your normal daily travel costs from your term time residence to university.

There are other allowances that may be applicable for some students. Details of all the allowances and the criteria for eligibility can be found in the latest edition of the Financial Help for Health Care Students which can be viewed on www.dh.gov.uk or www.nhsstudentgrants.co.uk, where you will also find answers to some of those frequently asked questions. The specific information on residency is also included in this website.

The Access to Learning Fund

Learning funds are made available by the government to universities to help students experiencing difficulty meeting essential living and course-related costs. This fund is for health care students on either diploma or degree courses defined as home students or students who have been granted refugee status and each application is considered within the criteria set down for management of the fund.

The government gives priority to the following groups of students:

- Students with children (especially lone parents).
- Other mature students (especially those with existing financial commitments, including priority debts).
- Students from low-income families.
- Disabled students.
- Students who are classified as 'care leavers'.
- Students from 'foyers' or who are homeless. (Foyers have been helping disadvantaged young people achieve independence since 1992. There are now 100 foyers in the UK, with many more in development. Each foyer provides affordable and safe accommodation, linked to employment and training opportunities, professional and peer-group support, and a range of other services. (For more information see http://foyer.net.)
- Final-year students.

The Access to Learning Fund can be used to help with the essential costs of being a student.

Other financial support

There may be other sources for financial support available in your university; your student advice centre will be able to tell you about these. There may be charitable funds, or special funds donated by benefactors, that you may be able to access in a crisis or emergency; a designated representative of the student support services will make sure you know what is possible in individual cases. Do ask for help if you need it. Most universities have a student services unit and many also have a Dean of Students. The key responsibilities of the student services unit and the Dean are to ensure the services for students fit the nature and options of the courses being studied. They will make sure you have details of all the resources, both financial and practical, that are available to help you. Of course, any information you share with the Dean or other members of the university (such as the students services centre) will be treated as confidential.

Learning together, working together

You might recognize much of your own experiences from Mya's circumstances (Case history 1.6). Many students are surprised by the volume of study they are facing and have difficulty disciplining themselves to make sure they use the study time effectively. Chapter 2 will provide some detailed guidance on how to be successful in studying, and will introduce you to some tactics that will help you get the best out of your learning.

One of the most effective ways of learning is to work with a small circle of friends who are going through similar experiences to you. In a sense, you will be creating your own community of practice, a community of peers that is aimed at learning from each other. From the research of Bradby (1989) and Spouse (2003), it has become evident that peer support is a significant critical factor in students' successful learning. From the Spouse (2003) study it appears that nursing students use social time to share three particular types of experience:

- *Experiences concerned with emotional challenges*: fear about inadequacy; knowing how to express emotions appropriately; fears of saying the wrong thing; responding to other people's sexuality; feeling isolated because the clinical staff are too busy.
- *Experiences that are confusing or unaccountable*: being shown how to do the same procedure differently by as many people; ethical dilemmas, such as whether a patient should be told of their diagnosis or be resuscitated; being older than the mentor and feeling inadequate; being asked to undertake tasks that are either well within or outside their capability; not feeling welcomed by the clinical staff;
- *Experiences that relate to formal learning*: having achieved a specific competency; being able to bring into use some previously learned but not fully understood information; excitement about having a personal caseload; specific aspects that relate to formal learning or that require some theoretical understanding.

Reflecting on practice with peers

Through regular meetings with a trusted peer group many students find they can increase their understanding by exchanging stories of their experiences (Figure 1.5). Sometimes these sessions provide insights that bring theoretical knowledge together with everyday practical experiences and provide the 'ah-ha' sensation. On other occasions, they allow group members to gauge their own progress against peers at the same stage in the programme and provide either an incentive to seek help, or to ask for specific experiences or to increase their self-confidence that they are on track.

With many students being preoccupied with a busy family life, meeting regularly with peers can be difficult. Having a sympathetic listener who is willing to hear you reflect on your experiences can also provide alternative perspectives that are helpful and developmental (see Case history 1.7). However, such listeners can sometimes misunderstand the seriousness and stress a nursing student is experiencing and consider them as 'drama

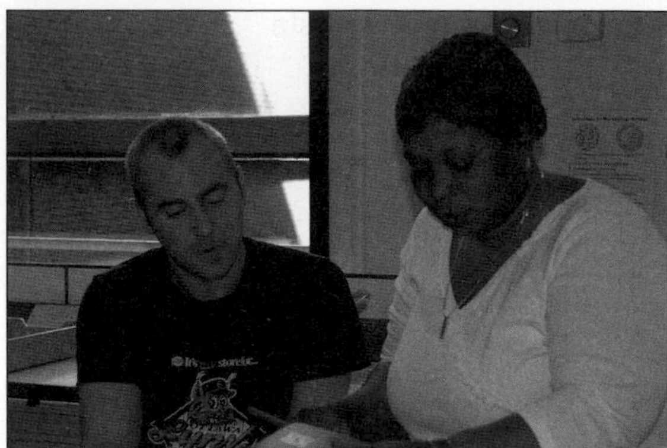

Figure 1.5 • Sharing learning and reflecting on practice.

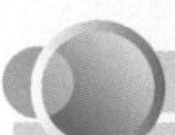

Case history 1.7

Jane's experience

Jane had not studied for some time although she had worked in the UK before taking an Access to Health Studies course. Jane got to know her personal tutor during the early modules and felt able to go and see her for advice. Jane had two children and sometimes missed classes as she had to care for them. She failed some examinations and was very upset as she had studied hard and thought she was ready. She saw her tutor and did manage to pass one exam but failed the other one for the second time. She was encouraged to ask for a third attempt as her son had been ill and Jane's dad had died just before the examination. She was advised to see the university learning support and counselling services to help her with her preparation. She found this all very helpful and could not help thinking she should have gone earlier as the advisors introduced her to a useful way of planning her work. Her personal tutor had previously suggested that she used this service but Jane had understood it to mean she was 'a dunce' and needed remedial help. Nothing was further from the truth as the counsellor also helped her with learning to live with her bereavement and taught her some relaxation skills.

queens', so having a network of nursing colleagues to talk to seems to be important to help you make progress.

Many students find they can get similar benefits from having a peer study group, where each person shares their learning and uses their peers as critical readers of their draft assignments. Through this activity, students can learn how to structure their assignments, how to reference and create a bibliography, how to express different concepts and how to apply them to personal experiences. Often having a good written model as a starting point helps students to get the hang of academic writing much more quickly than repeated attempts undertaken in isolation. However, this does not mean that students should imagine they will be successful with only one or two drafts of their assignments. The more an assignment is carefully crafted the more learning has been achieved.

Student services: practical help for academic work

There is a range of student services available to students to help with academic studying. For many people learning to be a nurse may be the first academically demanding course they have done for some time. Others may have studied in another country where the way of teaching and learning can be very different. So it is important to recognize that seeking help is a good strategy towards being successful.

Some students have special educational needs and there are support centres specifically intended to help students with a number of disabilities such as dyslexia (a difficulty with reading and writing certain words), hearing or visual impairment or supporting students whose first language is not English. You might feel concerned by the use of the word 'disability'. However, the Special Educational Needs and Education Act (2001) uses these terms in order to ensure that universities provide resources to help students achieve their aspirations and potential. If you find that you have difficulty in this way it is important to feel confident and access the support you might need and not to be concerned by these terms.

Every student has the right to make use of their university's student support resources free of charge. These resources include academic learning support, disability, student health and student counselling services. The way universities offer these resources will vary from institution to institution; you can check your own university website to identify what is on offer to you.

Academic learning support

These services are designed to help students increase the effectiveness of their study skills and achieve the best results. Students are helped to develop a study plan that meets their personal needs and learning style.

As a result of using this service you might be able to:

- Better understand your learning style.
- Understand how to benefit from tutor feedback.
- Prepare oral presentations.
- Learn revision and exam techniques.
- Develop writing skills.
- Improve note-taking and report-writing.
- Enhance your numeracy skills.

Using these facilities early in your programme can prevent you from getting into difficulty such as failing an assignment. As a university student you need to remember that your course is designed on the premise that students can take responsibility for their own learning and are able to plan their own study time. Identifying the way in which you learn and study will help you plan the approach that works best for you. You should not feel shy about assessing your needs long before you start to cope with the challenges of assessments. There are several books available on this subject (Cotrell 1999, Goodwyn & Stables 2004, Lewis & Reinders 2003, McIlroy 2003, Nicol et al 2004, Silviter 2004, Whitehead & Mason 2003) and you will find more information and help on this when you read Chapter 2.

Counselling services

Counselling services aim to help you address personal concerns that may be impeding your social and academic development. The service is confidential and free to university students. Many students use this service if they are struggling with coming to terms with a bereavement or if they have family or marital problems or other personal and emotional challenges.

Disability services

Disability services can offer advice to students with disabilities, including long-term medical conditions and dyslexia. Students can be helped to identify and access arrangements enabling them to get the most out of their time at university. This can include help with completing a disabled student's allowance application form or ensuring that appropriate arrangements for teaching and examinations have been made for the student by the university department.

Student health services

Student health services offer a range of resources advising on minor illness or injury, contraception and sexual health, as well as information and support on health matters. Students are advised to use this service to discuss managing their needs while at university.

There will be other services available to you in the university; details of the full range of services should be provided in the student information packs on offer.

Personal tutor

At the beginning of your programme you will be assigned a personal tutor. This person is normally a registered nurse on the branch of the Professional Register you are studying and is available to act as your advisor throughout the course. As in the case study of Jane (Case history 1.7), your personal tutor can advise and help you with your academic work and with personal problems that may affect your studies and your progress. A personal tutor can refer you to the university services that could help you with your progress.

Joining a community of practice

Communities of practice exist all around us in society and it is likely that you are already a member of several: perhaps as a parent with specific knowledge about parenting, or managing a home; perhaps as an enthusiast with expertise derived from a previous occupation or from studying a particular topic in depth over sufficient time for you to teach another person how to develop the same skills. So a community of practice is any group of people who share an expertise and which is often distinguished by specific terminology (a shorthand to describe quite complex concepts) and ways of working that can only be learned by engaging in the activities under supervision from a more experienced person.

University community of practice

As a nursing student studying in a higher education institution, you are a newcomer to several communities of practice. The first community of practice is the academic community of staff who will be teaching you and supporting your learning of the special skills and knowledge required to be successful in that setting. This includes learning how to learn efficiently as well as developing all the associated academic skills, such as using a library to access relevant information, creating an accurate bibliography that conforms to specific standards, reading texts critically and using the knowledge to support your arguments whilst acknowledging their sources. A more complex skill is learning to write assignments according to specific standards, ensuring you are observing academic conventions and at the same time demonstrating a profound understanding of the topic area and its relationship to your practice as a nursing student. Your grades will reflect the extent to which you have managed to develop such skills and acquire the relevant language, which is not only descriptive but also critical and analytical and shows that you can relate your reading to your clinical practice. Academic staff from the information centres (library, information technology staff) and the lecturers will be willing and available to help you develop these skills; you will find more information about how to develop such skills in Chapter 2.

Even if you have recently successfully completed a programme of study, you may find being a nursing student quite daunting. This is often because students don't expect to have to do so much study and to work; they usually assume that, with nursing being a practical subject, all their learning will take place with patients. Others think of nursing as an academic course because it is located in a university setting and they forget that nursing has strong practical, technical and emotional components. The complexity of nursing means that there is a wide range of associated topics to learn and a huge vocabulary that is probably unfamiliar to many newcomers. The range of topics that are likely to be included in a nursing course is shown in Box 1.1. Although this list is incomplete, it illustrates the complexity and range of disciplines that influence good nursing practice. Unlike many academic subjects, which are studied in relative isolation from everyday life, in nursing, all these topics are studied in relation to people's health and illness and their spiritual, social, mental and physical needs. So there are other major communities of practice that new nursing students enter when they enter the practical world of nursing itself. Each of these communities of practice have their different vocabulary, many acronyms and, more importantly, a code of professional practice that all students are expected to observe. You will find more information about the professional, legal and ethical aspects of being a nursing student and becoming a nurse in Chapter 4.

Box 1.1

Some of the subject areas you are likely to encounter during your nursing course

- Anatomy and physiology (pure and applied)
- Biochemistry
- Environmental health
- Ethics
- Forensic science
- Genetics
- Health education
- Human behaviour
- Infection control
- Information technology
- Interpersonal skills
- Law
- Management skills
- Microbiology
- Nursing care of patients experiencing a range of health care disorders
- Nursing theory
- Nutrition and dietetics
- Pharmacology
- Psychology
- Public health
- Research utilization skills
- Social policy
- Sociology
- Spiritual care
- Technical skills
- Therapeutics

Having a voice in the university and your programme

Being a nursing student at university offers a range of opportunities to influence the way your programme is organized and to have your voice heard. Every programme has its own committee structure and there are normally special committees for students to represent the views of their peers.

University governance and student representation

It is most important that you contribute to the university governance structure. You can contribute in a number of ways, but this depends upon you taking an active part in the process. It does not mean spending your precious study, personal and social time attending meetings, although you will be very welcome to be part of a number of committees and working groups. Student representation is critical to the life-blood of higher education and much of this is achieved through student union councils under the auspices of the National Union of Students. There are university-appointed sabbatical officers who are elected by students. Their role is to represent you as the student body in a number of different ways associated with such aspects as student welfare, publicity and social activities. Each university will have a student president who will be a voting member of the Senate and University Council which sets all the statutes and regulations governing your courses. Training is offered for these roles, with support provided through the institution; this will help you develop excellent skills that will be important for your career development.

Departments, faculties, institutes and schools of a university are very likely to have a student representative group of their own and have representation on the Student Union Council, determined by the proportion of students being represented. By engaging as a student representative you will be able to contribute to decisions being made which affect your life as a student.

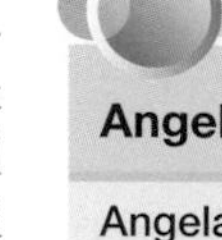

Case history 1.8

Angela as student representative

Angela started her programme 2 years ago and was elected by her seminar group to be their student representative at the programme forum. This entailed attending a meeting once each term. Meetings were chaired by one of the student members elected each year and other members included academic and administrative staff. Students found such meetings helpful as it enabled them to contribute to changes in the curriculum as well as to the curriculum that was being developed for introduction in a year's time. Being her seminar group representative meant that Angela needed to be confident that she had got the views of her peers and was representing them faithfully. To do this she canvassed her peers for their views before the meetings and fed back information. In all, the commitment took up about 3 hours each term. Others in her intake group were on the Students Representative Council, which was concerned with improving the overall conditions for students, or on the placement education committee and its subcommittees. Having gained confidence in contributing to these committees, Angela put herself up to be a nursing representative on the University Students Council which contributed to the university governance.

Student staff liaison committees and boards

There will be useful formal mechanisms for student/staff dialogue through student/staff liaison committees, programme management committees and boards of study. As a student representative, your voice is important and systems for student feedback will feature regularly during your studies (see Case history 1.8). The feedback will relate to a number of levels in the university, from an individual lecturer or class to a programme of study, a department or faculty, or an institution.

Each year students are invited to contribute to a National Student Survey. Students are also asked to contribute to strategic decisions locally and through reports submitted by your student union to the Quality Assurance Agency institutional audit.

Learning and working in a clinical placement community of practice

Standards for achievement

The nature of your placements will depend on which branch of nursing you plan to become registered in. During your programme you will be placed in settings that contribute to your development of a wide understanding of different areas of nursing, acquisition of core skills, knowledge and abilities to care for children or for adults and which are aimed at providing you with a comprehensive preparation for further learning once you have become a qualified nurse. Inevitably it is impossible for each student to learn all there is about their chosen branch of nursing. The most important skills are learning how to learn from experience, learning how to function effectively as a member of the health care team and learning how to be an effective practitioner.

Your nursing programme will be planned to ensure that you meet the requirements of your professional statutory organization. Normally, it is planned in two phases: the foundation year and the branch programme (normally 2 years). Practice constitutes 50% of the total hours in both phases. Successful completion of both parts of your programme depends on your ability to demonstrate that you can work as a safe practitioner for that stage of your programme and that you have developed the required level of knowledge. For the foundation year you will be expected to achieve all the learning outcomes for entry to the branch programme. Before you complete the branch programme you must have demonstrated achievement in all the proficiencies for registration (see Table 1.1). Each category has specified standards that each nursing student must demonstrate at different stages in their programme. As you read through this book you will find pointers to the relevant category.

An important aspect of demonstrating these specific activities is that you can perform them in different settings and under different conditions. Being able to wash a dummy in a practical room or skills laboratory is clearly not the same as washing an elderly person who is in pain from rheumatoid arthritis, or a confused and incontinent person, or a child in acute pain. Similarly, being able to help someone who is pretending to be confused in a classroom setting is very different to supporting someone in their home or on a busy ward who is being aggressive because of their confusion. The skill and artistry of nursing is in the ability to deliver care that is effective under a range of circumstances and to anyone who needs it whilst being mindful of the boundaries of personal responsibility. Maintaining your own professional knowledge enables you to achieve this and knowing how to access information and to document your practice allows you to demonstrate it to the professional statutory organization. This is why keeping a reflective diary and a portfolio of your professional development while a student is important to your professional development (see Chapter 11).

Table 1.1 Nursing and Midwifery Council professional requirements for registration

Standards	Foundation course	Branch programme
Professional and ethical practice	×	×
Care delivery	×	×
Care management	×	×
Personal and professional development	×	×

Sources of support in placements

Keeping accurate records of your achievements is essential and as a nursing student you will be provided with handbooks to record your achievement of specific skills and assessment schedules to demonstrate your performance while on placement. If you have any doubts or anxieties about meeting the requirements during your placement it is important that you seek and obtain help quickly, rather than wait and hope that 'things will get better'. Clinical staff are often busy with their main priority which is delivering and managing patient care. Students often take second place in the busy clinical world and staff forget how important your placement is to your progress. As a student it is important that you have your records witnessed by a responsible member of the health care team. Normally this would be a nurse who has specific responsibility for supporting you during your placement. In some settings, students receive support from other members of the health and social care team. The person who will be supporting you in your practice setting is normally called a 'mentor'; this person may be assisted by another staff member, called a 'co-mentor' or 'associate mentor'.

Preparing for your placement is an important part of your learning and makes it more likely that it will be a successful experience. Throughout your programme you are likely to go to several different placements, often in different NHS or independent sector settings. Programme developers try to match theory with practice so you are prepared for the kinds of nursing you will be encountering before you start in the placement. Sometimes you may find the connection between theory and the placement difficult to recognize, although having clear learning outcomes for each placement will help you. The following provides some guidelines about how to make the most of your placement.

In Chapter 6 you will find several activities that are designed to help you plan your learning, negotiate learning and working experiences and to keep records of what you have done. These help you to learn from your everyday practice and to begin to recognize its salience to what you have learned formally in the classroom or through your studies. Making use of your practical experiences as learning opportunities is the hardest challenge for many students, simply because there is so much going on, and without some sort of guide to translate what you are seeing and doing, it is often hard to understand what there is to learn.

You may also find it helpful to obtain a copy of the Royal College of Nursing (RCN) toolkit. This is a set of guideline standards for nursing students to use when first going to a new placement. You can download it from the RCN website (www.rcn.org.uk) if you are a member of the RCN students section.

Preparing for the first visit to your practice placement

Once you have details of your placement there are several things you can do to make the most of it:

- *Find out as much as possible about the placement.* Where can you get information? Does it have a website or is there information about the staff, the setting and any clinical specialist practice that staff are particularly skilled at? If it is a hospital setting you could check the hospital intranet. If it is a community placement you could check the Trust's website for information about the geographical area, the population age and social mix. You may find that there are specialist nurses working in that setting and with whom you could meet.
- *Educational links.* Does the placement have a nurse teacher or practice educator who links with the setting? How often do they visit the placement?
- *Mentor support, shift times, special expectations of students, welcome pack.* Many clinical placements send students a welcome letter as soon as they receive the allocation's information. Sometimes the information along with travel directions are available on a website. Alternatively, placements encourage students to visit the placement a week before the start date so they can meet their mentor, negotiate their attendance times so they can work alongside their mentor, and find out about the setting. Armed with such information it is good practice to read up about the clinical specialities that are nursed in the setting so you can match the knowledge against your educational needs and develop a learning plan for your placement. Arriving well informed and prepared at a placement creates a good impression. Staff welcome students who are interested in learning and are enthusiastic. It is the same as going on holiday in a foreign country: if you have learned some of the language and have taken the trouble to find out a little of the history, people feel more inclined to be extra helpful.

Wearing your uniform

If you are placed in a community setting, staff may expect you to wear clean and smart clothes that are discreet rather than wear a uniform. You will be there as an ambassador for both the university and your profession, so it is important that you check how your mentor expects you to behave when meeting people in their own homes.

Wearing uniform is a controversial subject and you may be familiar with nurses wearing their uniform in public places. You may have wondered what the person has been doing, whether they have been working with patients or whether they are about to go on duty. With so much discussion in the press about highly infectious bacteria, MRSA (methicillin-resistant *Staphylococcus aureus*) being one of them (see also Chapters 9 and 13), it is very inappropriate for uniforms to be worn away from the practice setting. Most hospitals have a strict uniform policy banning staff from wearing their uniform out of the hospital grounds.

As a student you are in a potentially dangerous situation when wearing your uniform in public places. A member of the public may ask for your assistance, which may entail responsibilities that are beyond your capability, such as giving emergency first aid to someone who has collapsed. If the situation goes wrong and you make a mistake, you become accountable for your actions and are at risk.

Wearing uniform in hospital tells people who you are, and the design of the uniform is intended to protect you from harm. Wearing jewellery such as rings, ear-rings and hair ornaments could allow bacteria to be harboured which could then be passed on to vulnerable patients; this is especially the case with hand-washing, which is notoriously poorly done, leaving bacteria hiding under wedding rings. So it is better to store pieces of jewellery in a safe place before you go on duty, preferably at home where they are not at risk of being lost or stolen.

Washing your uniform is also important, as bacteria can survive on uniforms for some time. Current advice is that you should wash your uniform at a temperature of 60°C. Inevitably this has cost implications, but following this advice could save lives, including your own or that of a family member.

Breaking the ice and making your entry

Entering a placement for the first time can be quite daunting for many people. It is rather like joining a party of strangers who know each other very well and work closely together. Each different placement consists of a community of practitioners with expertise in their area of nursing. As a newcomer you need a sponsor to introduce you to the community, its unwritten and written rules and codes of conduct (e.g. when people go to meal breaks, whether students go at the same time as the qualified staff, whether they go to a staff canteen or stay in the setting, such as in the staff room, and eat sandwiches). Usually your sponsor will be your mentor, who has accepted responsibility for supporting your learning during your placement. During your first day you should be shown around the setting, where the emergency equipment is kept and all the health and safety procedures that are relevant to the setting. Your mentor will also introduce you to other members of the team, especially the people you will be working closely with, or in their absence, and where any educational materials are kept, including policy documents. Many students find this induction process very important, helping them to feel welcomed to the setting and giving them confidence that their learning is going to be respected.

As a newcomer to the setting, it is important that you also play your part. Students who are the most successful are those who have organized their lives in order to free themselves up to concentrate on their learning. Being punctual and wearing the appropriate dress means checking these out beforehand and ensuring that you know the quickest route to the placement and have made any necessary arrangements for child care well in advance. Planning duty times so they fit in with your mentor or associate mentor is important. Even though you are a supernumerary member of the team, for the benefit of your learning you need to make sure you are available at times that match those of your mentor and that you use every opportunity to participate in care delivery activities, preferably alongside a first-level nurse.

Being supernumerary

As a student, you are not counted in the workforce numbers of your placement. This means that there are sufficient staff available to deliver the required care to each of the patients or clients in the setting without your presence. Very rarely are there extra staff available to support students, and so staff are undertaking their teaching activities in addition to their nursing workload.

As a student, your responsibility is to ensure that you undertake the prescribed number of clinical hours in the placement and use these hours to meet the curriculum requirements of the professional statutory organization to become a registered nurse. You will be aware that there is enormous competition for placements and so it is important that you make the most of each placement. Case history 1.9 illustrates how you may be learning and working in a placement setting.

Kate's plan included time working with Kevin and another nurse (Fortune) who would be her associate mentor so they can assess her core nursing skills and ensure she meets the requirements for successful completion of the module. After the second week on the placement Kate's confidence was quite shaken as she realized that many of the skills she had been practising as a care assistant were unsafe. She also began to realize that the speed of getting work done was less important on this ward and that she was expected to spend more time helping patients to help themselves. Kevin and Fortune had discussed this realization with her and were now satisfied that Kate was safe to give care to a small group of patients so she could practise her skills. Kate worked alongside her mentor once a week and with Fortune on the other two shifts. At the beginning and end of each shift they discussed how Kate had got on and went through the care she had given. It gave Kate a chance to ask questions about things she had noticed as well as to see whether she was making the right progress. By week 6 of her placement Kate was feeling that she was more comfortable with this new way of working and this was reflected in her midway discussion with Kevin. Together they wrote a summary of her progress and made a plan for Kate's next 4 weeks of the placement. Feeling more confident about her nursing care, Kate began to take more interest in her patients' medical and nursing history and started to read their notes and to ask questions about their drug therapy. She kept a pocket book of unfamiliar words and drugs so she could check them up when she was off duty.

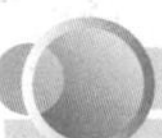

Case history 1.9

Kate learning and working in a placement setting

Kate is a 40-year old care assistant who previously worked in a private nursing home for older people. She is on her first placement for the pre-registration (adult) nursing programme, which is an acute medical ward. This particular allocation is over 9 weeks and Kate will spend 3 days each week on the placement. She will be coming back to the same placement for the following two terms, giving her some stability. Kate is particularly interested in diabetic nursing as many of the residents had this condition. When Kate met with her mentor she discussed her earlier nursing experiences and what she had found out about the placement. Her curriculum module required her to demonstrate a number of specific clinical skills (which she felt she was already more than capable of doing) and to write about her experiences in relation to the NMC competencies for entry to the branch programme. Because of her interest in the care of people with diabetes, Kate and her mentor (Kevin) agreed on a plan for Kate to get the necessary experience.

As an experienced health care assistant, Kate believed she would be able to get into the theoretical aspects of care-giving quickly, so she was quite shocked when she realized that she had to re-learn many technical skills she had taken for granted. You will note that, although she was supernumerary, she did spend some time working on her own giving essential care to patients. Her mentors had planned this with Kate once they felt confident that she was safe working on her own. They had also planned the kinds of patients Kate should nurse so that she was able to meet her learning outcomes and nurse a diverse group of patients. Clinical staff have a duty of care towards patients, which means they must be sure that anyone who is delegated responsibilities is capable of carrying them out safely and effectively. Working in this way gave Kate the opportunity to refine her essential technical skills and to feel that she was contributing to the work of the placement staff. This form of reciprocity often helps students feel more comfortable about seeking help. Importantly, it also exposed Kate to thinking about why she was giving particular forms of care and why patients were receiving particular kinds of treatment. This strategy of question framing and answering is a very powerful way for students to make links between their classroom learning and their practical learning. Most students believe this is more memorable than reading texts, but it needs both approaches to be effective learning.

If Kate had been a complete novice she would have needed more time working alongside her mentors to develop her nursing skills until her mentor was satisfied that she was capable of managing a small caseload of patients.

Watching, talking and learning in practice

Working under close supervision is a good way of learning from your mentor. Watching what they are doing and how they do it provides opportunities for learning the more subtle aspects of nursing. Seeing how an expert nurse helps a confused person, or talks to someone who has a hearing deficit, or helps someone move in bed when they are paralysed down one side or have a broken leg or persuades them to eat and drink when they are suffering from depression are all complex skills that are difficult to develop through trial and error. Sometimes the most obvious things get forgotten by a student because of their inexperience, and talking through the care you are planning to give a patient helps prepare you for the unexpected or the obvious. Similarly, to be able to debrief following a shift of working under distant supervision helps you to rationalize your care and so begin to make links between theory and practice. It also helps you to develop the necessary vocabulary of the community of practitioners that you are working with, which again helps with your learning. As you become more confident about talking and working with patients and their carers you will find it easier to notice some of the symptoms they are experiencing and to find out more about their health care problem and their nursing needs.

An essential aspect of learning to nurse is the opportunity to do the same kinds of nursing activities over and over again, until you have developed the technical skills as well as the interpersonal skills to conduct the activity safely and thoughtfully. This often means planning to work several short shifts rather than a few long shifts.

A study by Spouse (2003) indicated that nursing students were concerned with seven particular aspects of learning to nurse:

- Relating to patients and their carers.
- Developing technical knowledge.
- Learning to bundle nursing activities together.
- Developing craft knowledge.
- Managing feelings and emotions (both their own and responding to those of patients and their carers).
- Being therapeutic in their nursing care.
- Relating and functioning in the health care team.

Kate's experience (Case history 1.9) indicated that she already felt confident about relating to patients and felt comfortable talking to patients as she provided care. Many new nurses find this very difficult, often because they are too self-conscious to know how to put people at their ease. Kate had also developed a number of essential technical skills. Although she subsequently realized that she needed to re-learn some of them, she had learned how to prioritize her time and knew how to assess which patients needed her attention first and which she could leave for a bit longer. Learning these management skills takes some experience and sensitivity to patients' individual needs. Often students do not feel able to remember their theoretical learning until they feel comfortable in their performance as a member of the team and contributing to the workload (Spouse 2001). You will find some guidelines in Chapter 3 about how to manage feelings (both your own and those of your patients). Chapter 10 provides some information about being an effective team member and Chapter 11 discusses how to manage your workload effectively.

Preparing to leave your placement: assignments, recording progress

In the case study about Kate (Case history 1.9), she was going to return to the same placement the following term. This is not always the case and students often go to a new placement whenever they start a new term or semester. This usually means that specific learning outcomes must be achieved for each placement in order to progress through the programme. You read that Kate had a preliminary discussion about her placement, which was followed up with a plan of action. This was subsequently reviewed and documented as a result of her mentors' observations of her practice and their opinion of her achievements. This assessment cycle of assessment, planning, reviewing and documenting is important. If you find that you are not receiving verbal and written feedback then you must speak to your mentor or the placement manager. If this does not work then you should contact the practice educator or the lecturer who links with your placement or your personal tutor.

As a nursing student, it is important that you join a students' association either through the RCN or UNISON. Joining fees are quite cheap and in return you have access to a wide range of professional and personal services, including reading materials, indemnity insurance and solicitors' expenses if you make a mistake when you are in placement.

Conclusion

Joining the nursing profession brings an exciting and rewarding career. Inevitably there will be ups and downs and there will be times when you will question your decision. If you have a vision of what you want to achieve as a nurse, then it is a career that you will find satisfying and emotionally rewarding. The programme is known to be one of the toughest in universities, not necessarily because of the academic demands but because of the complex nature of nursing: as a student you will be at the forefront of care delivery, supporting people who are undergoing life-changing experiences whilst also learning how to respond professionally to such events in practice and in your own life. Once embarked on a career in nursing, you will face an exciting choice of career opportunities. You can practise in any one of a wide range of health care fields, and there are good opportunities for further academic development as well as career options in nursing management or in education.

References

Bradby M 1989 Self esteem and status passage: a longitudinal study of the self perceptions of nurses during their first year of training. Unpublished PhD thesis, University of Exeter

Bradby M 1990 Status passage into nursing: understanding nursing care. Journal of Advanced Nursing 15:1363–1369

Bradby M 1991 Getting to know you: a study of student nurse peer group formations. Journal of Advances in Health and Nursing Care 1(4):33–49

Cottrell S 1999 The study skills handbook. Palgrave, Basingstoke

Goodwyn A, Stables A (eds) 2004 Language and literacy. Sage, London

Henderson V 1966 The nature of nursing. Macmillan, New York

Lewis M, Reinders H 2003 Study skills for speakers of English as a second language. Palgrave, Basingstoke

McIlroy D 2003 Studying at university. Sage, London

Melia K 1987 Learning and working: the occupational socialization of nurses. Tavistock, London

Nicol M, Bavin C, Bedford-Turner S et al 2004 Essential nursing skills, 2nd edn. Mosby, London

Olesen VL, Whittaker EW 1968 The silent dialogue: a study in the social psychology of professional socialization. Jossey-Bass, San Francisco

Orem DE 1959 Nursing: concepts of practice (2nd edn, 1980). McGraw Hill, New York

Pearson A, Vaughan B, Fitzgerald M 2005 Nursing models for practice, 3rd edn. Butterworth-Heinemann, Edinburgh

Peplau E 1952 Interpersonal relations in nursing. GP Putnam, New York

Rogers ME 1970 The theoretical basis of nursing. FA Davis, Philadelphia

Roper N, Logan W, Tierney A 1996 The elements of nursing: a model for nursing based on a model for living, 4th edn. Churchill Livingstone, London

Silviter B 2004 The student nurse handbook. Baillière Tindall, London

Simpson IH 1967 Patterns of socialization into professions: the case of student nurses. Sociological Inquiry 37:47–54

Spouse J 2001 Workplace learning: pre-registration nursing students' perspectives. Nurse Education in Practice 1:149–156

Spouse J 2003 Professional learning in nursing. Blackwell, Oxford

Taylor M 1987 Self directed learning: more than meets the observer's eye. In: Boud D, Griffin V (eds) Appreciating adults learning. Kogan Page, London, p 179–196

Whitehead E, Mason T 2003 Study skills for nurses. Sage, London

Chapter Two

2

How to study and learn effectively

Ian Scott, Chris Ely

Key topics

- The importance of becoming a learner for life
- Planning to be a successful learner through use of time-management techniques
- Making good use of study time to focus your learning and improve your ability to understand
- Note-making and note-taking from taught sessions and from practice
- Reviewing your approaches to studying
- Reading analytically and critically
- Information gathering: using the Internet and using a database
- Learning from practice-placement experiences
- Using reflective practice
- Enquiry-based learning and learning in groups
- Learning the skills of academic writing, reflective styles of writing and referencing

Introduction

This chapter will help you gain the most from all your learning experiences both in the classroom and in placement settings, and will give you practical ideas and guidance that will help you succeed as a student. The focus is on developing the skills that will help you to learn for the rest of your life.

The value of learning for life

The rate of change that we face today is arguably greater than it has ever been in the history of the world (Barnett 2004), and along with the challenge of change also comes the challenge of coping with the vast quantities of information that the modern world is producing. Lukasiewicz (1994) used the phrase 'ignorance explosion' to describe this phenomenon and how it affects all of us in society, because no longer can anyone know everything about their subject let alone about several subjects. With large amounts of change and knowledge being generated how can we learn for such an unknown future (Barnett 2004)? This question has been grappled with in recent times, and the discussion has brought a new phrase and concept: 'lifelong learning'. Lifelong learning refers to the notion that an individual will engage with formal learning throughout their lives; what will be learnt will be determined by the needs of the individual in response to their own survival challenges and of society. To cope with these dramatic changes to our way of living and the volume of information around us, educational organizations have also been changing their approach to education. They are less concerned about ensuring students can repeat large volumes of facts and figures or transmitting knowledge, but are concerned more with helping students to discover how to learn for themselves. This chapter is about helping you to develop these skills. and so become accomplished at knowing how to learn.

As you have probably already discovered, learning is not only about sitting at a desk or reading a text. In fact, many would argue these are the least effective ways of learning. You will have learned a huge amount of information from using all your senses from watching, listening, tasting, smelling, doing and interacting with others. The trick is to be able to remember what the experience taught you and how you can use the knowledge again and perhaps in a different situation. Sometimes learning like this may happen without even recognizing it has happened (passive learning), such as learning the difference between sweet and sour; sometimes it may be as a result of a decision, for example to ride a bicycle, or to create something (active learning).

Learning nursing

You may have several reasons for continuing or returning to education. Learning to become a nurse is an opportunity for many people to study at university whilst also developing the knowledge and skills for their future career. With the rapid expansion in knowledge the important skills that all workers need to acquire are not concerned with learning facts but knowing how to learn independently so that they can adjust to rapid changes and uncertainty. Expectations of the general public and health care users have become much higher as people have become better informed. If you are to respond safely and effectively to this constant change you will need to learn how to adapt to the changes that new knowledge brings, to be responsive to the demands of your health care clients as well as to the inevitable changes in how health care is delivered as you progress through your career.

Planning to succeed

If you want to succeed then you almost certainly need to do some planning.

Your time is yours to spend as and how you like but recognizing how you use your time is important. There will of course be lots of different things that will be competing for your time; the trick is to decide what is important and what is not and how to allocate your time between these different priorities. Two important points to remember are: your time is yours to control and, if your goal is to become a qualified nurse, then you must dedicate time to that goal.

It is worth stressing that when you start a course in pre-registration nursing your life will change, often in ways that are often impossible to imagine before starting the course. As a result of the changes, the way in which you use your time will need to change also. If you already have a busy life you will need to spend time considering and planning how to make sufficient time and how to adjust your lifestyle to include time for attending university, travelling to your placements and doing your studies. The adjustments you make may affect your friends and family, so it is probably a good idea to share your ideas and plans with them.

Time budgets

You might like to think of time in the same way that you think of money, as a fixed income that needs to be planned and budgeted, so that there is enough for you to achieve all the things that *must* be achieved, with some to spare for fun and the unexpected. By thinking and planning your time at the beginning of your course you are less likely to run out of time.

Planning your time will include thinking about how to use all 168 hours of the week. During the course of a week you probably spend about 56

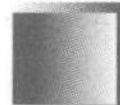

Time	Mon	Tues	Wed	Thurs	Fri	Sat	Sun
00:00							
01:00							
02:00							
03:00							
04:00							
05:00							
06:00							
07:00							
08:00							
09:00							
10:00							
11:00							
12:00							
13:00							
14:00							
15:00							
16:00							
17:00							
18:00							
19:00							
20:00							
21:00							
22:00							
23:00							

Figure 2.1 • Template for a weekly time–activity log.

hours sleeping, this leaves you with a balance of 112 hours to spend in a variety of ways. When starting a time budget it is worth examining how you currently spend your time by keeping a record of what you do with your time during one week. Include all the many routine activities that are essential, such as washing and dressing. You might find an activity log like the one shown in Figure 2.1 useful, and using symbols for different activities such as 'T' for travel, 'W' for work and so on might help.

To do this exercise effectively you need to keep a record as you go about your daily activities. When you change activities, record how much time you spent on the previous activity. At the end of each day think about how much time you spent on each activity. Is there any time that could be saved? Once you identify how you currently spend your time you can start to plan how you can find time for your course studies. Using this technique lets you see how you are spending time, and so can help you decide where your priorities lie and how you can save time. Knowing how you spend your time will help you to take control of your time, and being in control can help to reduce stress. Take a look at the list that Shona developed and see how it compares with your own (Box 2.1). Making this list helped Shona to recognize how her time was being spent and to fill in her chart.

There are some caveats to time management and these revolve around the fact that how we perceive time and the tasks we have to do varies depending on circumstance. Take a look at some of the sayings connected with time and tasks:

> *If you want something done ask a busy person.*
> *A job expands to fit the time available to it.*

These familiar and apparently contradictory sayings tell us what an unusual phenomenon time is, and how differently people use it, with some people able to achieve a lot more than others within the same amount of time. They also suggest that if we can focus and concentrate on a task it can take less of our time.

Box 2.1

Shona's list

- Sleeping
- Morning and evening wash
- Preparing and eating meals
- Spending time with Gus (partner)
- Collecting children from school
- Sport/exercise
- Travelling: to shops, to work, to school
- Watching TV
- Reading
- Shopping
- Talking to friends
- Washing clothes
- Working
- Playing with children

Prioritizing your study time

As you get into your studies, you will find that you need to manage your study time. During your studies you are likely to have competing demands for your time, and you will need to review your studies, complete assignments and reflect on practice. We have given you some ideas about how to budget your time; here, we are suggesting that you also need to identify priorities so that you can organize your life and particularly your career studies in an effective and efficient manner.

One method of time management is to prioritize tasks and design schedules. This can be a challenging activity for some people who are not by nature planners, whereas other people may be highly organized and skilled at planning every aspect of their life. If you belong to the latter group you probably will not need to read this section. However, if you are not by nature a planner you will find it helpful to learn how to manage your time so you can get more out of your life. Using lists and schedules and seeing study as a series of tasks is not for everyone and they may even find using lists and schedules positively stressful. It is therefore worth thinking about whether you do actually like to plan things. When designing schedules you need to decide which tasks are most important to achieve and when you will accomplish them.

Tasks you should include:

- Attending classes.
- Reviewing.
- Searching for information.
- Studying.
- Assignments.
- Seminar preparation.
- Presentations.
- Planning/scheduling.
- Meetings with tutor.
- Meetings with mentor.
- Reading.
- Practising clinical skills.

Schedules

One way to manage your study time is to use a series of schedules that relate to different periods of time and priority levels (Rowntree 1998).

Very important tasks

Make a schedule of very important tasks, indicate hand-in dates for all assignments and add other tasks as they occur. Give yourself target dates for all tasks and indicate which are the most important. It is worth remembering that when you write an assignment you are actually learning about your assignment topic, so using your assignment hand-in date as your deadline is not a good target date. You will need more time to reflect and refine what you have written once you have produced your first draft.

From the completion date of these tasks you should then work backwards to important points that lead to the completion of the task. If, for example, you need to produce an essay, an important point could be the completion of the search of the literature or delivering a first draft to your tutor. These events need to be given a completion date in your schedule. When managing a project these important points are often called 'milestones'. Once all your milestones have been logged and given a completion date you have your 'main schedule'.

Weekly schedule

The next level of planning is your 'weekly schedule'. This should be informed by your main schedule but needs to include basic study tasks such as reviewing, practising, searching for information, visits to tutor. You may need to form weekly lists of tasks to inform your schedule, indicating on which day you will complete each task.

When you form your schedule, allocate a certain amount of time to each task. In forming your weekly study schedule you need to pay regard to your overall time budget.

Daily schedule

It is also a good idea to have a 'daily schedule'. Each night or morning look at your weekly schedule see what you were meant to have achieved and how well you have done. Then schedule your day, prioritize the tasks using EIP (essential, important, postponable). 'E' tasks must be done that day. 'I' tasks have a high priority but not as high as those graded 'E'. 'P' tasks can be put off. 'E' tasks need to have a firm time when they will be tackled, everything stops for an 'E'. 'I' tasks should also have a firm time, 'P' tasks can be slotted in when time allows. Cross tasks off your list as you complete them; this will give you a good feeling of satisfaction.

Review your schedules

You must make sure you review your schedules; if you don't, you may not meet an assignment deadline, or you may fail to revise sufficiently. Your review needs to be done both daily and weekly. On a daily basis look at what you didn't achieve; if you feel you spent too little or too much time studying a particular subject, adjust the next day's schedule. Your weekly review needs to do the same, but also needs to be based on an overall view of how long particular tasks take. The time you take to achieve tasks will change as you become more experienced and if tasks that you need to complete become more challenging. When you do a weekly review, you must also bear in mind your overall schedule, in order that you remain on target.

But I hate schedules

People are different, and some people just hate lists and schedules. Nevertheless, you will have deadlines to meet and you will need to make decisions about your time. An alternative method of thinking about tasks and time is known as the 'pickle jar theory' (Figure 2.2). Here, you imagine that all your available time is represented by an empty jar. You first fill your jar with the big important tasks, the ones that are going to make a difference to your life and studies; each task is represented by a pickle, hence big important task, big item of pickle. But if you fill your jar with big pickles you will notice that there is still space; this space can be filled with the less important stuff. Hence, answering the last text message or e-mail will probably come into the small stuff category and should not encroach upon your big pickles. Try Activity 2.1.

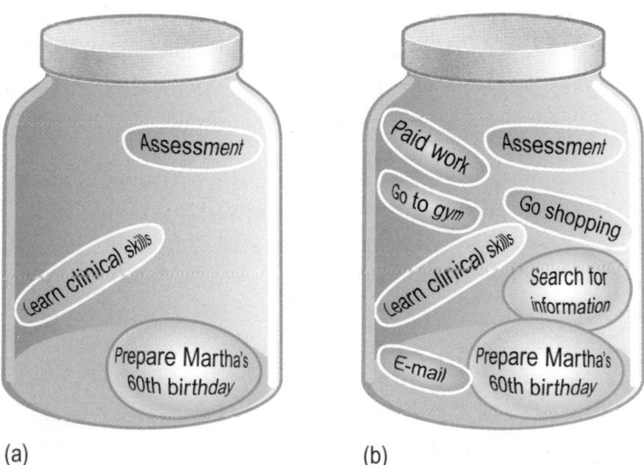

Figure 2.2 • The pickle jar theory. First fill the jar with big, important tasks (a), then add the smaller, less important, stuff (b). (After Wright 2002.)

Activity 2.1

Produce a schedule for your studies. Decide which targets are the most important, medium important, least important and so on. Next plan when you want to do the work to complete your targets according to their priority. Now develop your schedule for each week, highlighting priority tasks. Don't forget to reward yourself each time you have completed a target!

Using pictures

Another way of identifying your targets is to draw a picture showing your different goals and their importance to you. You can then use this to help centre your thoughts and focus on particular activities that have most prominence for you. From your picture, produce a weekly schedule, highlighting priority tasks. If you find images help you to remember things better than lists, you may find it helpful to stick or draw a different carton next to each of your targets, so that you associate the image with the target and so remember it better.

Making good use of your study time

Many people starting full-time study courses anticipate that they will have much more time for their studies than they expected. What many people do not realize is that they have to plan their time for this study, otherwise other things use the time up. Having found time for study in your schedule, you need to think about making the most of that time.

Quality of study

Some people can spend longer studying at any one time than others who can concentrate better by taking short breaks after say 20 minutes. By study, we mean focusing on learning something. You will find it helpful to find out for how long you can study before you become restless; is it, for example,

20, 30 or 50 minutes? Knowing what your concentration span is helps you to plan breaks between your periods of study. Breaks should last no longer than your concentration span and are better at about 5 or 10 minutes. When writing this section, for example, I find that I work for about 20 minutes before having a short break. You will probably find that, if you are studying subjects that are unfamiliar or you find difficult, you will only be able to concentrate for a short period. Conversely, if your studying involves activity such as searching for material or practising something, you will probably find that your ability to concentrate is extended. By knowing your concentration span for different study activities you are more able to plan and allocate your time effectively and to know how to use your breaks. You can improve your concentration span by using good note-taking techniques, which we shall be describing further on in this chapter.

Best time to study

When is your best time to study? Are you an early bird or a night owl? When can you fit your study time in around all your home activities? Some people study in the small hours of the night when their family are asleep, others prefer to get up early. Knowing what is your best 'time' to study helps you to study effectively.

Minimizing distractions

Regardless of how you study, you need to be focused on what you are studying; this means you need to be free from things that might distract you. What distracts us is very much an individual thing. Some people, for example, do not like studying in quiet rooms as they find silence distracting, whereas others prefer to have music in the background. Also recognizing what has been study and what has been learning through chatting with friends is important. Studying with friends can be very beneficial once the ground work of becoming familiar with the subject has been achieved. Sharing your understanding and testing out your use of unfamiliar terminology or ideas with a small group of trusted friends is very helpful and students who can work this way tend to be more successful.

Adjusting to new learning

Learning new words and learning about unfamiliar ideas can be challenging to newcomers to a course. The process many adults embarking on an unfamiliar subject area go through has been described by Taylor (1986) as a series of experiences that can be both uncomfortable but also exciting, suggesting that adult students initially feel overwhelmed and then angry with themselves and their course teachers. She called this phase 'disconfirmation' and it is associated with the struggle to learn the unfamiliar concepts and language of the subject. After this stage, once students had learnt the basic concepts and felt sufficiently confident to talk about the subject with other people, they could move on to the stage of 'exploration'. This is the stage in a learning process when adult students can acknowledge their struggles, share the experience with others and relate their difficulties to the course material. It also leads to the next stage when students begin to expand their knowledge and are able to relate it to their everyday experiences. This stage Taylor called 'reorientation'. We have described these stages because being aware that at times you will feel uncomfortable and struggle to learn will help you not to feel quite so isolated. If you don't quite grasp an aspect of any particular topic, there are some activities you could try (see Activity 2.2).

Activity 2.2

- Ask a friend or colleague if they have understood the topic. If they did, it is likely they will help you and this will improve their understanding even further. If they didn't understand, then you can work together to help each other. Either way you will feel supported.
- Read some of the articles that are in your course reference list and work through the SQR3 technique (we describe this further on in the chapter).
- Make an appointment to see your tutor to get additional help, making sure that you tell them beforehand what you want to discuss.

Using study techniques

In this section we introduce some ideas that will help you to study effectively and how to make notes that you can use both to help you learn and to use when you come to revising for assignments or examinations.

SQ3R

SQ3R is a system that was developed to promote detailed active reading, but it can also be seen as a system for studying. SQ3R stands for 'survey, question, read, recall, review' (Beard 1990). Although strictly the acronym should be SQRRR, it is usually written as SQ3R. The focus of the next sections will be the differences between each of the stages. The system will help you to make good use of your study time as it supports reading for understanding or taking a deep approach to your learning.

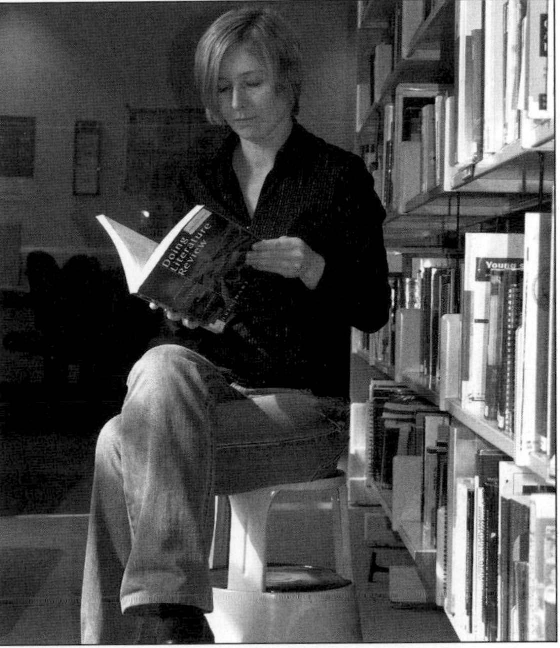

Figure 2.3 • Surveying texts.

Survey

The survey stage is the part of the SQ3R process that can take a lot of time as it involves asking not only the question 'What is this article/book about?' but also 'How is it structured?' and 'Which bits might be useful?'

Analysing a book or text

You probably started surveying this book by checking the title and then went to look at the contents page at the front and perhaps the index at the back (Figure 2.3). The contents page lists the chapters of the book and sometimes an outline of the material covered within each chapter. If you are interested in a particular subject such as intravenous infusion and you find a chapter on non-oral nutrition, it would be reasonable to assume that this information would be found in that chapter. If you cannot find the information in the contents page, then try the index. The index records the occurrence of topics in alphabetical order and lists the pages on which each topic occurs. Using the index is more efficient than simply flipping through the book hoping you will find your topic under a heading. You may need to be flexible and use your imagination to think of alternative headings for your topic. For example, information about an intravenous infusion could come under headings such as 'infusion', 'therapy', 'hydration', 'fluid balance' and so on. Sometimes a textbook will include a glossary which can provide some guidance as to the likely terms that are used in the text; this is often a good source of help. Other sources of information about a book and its usefulness are the introductory page, the foreword and the preface, which normally contain general information about how a book is structured and for whom it is written. Most books will have a bibliographic page before the main body of the text; this tells you information such as when and where it was published, who it was published by and what edition it is. In a field such as nursing, knowing the date of publication is particularly important as information quickly becomes out-of-date. Similarly, place of publication is important because there is considerable variation in practice, and the names of medicines and equipment, from country to country.

You can use the same kind of approach when surveying research articles and articles published in professional journals. The title, introduction and concluding paragraphs should be examined as good indicators of the content of such articles.

Skim reading

The next stage in the survey process is to skim read the journal article or the section of the book or the text that you need to understand. At this stage you are reading to get a sense of the content and what the text is about. Does it address the information you really need to know? How much time are you likely to need to read and understand the material? Are you already familiar with the key principles? If the text is right for you then you are ready to go to the next stage of SQ3R.

Questioning and preparing for reading

Before surveying for information, it is a good idea to make an association map using the actual phenomena you are interested in. The associations are words or processes, which are linked with the phenomena you are interested in. This process is similar to what is known as brainstorming or free thinking. In brainstorming you simply write down anything that comes into your head that may be connected to the subject that you are interested in. As you brainstorm do not stop to consider the relative merits of your suggestions, just carry on until you run out of ideas. Once you have done this you can then decide which of your ideas, questions and suggestions are linked to your subject; do not throw out your original list as you may want to refer to it once you have completed your reading. Brainstorming is most effective when carried out with other people and is a very good activity for a study group.

Once you have started your survey and begun to think about the significance of your findings to the subject you are interested in you have entered the questioning stage of the SQ3R technique. At this stage in the process you will need to focus on the type of information and what you want it for. Useful questions will be associated with the textbook or article itself and then with the content:

- Is this text of use?
- Is the article/book suitable for me?
- Does it give me the information that I am searching for?
- Is the content factual/opinion based?
- Is it new information or based on the interpretation of other people's work?
- What does the author think about this subject?
- What new technical terms are used?
- Can I make sense of what is being said?
- Is it written in a particular style?
- What are the key points of this text and do they relate to my quest?
- What questions am I trying to find the answers to?
- What am I trying to understand?

Your questions should be based on your association map from your brainstorm and your survey of the information in the text. Using this technique will help you to choose texts that meet your needs.

Reading

The reading phase at first sight seems obvious, and of course in order to complete the question phase you need to have done some reading. The distinction here is that in the question phase you need to be surveying the text quickly to get an appreciation of the content of the material, whereas in this reading phase you will be reading with much greater depth and focus with the intention of evaluating the material. Figure 2.4 illustrates the steps to take.

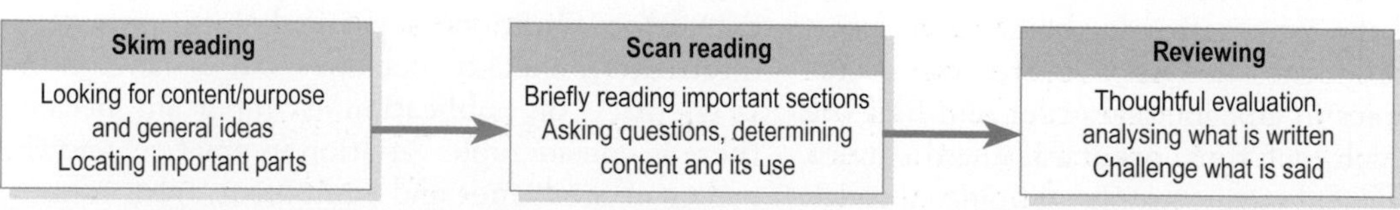

Figure 2.4 • Different forms of reading texts.

There are thus different forms of reading. In the survey stage of the SQ3R technique you will probably be skimming; in the questioning part, you might be looking in more detail at specific aspects and this might be called 'scan reading' (Payne and Whittaker 2000).

Deep reading is a skill that involves concentration. Rowntree (1998) suggests that at this stage taking notes should be avoided. This is because the process of note-taking can distract you from the main task of reading and understanding what is written.

When you read deeply you need to be sceptical and ask questions of what is written. The idea of deep reading is to try to engage and be an active reader. When you are reading at this deep level you are looking to find answers to specific questions. The term deep here is quite important because what you want to avoid is reading at a surface level. If you read at a surface level you will fixate on trying to remember what you read. Remembering is not the main point of reading at a deep level. The main point of reading deeply is to gain understanding because, if you understand why something is done in a certain way, remembering becomes very much easier. To achieve a deep approach to your reading you need to try to relate your reading to something you already know about, your own body functions if you are learning about body functions, or to your everyday experiences if it is concerned with sociology or nursing practice.

When you read, notice whether you can identify individual topics and ideas within the text. These can be generally signified by headings or be more specific and located within individual paragraphs. The survey stage of the SQ3R technique will have helped you to home in on the sections that are relevant to you. You may find it helpful to work with a highlighter pen or a pencil to mark the specific texts you think are important.

Just as each paragraph will normally carry an idea or concept, it may also carry illustrative detail. Following this detail can help you remember the main ideas; trying to remember all the detail will probably be difficult and unnecessary. Often texts provide examples to illustrate a specific point. Do either read through any examples or try to think of your own examples, as they will help you to understand and are often easier to remember.

Reading in a questioning or critical manner comes with practice. When reading in this critical way good starting questions are:

- Do I know this already?
- Is this information something I have never heard of before?
- Is it of use and relevant to the question I am trying to solve?

As you start to evaluate the content, you may ask some basic evaluative questions. These may initially be based on your current experiences and understanding of the subject:

- Does what I am reading match my experience?
- Does this writer's perspective match those authors of other text(s) I have read?
- Do I agree with the author?
- Are there any contradictions in what is being said?
- Where have the facts come from?
- Are the facts right?

As you read, you may also ask some more analytical questions:

- What are the ideas that support the author's ideas/argument?
- Do the facts support the conclusion?
- Are the facts true but is the conclusion wrong?
- Do all the examples support the author or are there other examples that do not?
- If some examples do not fit with the author's view why don't they fit?
- Is there an alternative conclusion?
- What happens to the idea/argument if some of the supporting facts are not true?
- How do the author's arguments/ideas fit in with those of other writers?
- Are the arguments good, but do others agree with them?

Finally, some utilitarian questions:

- Is this author's work worth remembering?
- Should I make notes?

- Do I need to be aware of this article for an assessment?
- Should I discuss this work with my tutor, friend or study group?
- How does what the writer suggests relate to my practice: will I change what I do?
- What have I learnt from reading this article?

Recall

Rowntree (1998) suggests that you are likely to forget about half of the ideas and concepts within what you read the moment you put down what you are reading unless you make an active attempt to recall it. We suggested that the reading aspect of what you do is best conducted without making notes. Making notes is best when undertaking the recall stage of SQ3R. To get the best results from your reading, you need to make use of it and relate it to your existing knowledge of the subject. This means that your note formation should be an active process. Using your reading in your note-making includes providing your own examples and comments on the reading and exploring what other ideas could relate to the information. Other good strategies to help retain the information is to discuss your reading with friends and getting their perspectives, putting what you have read into an assignment or trying to relate the information to your nursing practice experiences.

Recall can occur during the reading stage. For example, you might just pause to think about and make sense of what you have read, putting to one side what you are reading to make some notes. Knowing that you will do some recall will help you concentrate on what you are reading.

Recall takes practice; at first you may want to stop every one or two paragraphs. As you become more familiar with the concepts and language of the text so you become better at describing the content (meaning) to another person. The important aspect of recall is that you should make sense of what you have read without reading the original article. If you cannot recall and make sense of it then you must re-read it. Recall can take time, but it is an essential part of the studying process and has been shown to improve success at college and university.

Your notes should be based on what you initially recall (remember) from your reading. There is no right or wrong way of making notes but they do need to be made in such a way that you can link the notes to the text that you are reading. So making sure you have the full details of the text, (title, author, date, publisher) on each page of your notes and numbering the pages of your notes means you can trace the original text if you need to go back to it.

You could, for example, give a Cornell note page (see below) to each item that you read; each page can then be placed in a file under the particular subject or topic that it relates to. The most important and obvious thing is that you can use your notes at a later stage in your course and so they need to be legible and comprehensible. Some people find that creating a 'mind map' or a 'spider diagram' is a useful way of documenting the key points of a chapter or article (see below), and use them as a summary with page numbers for each key point. These tools are useful at the initial recall stage of SQ3R as they help you to recognize what you have understood and which sections of the text need further work. Using a mind map or a spider diagram as a record of your reading may require further notes if they are to be of use at a later date.

Review

The final stage of SQ3R is the review stage. This review stage provides an opportunity to go over the notes you have made to make sure they are suitable for the reasons for which you made them. In this stage, check back to the original purpose of your study, go back to the survey stage and ask yourself:

- What did I set out to achieve?
- What was the purpose of this period of study?
- Have I answered my questions from the survey stage?
- Do my notes make sense?
- What did I achieve?"
- What have I learnt from reading this article/book?
- Will I change what I do?

You may want to re-read the article(s) or book chapter, adding to your notes if you find you missed something.

Review your notes as your course progresses, checking that they still represent what you think about the subject and update them as you discover new material and as new research emerges.

Using the SQ3R technique for taught sessions and in practice placements

The SQ3R method is a structured approach to study and as you use it and become familiar with a subject you will find that many of the steps you can do without having to make lists of questions. Don't try to use the SQ3R approach too prescriptively as you will find that you can adapt the techniques to the type of reading that you are doing. For instance, if you are reading about how to perform a very well-defined and established procedure, you probably will not spend much time evaluating the content but more time questioning your own understanding.

SQ3R in lectures

The SQ3R was originally devised for reading texts, but it can also be used in other circumstances such as lectures and seminars and even when you are learning in practice. In the lecture situation, you will need to do some preparation beforehand. This stage is similar to the survey stage when you think of what questions you would like the lecturer to answer. Using active listening is akin to the reading stage of SQ3R. The recall and review stages are important to carry out at the end of the lecture so that you can begin to relate the content to your own experiences and thus integrate it with your existing knowledge.

SQ3R in practice placement experiences

In practice situations, you can use the SQ3R in several different ways. For example, you can go through each phase of the SQ3R to prepare yourself for your placement while learning about specific skills or patients' health care needs and for learning about health care delivery.

You can also use the SQ3R technique to prepare for developing a learning agreement or a learning contract for your placement experience. The survey stage is about preparation and finding out what a particular placement experience has to offer. The questioning stage is about focusing on what you want to learn about and the questions that you want answered, perhaps by staff or by patients. The read and recall stages can be used to read up about specific health care problems that patients nursed in the placement are experiencing, and investigations and procedures that they may experience. Using this approach helps you to be knowledgeable and able to learn successfully from your placement.

You can also use the SQ3R technique for preparing to give care or learning about a specific aspect of patients' health care problems. Your questions may also be related to your own personal development and what you can learn in the setting and how you want to develop. Both the questioning and reading activities can be used when reading patients' notes and records, or reading through a procedure or text about specific skills and techniques. Your review could be talking to patients to find out about their symptoms or their care and then relating your findings to your reading in your nursing textbook. In addition, you can use the recall stage to make notes about your activities during the shift so that you can review them with your mentor or with your friends, and check them out with your textbooks.

Note-making and note-taking

Note-making is valuable for a variety of reasons and people use note-taking under a variety of circumstances. Here are three principal reasons why you might take notes:

- To help you remember texts or experiences, or advice or instructions.
- To help you learn from texts or taught sessions.
- To create a formal record of interactions, events or conversations.

Styles with which notes are made vary and depend upon personal taste. Essentially there are three types of note-making: linear prose, outline summaries, and diagrammatic (Rowntree 1998). Most students start off using the prose approach but often find that they tend to write too much.

Research has shown that making notes is a very important part of the learning process (Kiewra 1985, 1987), especially when the note-making process builds on and extends the learning that has taken place. Note-making is best when it involves using supplementary materials from journals or textbooks that expand what you have learned in a taught session. By making time to reflect upon your taught session and expanding your knowledge, you will find you can remember the information much better. Working this way draws on the same skills that you learned with the SQ3R system.

Another important advantage of making notes is that it helps you to learn how to make accurate notes, which is an essential part of your professional life. You will want to make notes in your practice placements about patients or activities you have been undertaking so that you can create an accurate record. Note-making is thus a skill that is well worth perfecting. People often learn to create their own form of shorthand and to use abbreviations when writing notes. You will need to organize your notes so that you can read and use them easily for your intended purpose, as well as having a good place to store them so you can locate them when needed.

Notes, when used in the context of study, are an interim measure between finding new information and learning it and/or using the information for a specific end. Rowntree (1998) makes the distinction between making and taking notes. Taking notes may be passive when done to aid memory and to concentrate; making notes is usually an active process with a focus on expanding and organizing information and thoughts. There is research evidence to suggest that students who make notes perform better at assessments than those who do not (Annis and Davis 1978, Kulhavy and Dyer 1975).

The Cornell system of making notes

Using the Cornell system (Pauk 1993) can help you to make the most of the material that you are studying. The system provides opportunities for you to follow the SQ3R approach as you write your notes and so helps with your learning. You can use the Cornell system in different settings, such as taught sessions, lectures and seminars, as well as when you are studying texts and in placement settings. The system can also help you to become better at learning through the process of note-taking.

To use the Cornell system you need to divide your notepaper into columns and boxes so you can record specific kinds of information. Have a look at the example that Hannah created when she was studying part of this chapter (Table 2.1).

Hannah's use of the Cornell system helped her to create a short and succinct summary of her reading of this chapter up until this point. She included the main points about using the SQ3R method in the second column and then she made very brief notes in the first column in her own form of shorthand; this is called reducing the notes. It helped her to transfer the information into her own language, which is a very important step in helping her to take a deep approach to her studies. It is a good idea to do this as soon as you can after reading a text or attending a taught session.

The bottom section of the Cornell system can be used in different ways; here Hannah has reflected on how helpful the system was for reading a difficult and unfamiliar text. In the next section we shall be discussing how you can use the Cornell system for taught sessions, such as lectures and seminars particularly.

Using the Cornell system for taught sessions

You can use the Cornell system to prepare yourself for a taught session and to summarize what you have gained from the session.

Table 2.1 Hannah's notes for part of this chapter using the Cornell system

Recall/cue column[1]	Recording column[2]
SQ3R	A system for studying text materials particularly. Need to use five different strategies: survey, question, read, recall, record
Survey: skim read 2c if text is Ok 4me	Check text for relevance and quality of information; home into specific areas of interest, and so save time
Question: questions I need 2 find answers 2 in text	Prepare with some questions on subject I want answered (may be tricky if I don't know anything about the topic)
Read: intensive process	Taylor (1986) says getting to grips with unfamiliar information is difficult and uncomfortable, so I need to be patient with myself and plan enough time to read the first articles, until I feel I have got to grips with the language and ideas
Recall: check how much I understand, relate 2my experiences	After reading article, try to recall the main points; if I can't go back and read again, will need some memorization as well as application
Record: notes of content	Record summary of what I have understood and check against the text for accuracy; must remember to include reference information so I can find the article again if I need to re-read it
Plan time	Try out system in class next time and when on placement
Reflection and review	Used the process to make notes when reading a text on causes of Down's syndrome; it was a tough text but the system helped, especially when I came to write up the summary of what I had learned. I found that I could use the new words that I had learned in the class when we discussed the text. This increased my self-confidence
Source of notes	Pauk W 1993 How to study in college. Houghton Mifflin, Boston Scott I, Ely C 2007 Learning how to study and learn effectively. In: Spouse J, Cox C, Cook M (eds) Common foundation studies in nursing. Elsevier, Edinburgh

[1] for reviewing the lecture notes and writing short summaries; helps with organizing your thoughts
[2] for recording ideas, explanations and examples using a suitable form of notes

Preparation: survey and question

Before you go to a lecture it is a good idea to think about its title and likely content. In the second column write some questions that come to mind.

Read (listen)

When you attend the lecture, use the second column for notes taken during the lecture. Focus on the ideas and explanations and the examples that have been used to support them.

Recall

After the lecture, work on reducing your notes. Do this by asking questions; these questions should be based on the content of the lecture. Put these reduced recall notes in the first column. This process should be completed as soon as possible after the lecture. Reducing the notes in this way will help you sort out the meaning within the notes, and to make sense of them. It will force you to revisit the lecture you have just had, and will help you to recall your learning from the lecture at a later date.

Recite and reflection

The next step is to use what you have written in the recall column to go over what was said in the lecture. At this stage, look just at the recall column not the actual notes. This stage is known as the 'recite' stage. Getting together with friends and discussing your understanding is an excellent way of learning and remembering important material. If you can arrange to meet up with others after a taught session in, for example, a study group or during break time, it is a good idea for each of you to describe, using your recall column, what you think the lecture was about and what you think you learned. You may be surprised at the differences between your notes and those of your colleagues.

You may find it helpful to make some notes in your first column about your preparation for the taught session and what you could do better next time to prepare.

Reflection or critical analysis

Now that you are clear on what the session was about, you can start to think critically about the content of the session. How well did the information you heard match with what you had previously read or experienced in other sessions? How logical was the information: was it the way the information was organized and presented or were the underlying concepts incoherent or described wrongly? How well were the arguments supported by examples? What are you going to do with the information that you gained from the session? What suggestions did your lecturer make about the relevance of the information to your placement or to your course? Your answers to these questions can go in the last box at the bottom of the columns.

Using the Cornell system of note-making

Some writers suggest that one of the advantages of the Cornell system is that, once the notes are written, they do not need to be revisited; however, we have found that most students need to review their notes. The last stage in the system is thus to revisit your notes periodically to review them. Reviewing your notes now and again, and especially if you come across an experience that relates to them, will help you to remember the contents. It also allows you to add to your notes and expand them as your understanding of the topic increases as a result of your reading or your practice experiences and to expand your understanding. In Table 2.2 you can see how Jolene made a Cornell note on a taught session on pain management.

Charting information

When using the charting method you need to have done your preparation for the session and have a good idea of the main themes that will be covered by the taught session. You then divide your notepaper into columns that represent each of the themes, and as the session progresses make a record in each column according to the theme being discussed. You will have quite narrow columns, so your note-taking will be restricted to keywords and phrases; this will limit the amount of writing that is required. This approach is useful for discussion and seminars; also it will help you to make connections between different ideas. Figure 2.5 is an example of a student working in the biology laboratory and making notes of her observations.

Diagrammatic methods for note-making

There are several different names given to diagram notations, such as spray diagrams, spider diagrams

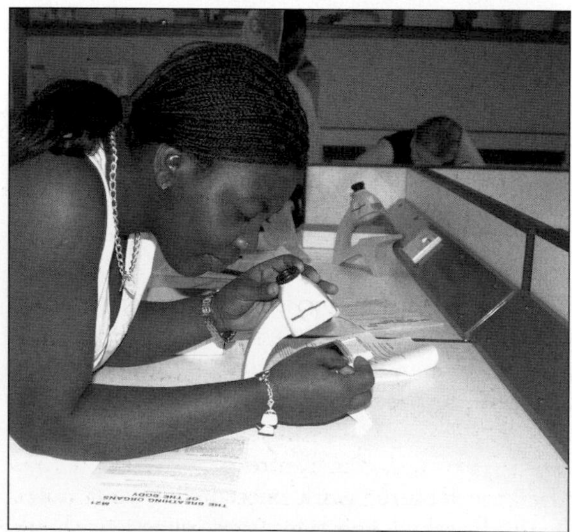

Figure 2.5 • Note-making and charting.

Table 2.2 Jolene's use of the Cornell system to make notes on pain management

Recall/cue column	Recording column
Aim is to reduce suffering	Pain management is about reducing the experience of pain
Why? Uncomfortable, distressing, also many consequences on rest of life (whole)	Pain can affect many aspects of a person's life. Examples: mobility, social activities, mood, confidence and ability to concentrate. It can change relationships, affect sleep patterns or/and how much they enjoy life
We do not have a complete understanding, sometimes direct; cause and effect. Gate theory useful	Pain is an unpleasant sensory and emotional experience associated with actual or potential tissue damage
Different types of pain occur; important division between acute and chronic	Contradicted by the gate control theory of pain. Melzak & Wall. Focuses on different pain states at the brain, rather than at the site where the brain perceives the pain to be. Pain is really a perception, and not an objective state of a body
Acute pain responds well to drugs (analgesics: what type of drugs are these?)	Pain can be either acute or chronic. Acute pain does not last long, it is short term; normally the pain and the cause of the pain are directly linked; it tends to be sharp (not always). Medicine-based treatments are very effective
Chronic pain difficult to treat; alternative therapies	Chronic pain is longer term and often more diffuse, less sharp, not always linked strongly to source. Although not often sharp, it can be very debilitating
Pain can be classified based on tissue of origin	Chronic pain does not always respond well to medicines and habituation to drugs can occur; some concern about addiction to opiate-based analgesics. Alternative therapies (acupuncture, hypnotherapy) found to be effective
Not really sure what was meant; is this linked to gate theory?	Chronic pain management often combines physical, emotional, intellectual and social approaches to help the individual regain control of their life Pain can also be classified based on tissue type: somatic, visceral and cutaneous, also neuropathic Chronic pain does not seem to have a reason
Reflection and review	Pain is very important to patients. Sometimes it is difficult to know what to do for patients with chronic pain; many have 'tried everything'. Wide range of alternatives to drugs available. Need to explore gate theory and clarify why chronic pain does not seem to have a reason. I'm not sure what use the classification of pain into tissue of origin is: does this help in the therapy, does pain from different tissues respond differently?
Source of notes	Lecture notes from Miss Anthrope, June 2006

and mind maps. The use of such diagrams requires active engagement with the materials as the idea of these diagrams is that related concepts, facts and examples are linked together. These diagrams tend to start off with a general issue written down, normally towards the centre of a page and then lines are radiated from the centre for each major theme as it is developed. Each branch from the centre is labelled. Sub-branches can be developed as issues become more specific or less important to the central theme. Each sub-branch is itself labelled: in Figure 2.6 you will see how Benjamin started to create his notes on types of stress. Some individuals will like to use boxes to put their themes and sub-themes in and then link these with lines where the various themes are connected. These diagrams are similar to those known as mind maps (see Chapter 6).

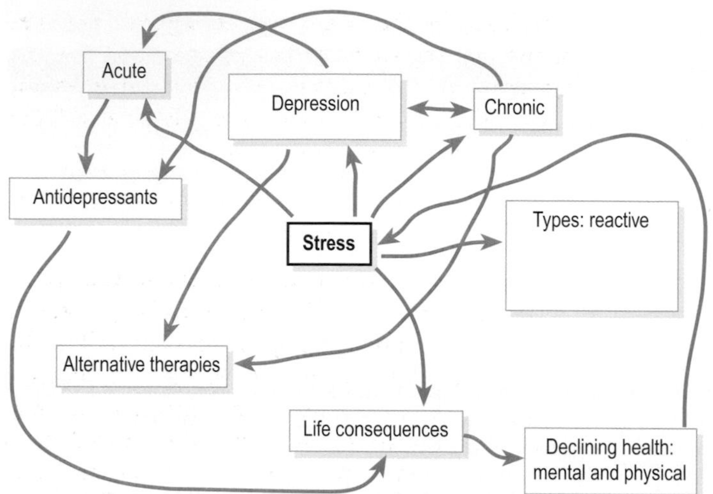

Figure 2.6 • Benjamin's mind map for note-making about stress.

The advantage of a diagrammatic approach is that it provides a visual record of a lecture/seminar, and such records are often more helpful if you are one of those people who is a visual learner (Garder 1993). This approach of recording information is good in most study activities such as recording your reading or when preparing for an assignment or an examination. Using diagrammatic note-making also highlights the important issues of your learning. Using this approach will help you to see the connections between the various points more clearly. If you use this approach when reading a text it is helpful to include the page number for each core theme; this will help you to find the specific information at a later stage.

Some people find that normal-sized notepaper does not provide sufficient space and that the page becomes too full of information. An alternative strategy is to use smaller squares of paper to write key concepts on and then attach them to a larger sheet in the order that you want. Whatever approach you choose, make sure you enter all the information (data) that you need in order to go back to the original text at a later stage if necessary, or to quote the reference in assignments.

Making notes in taught sessions

Most people will need to take notes during lectures and seminars. For some people, taking notes can help you to focus on what is being said and at a later point in time serve to help you remember and recall the ideas and the content. Many lecturers will provide handouts of their lectures; they may be quite simple or very comprehensive. Studies suggest that students who do well are those who expand on their lecturer's notes with additional information (e.g. Kesselman-Turkel & Peterson 1982, Kiewra 1987). Thus it is a good idea to actively search out your lecturer's notes and to use them. If you are able to develop the skill of making accurate and succinct notes in one of the ways we have described above, you will find that your learning is more successful.

Text and taught sessions

You need to think about what you can gain from a lecture that it is difficult to find elsewhere (see Activity 2.3). For instance, you will probably be able to obtain factual information relatively easily from textbooks. A good lecture will give you insight and understanding, and provide a structure that will help you organize your thoughts. It will also help you to develop a sense of your subject and how experts seek to understand its nature. You may want to focus your notes on these factors rather than on noting down factual information. If, when looking at your notes, you find they are of little use (either they do not make sense or they

Activity 2.3

Question: What are the differences between learning through a lecture and learning through a text book?

Answer: Here is a list of some of the benefits students say that they get from lectures:

- Socializing.
- Information.
- Understanding.
- Knowing what to do.
- Getting notes.

Put these in order with the item that is most important for you first and the one that is least important last.

---

lack detail and structure), you will need to think about how you take notes and consider the method that you use. We have described several systems and strategies for producing notes. The evidence base to determine whether one method is superior to another is practically non-existent. We favour the Cornell system of note-making as it is a system that helps you to prepare for your sessions as well as to follow up with a review. The Cornell system can be used to fit with different note-taking strategies.

Whichever system of note-making and note-taking you use, it is worth remembering that by turning up at a taught session you are choosing to go to it and therefore you must have a reason for attending. So, the first part of any successful note system that is going to help you learn is, in fact, to think about why you are attending. The sorts of reasons that students give include:

- To learn.
- To make sure I know what I need to (so that I can pass).
- Because the lecturer is good.
- To be entertained (the lecturer is funny).
- Because I feel I should do, and because my friends do.

Not one of these reasons is mutually exclusive, but the important point to remember is that the majority of the responsibility for gaining something from a taught session lies with you. If you prepare well you should be able to gain something from a lecture or seminar regardless of how good or bad the presenter is. When you know why you are attending a lecture, you will be in a better position to focus on learning and your note-taking.

Note-making in practice

When you are learning and working in your practice placement you will still need to keep notes of what you are experiencing and learning. All of the systems for note-taking can be used in practice situations. You are likely to encounter issues and to experience events that you will wish to discuss with your mentor, preceptor, supervisor or tutor, usually at some time after the event. There will also be experiences that you want to remember so that you can use them for your own private reflections. In most practice situations there will also be some occasions when you will be expected to make notes (e.g. at 'handover' on ward-based placements) or use notes (e.g. in case conferences). When recording notes in practice situations you will probably need to adopt a style that is relatively rapid yet still provides sufficient detail to allow for recall.

Keeping a small pocket notebook is useful for recording your observations and making notes using diagrams, charts or prose notes. Many students find it helpful to keep a note of any questions that come to mind so they can look up the answers when they have the opportunity. If they get stuck and can not find an answer, they can then ask a staff member for help. Educational theory suggests that you are much more likely to remember and understand phenomena if you are forced to discover the answers for yourself (Entwistle 1997).

Over the course of your practice experience you will come across ideal opportunities for note-taking; one of them is when staff from one shift hand over their patients and report to the staff on the next shift. In the early stage of your course you will encounter a lot of unfamiliar terms and acronyms, especially at this handover period, so it is a good idea to make a note of them for later research.

Note-making and confidentiality

Whenever you make notes in a placement setting, such as at patient handover and at case meetings, it is vital that you remember to respect patient confidentiality. A breach of confidentiality will occur if you use information that identifies an individual patient. Any notes with patient's details *must* be destroyed immediately after use on that shift. No information of a highly confidential nature should be made on scraps of paper that may cause an inappropriate disclosure of patient details. Any written information about a patient, however much in note form, can be used as a legal document. When note-taking during handover, it is a good idea to observe the following:

- *Noting patients' details*. You should note patients' problems and proposed investigations and treatments.
- *Using abbreviations*. This is not good practice for various reasons, although it is often the common shorthand of placement settings. Most importantly, never use abbreviations if you do not know what they stand for.
- *Confidentiality issues*. Be careful what you write about patients. If you have a notebook for looking up material, always use a fictitious name or preferably just a letter, such as Mrs X.
- *Checking and confirming information*. This should be done with the registered nurse or other health professional supervising at the end of report.
- *Preparation for meetings*. Make notes with regard to any questions you have about patients.

While on placement, you may be asked to visit other departments where patients undergo investigations or treatments. It is a good idea to keep short notes about these departments, the visits you make and include notes on how staff provide care to patients. It is also helpful to include a note on any similarities and differences there are with other areas to which you have been placed or you have visited. This will help you develop your skills of analysis as well as your understanding of what health care experiences patients undergo. It is also a good idea to try to reflect on the role of any other professionals that you meet and who support patient care and treatment. All this contributes to increasing your understanding of each patient's experience.

Reviewing your approach to studying

When studying, it is important to build in review periods. A review period is when you put your study materials aside and really think about what you have learnt during your last period of study. You can review what you have learnt during a break, while you exercise or even on the bus. You should also be prepared to test yourself; this is important for recalling information that you need to remember, or for making sure you can execute a practice procedure correctly. Most importantly, if your study strategy is working, you feel an increase in your confidence, a better understanding of what you encounter in practice placements and an increased interest in your career choice, which will in turn make your studying easier and more satisfying.

Lectures and seminars

Lectures and seminars are places where the content that particular courses cover is outlined and made clear. The idea of a lecture is to give students an introduction to a subject and some key concepts; rather like the body, which has a skeletal framework that is 'fleshed out' and has content in the form of organs and systems of nerves and blood vessels, so a lecture is aimed to give you the basis for further study to 'flesh out' the subject. By the end of a lecture you should have a structure of the particular subject that will help you to learn and understand further.

Seminars are often places where topics and themes are developed and expanded upon. They provide a useful opportunity to help you review your level of understanding and have your thoughts changed and altered when talking to your colleagues in discussion sessions or during activities involving problem-based learning. Going to seminars and lectures is important, because research indicates that students who are good at attending taught sessions do better than those who do not attend consistently (Astin 1993, Pascarella & Terenzini 1991).

Through the taught sessions you will gain more insight into what it is to be a professional nurse and what professional practice means from the insights, explanations, examples, behaviour and anecdotes given by your lecturers. These taught sessions often include important information about your course, such as changes to assessments, seminar rooms, important resources such as texts, journal articles and audiovisual materials to use. If you are unable to attend, you will need to make sure you get the information from your friends or the lecturer so that you are not seriously disadvantaged by your absence.

Making the most of a lecture

Many taught sessions that you will be attending are in the form of lectures. Lectures are sometimes regarded as passive learning events (Ramsden 1992). The art of getting the most from your lecture is to be an active and engaged participant. This entails being able to listen and to concentrate during the session and afterwards to think about how you make and form your own notes following it. You will come across both good and bad lecturers, but, as a student, you need to learn from both.

Enhancing listening and concentration

When we discussed the art of note-taking for lectures, we urged you to prepare for your lecture by thinking about the title and the content. These activities raise your motivation and, if you are motivated to attend, you are more likely to listen and be able to concentrate and thus learn from the event. Planning for the lecture makes it easier to hear and learn from what is being said. If, for example, your lecture is about communication skills, spend 10 minutes (perhaps on your journey to the lecture) thinking about different forms of communication, verbal, non-verbal, images, sounds and so on. If you do this, you are already starting to tune into the session and you are more able to be focused during the session, and remembering the content and the ideas from the session will be that much easier.

Where you sit in the lecture theatre makes a difference to your ability to concentrate on the session. Try to sit in a place where you can hear the speaker easily and other distractions are few; this will normally be in the middle of a room or at the front (speakers tend to concentrate on the middle and back rows rather than the front rows).

Listening is an important skill for a nurse and is quite a hard skill to do well as it requires deliberate effort that needs practice. A lecture can be a safe environment to practise this skill of active listening, which requires effort and concentration. Concentration is the act of dedicating most of your energy and effort to a particular activity and avoiding distractions whatever the source. Distractions can be external (e.g. noise, change in lighting, a particularly handsome or odd-looking lecturer) or internal (e.g. worries, dreams or thoughts of other activities).

Developing skills of concentration

One idea to help you think about concentration is to make a concentration score sheet. On this score sheet keep a tally of the number of times you have been distracted. Students have found that the very act of keeping a score sheet helps them to concentrate (Pauk 1993). If you also record the type of distraction, you get a picture of the factors that are disturbing you, and you can use this information to take action to reduce the distractions.

A similar approach is to keep a 'worry diary'. In a worry diary you record during the day the things that worry you as you go about your daily activities. When you look back at the diary it will help you identify the main things that are blocking effective study and you can then think about how the issues can be resolved or reduced in size.

Learning from a taught session

Just as we discussed about taking Cornell notes for note-making in taught sessions, the same principles apply to attending a lecture. You need to listen for the main ideas or concepts of a lecture and make notes of the facts that are used to support the speaker's arguments, summaries and conclusions. The kinds of things that will help include:

- *Use of key or signal words*. An important fact is often signalled by the lecturer who will key or signal words as an introduction to a section of the lecture. For example, if talking about hospital-acquired infections, the lecturer will probably use the heading 'universal precautions'; this word is a signal or keyword and will tell you that there are a series of precautions that will fit under this heading.
- *Breaks and pauses after a summary*. A lecturer will make a small break or pause between different topics. Often this will follow a summary. With a good lecturer there will be a summary that brings the whole lecture together at the end.
- *Significant or leading phrases*. These phrases are used by lecturers to emphasize significant points of interest. Try listening out for important phrases and, as you become a more accomplished listener, you will start to spot them on your own.

Controversy and debate

Some lecturers enjoy raising controversy and debate, and their sessions are often designed to encourage students to develop their ability to think critically and analytically. Sometimes students are encouraged to engage in debate, whereas other lecturers prefer students to listen and discuss the issues at smaller seminar sessions. If your lecturer says something that you do not agree with, try to think about what was said, and why you disagree. Note the point and then at a later point justify why you did not agree and go over the speaker's argument. Even if you agree and understand what the speaker is saying, check the points and argument mentally during the lecture, and on paper afterwards. Using these techniques can transform you from a passive listener to an active listener and learner. The term 'active listener' really means that, not only are your ears detecting the sound, but also your brain is thinking about what you are hearing.

As we suggested with preparation for reading a text and preparation for your taught sessions, you need to be asking questions about what you hear and relate what you hear to what you know. Box 2.2 lists a series of questions that active listeners might ask.

Your note-taking will help both with your concentration and with your listening. However, you need to be sure that your note-taking does not distract you from the taught session and that you do not miss important points. You are very

Box 2.2

Questions that active listeners might ask

Questions that will help you connect with the way the lecturer is thinking

- What is the structure of the lecture?
- How is this session being put together?
- Where is it leading?
- How does it fit with what I know already?

Questions about the content of the session

- What are the main ideas?
- What is the information that supports these ideas?
- What are the main signal or key words (important phrases or words)?
- Am I finding answers to things I have not understood?
- Are the arguments logical?
- Are the conclusions valid?
- Is the material worth making notes on?

Questions focused on you and what you want to gain from the lecture

- Are there things in this lecture that I do not understand?
- What questions do I still have?
- How am I going to use the information from this lecture?
- What does the lecturer want me to do with the information (e.g. remember it, understand it, use it in practice)?

Adapted from Rowntree (1998).

likely to find much of the material, particularly the factual material of a lecture, elsewhere (e.g. in a textbook). Your lecture notes should therefore be brief, allowing you to focus on the lecture, but you must be prepared to make full notes when you can. Lecture notes are not the finished product; they should be seen as an aid to concentration and a basis for further study.

Reading analytically and critically

Being able to read texts and decide if the authors' arguments are valid (true) is an important skill and one that helps you wherever you are, and is essential as a student and as a professional. All the authors whose texts you read will be trying to tell you something and your task is to decide what they are trying to tell you and whether or not they are giving you the correct information. Being able to analyse, evaluate and critique other people's ideas is an important part of most written assessments when studying at university or college. You probably have a favourite newspaper and it may be worth pausing for a moment to think why you choose one newspaper in preference to another. Is it because you have more faith in the way the journalists view the world? Do they promote one political perspective over another? Making choices about which newspaper to read suggests that you are already thinking critically about what you read, and as a student and a professional you need to develop these analytical and critical skills further.

When reading textbooks or journal articles most writers are trying to persuade you to see the world from their perspective. Perhaps a writer is concerned to change certain aspects of practice such as hand hygiene, or, as in this book, to persuade you to adopt certain approaches to studying. Academic writing is often written in the form of a rational argument and this is not the same kind of argument that may occur between individuals in dispute (which may not be rational). Good academic arguments provide a reasoned view or position based on conclusions formed from referenced, factual information that is provided as evidence. Conclusions follow logically from statements (premises) based on sound evidence and the reader is able to see how the arguments led to the conclusions. Using evidence based on carefully documented fact (empirical evidence) distinguishes a rational from a non-rational argument. Within rational arguments you will notice that the statements are designed to persuade. In some texts you may find that even after careful reading the evidence does not support the statements, and the factual information is insufficient to support the arguments and the conclusions. Noticing this is what makes a good critical reader. Sometimes an author may acknowledge that supporting information is scarce and that the arguments have been developed from the best material available.

Judging the arguments

Reading through a text and deciding which are the arguments and whether they are supported sufficiently is a skill that takes practice to learn and refine. Often you will need to read several texts on the same subject so that you have developed your own understanding of the topic. Then you will be in a better position to judge the strengths of one writer's arguments over another's. Also you will be in a good position to judge if the factual statements are true and if the conclusions are correct. When reading, look carefully for contradictions and discrepancies in the text as well as for any statements that do not seem logical. Look out for any taken-for-granted statements, or assumptions that underpin any arguments and check whether they are reasonable. Reading in this way helps you to develop critical thinking skills. For example, arguments for good hand hygiene are underpinned by the assumption that an important cause of the spread of pathogens is physical contact. When looking at the arguments it is worth looking for potential alternative perspectives that can also explain the phenomena or thing that is being investigated. Evaluating and analysing arguments is not always straightforward; it is a skill that improves with practice (try Activity 2.4). If you would like to find out more see Part 3 of Fairbairn & Winch (1998).

Activity 2.4

A useful exercise to help develop the skills of analysis and evaluation is to select a page of writing from a nursing journal and focus on identifying the various components. Read the article, then using a highlighter pen identify the premises (statements of evidence to support an argument). Then using a different coloured pen identify the sentences that you think are there to persuade you. Finally, identify concluding statements; these kinds of statements are not just found at the end of articles but tend to occur after some supporting statements have been made.

Arguments are not always put in a straightforward manner. Look at the examples below; we have numbered each sentence to aid with the analysis (all the citations are fictitious).

1 Improving the hand hygiene practice of health care professionals is a quick and easy way of decreasing the number of hospital-acquired infections that occur every year.
2 Significant numbers of patients acquire infections during stays in hospital (Bloggs 2005).
3 Hospital-acquired infections cost the health services millions of pounds each year and cause an unnecessary burden on staff (Smith 2005).
4 Tackling hospital-acquired infections should be a priority for the health services and it is therefore essential that increased effort be put into the hand hygiene education of health care professionals.

The first three sentences are premises; they are statements to support the argument. The last sentence (4) has two parts (separated by the word 'and'). The first part of the sentence is an aspiration, a hope, a demand; it is therefore not a supporting statement. It could be a conclusion if it were a sentence on its own, but read with the second half of the sentence it is clearly an attempt to persuade us of the validity of the conclusion which is in the second half of the last sentence. When you have identified the components of the argument (analysed it), you now need to do some evaluation. Look at the supporting statements (sentences 1, 2 and 3). Are they evidenced-based? Sentences 2 and 3 have referenced sources; also statement 3 follows from statement 2. *If significant numbers of patients get hospital-acquired infections then it is bound to cost money to treat them and use staff time.* In sentence 1 there is a claim that improving hand hygiene is 'quick and easy'; this statement has no reference and also does not seem to ring true. Surely if improving hand hygiene were quick and easy it would have been done? We would evaluate this supporting statement as being weak and we could even regard it as purely persuasive or even deceptive. Sentence 4 contains the conclusion. When judging conclusions we need to make sure that they follow naturally from the premises. In this case, there is in fact no connection between the premises and the conclusion. The conclusion contains the unsupported assumption that increasing the amount of hand hygiene education will result in better practice. The conclusion is thus spurious.

Do be aware that not all subject disciplines will agree on what constitutes evidence (Tapper 2004), and therefore what may seem a reasonable argument to a sociologist may sometimes be a poor argument for an historian or biologist.

When you approach an article that you are going to read for the first time you may want to use a framework to help you focus your reading. You may want to look for answers to the following questions:

- What is the main reason why the author has written the article?
- Are the assumptions realistic and evidence-based?
- What evidence has been used to support the conclusion? Is the evidence good?
- What is the main conclusion? Is it realistic? Is it based on the evidence that has been presented?
- Is there other work that supports the author's conclusions?
- Would I apply the findings to my practice? If not, why not? What are my doubts?

It is important to remember that whatever your method it is up to you to make the judgement on the quality and applicability of any particular article. Simply because a piece of writing has been published does not mean it is correct.

Information gathering

The main function of universities and colleges is the creation of knowledge and its distribution to the wider community. Universities are vast repositories of information and as a student you will certainly want to use that information and may even contribute to that knowledge. Finding and using information is a very important skill to learn. It is a vital skill for you to acquire if your practice is to be based on evidence and up-to-date. It will also help you to learn and develop your professional knowledge throughout your career.

As a nursing student you will be introduced to ways of obtaining information from a wide variety of sources; this will include sources such as printed materia. electronic media, practice experience, lectures, seminars and tutorials. This section will look at obtaining information from web-based material and from other forms of databases.

An important task is to learn the strategies to locate and sort through the information that will be of use to you. Computer databases have many advantages; not only do they offer easy access to large amounts of information but they are often accessible from anywhere in the world. This gives you the choice of where and when you wish to use them: home, library, Internet cafe and so on. Most databases provide an abstract or summary of each journal article, but some will link you to the full original article. At the end of your search you can e-mail the results of your search to your personal Internet account.

Using the Internet

Introduction

The Internet is a network of interconnected computers that no one individual owns. The computers are connected electronically and they communicate with each other. As many thousands if not millions of computers are attached to this network, the capacity of the system to store information is very great. You can normally access the Internet at your university, in your workplace or in your home. The Internet is often referred to as the 'web'. To access the Internet from home, you will use a modem and an Internet service provider (ISP). The ISP is normally an organization that allows you to connect to a special computer called a server. The server is attached to the wider Internet. When you use the Internet at university, the university is acting as the ISP.

At most universities you can get help from the university librarians who run special classes to teach you how to get the most from the Internet. These classes will teach you how to access the Internet and how to use the various search engines and databases. Your university library will advertise the times and dates of these sessions, which often take place at the beginning of each academic year. In the next few paragraphs we shall introduce you to some of the principles of using the Internet and the world wide web.

Accessing the Internet

If you are using a home computer, rather than one at your university, you need to check that it has an appropriate software programme, called a browser, which will allow you to access the Internet. Currently, there are two main programmes on the market: Microsoft Explorer® and Netscape Navigator®. They are similar to each other, and at least one and sometimes both can be found on most personal computers (PCs) or Apple Macintosh computers. Browsers read and translate Internet files so that you can view them from your computer. Browsers also make it possible to find and read different Internet files and pages by allowing you to move between Internet files and pages with relative ease.

Hypertext links

Most Internet pages are written in a special computer language called hypertext mark-up language (HTML). One of the advantages of this is that Internet pages and files can be linked to each other, rather as a spider's web makes links between different strands of mesh and allows the spider to travel easily from one part of the web to another.

Drawing on this analogy, the original developers created the world wide web (of sources of information), mostly in the form of web pages using what are called hypertext links. These links connect you to other parts of the web page you are currently using or to other web pages. A hypertext link (text) tends to be highlighted on a page either because it is underlined or distinguished by some other form of highlighting. In addition, hypertext links can also be images and figures. You can always tell when your cursor is on a hypertext link because the cursor symbol will change from an arrow to a pointing finger. When you go onto a web page you will find something similar to the web page for Elsevier Health shown in Figure 2.7.

Internet pages

The two browsers (Microsoft Explorer and Netscape Navigator) have a similar layout: they have a navigation toolbar at the top, and also a dialogue box where you can write the address of web pages

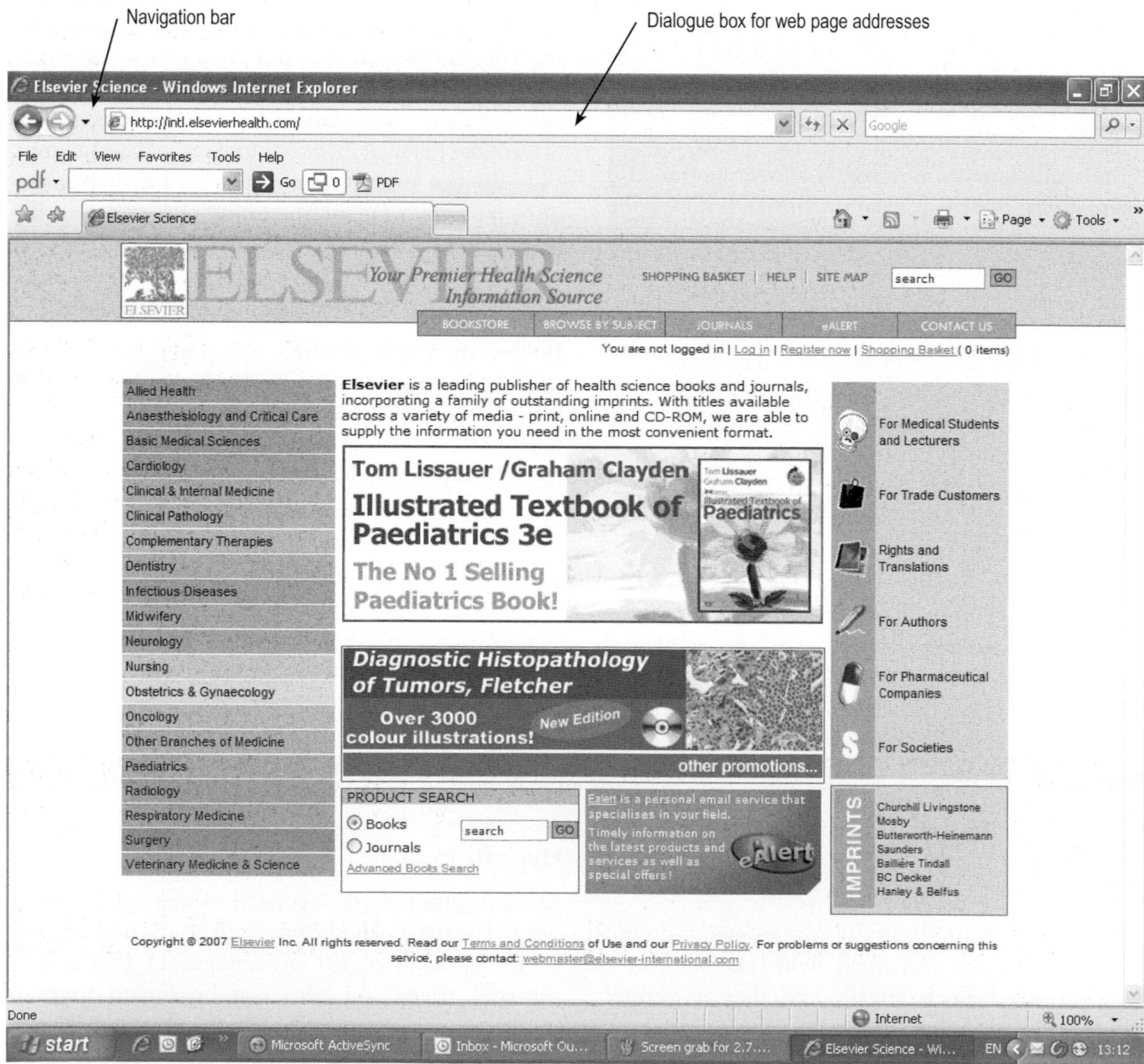

Figure 2.7 • Example of a web home page.

that you may wish to visit, such as the web page illustrated in Figure 2.7. The navigation toolbar has a series of buttons that help in managing your ability to move (sometimes called surfing) through the Internet. If you know the name (address) of the site you wish to visit, type its details into the dialogue box and then press enter on your keyboard or click on 'Go'. The buttons on the navigation bar provide easy access to a range of functions, the most useful of which are described below.

Our illustrations are based on Microsoft Explorer (as mentioned above, Netscape Navigator looks similar and has a similar navigation bar). Web pages do not all look alike; the web page in Figure 2.7 is designed for the public accessing Elsevier journals related to health. Like most pages it has many hypertext links that will connect you with other pages, which will themselves have links to other pages. If you can imagine a series of pages all linked together it is possible to understand how the term 'web' came about, although it is probably harder to imagine how all these pages can be accessed and linked both nationally and internationally. It is easy to become lost within the web, and this is where your 'Home' button comes in useful (Figure 2.8). This key button will take you back to the web page with which your browser automatically starts.

Your university or college will normally set the home page. This is usually the first page of the university website or, if you are using a home computer, it may be the home page of your ISP. If you are using your personal computer, you can choose a home page that suits your needs. Normally, when you first buy a computer, the home page will be set by the manufacturer; you can then decide whether or not you want to change the home page yourself (or get a friend to help).

Searching the Internet

To search the Internet, a device called a 'search engine' is used, which can normally be accessed from your home page. The most commonly used search engine is Google (http://www.google.co.uk); other well-known search engines are Yahoo (http://www.yahoo.co.uk) and Ask (http://www.ask.co.uk). Most search engines ask you to enter a keyword or phrase. They will then search across the Internet and produce a list of web pages and websites containing your keyword. Each website listed in the results is referred to as a 'hit'. The mechanism used by the different search engines varies (Yahoo, for instance, puts the results into a hierarchy of categories), so you might find that one search engine yields more relevant hits than another even when you enter the same keyword(s).

Using commonly words will tend to produce very long lists of possibly relevant websites. When we entered the word 'cardiac' using the Google search engine, we came up with over 4 million hits. When we entered the phrase 'care of the elderly' just 72 400 hits were made. Although even 72 400

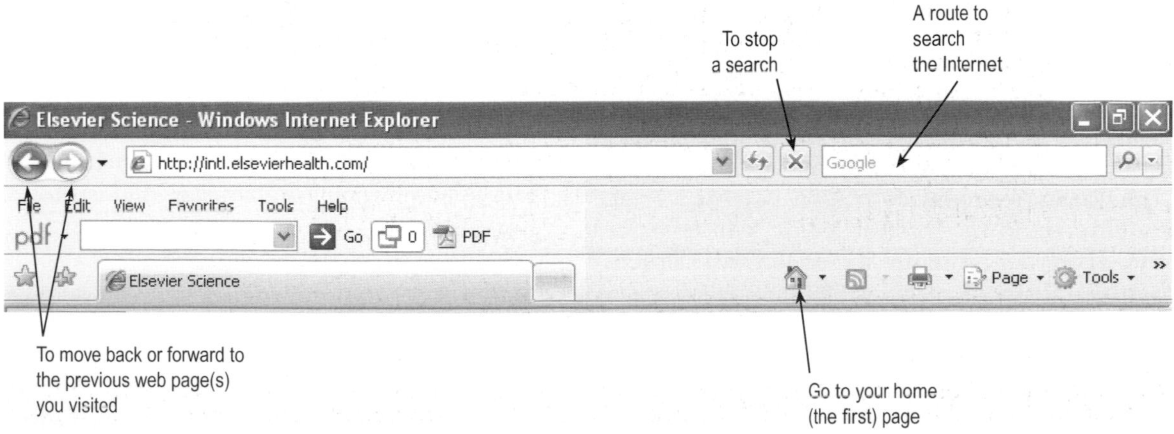

Figure 2.8 • Example of an Internet tool bar.

hits may be excessive, the search engines rank the sites in order of 'perceived relevance'. Don't worry how this is achieved, but normally the relevant information that you will need can be found within the first 0–50 sites listed, although you do need to choose the search word or phrase carefully. Generally, Internet searches can be made more specific by adding more words because the search will be restricted to those sites that contain all the words that have been used. This is as if you were using a Boolean operator such as the word 'and'. Boolean operators provide a means of stringing several seemingly unrelated words together and instructing the Internet search engine to find texts that match the key words (i.e. words other than the connecting Boolean operators). Most search engines within their advanced facilities do support the use of Boolean operators. Using a phrase and enclosing it within inverted commas restricts the search to those sites using that exact phrase. In addition, some search engines will let you confine your search to certain domains (see below).

You will find that most search engines are not case-sensitive, so searching for 'NURSE' or 'nurse' should get you the same results. Some search engines allow you to browse through by subject category. This is the basis of Yahoo, and can also be carried out within Google's advanced options. Category-based searches are a good idea if you are not sure about which keyword to use.

Internet and quality

One important issue about the Internet concerns the quality of information that it contains. Quality is an issue for the Internet because anyone can post information to be retrieved by others, and because unlike other media it is relatively easy to give an impression that the material has come from a high-quality source. Information is posted on to the Internet in the form of 'pages', which can be viewed on your computer screen and are analogous to pages of a book.

Unlike books and journals for which an editorial team has usually made a judgement on the quality and accuracy of the content, no such safeguard is in place for the majority of information and material placed on the Internet. Therefore, when using the web, you are the person who needs to make a decision about the reliability and suitability of the material you are using. Now, it is true that you also need to make decisions about other forms of information, but, unlike books, journals and magazines, it is often not clear from web pages who or what organization has actually produced the material. Indeed, it is quite easy to find pages on the web where the organization responsible for the material is deliberately trying to be obscure. Much web-based material is highly subjective (biased) and can be misleading, and in general should be treated with caution. In the following section, we give some guidelines to help you make decisions about how accurate and impartial web-based material is likely to be.

Judging quality of search finds from web-based material

In this section, we will be discussing web pages and material that has been specifically generated to be used with the web.

Identification of author or source

When you find a web page that interests you, there are several questions that are worth asking:

- Who is the author? Someone is less likely to put their name to work if it is incorrect or possibly libellous.
- Are contact details available?
- Do the contact details work?
- Is it an organization (e.g. Department of Health)? Can you contact the organization?
- What are the benefits to the organization or the author of having this material published on a website?
- Is the material impartial or is it promoting a particular viewpoint or campaign and is this appropriate?

Type of site

Sometimes you can tell the origin of a site from its address. An Internet address is called a URL (universal resource locator). Elsevier's website address relating to health sciences is http://www.elsevierhealth.com. The first part of the address tells computers what language the computer file is written in ('http' stands for hypertext transfer protocol). The next part of the address ('www') stands for 'world wide web'; this tells the computer what network the file page is on (in this case the world wide web). Next, the address indicates the server, or at least a name given to the server by the owner; in this example, it is called 'elsevierhealth'. The name of the server is followed by the part of the address that indicates the type of organization to which the site belongs ('com' indicates commercial, so it is a commercial institution). Finally, there may be an indication of the country where the server is based (see below). Taken together, the part of the address 'www.elsevierhealth.com' is known as the 'domain'. In the example of our publisher's website, we therefore know that we are dealing with a world wide web page that is owned by an organization that has called its server elsevierhealth, which is the division of the publishing company that is concerned with health.

Types of organization code

From the web address it is possible to get an indication of both the name of the organization and the type of organization it is (see Box 2.3).

Box 2.3

Organization codes used in website addresses

ac: higher-education establishments in the UK

co: a company normally based outside of North America

com: a commercial company often based in North America

edu: usually educational establishments in North America and in Australia

gov: government linked sites

net: a network site

nhs: UK national health service (NHS) organizations and trusts

org: usually organizations such as charities and not-for-profit organizations

uk, ca, nz, fr, etc.: country codes, which are numerous

However, do be aware that servers might be given names that do not relate to the name of the organization, and are sometimes given an 'org' code when it should in fact be a 'com'. Codes can help but do not rely on them.

The organization that is promoting the site is important because this will affect how impartial or biased the information is likely to be. You would not expect anti-abortion and 'pro-choice' sites to give you the same information in the same way. However, do not expect sites to be up-front about which camp they are in; caution is always required. The country of origin can also have an impact on the information. In relation to health issues, different countries, as in most things, have differing cultures; in France, for example, the use of enemas as a means to deliver drugs is common whereas in the UK it is less common.

Authority

By authority we mean what makes the individual (and so the web page) believable and trustworthy. Why are they likely to know the truth more than the next person is? If you read the introductory pages of this book and read the brief biographies of the authors, you will have learned that the authors of this chapter are both lecturers in universities and have experience of working with students who are starting their studies in higher education.

Another aspect of authority is the quality-assurance process established by the publishers. The proposal for this book went through a review process before it was agreed to commission people to write the chapters. Each author was selected for their expertise; then, when each chapter had been written, it was reviewed and edited by the book editors and then reviewed by external reviewers employed by the publishers. Altogether, these factors give this book authority on the different subjects listed in the contents section. However, it is important not to make assumptions about the rigour of anything that has been published, even if it has been peer-reviewed, and you should check through the publisher's information about their quality-assurance processes. Journal articles for peer-reviewed journals go through a similar rigorous process before they are published.

When considering materials obtained from a web page it is worth asking what gives the web page the same authority. As you become more experienced at analysing and evaluating information, authority will become less important to you, because you should be able to evaluate the quality of the arguments for yourself. Looking for authority is a good starting point, but sometimes even under the most rigorous processes mistakes can happen.

As well as an individual's authority, we can look for an organization's authority. Here, you should be looking for the status and integrity of the organization and its reputation. For example, sites that are maintained by organizations such as the World Health Organization (WHO), the NHS (National Health Service) and professional bodies are likely to contain information that has been scrutinized for accuracy, but be suspicious about sites from organizations you are not familiar with and always ask the question 'What gives this organization authority?'

Using healthy scepticism

As you will have read, anyone can put what they like on to a web page and broadcast it for the world to read. Once you feel satisfied with the source of information, the next thing to consider is the content. Try asking these straightforward questions:

- What has this web page been created for? (Possible answers could be: to sell me something, to entertain, to persuade, to inform, to promote).
- Are there important things that it does not say?
- Does the site express opinions, is it ambiguous, does it use emotional language?
- Are statements of facts supported by references to the source of that information?
- Are the sources accurate?
- How old or how current is the site?

The next step is to check the information against other sites. You will find that information that is accurate will often be repeated on other sites.

Construction

The last clue to quality is the construction of the site. By construction, we do not mean does it look nice but does it work. Is the site organized well? Does it follow a logical path? Are any arguments constructed well? Do the hypertext links work? Is the site's use of English correct or does the site have lots of spelling and grammatical errors? Try Activity 2.5.

Activity 2.5

Choose a topic that you are interested in, such as nursing history, therapeutic touch, dealing with aggressive behaviour. Connect with your ISP and, using their search engine, conduct an Internet search using your chosen term(s). Briefly, review the sites you have found; select three sites and evaluate each site using the ideas described in this section. Compare each site and identify similarities and differences. Score each site from 1 to 5 (5 = highest score) for each of the following attributes: authority, ease of location, the source, accuracy, design.

Treat all sources of information with healthy scepticism. Treat Internet pages with even more scepticism because in general there is even less control on what gets onto the Internet than into other (text-based) media. Remember, you are the ultimate judge of the quality of sources of information.

Databases

Bibliographic databases normally have stored within them information about the content of many thousands, if not hundreds of thousands, of articles. They can cover things such as textbooks, research journals, trade journals, magazines, newspapers and even conference proceedings. Within bibliographic databases articles are listed under headings that are designed to help you search for the information you want. Common headings in a database are: subject, author, date of publication, title, type of publication and keywords. For example, an article such as 'Depression, alexithymia, and pain prone disorder: a Rorschach study' by Acklin MW and Bernat E, published in the Journal of Personality Assessment, may be stored in a database under the following headings: author, date of publication, title of text, subject of text, type of publication that the text was published as (journal article, report, book and so on). Table 2.3 provides an example of how you could create a database of this article.

The database is likely to contain more information than is displayed in Table 2.3. For example, it will probably contain a summary of the findings of the paper, keywords and exact publication details (e.g. volume of the journal and page numbers). It is important when searching databases to hold in your mind an idea of how the data are laid out.

Most databases do not contain the full text of articles, but only a short summary, sometimes called an 'abstract'. The abstract tells you in a few paragraphs what the article concerns and what its conclusions are. You can read the abstract and use this to decide if you then want to go off and find the article. You can often obtain online access to the article if your library subscribes to that particular journal.

Most databases are now accessed via computer (Figure 2.9) and many can be accessed from anywhere in the world (using the Internet). Examples of some of the most common databases used by students of nursing are Nursing Collection, MEDLINE, Child Data, PsycINFO, and Cochrane Library.

When searching for information it is often worth looking beyond just databases concerned with nursing. This is because different fields of study may look at the same topic from differing perspectives (e.g. BIDS, ZETOC, ISI Web of Science, and Butterworths Law Direct); sometimes a different perspective can give us new insight.

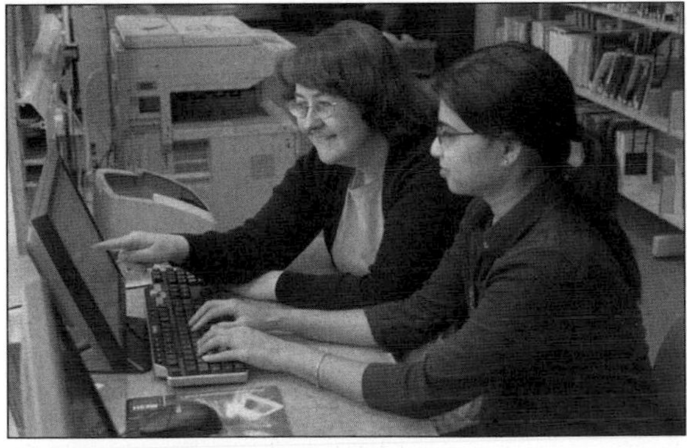

Figure 2.9 • Searching electronic databases.

Searching databases

Computer databases give great flexibility and a search tends to fall into the category of searches based either on a subject of interest or on a particular author. It is also possible to perform searches based on the contents of a particular type of publication or even on a single journal title (e.g. Nurse Education Today).

The detail of how you go about searching an individual database will depend on the database in question. Your university or college will provide you with the specifics concerning the databases that they support. It is not possible in this chapter to look at how individual databases allow searches to be constructed; instead we will discuss principles and give some useful tips and hints.

Some databases are easier to use than others. However, it is not a good strategy to restrict your search to those that are easy to use; if you do, you could miss valuable information. We would recommend trying the British Library database ZETOC, if you have access to it, as it is a very user-friendly starting point.

Table 2.3 A bibliographic database

Author(s)	Title	Subject	Date of publication	Type of publication
Acklin MW, Bernat, E	Depression, alexithymia and pain prone disorder: a Rorschach study	Mental health	1987	Research journal

Search strategy and learning

When you search, consider how you will be storing the information (see Table 2.4); this can help you build a 'search strategy'. The art of searching for information is to find a way through to the information that is useful to you. Normally this means trying to find a method that does not provide too much information or too little. Searching for information can actually help you to focus your thoughts on what you are actually interested in. Before starting a search it might be worth considering the questions listed in Table 2.5.

A strategy should summarize the way in which you are going to go about your search. You might, for example, consider starting broadly and then narrowing your search. Alternatively, you might go for the specific area of your interest. Using well-known authors as a focus for searches can be a good starting point, but doing a subject-based or keyword search may bring you a broader perspective.

The way you search the database can help you learn more about a subject. For example, you may be interested in mouth care. By using a broad search to begin with you may locate information about different types of mouth washes, the kinds of problems people may have with their dentures or gums, the influence on oral health of taking antibiotics over a long time or of poor nutrition. You may learn about the impact of some oral infections on a patient's ability to eat and their nutrition and consequent recovery from illness. If you are interested in forming your own view or finding out how a particular practice came about, you may wish to focus on primary source material (i.e. the research that led to the knowledge), in which case your search strategy would have journal articles as a focus. These articles will normally

Table 2.4 Recording search materials

Author	Reference information	Key points	Topic relevance	Evidence base?
Acklin, MU & Bernat, E	Depression, alexithymia and pain prone disorder: A Rorschach study (1987), Journal of Personality Assessment, Vol. 51 (3) pp. 462–497	Patients with **lower back pain**, differ in the type of depression they suffer from than that suffered by patients in hospital	Chronic pain and incidences of depression associated pain	Quasi experimental design study: Sample = 33 people

Table 2.5 Questions to use when searching databases

Question	Example
Am I looking for general information or something more specific?	I am interested in general information about patient assessment or specific information about Roper's model
Do I want information from particular types of publication?	I just want research articles
Am I interested in specific groups of people?	I am interested in anorexia, but only in European males aged between 15 and 30 years
Do I want only information published over the past year, 2 years, 5 years, or is date of publication not important?	I am interested in the development of hand hygiene practice, so I want current and historical data
Do I know the names of any key writers or researchers in this subject area?	Dinah Gould has written quite a number of articles about hand hygiene

have been written and reviewed by people who are experts in their field.

Searching by author

Most bibliographic databases will allow you to search by author. Searching by author is useful when you have some information about the key individuals working in a particular subject area. If author searching is supported by the database you are using, there will be somewhere on the computer page you are using where you enter the author's name (you can also find articles written by more than one author).

Most databases search using the author's family (surname) name and the initials of their given (first) names. So be as specific as you can, using both the family name and as many of the given names as you can. The database will normally give you guidelines about how it wants you to enter the name, and take care to follow exactly the pattern (syntax) that is required. Take care to place commas and spaces in the correct position. The most common problems people encounter when undertaking author searches are caused by either not following the syntax or by making spelling errors.

Searching by keyword

Searching by using a keyword or a phase is probably the most common type of search you are likely to conduct. The search normally operates by looking for the word you specify within the title of the article, its abstract or within a set of keywords specified by the author. When you search using a keyword, the more general a keyword the more articles (hits) you will find. So you must use keywords that are as close as possible to the type of information you are searching for.

It is a good idea to consider the different words and expressions that may be used to describe and discuss the same or similar phenomena. If you are interested in those who work in the sex industry, you may want to perform searches based on the keyword 'prostitution' but also 'sex industry worker'. It is often worth using as search terms any abbreviations that can be used for the phenomena that is of interest (e.g. HIV as well as human immunodeficiency virus).

Quite often at the bottom of the abstracts of research articles you will find that the author has listed keywords. Authors are asked to think of keywords that they consider represent the topic(s) of their article. Using these keywords can often help you locate other similar articles.

Using article and book reviews in a literature search

Review articles, as well as being interesting to read, can be very useful when conducting literature searches. Review articles are concerned with discussion and summary of the most current and important articles relevant to a specific area of research and provide an overview of the research and thinking on a particular topic. As such it is possible to obtain not just summary information of articles but also the key references to those articles. The review author might also have commented on and performed some analysis of individual articles. In some respects a review article might be considered as a database with commentary.

Learning from practice experience

Information gathering from practice is closely linked to learning and understanding, as indeed is information gathering from taught sessions (Figure 2.10). Learning from practice experience has a long history and is linked to the general idea of

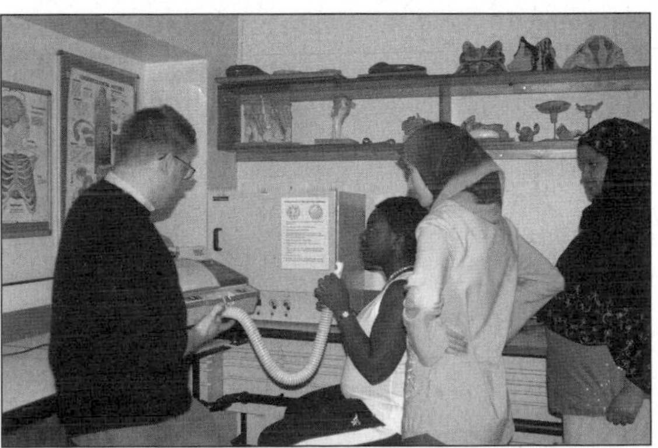

Figure 2.10 • Bringing practice into theory.

experience-based learning. We learn in many ways, but it tends to be generally acknowledged that most of our understanding is derived from experience. We can learn from a whole variety of experiences, such as our social life, sporting activity, family life, voluntary activities, work and even holidays. One of the issues with experience-based learning (experiential learning) is that it can be very inefficient and unpredictable. Sometimes we will have experiences that we do not learn from. A lot of our experiences (e.g. making toast) are learning experiences the first time we do them, but not when we do them for the hundredth time.

Experience-based learning can be informal or incidental (not arranged or planned) or formal (learning that has been planned and directed). When we have a formal and planned learning experience we aim to capture the essence of what we learnt through experienced-based learning but at the same time illuminate the inefficiencies that can occur when experience is not focused or channelled to help learning (Colley et al 2003). This is not to say that all your experiences in placements will be planned; in fact, many will not be. What is hoped is that the formal processes established to support learning will allow you to learn from all the potential learning experiences available to you in placement.

Experience-based learning is different from other forms of learning because the learning is gained through our own senses and therefore, as our brains gather information, that information interacts with our emotions. The way we make sense of and understand that information belongs much more to ourselves (intrinsic) than to others (extrinsic). Experiential learning is without doubt an important part of learning in health care education. Your experience will become vital in helping you to determine the correct approach to care for your patients and clients (Hull et al 2005). To use your experience effectively you need to develop the ways you learn from it.

Reflective practice

On the grand scale, in our society when things go wrong, the government often orders an inquiry. Events are examined and lessons are hopefully learned. On an individual basis, one can learn from exploring events that were not straightforward at the time. In the ever-changing world of nursing you need to be aware of how and what you have learnt from new experiences. Skills related to self-development equip you to cope with new and difficult situations. As a registered professional you must be answerable for your practice; therefore you must ensure through self-analysis that your practice is appropriate and current. An essential aspect of being a professional is to respect information that is confidential in nature. When you look back on your time in a clinical area, some of your experiences may seem perplexing and, given the nature of health care, they might also be distressing. Coming face to face with harsh realities can be upsetting. However, you can sometimes help resolve your feelings and grow personally and professionally by the process of reflection. Recognizing all that you have learnt from a particular experience requires a bit more thought, and trying to relate that experience to theory and even develop theory from the experience is a little more challenging still.

Reflection is a tool that can be used to help you make sense of, and learn from, your experience. Using reflection encourages you to take an objective and sometimes dispassionate look at your experience. This way you can learn from your experiences and establish what you have learned from experience as well as identify your learning needs.

When reflecting on past events and seeing, perhaps from a different perspective, how things occurred, you are analysing your actions and those of other people. You can then make some deductions about what happened and perhaps why they happened. Learning from experience in this way helps you to do things differently and more effectively. Reflection is about re-framing and re-interpreting experiences so that they can be examined in the light of theoretical knowledge. Sometimes it is good to use reflection with a more experienced colleague who, because of their greater experience, can debrief you from an experience and help you arrive at new understandings.

Another way of using reflection can involve examining your own experiences through keeping a journal. You do not need to use any rigid conventions, but it often helps to use a framework or a structured approach. There are several models or frameworks that are available to help us use reflection. Two popular models are those of Johns (1995) and Gibbs (1988). Johns's model is linear in its nature whereas Gibbs's model is always described as being a cycle, although it should really be seen as a spiral. Despite their structural differences, Johns's and Gibbs's models are similar in character and have the same core components:

- A description of events.
- An evaluation of your feelings (and those of others) about the events.
- An analysis of the events.
- Thinking about future needs or developments.

Sometimes it is difficult to start the reflective process, but if you maintain a diary during your practice you will find that you will remember events more clearly. From your diary you should be able to draw out events or experiences that seemed, at the time, significant to you; the events do not need to be good or bad, just significant. This experience may be something that you did, a training session that you attended, or events that you witnessed. The only important aspect is that they are part of your experience.

You may actually want to start by breaking down an event or experience into sections that relate to different activities, or perhaps into descriptions of what various individuals in the event were actually doing. The process of thinking about the component parts of an event will help you when you go to analyse the experience.

For example, if I am reflecting on a lecture that I have given, I may think about this event in terms of preparation, introduction, middle, conclusions, resources, and questions asked by students. In a practice situation, you may think of an event in terms of the part you played, the part the patient/client played and the role of other health care professionals. Alternatively, you could take an approached based more on the chronology of the event, such as preparation to deliver care, initiation of patient contact, delivery of care, evaluation of immediate impact, and leaving the patient. There is no correct way to break down the description of an event, it simply helps when it comes to an analysis. When you are describing the events for others (e.g. as part of an assignment), you may simply recall the event as a narrative; however, it is still a good idea to break down the description, even if you do not reveal that description to anyone else.

Reflection can also be helped if you initially outline what you think you have learnt. You may want to break this down into convenient areas such as:

- Knowledge/understanding.
- Skills.
- Values and attitudes.

For each area, you might like to think of answers to the questions How? What? Why? When? Where? Thinking in this way will help you to identify what your experience was and what you have learnt from it. Sometime it helps to conduct these preliminary phases working with a colleague or friend.

Having conducted the preliminaries, you can now return to your chosen model (i.e. Gibbs' or Johns'). After describing the events, probably as you would a story (narrative), you may now want to consider your feelings and emotions. What were your emotions (e.g. compassion, anger, fear, warmth) and why do you think you had those emotions. Johns' model suggests it is a good idea to consider the emotions of your patient and how you knew what their emotions were.

Having considered emotions, most reflective models move towards an analysis phase whereby the reasons for particular decisions can be critically evaluated, bearing in mind the internal and external factors that led to the event being considered. Events and actions should be compared to existing theory and knowledge. Using theory to understand and perhaps explain your experience of an event can be a helpful way of gaining insights, even to challenge existing practices. Alternative actions can be explored and their possible consequences discussed. This process of analysis should be a learning experience in itself. As you move out of the analysis phase and think about future developments, you should consider what you have learnt and what the implications are for yourself and your area of practice. Finally, consider how these developments can be implemented. You may want to write down your own action plan or discuss your conclusions with your personal tutor or your placement supervisor.

Learning in groups and enquiry-based learning

Working within groups is now a feature of many educational courses and programmes. Identifying how to learn within a group is therefore an important skill. Group learning can have similarities to team working in clinical settings. When you are asked to learn within a team you may want to also think about how teams work and the roles that you take within a team (see Chapter 10).

Small group sessions are often known as seminars or tutorials. The purpose of group working will vary both between and within educational institutions. In general, however, it is thought that students learn differently from working in small groups than from large lectures. Sometimes in a seminar you will have a more intimate lecture-type experience with more opportunity to ask questions. At other times, your group may be asked to decide what you want to learn about and how you are going to do it.

Important aspects of small group work are:

- Discussion.
- Listening.
- Testing ideas.
- Practising communication skills.
- Evaluating the ideas of others.
- Developing relationships.
- Team working.

One of the difficulties with group learning is that you do not choose the individuals who form your group, but then in the clinical environment you will not choose the individuals that make up your team either. Understanding how you can get the most from your group and how groups function is thus an important skill for working in the clinical environment.

Learning in groups requires active listening because, if you are going to discuss a topic with someone, you need to know what they have said. It is important, however, to think about what active listening really is. It is not only hearing but thinking about what was said. So, if you find yourself finishing people's sentences for them, or thinking of what you are going to say as other people are speaking, then you are probably not listening. You can test your listening skills by seeing if you can recall what people have said in your own words to their satisfaction.

Enquiry-based learning

A particular form of group working known as enquiry-based learning (EBL) or problem-based learning (PBL) is often used at universities and colleges. This type of learning is based on the group being given a scenario based on real life to stimulate their learning. In PBL, the goal of the group is often to find a solution to an issue within the scenario; in EBL, the issues and solutions are often less clear. What EBL and PBL have in common is that it is the group (the learners) who must decide what they need to know/understand in order to get to grips with the issues within the scenarios.

The lecturer often takes the role of facilitator, which is to try to keep the group focused and working well. The facilitator may ask questions to stimulate the group, suggest sources of information, but will seldom give direct answers to questions. The educational philosophy of EBL/PBL is about giving students ownership of the knowledge and to promote a deep approach to learning. When students need to decide for themselves what they need to know and then go and find the information, research suggests they are much more likely to both understand and remember that information (Morton and Säljö 1976).

EBL/PBL requires students to organize themselves into a learning unit, to set goals and to decide how to learn about the issues they have identified. At the end of each EBL session each member of the group will have tasks to accomplish; when the group reconvenes, this information must be shared amongst the group. Thus EBL/PBL requires students to be organized, to be prepared to share their research with others and to be able to present their findings.

If you are asked to be part of an EBL/PBL group, it is a good idea to think about what you wish to get out of the group. Ensure that the group sets working rules that you are happy with. The group should think about rules in relation to things such as confidentiality, participation, respecting others views, and absenteeism. One issue that most groups need to deal with is how to respond to those members who do not play a full role yet wish to share the group's learning. There are no quick and easy solutions to this problem, but making decisions is much easier if the group has decided what it will do before such events happen. Making a record of the agreed rules is helpful when disputes do arise.

Individuals within groups will take on different roles. Some of these roles are formal (e.g. most groups will need a chair and a scribe), but such roles can rotate. Other roles are more in relation to the needs of groups in general and our own personalities. For instance, most groups will have natural leaders, idea generators, team maintainers and implementers. Groups will take time to settle while roles are established; once this is done, the team will start to work more efficiently. It is important to try to establish the type of role you normally play and sometimes to try to take on different roles. When working in an EBL group, make sure that the group is working towards a clear target and that the following are also undertaken:

- A summary is made of what has been done and what needs to be done.
- There is a flow of facts and information.
- Alternative ideas are given consideration.
- There is a strategy to prevent certain individuals dominating.
- The group receives feedback on how well it is getting on with the task.
- The workload is organized.
- If there is a group assessment, there is collective responsibility.
- The group does not rely on your facilitator to organize your group or learning.

Do make sure that you use EBL as an opportunity to learn about something you want to in a way that you want to. Even if your group does not work well (dysfunctional), you can still use EBL as an exciting opportunity to learn. When taking part in EBL/PBL it is often helpful to keep a reflective diary so you can remember key events or insights and learn from them. An important bonus of EBL is learning about group and team working and particularly your own contribution and role as a member of the group and team member.

Academic and reflective styles of writing

You will hear people talk about academic writing. Essentially, academic writing is a particular style of writing that occurs widely in the academic and research world. It is an approach you will be expected to learn in order to pass your assignments and to complete your course in higher education. The academic style helps you to discuss unfamiliar ideas and thoughts in an objective way. Academic writing style is used because it infers that the writer is being objective (has considered all of the evidence without being biased) and personal bias has not influenced the outcome of research or investigation. The passive voice (third person or impersonal) is often used in relation to academic writing style. Academic style is formal and, as such, it avoids trying to be funny, light-hearted or emotional; this is because the intention is to present knowledge and help others to understand rather than entertain.

Academic writing style tends to have the following characteristics:

- Formal.
- Objective (unbiased).
- Analytical (breaks down issues into their component parts).

- Rational (based on the logical use of factual information).
- Balanced (doesn't give undue weight to a particular view).
- Logical.
- Normally written in the third person, but can be in the first person when the subject relates to reflections on personal professional practice.
- Avoids the use of colloquial English.
- Uses 'standard' English.
- Systematic (tends to follow a predictable pattern of development).
- Uses scientific terminology.
- Evidenced-based (opinions and views are based on established facts).
- Assertions are referenced to original authors or to authorities on the subject.

Writing in the first, second or third person

We have noted how formal writing is often characterized by being written in the third person in order to present an impersonal or dispassionate voice in the text. You will read this form of writing in scientific or medical research reports. The third person is impersonal, but what about the first and second persons?

The 'first person' is used when you are referring to your own actions or those of a group that you belong to. When using the first person it is common to use the words 'I' and 'we'. In other words, you are describing the world from your own point of view. The 'second person' is a term used when the writer is talking to the reader. In this book, we have used the second person when giving suggestions or recommendations; for example, when we suggest that 'you should always arrive on time for lectures' we are using the second person.

The 'third person' is where the subject (in grammatical terms) is not an identifiable individual and is often replaced with pronouns such as 'it', 'he/she' and 'they'. For example, when describing an experiment I could write:

I put the water in the test tube.

But when writing in the third person:

The water was put in the test tube.

Note how, in the second version, the reader does not really know who put the water in the test tube, whereas in the first it is clear that it was me.

By removing any personal reference, writing in the third person, or using words such as 'I', 'we', 'they', 'he', or 'she', renders the text dispassionate. However, the use of the third person in academic work is being challenged, as to some it does seem arcane and perhaps even dishonest. However, the style does give power to sentences; note the difference between the following sentences:

Free health care, at the point of delivery, is essential for all children.

and

I think free health care, at the point of delivery, is essential for all children.

The first sentence, as well as being forceful, also sets one off looking for the evidence; I want to know how this conclusion was come to. In the second version, this is not the case, and I am inclined to believe it is simply the writer's view. This point is important because the most important feature of academic writing is not that it is written in the third person but that evidence or references support statements. Academic writing, for example, would avoid statements such as 'All doctors are poor at hand washing' or 'Nurses are good at communicating bad news' unless there was evidence to support these statements.

Referencing

In general, when writing academically we use references or actual data to back up what we are saying. In a passage of text where the writer is drawing on evidence from a published author to support arguments, the reference or citation identifies the name of the author and the date of the work published. At the end of the writing, in the reference list or bibliography, this author's details should be documented. You will see we have used this approach when citing authors to support our claims in this chapter. The references refer to the sources of the information we are using and should allow you, the reader, to track back to where the original idea or information came from. Referencing is also important because it identifies which ideas are not our own. It acknowledges the source of the original ideas and provides you with the information to read the original source. Not to acknowledge another person's idea through referencing is a form of theft known as plagiarism. Note in the excerpt below how each fact has been referenced.

> *Although inserting a peripheral cannula is under most circumstances easy, some complications such as phlebitis and extravasation can occur (Gobbi 2000). It is then necessary to resite the cannula to continue the intravenous infusion (Dougherty & Mallett 2000). The cannula should be made from a non-irritant material as, according to Dougherty and Mallett, citing Payne-James et al (1991), this reduces the incidence of thrombosis formation.*

Practising academic writing

As with most skills, you can improve your ability to write academically by observation, experience, practice and review. If you want to improve your ability to write in the third person, you must ensure that there is no reference to you, the writer, in the sentences. Thus, 'It it seems to me that schizophrenia is a treatable syndrome' becomes 'It seems that schizophrenia is a treatable syndrome' and 'I think observation is central to the nursing process' translates to the third person as 'Observation is central to the nursing process'. When writing academically, remember that evidence is important, so you must constantly ask yourself questions such as 'Who said that?', 'Where did that thought come from?' and 'Where is the material to support that statement?' It is also important to remember that academic writing should flow logically and that evaluations are based on an analysis of the evidence. Lastly, if something really is just your opinion say 'in my opinion'.

Try to read two research-based articles per week. These need not come from the main academic journals, but could come from professional magazines such as Nursing Times or Nursing Standard. Choose articles that are from the research sections rather than 'news' articles. As you read the articles, note the writing style and how and when it changes. See if you can spot where the author has an opinion but has used the third person.

When you are comfortable reading such articles, move on to articles from research journals. This will help to improve your ability as a writer as well as helping you discover new ideas about nursing practice (if you travel to college or your practice area by train or bus these could be times when this type of reading can be done). Try practising converting first person to third person and third to first (harder). Lastly, when you have written an assignment or report, let someone whose writing you respect read it over. This helps you to ensure that your arguments flow logically and make sense to someone else. It also helps to have another person to spot the grammatical or spelling errors that creep into everyone's writing.

Reflective style

You will recognize that writing about personal experiences should not be done using the third person. Writing about reflective activities, where you are trying to make sense of and have learnt from personal experiences, needs to be a personal account. Learning how to write in the first person whilst combining the academic approach (third person) and the reflective can be challenging.

If you are asked to reflect on your own experience in an assignment, it is acceptable to write in the first person. Some of the rules of academic style still apply, such as not using slang or informal terms. When reflecting on professional practice, it is acceptable to use the first person; this is demonstrated in some books and journal articles written on reflection and professional practice. An essential issue when writing as a health care professional is when to write in the first person and when to write in the third person. In general, when writing reflectively, description of events and of emotions should be in the first person. Analysis of events should be written in the third person. If you are writing for an assignment, it is always a good idea to ask your tutor to confirm what their expectations are.

Which tense to use?

Deciding on which tense to use is sometimes difficult, particularly if a mix of reflective and academic styles is being used. Reflective activities always tend to start with a description of an event, so clearly this type of writing should start in the past tense. This is also the case when describing procedures that you have taken part in or witnessed. When writing about the work of others where conclusions have been made, the past tense should be used. For instance, 'Johnson and Johnson (1909) found that massaging with certain oils made the skin feel much smoother.' Here you are reporting the findings of others; these findings have been made in the past and so the past tense is appropriate. However, it is common to use the present tense when introducing established ideas and concepts, such as 'chicken pox is a common childhood illness'. The present tense can be used in this manner where there is no dispute about the fact of the information (Powell 1999). The present tense is normally also used when writing a set of instructions or giving a description of something.

When reflecting, the past tense will be used for describing events, emotions, analysing and relating them to theory; however, as you move through the reflective cycle you will start to consider what has been learnt from your experience, and how this will affect your future practice and learning. In this final stage, you will start to use the future tense as you forecast what developments will occur.

Some styles to avoid

There are some features of language that it is best to avoid when writing as a student or registered nurse; we discuss a few below. Communicating ideas and information is the prime reason for writing and thus being clear when we write is very important.

Jargon

Some aspects of language are best avoided when trying to discuss professional practice or to demonstrate understanding. We mentioned above that you should not use colloquialism; a similar phenomenon to colloquialism is professional jargon. Professional jargon is really colloquialisms that belong to a particular profession. Nurses may talk, for example, of a particular drug being given 'sub-cut'; this is shorthand for a drug being given by injection sub-*cutaneously*. It is important to recognize the difference between jargon and that of specialized technical terms. Specialized technical terms are used to ensure precision and tend to be recognized by health professionals across the world. Jargon tends to evolve out of linguistic shortcuts and tends to be recognized relatively locally.

Quality not quantity: on writing too much

Writing in an academic style does not mean that you should write extended sentences using the longest words you can find. If possible, stick to short sentences and short words. If you do this the meaning of your sentences will be clear, and you will need to use much less punctuation. Look at the following sentence:

> *At this moment in time we are now in a position to refocus the remuneration scale, such that employees will observe a substantial elevation in their take-home pay; this will be actuated from the first day of next month.*

Put more simply:

> *From the first of next month, all staff will receive a big pay increase.*

Note how much more pompous the first sentence is than the second. The first sentence has used phases where a single word would do, and has used longer words where a smaller one would do. Words that have the same or similar meaning are called synonyms. They can be used to keep the language that we are using interesting. The English language has so many of these that special books are available called thesauruses. Thesauruses indicate words with similar meanings. Not all synonyms are interchangeable and context is very important. In the first sentence, the word elevation has been used as a synonym of rise. But in a different sentence we can not necessarily use the words interchangeably (e.g. The house had an elevation of 6 metres).

Try to avoid the trap of being over-complex, and thus seeming pompous, by always reviewing your work to see if it can be expressed with greater simplicity. Given a choice of words to use, select the word that is used more commonly and normally the smaller word. Fairbairn & Winch (1996) provide some good and amusing examples of pompous and rather long-winded writing.

Conclusion

As a health care professional, you will need to and be expected to continually improve your knowledge and skills throughout your career. To make most use of your time and resources you need to be able to make the best use of the study and development opportunities available to you. By mastering the skills and approaches described in this chapter you will be able to learn effectively using a range of tools that will help you make sense of your studies, training and experience. You will be well on the way to becoming a lifelong learner.

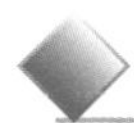

References

Annis L, Davis JK 1978 Study techniques and cognitive styles: their effect on recall and recognition. Journal of Educational Research 71:175–178

Astin AW 1993 What matters in college? Four critical years revisited. Jossey-Bass, San Francisco

Barnett R 2004 Learning for an unknown future. Higher Education Research and Development 23(3):247–261

Beard R 1990 Developing reading, 2nd edn. Hodder & Stoughton, London

Colley H, Hodkinson P, Malcolm J 2003 Informality and formality in learning: a report for the learning and skills research centre. Learning and Skills Research Centre, Leeds

Entwistle N 1997 Styles of learning and teaching: an integrated outline of educational psychology for students teachers and lecturers. David Fulton Publishers, London

Fairbairn GJ, Winch C 1996 Reading, writing and reasoning: a guide for students, 2nd edn. Open University, Buckingham

Garder H 1993 Frames of mind: the theory of multiple intelligences, 10th edn. Basic Books, New York

Gibbs G 1988 Learning by doing: a guide to teaching and learning methods. Further Education Unit, Oxford Polytechnic, Oxford

Hull C, Redfern L, Shuttleworth A 2005 Profiles and portfolios: a guide for health and social care, 2nd edn. Palgrave, Basingstoke

Johns C 1995 The value of reflective practice for nursing. Journal of Clinical Nursing 4:23–40

Kesselman-Turkel J, Peterson F 1982 Note-taking made easy. Contemporary Books, Lincolnwood, IL

Kiewra KA 1985 Learning from a lecture: an investigation into note taking, review and attendance at a lecture. Human Learning 4:73–77

Kiewra KA 1987 Note taking and review: the research and its implications. Instructional Science 16(3):233–249

Kulhavy RW, Dyer JW 1975 The effects of note taking and test expectancy on the learning of text material. Journal of Educational Research 68:363–365

Lukasiewicz J 1994 The ignorance explosion. Carlton University Press, Ottawa

Morton F, Säljö R 1976 On qualitative differences in learning outcomes and processes. British Journal of Education Psychology 46:4–11

Pascarella ET, Terenzini PT 1991 How college affects students: findings and insights from twenty years of research. Jossey-Bass, San Francisco, CA

Pauk W 1993 How to study in college. Houghton Mifflin, Boston, MA

Payne E, Whittaker L 2000 Developing essential study skills. Pearson, London

Powell S 1999 Returning to study: a guide for professionals. Open University Press, Buckingham

Ramsden P 1992 Learning to teach in higher education. Routledge, London.

Rowntree D 1998 Learn how to study: a realistic approach, 4th edn. Time Warner, London

Tapper J 2004 Student perceptions of how critical thinking is embedded in a degree program. Higher Education Research and Development 23(2):199–223

Taylor M 1986 Learning for self direction in the classroom: the pattern of a transitional process. Studies in Higher Education 11(1):55–72

Wright J 2002 Time management: the pickle jar theory. A List Apart issue 146. Online. Available: http://alistapart.com/articles/pickle/

Chapter Three

3

The emotional labour of nursing

Pam Smith, Maria Lorentzon

Key topics

- Becoming a nurse
- Learning to become a professional
- Emotional labour and feeling rules
- Learning to do emotional labour
- Learning and managing the emotional labour of cancer care
- Practising emotional labour in everyday practice of: intimate physical care; emotional care; coping with emergencies; dealing with confidential information and patients' questions; defusing aggression; responding to joy and sorrow

Introduction

When asking nurses why they have chosen nursing as a profession, responses such as 'I wanted to work with people' or 'I wanted to do some good' are often given. These kinds of replies are in our experience more common than a response such as: 'I was fascinated by nursing science'. Although reasons for human action are complex and seldom arise from one cause only, there would appear to be a strong 'people-centredness' in the personality profile of most people who enter nursing courses and who remain in nursing practice.

Candidates applying for places on a nursing programme often explain their career choice as being because they liked people. Other candidates argue it was because nursing is a 'good job' rather than a vocation. Often such candidates resent patients who see them in a vocational light, referring to them as 'angels' (Smith 1992). Over the last 20 years nursing programmes have changed considerably, but reasons for choosing nursing as a career have not, although, for many, studying at university has an added attraction or because they see themselves joining a profession (Smith et al 2005). Most applicants choose nursing because they believe they want to work with people or they feel the need 'to do some good'. Doing nursing and being a nurse are different facets of the same role.

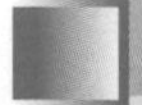

Engaging with people in their most vulnerable moments and with those who are disturbed, mentally or physically, and being able to respond in a sensitive and therapeutic manner are things that all nursing students need to learn if they are to be effective practitioners. However, these are also probably the most challenging aspects of learning to nurse. By drawing on examples taken from research into nurses' professional development, this chapter provides some guidelines about how to go about developing the skills of people-centredness whilst maintaining your personal integrity and humanity.

Becoming a nurse

Earlier chapters in this book demonstrate that learning to become a nurse means balancing life between being a student in a university and being a member of a clinical team. Some of the images on recruitment posters are concerned with 'the price of nursing' (seen on a 2005 recruitment poster), the answer in the poster being '£20 000 a year starting salary and a university qualification'. Would this be the message that attracted you to nursing? Other images are related to the idea of nursing being a vocation. An explicit example of this was a recruitment poster in the early 1990s, which asked the question 'Do the financial rewards match the emotional ones?' The answer (unlike the 2005 poster described above) gave a mixed message, on the one hand reassuring prospective nurses that, although they were unlikely to be attracted to the job for the money, they could expect emotional rewards as well as financial ones. The conclusion here was that the emotional rewards came as an added extra for working in one of the most 'emotionally satisfying careers' (Smith 1992, p 11). Even earlier images of nurses described the nurse as a 'young lady' or a 'good woman', and Nightingale's descendants were identified as vocationally motivated, obedient and subservient to both medical and nursing superiors (Smith 1992, p 21). This image is exemplified in early extracts from the Nursing Times (see Box 3.1).

These early letters from the Nursing Times illustrate the emphasis on emotion in the ideal type of the 'reformed' nurse in the early 20th century. It would seem clear that the desirable nurse was also the ideal woman. Her virtues were womanly – kindness, even 'love' – as well as loyalty and obedience. It is interesting to note that ideally nurses should be socialized into the role through 'love', although in most cases 'discipline' was also necessary.

One hundred years later this image of a nurse is clearly outdated, but you might like to critically reflect on the extent to which this is still the case. Some may believe that subservience is no longer advocated, although 'vocational motivation' has

Box 3.1

Letters relating to nurses in the British nursing press

[Anonymous] 1905 An open letter to a nurse by a matron. Nursing Times 6 May:42

But of character building and the primal necessity for the fundamental virtues I say little on lecture nights, for of this each must know for herself the various graces that make for perfect, wholesome womanhood . . .

Comment: The perfect woman is equated with the perfect nurse . . .

[Anonymous] 1905 An open letter to a matron from two nurses. Nursing Times 17 June:114–115

Discipline is the very salt of training. It is the enthusiast only who dares to think kindness, courtesy and discipline may be combined . . . most young girls are ready enough to give the gifts matrons demand from probationers: respect, reverence, kindness (or love) and loyalty . . .

[Anonymous] 1911 Discipline and nursing by an ex-matron. Nursing Times 6 May:432

Discipline aims at the removal of bad habits and the substitution of good ones, especially those of order, regularity and obedience . . . I have always had nurses who could be ruled by love . . . but, I always had some of the other kind – those in whom the compelling force of love was far from sufficient to keep them in the straight line of duty . . . They proved in various ways that they were true daughters of Eve . . .

Comment: Just as the 'good woman' is equivalent to the 'good nurse', the 'bad nurse' is a 'daughter of Eve' and far from perfect . . .

perhaps been too easily discarded, often being viewed as an emotional tool used by management to make nurses work for low salaries; see Abel-Smith (1960) and Davies (1980) for further discussion on this topic.

Pause to ponder

What first attracted you to being a nurse? Was it recruitment posters, adverts or television programmes such as ER and Casualty? Or was nursing something that you thought would give you both a university education and skills that would increase your chances of future employment?

In a recent evaluation of part-time nursing programmes, it was found that students attracted to these programmes were described as 'non-traditional'. The students were also very clear that they were attracted to nursing as a profession rather than as an academic career (Smith et al 2005). By 'non-traditional' the researchers meant that the 'typical' student was older than the 18-year-olds of Smith's earlier study. Often, 21st century nursing students were found to be female, with at least one child, and individuals who had already done a variety of jobs, often as a health care assistant. How does this profile relate to your own?

To some extent, the student's profile was reflected in the literature. One such study described the 'non-traditional' student as over 25, male, having English as a second language, belonging to an ethnic or racial minority and having dependent children (Jeffreys 1998). Given that nursing is predominantly a female profession, this is a significant change.

Students from a lower socioeconomic group (i.e. typically described as 'working class') have also been considered as 'non-traditional' for a variety of reasons, some being that they may be at a disadvantage in terms of understanding the 'culture' of higher education and are also more likely to struggle financially. Additional criteria include being a commuter (Bean and Metzner 1985) and having domestic responsibilities other than children/spouse (e.g. being a carer for a parent). The important factor here is that the so-called 'non-traditional' student has responsibilities outside of the programme.

Can you identify with any of these factors? Certainly any or all of these characteristics may add to the emotional demands of being a nurse. On the positive side they may also assist students to understand some of the concerns faced by patients and their families.

In Chapter 1, Spouse aptly portrays the position of new nursing students. She stresses the need for 'selflessness' and academic ability, also pointing to the mixture of 'anticipation and trepidation' with which new students approach their chosen career path in terms of academic requirements, clinical skills and emotional input, and the mixture of emotions experienced by the new student nurse.

Another group who need to be considered here, from the perspective of both patients and staff, are internationally recruited nurses, who add to the multicultural, ethnically mixed background within which NHS nurses work. In 2003/04, for example, nearly half the new nursing registrants with the Nursing and Midwifery Council were nurses who had trained overseas. A study in which the experiences of overseas recruits are explored revealed that they reported having a hard time feeling accepted within British culture, either at home or at work (Allan and Larsen 2003). When it comes to emotional labour, there were heavy demands placed on overseas staff to conform and often they felt that their motivations, abilities, knowledge and skills were either misunderstood or went unrecognized and unrewarded. As new student nurses, they also found themselves on a 'roller coaster' of emotions.

Learning to become a professional

Concepts of professionalism in nursing

Professionalism, especially as it applies to those areas of service work, where women traditionally are more numerous than men, has tended to emphasize altruism more than professional control through statutory means and the protection of a body of knowledge, claimed as 'unique' to the particular profession. Lorentzon (1990) developed a concept named 'feminine professionalism', components of which are similar to emotional labour in that 'self-giving' is emphasized over power-seeking, within an altruistic model, which was traditionally described as 'vocational' in nursing. The term 'vocational' is now more frequently used to denote a 'practical' rather than 'academic' qualification and is less frequently applied to qualified nurses. Lorentzon (1990) points to gender-typing of altruistic service which is more frequently associated with female biology, and women's choice of occupation was traditionally seen to be influenced by such biological factors. Such gender stereotypes of women as 'natural' carers have been challenged by feminist thinkers.

This female model of nurturing fits well with the functions of what were described as 'semi-professions' (Etzioni 1969). These included occupations such as nursing, social work and school teaching; that is, less influential groups than the traditional professions such as medicine and law, which have tended to be dominated by a majority of male members. Lorentzon argues that the former 'semi-professional' workers might more positively be described as practising 'feminine professionalism', with a strong emphasis on altruistic service. Both women and men could exercise this function, as it would denote an 'ideal type' (Weber in Runciman 1978), rather being necessarily linked to being biologically female or male. The person-centredness of this mode of giving professional service clearly resonates with current conceptions of emotional labour.

Analysis of data from probationer registers during the late 19th and early 20th centuries, maintained in both voluntary hospitals and poor law infirmaries, revealed that the most commonly occurring description of probationers was 'kind'. This was related specifically to interaction with patients (Lorentzon 2000, 2001, 2003). At best, the nurse operating in the Nightingale style was genuinely patient-centred in terms of general kindness. However, in-depth communication with patients, relatives and colleagues was discouraged if such activity interfered with the practical running of the wards and availability for immediate response to the commands of doctors and senior nurses. It was also feared that an overly friendly nurse might be conducting herself inappropriately, and so fraternizing with patients (as it was interpreted) was forbidden (Maggs 1981).

Nursing or medical tours of the patients (the rounds) were often conducted in a perfunctory manner and from the bottom of the patients' beds, denoting that doctors and nurses were very busy people. It might be argued that such 'guarding', which protected nurses from the real feelings of patients, avoided having to do too much emotional labour. In the 21st century health service, patients are in and out of hospital much more quickly than they were 20 years ago and so their opportunity to get to know their nurses occurs less frequently. However, this is counterbalanced in primary health care settings, where the same team of nurses may look after certain patients and their families for many years. With increased understanding, health professionals and nurses in particular are much more inclined to value 'quality time' with patients and relatives.

The hidden curriculum of nursing

You may not be familiar with the term 'hidden curriculum'. This refers to the informal learning that is not included in any written programme specification but is nevertheless taught. The hidden curriculum is often concerned with attitudes, values and beliefs that are expressed by the people with whom students come into contact, the environment they learn in and the manner in which the programme is delivered. It is called the hidden curriculum simply because it is difficult to articulate, and 'teachers' (who will be practice staff as well as lecturers) may not even be aware that they are teaching a newcomer these attitudes and values. The attitudes that are conveyed through this hidden curriculum are often about nurses and nursing or patients and patient care and are communicated in subtle and often subliminal ways. The hidden curriculum may be taught through everyday encounters with academic staff, personal tutors and other students. It may be more subtle, for example the quality of the furnishings of the classrooms and the available resources, which communicate the extent to which the students and the programmes are valued by the university. But it is not only through university-based activities that you will be exposed to the hidden curriculum. It is often what nursing students learn in their practice placements that has the most impact, and they learn this through watching and listening to other nurses undertaking their daily activities, seeing them interact with patients and their carers, seeing how other health care professionals interact with nurses and how nurses interact with each other. It is these learning experiences that provide the most enduring influence on newcomers, as Mark's experiences illustrate (Case history 3.1).

From their brief conversation, you can begin to see that these two students have learned quite a lot that was part of the curriculum (e.g. seeing how people from different income groups live and manage). What perhaps was more implicit, or part of the hidden curriculum, was the relationship that was being developed by the two students from different professional groups through having the opportunity to share experiences and perspectives. They also had an opportunity to see how an experienced professional works collaboratively with her clients and is able to develop an effective professional relationship, and that that relationship is a long-term one. The kind of work the health visitor was undertaking was the emotional labour of developing a strong and supportive relationship so that she could befriend the young mother and her baby and thus reduce the likelihood of them encountering serious difficulties despite living under challenging circumstances.

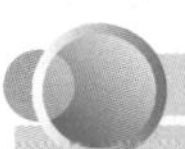

Case history 3.1

Mark's experiences of a professional relationship and the hidden curriculum

Mark is a first-year nursing student on placement in the community with a first-year medical student (Annette). The aim of this placement is to develop an appreciation of the role of community care staff and to understand how different families understand health and healthy living. This morning they have been visiting their family with the health visitor (Maisie) and are discussing their experiences in the debriefing seminar.

Mark: *I was quite shocked at how such a young family can have a normal lifestyle living in a caravan. They did have running water and electricity, as well as proper sanitation, but the caravan itself was damp and that cannot be good for a baby. It must be such a struggle for the Mum, with her being only 19.*

Annette: *Yes, I was shocked as well, as I had never imagined people trying to live under such conditions; it makes you realize how privileged you are. I was particularly impressed by the health visitor. Clearly she has a good relationship with the mother and she seems to almost treat her as a mum. With the baby being 9 months now, they have had a chance to get to know each other.*

Mark: *Yes, I was struck at how friendly the relationship seemed between the mother and Maisie. Maisie seemed to know a huge amount about the family and clearly saw them frequently, which must be quite hard work for her as the caravan park is quite difficult to get to.*

Annette: *Yes, and that must make it difficult for the Mum to get her shopping or to have any social contact. She must feel very isolated living there, which must be hard with a young baby.*

Professional work as emotional work

Nursing work inevitably involves the emotions. Mark and Annette (Case history 3.1) were possibly quite affected by the experience of visiting this young mother in her poor housing conditions and social isolation. Working as a nurse involves a whole range of emotions. Such emotions experienced by nurses was powerfully portrayed in the research by Lesley Mackay in her book 'Nursing a Problem' (Mackay 1989). Mackay described nursing in the late 1980s as being 'in crisis', due to poor recruitment and retention rates, low pay and unsatisfactory conditions of work. Yet many of the nurses she interviewed expressed love for nursing work in spite of problems identified. In the extracts from interviews with clinical nurses given in Box 3.2, strong job satisfaction is expressed, although some nurses clearly had a sense of being both exploited and misunderstood.

Despite the mixed emotions reported by the research participants of Mackay (Box 3.2), they appear to have derived considerable job satisfaction from having contributed to their patients' recovery or to their peaceful death and from the human relationships, expressed as 'love' by one respondent. This notion of nursing being a labour of love reflects work by writers such as Campbell (1984) and Jourard (1971), who both argue that, to be

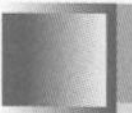

Box 3.2

Extracts from interviews with clinical nurses (from Mackay 1989)

The patients . . . on a good day when they respond. After two years and they get your name right, it's fantastic . . . They all ate with spoons in here when I came on in the beginning of January and now they all use a knife and fork.

(Staff nurse)

I enjoy it, sometimes I'm fed up, but on the whole when you nurse somebody, especially down here when they are really ill and then you see them when they are getting better and then they go on to the ward and they come down to see us before they go home, really well, it's good.

(Staff nurse)

It's just the patients, I love the patients. It's not that I feel . . . I don't feel sorry of them, I don't feel I'm here to change their lives. Just to be here to make things a bit easier, a bit more comfortable.

(Enrolled nurse)

I feel it's something worthwhile that you are doing. And you do get rewards, hopefully seeing patients get well and going home or make the death as easy as possible. I feel that it is something worthwhile.

(Sister)

Although patients rate highly the attentions and kindnesses of nurses, calling them 'angels', the status accorded to nurses falls short of that accorded to members of the medical profession. Of course, at the same time nurses are seen, because they are women, as simply doing what comes naturally to them.

truly effective, people working in caring professions need to undertake their work in a loving manner. Jourard (1971) argues that it is only through self-knowledge and a willingness to be open and honest can practitioners become therapeutic. Campbell (1984) builds this argument further by advocating 'skilled companionship' as a means of 'working with' and 'being with' clients or patients as they progress through 'their own journey' towards recovery or death. He argues that skilled companionship is expressed through sensitivity to the person's needs and a willingness to engage with these, whilst retaining objectivity and professional boundaries. Rawnsley (1980) suggests that, in order to relate to others at an emotional level, practitioners need to grasp the mystery of the human condition.

Emotional labour and feeling rules

Emotional labour is often described as a form of being present with patients at a psychological and emotional level that responds to their human condition. Smith & Gray (2001a) draw on Hochschild's (1983) work to use the term 'emotional labour' to describe the intimate nature of care that draws on emotional work, and, along with Aldridge (1994), recognize that therapeutic relationships of this nature can be stressful and that practitioners as well as students need structures and processes designed to help and protect them from the consequences of engaging in emotional labour. Similarly, Graham (1983), in an account of women's work, describes caring as both labour and love, caring for and caring about another person, doing and feeling. Although Graham's work is focused on women's work, it is not intended to exclude men, and the number of men in caring activities and in nursing is significant. The traditional view that nursing is essentially 'female', and to a great extent an extension of mothering, has now been revised, not least because it makes little sense to male students (Lorentzon 2004). This oversimplistic notion, that 'maternal' equals nurturing, without acknowledgement of similar behaviour by men, and that all women actually have such an 'instinct', has been seriously revised. There is clear awareness that, while most candidates for nurse education are likely to be persons of good will who want to work with people, specific techniques and behaviours may need to be learnt. Following earlier research on 'feminine professionalism' (Lorentzon 1990), one of the authors is now aware that this concept resonates with 'emotional labour' as described by Hochschild (1983) and Smith (1992). Both of these concepts can be seen as pointing to the connection between emotions and clinical care and as an essential part of professionalism. Perhaps the most important element of learning to provide emotional care is dependent on finding suitable role models. For many students, their first role models are familiar caring figures such as 'mother' or 'parent'. As students progressed through their 3-year education, their perspectives were found to mature, and the roles of staff, lecturers and clinical leaders were mentioned more frequently as helping to develop the student nurse's view of emotional labour and the job of nursing (Smith & Gray 2000). Case history 3.2 is an example of how one student, whom we have called Sally, developed her understanding of how to provide emotional support (try Activity 3.1).

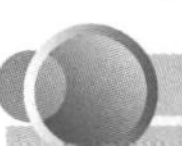

Case history 3.2

Sally's experiences of 'feeling rules'

When I first started on the ward I was nervous and really did not know what patients wanted from me. I was quite nervous about spending time on my own with any one patient in case they asked me something I could not answer. In one of my earlier placements, I was upset at how indifferent the nurses seemed when a patient was suffering or had died. But later I realized they were just bottling up their feelings because they had to get on with the work. They could not afford to go and hide in the office while they let go of their feelings.

Learning how to cope with these situations was by watching what my mentor did in such cases, or watching another staff member whom I thought of as a good nurse. I would notice how they answered some questions and not others. I also drew on my memories of how my parents dealt with similar incidents. Gradually I got the hang of feeling my way into the patient's question, so rather than make a quick response I would explore what their question was really about. Sometimes I realized they really had the answer; they just wanted a different one or to have their own views confirmed.

Activity 3.1

Sally's account (Case history 3.2) reflects the experiences of many new nursing students. So, as you read the account, consider whether it relates to any of your own experiences, and, if it does, whether it influences your perspective of emotional labour. How does this relate to your own learning needs?

Emotional labour and professionalism: theoretical perspectives

Over the past 30 years the volume of research into and about nursing has increased significantly and has provided a basis for our understanding of nursing. Many studies have focused on the education and practice of nurses and the impact this has had on patient care. Working in the 1980s, Smith began her study with the question 'How do student nurses learn to care?' She very quickly discovered that the emotional style of the ward sister or charge nurse who managed the ward was crucial not only to how the students learnt to care but also to the quality of care that they were able to give to patients. In turn, patients judged the quality of care by the emotional style in which it was given.

A theoretical framework for emotional labour

Emotional labour was first described by the sociologist Arlie Russell Hochschild, who produced a key text on the emotion debate in service occupations (The managed heart: the commercialization of human feeling, 1983, 2003). In Hochschild's book, which is based on research involving flight attendants employed by a United States airline and research on individuals involved in debt-collecting, she describes the 'uncosted' labour related to dealing with positive or negative emotions when fulfilling the requirements of a role. Using the term 'feeling rules', Hochschild described emotional labour as when actors manage to balance actions with feelings that are genuine, and feelings and actions that are insincere but required in order to fulfil the role demanded by the job. The key factor is that the audience or the recipient believes in the actions and the sincerity of the feelings. Being congruent in action and feeling can be hard. If the individuals displaying such feelings are unable to reconcile the emotional content of such feelings, they experience dissonance and strain or self-destruction. As a result, actors develop coping strategies that can lead to what is known as 'emotional burn-out'.

Box 3.3

Feeling rules of emotional labour

- Actors manage to make actions congruent with personal feelings.
- Feelings and actions may not be congruent but the actions are necessary to fulfil the role demanded by the job.
- The audience or the recipient of the interaction believes the feelings and associated actions are congruent.
- Congruence between action and feeling is often difficult for the actor.
- If the actor displays feelings that create conflict with their emotional content, they will experience dissonance and strain or self-destruction.
- The actor either develops coping strategies or will suffer emotional burn-out.

Hochschild's concept of 'feeling rules' illustrates the different levels of depth at which an actor or an employee may be required to identify with the role set by employers (see Box 3.3). She talks in this context of deep acting and surface acting. In deep acting, the employee learns to really feel the emotions of the customer or client, whereas surface acting is more superficial and allows the employee to feign the feeling. A most obvious example of surface acting is in the culture of fast food restaurants where almost every assistant wishes you to 'have a nice day'.

Hochschild draws her examples from the commercial world, hence her reference to 'commercialization' of an image that sells flight tickets or pays bills. In fact, for most of us it is the manner in which a service is delivered by the employee that is attractive. Many of us, especially those who are nervous of flying, value the 'smiling courteous attention' of flight attendants, or the helpful friendly shop assistant or waiter. These service roles may be cynically dismissed resulting in under valuing the expertise required to wait at table; giving a service rather than being servile. Indeed, much of nursing in the past can be viewed in similar terms. Yet, all these expert service providers, including nurses and flight attendants, know that they are 'adding value' to what, superficially, appears to be mundane, practical tasks. Using the concept of 'emotional labour' to understand the interpersonal processes that are vital to successful delivery of a service, including nursing care, helps us to appreciate how important a supportive environment must be. Creating this kind of environment in a health care setting can best be achieved through the influence and management style of clinical managers. Smith & Gray (2000) found that values of supportiveness and warmth underpin effective nurse–patient relationships and thus expose nurses to the same kinds of emotional labour that Hochschild described.

Hochschild compared the warmth of the airline hostess with that of debt collectors, who managed the unpleasantness of their jobs, and thus their emotional labour, by maintaining a hierarchical and distant relationship with the debtors. Thus they were able to instil fear and thus compliance on the part of debtors, ensuring compliance in repaying debts. This relationship Smith (1992) equated with traditional ward sisters and their students and which made working in an emotionally supportive way with patients very difficult. Smith's study indicated that, when students and staff nurses felt appreciated and supported emotionally by the ward sisters, they not only had a role model for emotionally explicit patient care but they also felt able to care for patients in this way. According to both Hochschild and Smith, emotional labour needs to be factored into the equation of nursing. The argument can be made that the actual work expanded into 'absorbing' and 'defusing' the positive and negative feelings of the 'recipients of care' are provided as part of the overall quality of service. The emotional cost to the service providers may be personally significant and cannot easily be assessed in financial terms.

Having a clearly identifiable way of describing the emotional work that makes caring more likely to be successful provides an analytical device that helps us to distinguish the different occupational groups and the kinds of emotion work they entail. In general, there are relatively few studies, but those of medical students (Smith III & Kleineman 1989) and of nurses working in a variety of clinical contexts, such as bone marrow transplant for

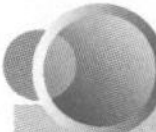

cancer (Kelly et al 2000), palliative care (James 1989, 1993, Kelly et al 2000) and gynaecology care (Bolton 2000), provide a firmer basis for describing what emotional work entails and this enables it to be recognized.

Learning the feeling rules

Hochschild points to the obvious fact that, 'even when people are paid to be nice, it is hard for them to be nice all the time' (Hochschild 2003, p 118). Therefore, a set of 'feeling rules' must be learnt and applied in order to manage the 'emotional load' that each day brings. How helpful do you find the following observations that nurses are expected to be 'nice' at all costs and that it is possible to learn a set of 'feeling rules' to manage these difficult situations through a process of 'transmutation' of feelings as described by Hochschild below?

- Emotion work is a public act, undertaken on behalf of others to ensure a service is delivered effectively.
- Feeling rules are an accepted way of delivering a service; developing the necessary skills and attitudes is or should be part of the training programme.
- Social exchange is forced into narrow channels; there may be hiding places along the shore, but there is much less room for individual navigation of the emotional waters.

Hochschild's research was based on two very different forms of work undertaken by flight attendants and debt collectors. The former are required to be generally friendly and to promote trust and reassurance, whereas the latter are meant to induce a degree of fear and obedience in debtors, inducing them to pay up. Each of these groups of workers inevitably require a different set of attitudes and approaches to their clients if they are to be successful in fulfilling their roles.

Smith relates the students' experience of 'just learning' or 'just picking it up' in relation to feeling rules and points to the tacit nature of learning in the practice setting rather than in the classroom.

Several researchers of nursing and student experiences indicate that facing people who are dying or have died may be one of their top concerns (James 1989, Kelly et al 2000, Smith 1992). Death has long been a taboo subject in modern Western society, although the hospice culture is going some way towards confronting this inevitable human process in a more positive manner. The short case history described here (Case history 3.3), summarizes many nursing students' experiences of their first encounter with a dying patient.

Case history 3.3

Learning to adjust to death and dying

I remember feeling very upset about the death of one patient I had nursed, and spent ages talking about it to my friends who were also nursing students, and later with my mentor. It helped me to put things into some sort of perspective and not to feel quite so sad about it all. This helped me cope better the next time a patient died and to be more open to her relatives without wanting to go and hide.

For a nurse, being able to debrief from a situation when a patient has died, whether or not they were present, is important. With nurses working closely with people in their care it inevitably means there is a bond that can become disturbing if opportunities to discuss situations are not made available, as Case history 3.4 illustrates.

Naomi's experience may be different to your own experiences as a nursing student in your foundation year, but it illustrates how closely nurses and health care support workers relate with patients and clients and their carers and that it is important to recognize that experiencing grief and sadness is natural even for the most experienced practitioner. It also illustrates the importance of receiving good support and guidance from either a counsellor or a more-experienced colleague. As a student, you will encounter people dying in a wide range of settings and situations. Sometimes death can be anticipated and the role of the nurse is to support the patient and their carer during the last hours, making sure this time is spent as comfortably and peacefully as possible. On other occasions, death comes unexpectedly, sometimes

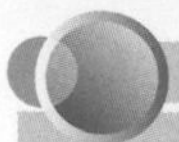

Case history 3.4

Coping with death and dying

Naomi is a care assistant working in a home for people who have learning disabilities. She has been working there since it first opened and when most of the five residents were transferred from the big institution 10 years ago. One of the residents, Brian, a 70-year-old, had developed cancer of the lung 6 months previously. He had been a heavy smoker despite undergoing anti-smoking treatment for some years. Brian had received radiotherapy at the local hospital; this had reduced his symptoms. He was now very weak and finding it difficult to breathe without the aid of oxygen. He was also receiving regular doses of a pain-relieving mixture that contained morphine, which helped his breathing. Everyone in the residence knew Brian did not have very much longer to live and were anxious that he should be looked after in his home. Both residents and staff were very much involved in sitting with him and keeping him company and generally looking after him. He had a special friendship with Naomi as she was the person who had been with him the longest. She had not cared for anyone who was dying before, nor had any other staff member, so it was hard to know what to do for the best. Fortunately, the manager of the residence had been able to arrange help from the Macmillan Nursing Fund, and their nurse had been in every day to support and advise the staff on the best means of making Brian comfortable. She had also provided group sessions for the staff and residents to work through their feelings about what was taking place.

The weekend Brian died was the first weekend Naomi had had off for a month and it was also the occasion of her youngest son's wedding. Before Naomi returned to duty on the Monday the manager of the home contacted her to let her know that Brian had died so she would have some time to prepare herself. The manager realized that Naomi would be very distressed that she had not been with Brian when he died and that Naomi needed to grieve for Brian. Naomi was offered compassionate leave, but preferred to stay at work, so the staff arranged for her to be looked after. She did go to see the bereavement counsellor for several sessions so she could talk through her feelings with someone outside the home.

leading to an emergency response, which may or may not be successful. Whatever the outcome, many of the patients sharing the same clinical area will also need support and comfort, which may be hard for the staff who are also coming to terms with the loss.

Learning how to care for the families of patients who are dying and the patients themselves is perhaps the most challenging role for nurses and much depends upon their own beliefs about pain, death and health care. Medicine and nursing are aimed primarily at promoting recovery from illness, often under heroic circumstances. Many nursing models also include statements relating to promoting a peaceful and dignified death. For Naomi, it was like caring for a close friend and thus all the more challenging, both during Brian's illness and learning to accept that he had gone whilst she continued to work with the other residents in the home.

Learning how to deal with personal grief is also a challenge that nurses need to achieve, as we saw from Naomi's story. She was fortunate in being able to have regular meetings with a bereavement counsellor. For many nurses, such services are not available or they choose not to use them, and they are left to manage their feelings alone. Sometimes feelings of distress may not be faced and 'managed', but simply bottled up, which if left unattended may eventually lead to stress and burnout. This is why, as we discuss below, systems of clinical supervision and mentorship are so important to assist nurses in dealing with such situations. Bottling up feelings is now acknowledged as a risky enterprise in the long run. You may find that nurses need to withdraw to a safe space, away from the business of everyday activities; maybe they delay full expression of their feelings, but they have to be dealt with otherwise the pressure will build up over time and unbearable stress could result. Having a counsellor, either a formally trained one or a clinical supervisor or a friend to talk over your experiences, is a vital part of being an effective nurse.

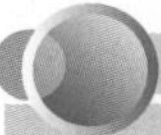

Many placement areas have a 'link lecturer' who is able to provide continuity between educational and clinical contexts and to foster reflective learning and informal emotional support. Quite frequently reflective sessions provide opportunities for students to discuss experiences that they have found hard to cope with or puzzling. These debriefing sessions are important. Similarly, sharing these kinds of concerns with your mentor is also important, as it helps your mentor to recognize what your needs are. By undertaking the emotional labour of working with either your mentor or your link lecturer you are more likely to learn to cope with the kinds of experiences that all practitioners find challenging or even painful.

With greater emphasis in the nursing curriculum on how to respond effectively to emotionally challenging experiences, Williams (1999) argues that nursing students will be more able to communicate with sensitivity, and to reflect with insight upon those interactions that they themselves perceive as meaningful and as a result develop greater self-awareness. Morrison & Burnard (1997) argue that self-awareness is an essential aspect of reflection. Reflective practice has been adopted in most professions as an important tool for developing professional knowledge, but it is also probably the most challenging skill to learn.

Some studies indicate that nursing students go through a series of steps before they become effective in using reflective practice (see English National Board 1994). Williams (1999) suggests that one of the possible reasons for their poor reflective powers may be the result of deliberately suppressing issues that are painful. There are also ethical issues related to ensuring students receive appropriate emotional support, especially when the purpose is educational rather than therapeutic (Mollon 1998). Sometimes, the reflection brings back painful and unresolved memories that require special help. On other occasions, particular situations arouse strong reactions that may cause us to respond in a way that changes the relationship and could even inhibit effective therapeutic actions, as Case history 3.5 highlights.

Case history 3.5

Ahmed

Ahmed came into nursing after qualifying as a primary school teacher. He is married and has two children aged 12 and 9 years. Changing career at the age of 40 years is a significant achievement. Ahmed chose to become a mental health nurse and is nearing his final placement. He is working on the adolescent unit where he is supporting a family with a severely disturbed daughter. He has a mentor who is an experienced and able mental health nurse called Angela. She is becoming worried about Ahmed's close involvement with this family as she sees him losing professional distance and thus his ability to work therapeutically with the family. She decides to discuss this with Ahmed having first talked through her concerns with Ahmed's personal tutor and the link lecturer of the ward. They decide that Angela should broach this in the team meeting which works like an action learning circle. During the conversation, Ahmed acknowledges that his relationship with the family is closer than normal. Almost as an aside he mentions how much his younger sister resembles the child he is caring for. His mentor invites him to explore this further and gradually Ahmed realizes that his close association with the family represents his own forgotten feelings of guilt and loss about his favourite sister. With careful support from the placement team he identifies that he has been subconsciously trying to compensate for the failure of his family to resolve the problems of his sister's illness through this family.

Recognizing this enables Ahmed to find the necessary emotional space that helps him to withdraw his emotional closeness whilst increasing his therapeutic approach, which the family needs.

Ahmed (Case history 3.5) expressed relief at having been able to explore the possible reasons for his exaggerated involvement with his patient and being facilitated by the group to 'normalize his feelings'. This example shows the benefit of dealing with suppressed and displaced feelings in a protective environment. The question inevitably arising from Williams' work is: Can this kind of emotionally supportive learning environment be provided by clinical staff for nursing students on busy placements in contemporary society? If you feel that the answer is 'no', then it is often advisable to discuss your concerns and feelings either with a counsellor in the university occupational health department or with your personal tutor. Williams argues that the nature of the relationships that you are likely to experience in academic settings and placements should reflect the same kinds of relationships you are expected to develop with your patients and clients. This should include respect for your needs for personal space and privacy as well as emotional security and psychological safety. It is only in such settings that you can engage in reflective practice on a voluntary basis (Williams 1999). Using reflective practice in a protective environment such as that illustrated in Case history 3.5 can be helpful in dealing with your emotions, be they happy or sad; but not all clinical settings have staff who are able to explore their own emotional needs and these staff members are less likely to recognize the needs of their students. An alternative setting is to join a reflective student group where you may feel more comfortable in experiencing and expressing such feelings together with peers who are going through similar experiences.

Learning and managing the emotional work of cancer care

Intense emotion work needs to be undertaken by both nurses and doctors in cancer and palliative care settings. James (1993), an important contributor to this field of research and clinical practice, describes how cancer requires considerable emotional effort on the part of the carers and is thus a significant area in which to learn how people cope. Cancer is, as she says, 'difficult to hide', which means that all staff involved in delivering care have at some level to explore and manage their feelings. In some cases this means having to work on maintaining the belief that everything is 'normal' in the patient's life and in other cases may mean being faced with the uncomfortable task of disclosure.

Doctors' emotion management is often influenced by the natural science approach to medicine on which their knowledge and skills are based. Specialities are divided up along biological lines and their training encourages them to maintain a sense of distance and objectivity. Doctors are the ones who own the diagnosis and are the keepers of patient information, even in the hospice where James undertook her study in the 1980s. A recent review of the treatment of leukaemia using bone marrow transplants showed that doctors continued to emphasize cure when a significant number of their patients would die (Kelly et al 2000). Nurses, on the other hand, have to manage the uncertainty and hopelessness as the patient slips from a curative to a terminal track. This approach contrasts with how nurses are educated to develop good communication skills, effective relationships and holistic patient care (Armstrong 1983).

The physicians' styles of emotional labour using distance and objectivity have their origins in their medical training (Smith III & Kleinman 1989). Whilst the style and content of medical education will have changed substantially since their article was published, the spirit remains the same. Smith III and Kleinman (1989) describe how medical students learn to suppress their feelings and adopt strategies to manage emotions in stressful clinical situations in order to deal with uncertainty and the pressure of making mistakes. Medical students learn to navigate their way through profound emotional experiences which they have to manage and make sense of. They use a repertoire of emotion management strategies shaped by the 'hidden curriculum' and practical procedures and routines designed to distance them from patients. These procedures and routines include dissection, autopsies, clinical examinations and investigations. 'Gallows humour' provides an acceptable format to contain problems and relieve tensions (Smith III and Kleinman 1989).

Practising emotional labour

So far we have explored some of the challenges that you may face as a student nurse and which many nurses fear. In this section, we discuss a number of everyday situations in which emotional labour is undertaken by nurses, midwives and other health professionals. These include emotional labour:

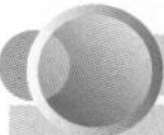

- In intimate care situations.
- When responding to emergencies.
- When dealing with difficult questions and confidential information.
- When seeking to defuse aggression.
- When sharing joy and sorrow, with patients, relatives, friends and colleagues.

Emotional labour and intimate care situations

In her book 'Nursing intimacy: an ethnographic approach to nurse–patient interaction' (Savage 1995), Savage touches on areas that are relevant to emotional labour. Savage draws on work by Leiniger who notes that care has been seen as 'the essences [*sic*] and the central unifying and dominant domain to characterize nursing' (Leiniger 1988). Yet, as a concept, caring is elusive, complex and open to a range of interpretations (Bartle 1991, Brykczynska 1992), to the extent that its meaning remains unclear (Swanson 1991). We have already pointed to the important distinction between 'caring about' and 'caring for' someone and Savage refers to the work of Chipman (1991) to further reinforce this point. 'Caring for' appears to predominate in emotional labour although caring for people is made easier and more pleasant if we genuinely 'care about' them. However, if intimate caring is not carefully managed it can obviously create problems in service work, including nursing, as it may cloud objectivity. We can see this in the example of Ahmed (Case history 3.5), where he over-identified with a child patient.

Intimate care situations are 'privileged' in that the persons being 'cared for' may perceive themselves as vulnerable, whether physically and/or emotionally, and are thus highly dependent upon the thoughtful and sensitive support of their carer. As a nursing student, it is important to be sensitive to this vulnerable state and to work collaboratively with the patients and their carers whilst retaining awareness of one's own needs and emotional safety.

Physical intimacy is experienced very differently by individuals. Some people fear being touched except perhaps by one or more chosen individuals. Being physically exposed as is likely to occur when being nursed may cause such people genuine distress. Some cultures have strict rules about exposure and physical contact, especially by someone of the opposite gender. In the multicultural setting of present-day Britain, nurses must take into account their patients' and clients' different expectations in relation to intimacy amongst their patients and colleagues. Case history 3.6 illustrates this.

Case history 3.6

Mr Stapleton and the bath

Mr Stapleton is a 70-year-old retired miner whose wife died 10 years ago. He is house-bound and has severe arthritis which makes it difficult for him to maintain his personal hygiene. He has two visits weekly from a health care assistant who helps him in and out of the bath. Mr Stapleton has asked for a male nurse to help him with this procedure as he finds it too embarrassing to have a female helping him. One day there was no male nurse available so Susan the local district nurse went to help him with his bath. He was horrified when she arrived and explained that he had never been washed by a woman. Not wishing to put Mr Stapleton into a difficult situation she made two suggestions: that he delayed having his regular bath until the male nurse returned from holiday or that he tried to imagine her as a professional carer, who was gender-free as indicated by the nurses' uniform which she was wearing. Fortunately, this suggestion fed into the patient's image of nurses as Florence Nightingale's 'lady with the lamp' and he agreed to have his bath. The uniform had proved useful in giving this man the privacy needed in order to accept intimate physical caring.

It is important for a nurse to make the connection between the formal uniform and the protection it can bestow, and although in Case history 3.6 the patient was a male with a female carer it is often equally problematic for female patients to be cared for by a male nurse. Providing patients with a genuine choice about their carer is important and a patient's preferences should be documented in their nursing care plan and respected. This choice should be offered to all patients, irrespective of their sex or cultural origins. Some communities have very clear symbols of the importance of privacy and discretion such as the veils and robes worn by Muslim women as it is forbidden for them to be seen by any man other than their husband. Research by Poya (1999) shows the more positive aspects of Muslim dress as a way of promoting women's identity and safety against the potential hostilities of the external world.

Emotional intimacy and the nurse relationship

In her discussion on intimacy, Savage (1995) refers to the shift towards 'new nursing' where the focus of the nurse–patient relationship moves towards emotional intimacy. May (1992) believes that this change in nurse–patient relationships raises interesting issues of power and control. He suggests that by nurses encouraging patients to reveal their innermost fears and emotions they are potentially putting the patients into an emotionally vulnerable position, which may not be addressed by the nurse. When patients are in a physically vulnerable situation they are dependent on the health care staff and so need to comply. The same situation applies to patients receiving mental health care. May argues that the greater a patient's frailty is the greater their dependency on the nurse–patient relationship. This raises an interesting aspect of 'intimacy'; that is, a kind of 'emotional nakedness' on the part of patients, who perhaps in the past were only asked to expose themselves to physical intimacy, which is inevitable in receiving hands-on health care. What emerges from May's argument may be a kind of 'emotional imperialism', exercised by health professionals, albeit with benevolent intent. Consent is as necessary before delving into the depths of a patient's or health professional's intimate, and maybe hidden, emotions, as it would be in the case of invasive physical therapy. The consequences for nurses of functioning within this 'new nursing' context is explicitly addressed by Savage (1995) who argues that the new 'closeness' with patients requires intimate emotional involvement and this substantially increases personal stress for the nurses. She found that factors contributing to this form of 'close' relationships with patients tended to be higher when:

- Nurses 'opened up' to patients. The assumption here seemed to be that these nurses were willing to be emotionally intimate with patients, and that this was generally reciprocated by patients.
- The nurses used a relaxed posture and informal uniform styles.
- These nurses felt supported by senior staff.

In such situations where nurses were willing to engage in a professionally emotional relationship with patients (and their carers), the relationships were not necessarily emotionally deep, but when deeper than average relationships did occur, nurses did not express particular 'support needs'. Predictably, 'closeness' with patients developed more readily in clinical environments where nurses felt supported by management styles and attitudes than in settings where this was not the case. Working in such environments often means that nurses are more in need of emotional support for themselves. Often in clinical areas that demand a high level of emotional labour, such as cancer care wards or children's wards, there are regular group sessions facilitated by a specially trained worker for staff wishing to engage in them. Clinical supervision sessions also provide nursing staff with support from peers as well as more experienced colleagues. In addition, many hospitals now provide professional counsellors for their staff through occupational health departments.

Social systems as a defence against anxiety

One of the ways in which nurses protect themselves against stress was identified as long ago as 1962 by a British psychoanalyst, Isobel Menzies (1962/1970). She demonstrated that, by passing on responsibility to increasingly more senior colleagues, nurses could reduce their own stress. Another strategy was through the system of care delivery. In settings where care was broken down into a series of tasks undertaken by different members of staff, patient relationships were fragmented and so emotional involvement was minimized. At the time of Menzies' study, most patients were hospitalized for several weeks and so it was more likely that close relationships could develop. Since that time, the average length of patients' hospital stay has been reduced to a matter of days for many surgical procedures. In contrast, more patients with long-term disorders are being cared for in their homes and the community nurses are particularly vulnerable to emotional burnout. Several pioneering research studies published by the Royal College of Nursing around the time of Menzies' study indicated that patient care in the 1970s and 1980s was less effective and was even harmful. This led to the introduction of patient allocation through team nursing or primary nursing (Manthey 1980) with the aim of providing care that was patient-centred and holistic. By working in a team it was anticipated that peer support would be sufficient to protect staff from emotional stress.

Emotional labour and emergency situations

As a foundation course nursing student you are unlikely to be placed in settings where you will encounter a severe major emergency until later in your programme. However, in many clinical settings emergencies may occur and it is often helpful to think about your own possible response beforehand. Some programmes include opportunities to role-play difficult or challenging situations. The aim is to provide you with an experience that helps you to prepare yourself both technically (what to do) and emotionally (what it feels like). Perhaps one of the greatest challenges that you will encounter is finding the ability to give an impression of being calm and knowledgeable about what to do despite any anxieties bubbling away beneath the surface. In emergency situations it is important to be able to convey calmness and confidence to people. In the early stages of your programme many situations that later become part of everyday nursing often seem urgent and create sensations of panic. Situations that often challenge foundation courses nurses could be times such as when a patient suddenly wants to vomit, or has a fall, or shouts at you. These events can create a turmoil of indecision, but gradually you will learn what to do and how to respond in an effective manner. One way is to watch how other colleagues deal with such events; another way is to remember and draw on your clinical skills sessions, or sessions addressing ways of responding to aggressive behaviour.

Taking a deep breath can be steadying, as it has a physiological effect that reduces the adrenaline rush that can cloud thinking. It also gives you a few seconds 'out of the situation' to let your learning come to the fore and inform your actions. Learning routines also helps with this process, which is why frequent practice in a skills laboratory is so important. Being able to set aside your own personal fears needs to be learned, but it is also essential to ensure that you have an opportunity to debrief those involved about their fears when the event is over. Case histories 3.7 and 3.8

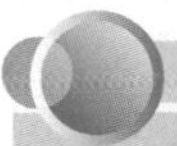

Case history 3.7

Responding to an emergency: cardiac arrest

It is mid-afternoon and things are quite slow on the ward today; many of the patients are having an afternoon sleep or have visitors. The afternoon staff are having an extended handover in the office and the morning shift staff are carrying on with general care activities. Suddenly, there's an urgent shout from the side-room. It's the first-year student nurse Hazel, who sees the patient appearing to have a fit. She has pulled the emergency bell and a staff nurse responds immediately: 'Call the crash team', she shouts. While they are being summoned, Brian, one of the care assistants, rushes the crash trolley into the room and sees that the staff nurse has started cardiac massage while the student is giving mouth-to-mouth respiration. Brian starts getting the necessary equipment together and begins timing the situation. The resuscitation team arrives within a few minutes and takes over the resuscitation; this time they are successful in bringing the patient back to life. Once the patient is made comfortable and everything is cleared up, Hazel is asked whether she would like to stay and help the staff nurse care for the patient when he is moved into the main ward area. The staff nurse and Hazel work together and talk about the situation with the patient, with the staff nurse taking him through what happened. The student has the opportunity to explore what had actually taken place and to express her feelings of tension and relief, as well as pride at being able to act promptly and effectively.

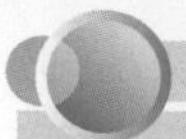

Case history 3.8

Responding to an emergency in a mental health placement

Tony is in the fourth week of his first mental health placement and this week he has been working with his mentor for the past three shifts. Today he is going to take Maisie as a patient of his own, after having cared for her with his mentor earlier in the week. They have discussed the plan of care with the patient and all seems to be going well. The patient has a history of self-harming and needs help with essential care. When Tony returns from his lunch-break he notices that Maisie is nowhere to be found on the ward. Tony feels a sense of panic and guilt and fears that she may have left the ward to self-harm. He goes to find his mentor, but she has been called away so he decides to go and search for Maisie. As he feared, she is sitting on a bench in the grounds and has a blade. Tony goes and sits next to her, and talks gently to her in an attempt to persuade her to come back to the ward and to give him the knife. At the back of his mind Tony is praying that a staff nurse will see them and come and provide some support, but at the same time carries on talking to Maisie as a means of distracting her. Shortly, Tony's mentor comes up and sits down and joins in the conversation, until Maisie eventually agrees to go back to the ward and to give Tony the blade.

In the debrief session, Tony's mentor praises him for his calm response and the style of his action. Tony confesses that it was something they had practised in the school skills lab; he had rather dismissed the session, but he could now recognize how much it had informed his thinking while he was trying to find Maisie.

provide examples of emergencies that could happen.

The incidents described in Case histories 3.7 and 3.8, although specific in details, will have a ring of familiarity to most hospital nurses. Calm waters can be ruffled in an instant by such emergencies in situations where acutely ill people are being cared for. The action taken by nurses on site is, indeed, crucial. The cardiac arrest (Case history 3.7) needed to be handled with efficiency and speed to save the patient's life because they will be at risk because of oxygen deprivation. This was not a time for openly 'expressing emotions', and internal feelings had to be contained in order to give an external appearance of calm and to deal with the practical management of the emergency. In this example, the student and the staff nurse had the opportunity to discuss the emotional aftermath.

Dealing with confidential information and patients' questions

As a foundation course nursing student, you will inevitably come across situations that involve learning to become confident in responding to confidential information. This could be information that you receive as a member of the placement team and may be related to the patient's diagnosis or the anticipated outcome of their treatment. Current practice recommends that patients and their carers are fully involved in decision-making about their treatment and diagnosis, although there may be times when this does not take place. In such situations, a considerable responsibility is placed on the nursing staff who are working closely with patients and their carers. Knowing how to respond in a professional and ethical manner is part of what we call emotional labour. Your response needs to reflect the policy or decisions made by the health care team caring for the patient, and it may include you saying that you 'do not know the answer' or that you are not in a position to answer the question but that if the patient wishes, you could tell your mentor and get their advice.

In many health care settings, decisions about how to respond to difficult questions are either decided upon by medical consultants on their own or in collaboration with all the relevant members of the health care team in consultation with the patient's carers. There is always the uncertainty about diagnosis, but, even when it seems certain that the condition is mortal, the period prior to death is often hard to assess. There is also the issue of deciding whether the patient actually wants the truth. Sometimes patients ask questions such as 'Am I dying?' in order to seek reassurance that all is well, or to confirm their own interpretation of their illness. Learning how to address such questions requires considerable expertise and knowledge of the patient. One of us (ML) recalls a hospital situation in which a terminally ill patient asked a house officer 'Am I going to die?'. He clearly had a fair idea of what the situation was, as he mentioned wanting to 'set his affairs in order' if he was likely to die soon. It did appear that he would like to hear the truth and he was given the bad news. Alas, the doctor had misread the cues, or at least the consequences of giving such bad news to the patient. Rather than accepting his fate and adopting a practical approach to preparing for death, all the patient had wanted was reassurance that he was not dying. Consequently, he reacted badly to his poor prognosis and the nurses and doctors were totally unprepared for this.

Chapter 5 provides some guidelines for dealing with similar situations. Inevitably, as a nursing student caring for a patient whilst being supervised by a mentor, you will come across situations that require counselling skills which are outside your current expertise, so seeking help from your mentor is good practice. The best learning comes from being able to witness how your mentors deal with such situations so that you can learn from their example. It is also a good idea to explore as honestly as you can your own attitudes and beliefs about death, serious illness or disability and uncertain diagnosis and prognosis. You might find it helpful to read as widely as possible, drawing on novels as well as films and texts so that you can learn about the subject and people's different responses. Another source of information is to explore the teachings of different religions and how these prepare people for uncertainty as well as death. Your reading will help you to discover and define your own attitudes, which will help you to be more effective as a nurse.

The emotional labour of responding to aggressive behaviour

You may have come across notices on buses, railway platforms and various other public places stating in effect that staff members have a right to work free from violence and that the management will deal firmly with anyone who is verbally or physically abusive. Facing aggression has become a major problem in all public areas of society, and health service workers need to develop the necessary skills of identifying situations that may lead to either verbal or physical abuse and of preventing such situations. In the health service, such situations are more likely to occur in areas where people feel they are being ignored or neglected, such as waiting rooms, or where people who are being attended to are affected by alcohol or non-prescription drugs. Other situations may arise when a patient is confused from lack of oxygen to their brain or as a result of illness.

Learning how to prevent someone's anger or confusion escalating into an attack is an important skill, as is learning how to recognize potential situations and to minimize any such risk. Another skill to learn is how to defuse someone's anger, by not getting angry yourself but acknowledging that the person is angry and that you are listening to the grievances expressed. Not engaging in an argument is important, and learning how to use your body language in an open and supportive way (despite any inward fears) can help defuse aggression. Various techniques designed to calm such individuals can be learnt, but safety must be maintained, and a strategy of saying to the aggressor 'I am a student nurse and I am unable to be of help but I will get someone who can' and then to retreat cautiously and courteously to obtain help is often the best action to take. Taking unwarranted personal risks in such situations can lead to escalation of the situation and cause harm.

The emotional labour of responding to extremes of emotion: joy and sorrow

As a nursing student, you are likely to encounter situations that are either happy or sad; you will also come across situations that appeal to your sense of humour or you want to use humour as a means of encouragement and support. Using humour to encourage patients to deal with a challenge such as learning to walk after an injury requires skill and sensitivity, but can free them from anxiety and so promote progress (Åstedt-Kurki & Liukkonen 1994).

Learning your role as a professional includes learning how to use these emotions in a positive and constructive manner. Being faced with sadness, as well as at times with joy, involves much personal effort as it is indeed emotional labour. Rejoicing at the birth of a baby and even to the point of tears of emotion and relief that the delivery has progressed safely takes as much courage as it does to cry alongside a patient who is coping with unbearable challenges. Being emotionally sensitive to patients includes recognizing your own boundaries and needs, and finding ways of having them met through contact and support from friends and colleagues. Support by colleagues makes for a positive work environment in general and a nursing environment in particular. It also facilitates the sharing of patients' anxieties and pleasures. Again, these may vary greatly. Taking time to look at photographs of patients' sons or daughters, and hearing about the details of happy events such as weddings, holidays and birthday parties, may be more therapeutic than sedation. Ways of dealing with patients' fears is clearly an area requiring the highest degree of emotional skill. We must always be prepared for the possibility that even our best efforts may sometimes fail.

Humility is important in all human relationships. If we have hurt someone, wittingly or unwittingly, it is important to be able to recognize this in order to be prepared to apologise and express regret. The fear of litigation has often inhibited health professionals in this area, as an apology may be viewed as admission of guilt. In fact, many accounts of unresolved patient complaints, which eventually end up on the Ombudsman's desk, include the complainants stating that they would never have complained in the first place if an apology for what occurred had been provided, freely and with honest regret.

Discussion and conclusions

In this chapter we have introduced you to some of the situations that are frequently encountered in nursing practice and that we have identified as emotional labour. By drawing on the work of Hochschild who studied the working life of airline stewards and debt collectors in the USA (Hochschild 1983), and the research of Smith who investigated the learning experiences of nursing students in the UK (Smith 1992), we have provided some of the theoretical background to emotional labour. Another aspect of what could be described as emotional labour is a form of professionalism that is typical of service professions (Lorentzon 1990). Mackay's study demonstrated that, in spite of difficult working conditions and low pay, nurses in the 1980s rated the job satisfaction derived from nursing very highly (Mackay 1989). Other studies from the subsequent two decades indicated that there were personal 'emotional costs' associated with nursing (Smith 1992, 2001) and that these were not generally fully acknowledged by managers in public and private services. However, in the 1990s, the British government began to introduce policies designed to make the needs of patients/clients central to health care delivery through the introduction of patient advocacy services and the requirement that each health care provider should include service users in their policy-making and structures (Department of Health 1997, 1998, 1999). The government also recognized that staff needs had to be addressed, and policies such as the 'Improving working lives standard' (http://www.doh.gov.uk) were designed to introduce family-friendly working conditions. Lorentzon's (1990) theory, that service occupations in which women traditionally are more numerous and sometimes described as 'semi-professions' (Etzioni 1969), are characterized by a high degree of altruism, does not preclude the likelihood that many such workers (e.g. nurses and teachers) operating in private sector areas behave in a similar manner. Hochschild's flight attendants operated in the private sector, where the profit motive is overt. However, the individuals were salaried and not personally rewarded financially for every smile and kind action.

Personal motivation is private, to a great extent, whether service is provided in the public or private sector. The division between the public and private sectors has become blurred with the introduction of private finance initiatives and use of the independent sector to deliver health care on behalf of the NHS. New hospitals and other capital investments have been made possible by bringing together mixed funding sources so that private funds can be used to finance public projects. It is worth speculating on the impact of introducing the private factor into the public sector and the long-term implications.

Although the private sector may be viewed with a degree of suspicion by public sector workers, the observation is often made by nurses working in the private hospitals that the perceived or reported lower stress levels in such hospitals allow them to 'care properly' for patients. Similar remarks are made by teachers transferring to private schools and the joy of teaching smaller classes.

The art of what we now describe as emotional labour in nursing has, traditionally, been linked to women's work and its association with the 'maternal instinct', a trait which all female workers are assumed to have. Extracts from early issues of the Nursing Times inferred the prevalence of such attitudes among women in general, as did remarks made by matrons concerning probationers in registers from the late 19th and early 20th centuries. With the transfer of nursing education into higher education and public concerns about the quality of care, the Royal College of Nursing (RCN) at its Annual Congress in 2004 debated a resolution put by one of its members: 'That this meeting of the RCN Congress believes that the caring component of nursing should be devolved to healthcare assistants to enable nurses to concentrate on treatment and technical nursing'. Delegates from across the country voted overwhelmingly against the resolution, with 95% voting against and only 5% for the resolution. One commentator, Scott (2004), argued that, if the vote was representative of general nursing opinion, then the profession needed to make their views clear in order to prevent 'politicians from interfering in the nursing role'. With the introduction of the government's review of professional roles with its policy document 'Agenda for change' (Department of Health 2003), there is a risk that those nurses who expand into medical and technological domains will be the ones who are financially rewarded (Scott 2004).

Freshwater & Stickley (2004), for example, wrote about the need to balance 'the rational and the emotional' in nursing, and argued that it is only through emotional intelligence that high standards of holistic care can be provided. This is reflected in studies of midwives who have worked as autonomous practitioners in the UK since 1902 when they were recognized through their own Midwives Registration Act, some 17 years before nurses. In a study by Hunter (2004), a small number of student midwives were interviewed about ways in which they experienced and managed emotions in their work. Interestingly, findings demonstrated a variety of views on midwifery practice, as does the current debate about balance between 'caring' and 'technological interventions' in nursing practice. Hunter concluded that it was the conflicting ideologies about midwifery that created dilemmas for the midwifery students rather than the client–midwife relationship.

It would seem clear that learning the art of emotion work is crucial, both in terms of serving patients/clients and in negotiating a balanced way of working for the nursing and midwifery professions, in which the cared-for person receives balanced attention from health professionals responding to both clinical and emotional needs. There is no 'either/or' in this regard. Technological intervention provided without sensitivity can be seriously damaging to vulnerable individuals. Likewise, extremely sensitive care given by persons who possess insufficient technical skills can be life-threatening at worst, and potentially damaging in less extreme cases.

The codification of patient-centred care by government policies endorses good practice that has been advocated by nursing and midwifery practitioners for many years. However, it is important to ensure that all aspects of patient care are considered and the balance between these elements must be safeguarded as part of comprehensive professionalism, to which patients, clients and their carers have a right. This art needs to be learnt and perfected in practice, to ensure the continued combination of 'caring' and 'technical' ingredients.

Learning the art of emotional labour involves dealing with specific situations, as described throughout this chapter. This includes responding to difficult questions, handling demanding situations which may incorporate an element of risk for carers, and sorting out problems that may arise due to the intimacy of the care situation. There is particular need for nurses, midwives and other health professionals to be aware of both patient/client and colleague needs for emotional care and this is what, in this chapter, we have endeavoured to describe and discuss.

Work with vulnerable patients/clients makes collegial support extremely important. As a nursing student, you will find it through your peers, with whom you can share your everyday experiences and learn from each other. Another source of collegial support can be your personal tutor and, in your placement, from your mentor. The general principles we have described in this chapter provide a basis for further study and consideration. Throughout the text we have urged you to learn from your observations of good practice and consolidation by reading widely so that you can develop your own professional knowledge base to pass on to the next generation of learners. Providing skilled professional care, including technical, spiritual and emotional aspects, is symbolic of an emotional labourer/practitioner of the highest integrity and represents the real heart-and-soul qualities of human beings.

References

Abel-Smith B 1960 A history of the nursing profession. Heinemann, London

Aldridge M 1994 Unlimited liability? Emotional labour in nursing and social work. Journal of Advanced Nursing 20:722–728

Allan H, Larsen J 2003 Give us respect. Royal College of Nursing, London

Anonymous 1905 An open letter to a nurse by a matron, Nursing Times 6 May:42

Anonymous 1905 An open letter to a matron from two nurses, Nursing Times, 17 June:114–115

Anonymous 1911 Discipline and nursing by an ex-matron, Nursing Times, 6 May:432

Armstrong D 1983 The fabrication of nurse–patient relationships. Social Science & Medicine 14:3–13

Åstedt-Kurki P, Liukkonen A 1994 Humour in nursing care. Journal of Advanced Nursing 20:183–188

Bartle J 1991 Caring in relation to Orem's theory. Nursing Standard 5(37):33–36

Bean JP, Metzner BS 1985 A conceptual model of non-traditional undergraduate student attrition. Review of Educational Research 55(4):485–540

Bolton SC 2000 Who cares? Offering emotions work as a gift in the nursing labour process. Journal of Advanced Nursing 32(3):580–586

Brykczynska G 1992 Caring: a dying art? In: Jolley M, Brykczynska G (eds) Nursing care: the challenge to change. Edward Arnold, London

Campbell AV 1984 Moderated love. SPCK, London

Chipman Y 1991 Caring: its meaning and place in the practice of nursing. Journal of Nursing Education 3(4):171–175

Davies C (ed) 1980 Re-writing nursing history. Croom & Helm, London

Department of Health (undated) Improving working lives standard. Department of Health, London (www.doh.gov.uk)

Department of Health 1997 The new NHS: modern and dependable. HMSO, London

Department of Health 1998 A first class service: quality in the new NHS. HMSO, London

Department of Health 1999 Making a difference: strengthening the nursing, midwifery, health visiting contribution to health and health care. Department of Health, London (www.doh.gov.uk)

Department of Health 2003 Agenda for change. Department of Health, London

English National Board 1994 The current teaching provision for individual learning styles of students on pre-registration diploma programmes in adult nursing (ENB Research Highlight 9). English National Board, London

Etzioni A (ed) 1969 Semi-professions and their organization. Free Press, New York

Freshwater D, Stickley T 2004 The heart of the art: emotional intelligence in nurse education. Nursing Inquiry 11(2):91–98

Graham H 1983 Caring: a labour of love. In: Finch J, Groves D (eds) A labour of love: women, work and caring. Routledge & Kegan Paul, London

Hochschild AR 1983 (20th anniversary edn 2003) The managed heart: commercialization of human feeling. University of California Press, Berkeley, CA

Hunter B 2004 Conflicting ideologies as a source of emotion work in midwifery. Midwifery 20:261–272

James N 1989 Emotional labour, skills and work in the social relations of feeling. Sociological Review 37(1):15–42

James N 1993 Division of emotional labour: disclosure and concern. In: Fineman S (ed) Emotion in organizations. Sage, London

Jeffreys MR 1998 Predicting non-traditional student retention and academic achievement. Nurse Education 23(1):42–48

Jourard SM 1971 The transparent self. Van Nostrand, New York

Kelly D, Ross S Gray B, Smith P 2000 Death, dying and emotional labour: problematic dimensions of the bone marrow transplant nursing role. Journal of Advanced Nursing 34(4):952–960

Leininger M 1988 Leininger's theory of nursing: cultural care diversity and universality. Nursing Science Quarterly 1(4): 175–181

Lorentzon M 1990 Professional status and managerial tasks: feminine service ideology in British nursing and social work. In: Abbot P, Wallace C (eds) The sociology of the caring professions. Falmer Press, London p 53–66

Lorentzon M 2000 Nurse education at the London Homoeopathic Hospital, 1903–1947: preparation for professional specialists or marginalised cinderellas? International History of Nursing Journal 5(2):20–27

Lorentzon M 2001 Grooming nurses for the new century: analysis of nurses' registers in London voluntary hospitals before the First World War. International History of Nursing Journal 5(2):20–27

Lorentzon M 2003 'Lower than a scullery maid': is this view of the British Poor Law nurse justified? International History of Nursing Journal 7(3): 4–16

Lorentzon M 2004 The way we were: sublimate your maternal instinct. Georges, Alumnus Magazine for St George's Hospital Medical School, p 12–13

Mackay L 1989 Nursing a problem. Open University, Milton Keynes

Maggs C 1981 Control mechanisms and the new nurses 1881–1914. Occasional paper 25. Nursing Times 77(36):97–100

Manthey M 1980 The practice of primary nursing. Blackwell Scientific, Boston

May C 1992 Individual care? Power and subjectivity in therapeutic relationships. Sociology 26(4):589–602

Menzies IEP 1962 A case study of the functioning of social systems as a defence against anxiety. A report on the study of a nursing service of a general hospital. Human Relations 13:95–121 (reprinted 1970, The functioning of social systems as a defence against anxiety. Tavistock Institute, London)

Mollon D 1998 False memories: finding a balance. Advances in psychiatric treatment, vol 4. Royal College of Psychiatrists, London

Morrison P, Burnard P 1997 Caring and communicating the interpersonal relationship in nursing. Macmillan, London

Poya M 1999 Women, work and Islamism ideology and resistance in Iran. Zed Books, London

Rawnsley MM 1980 Toward a conceptual base for affective nursing. Nursing Outlook April:244–247

Runciman WG 1978 Weber selections in translation. Cambridge University Press, Cambridge

Savage J 1995 Nursing intimacy: an ethnographic approach to nurse–patient interaction. Scutari Press, London

Scott H 2004 Are nurses 'too clever to care' and 'too posh to wash'? British Journal of Nursing 13(10):581

Smith III AC, Kleinman S 1989 Managing emotions in medical school: student contact with the living and the dead. Special issue: Sentiment, affect and emotions. Social Psychology Quarterly 52(1):56–69

Smith P 1992 The emotional labour of nursing. Macmillan, Basingstoke.

Smith P 2001 Emotional labour costs. Exploring health and illness care K203 B3, offprint 19. Working for health. Open University, Milton Keynes

Smith P, Gray B 2000 The emotional labour of nursing: how student and qualified nurses learn to care. Unpublished report. South Bank University, London (available from: p.a.smith@surrey.ac.uk)

Smith P, Gray B 2001 Re-assessing the concept of emotional labour in student nurse education. Nurse Education Today 21:230–237

Smith P, O'Driscoll M, Magnusson C 2005 Evaluation of the Diploma in Higher Education Nursing Studies (Adult) Pre-registration Nursing Programme. Unpublished report. Centre for Research in Nursing and Midwifery Education, University of Surrey, Guildford (available on request from centre-rnme@surrey.ac.uk)

Swanson K 1991 Empirical development of a middle range theory of caring. Nursing Research 40(3):161–166

Williams S 1999 Student carers: learning to manage emotions. Soundings 11:180–186

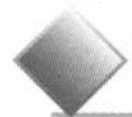

Further reading

Mann M, Cowburn J 2005 Emotional labour and stress within mental health nursing. Journal of Psychiatric and Mental Health Nursing 12(2):154–162

Nightingale F 1876–1884 Letters to nurses. Nightingale Collection, London Metropolitan Archives, London

Skilbeck J, Payne S 2003 Emotional support and the role of clinical nurse specialists in palliative care. Journal of Advanced Nursing 43(5):521–530

Smith P, James T, Lorentzon M et al 2004 Shaping the facts: evidence-based nursing and healthcare. Churchill Livingstone, London.

Chapter Four

4

Professional standards and rules:

the professional regulatory body and the nursing student

Isabelle Whaite

Key topics

- **Health care ethics and the moral character of the health care professional**
- **The responsibility of acting morally well through exercising the virtues in the delivery of care**
- **The relevance of a profession's values, standards for conduct and performance and ethics to health care practice**
- **How the 'Nursing and Midwifery Council (NMC) Code of professional conduct' can be used as a guide for acting morally well in practice**
- **Discussion of case studies of experiences encountered by nursing students**
- **The value of using different sources of knowledge and theory to explain and support decisions**

Introduction

Health care professionals have the potential to do much good but also the potential to do much harm to those to whom they deliver care. Health care is a moral endeavour, in that the aim of practice is to maximize health and well-being. This chapter concentrates on the human side of health care ethics and what we know of human nature whilst recognizing that health professionals are both fallible and vulnerable at times. It provides an initial framework for the student embarking on a study of ethics and its application to everyday health care practice. The focus is on you as a person, at the beginning of your journey to join a profession of practice, and the personal characteristics you need to nurture as an emerging professional. The view being promoted here is that, knowing the kind of person you are now and the person that you aspire to be, will make a difference to the potential you have to do good or to do harm to others. This will make a difference as to how your behaviour in practice is experienced by others, whether it is viewed as life-enhancing or life-diminishing by them as individual, worthwhile persons.

This chapter is about you taking responsibility for acting in the right manner, in the moral sense of rightness and wrongness, demonstrated in the way you are being with others and behaving towards one another. It is about being familiar with the rules for professional practice and developing understanding about the sources of the rules and standards for professional practice. In the third part of the chapter you will be invited to join the 'virtual' ethics class of a group of foundation students, and to consider their stories about practice experience. You will be able to participate in learning how to engage in the complex process of ethical enquiry. You will also be able to consider how the profession's rules and standards might be applied to inform standards of practice in general, as well as to consider the specific guidance on how to deal with difficult situations in practice. At this initial stage in your study of ethics it is less about taking the responsibility for ethical decision-making in practice and more about deciding what is the right course of action. This will engage you with the study of ethics as an academic discipline, including a detailed study of moral theory and the application of reasoning and logic in making judgements about the 'right' course of action to take from a range of possible options. It will become an important part of your study of ethics for practice as you progress to the next stages of your educational programme and as you acquire more experience in the practice of health care and further develop your thinking and reasoning abilities.

To assist you in developing this knowledge the chapter has been divided into three sections. The first section provides you with an overview of moral endeavour and ethical conduct. The second section is concerned with professional statutory regulations and how they provide a guide to practitioners and to students about their professional and everyday conduct. The third section is the 'virtual' discussion group mentioned above, in which you are invited to participate and where nursing students are exploring case studies from their own practice experiences and seeking resolution to issues they found problematic.

An introduction to principles of moral endeavour and ethical conduct

Ethics is a complex form of enquiry in pursuit of some standard with which to judge the rightness or wrongness of our actions in the moral sense. In deciding wrongness of our actions we can evaluate our behaviour from a number of points of view, of which morality is only one (Rowson 1990). We judge the rightness/wrongness, goodness/badness of our actions using a range of standards. For example, a judgement of what is right or wrong in the legal sense can be supported with evidence from the statute book. A judgement about what is right or wrong to do from the perspective of social convention can be supported with evidence from cultural codes, professional codes and standards of conduct, rules and etiquette. A judgement of what is right or wrong to do from a practical point of view can be supported with scientific evidence, evidence of best practice that is tested and proven in experience. These different sources of evidence are not sufficient standards in themselves to support a judgement of what is right or wrong to do in the moral sense. The standard by which to judge rightness or wrongness, goodness or badness of action in the moral sense requires different evidence.

Ethics as a complex process of enquiry

The more traditional approach to health care ethics involves health care professionals using reason and logic from moral philosophy in the analysis of complex arguments in order to defend judgements about what is right action in health care. It is a highly complex process and requires nurses to engage with in-depth study of different sources and kinds of knowledge in order to develop advanced levels of understanding across a range of subject disciplines. These include concepts and theories of health, nursing, law, politics, philosophy and moral theory which are beyond the scope of this chapter, but we have provided some suggested further reading at the end. Much of the ethics literature for health care professions is about the moral theory of the traditional philosophers and its application in the quest for the 'right' answer to an ethical dilemma in practice. As well, there is a tendency to dwell on the more dramatic life events such as whether or not to continue artificial feeding for a person with severe brain injury, arguing the rights and wrongs of genetic engineering and cloning, and euthanasia. These are discussed at great length in the public and political domains and are sometimes brought by health care professionals to the attention of the courts for legal judgement. In contrast are the everyday issues occurring in health care settings such as the challenge for nurses finding sufficient time to spend with patients, feeding and washing highly dependent patients and in promoting safe infection-free environments through a range of measures including hand-washing (Gould 2004). These are given less attention in the literature and can go unnoticed despite the fact they do matter to patients and their carers. Hand-washing is a simple procedure that is critical to the prevention of health care associated infection, including methicillin-resistant *Staphylococcus aureus* (commonly known as MRSA). MRSA can have devastating results for patients who become infected and there is a growing evidence base to inform health care practitioners about best practice to prevent this. Yet, despite knowing the facts, several studies have reported nurses do not always practise hand hygiene either by hand-washing (Boyle et al 2001) or the use of antiseptic wipes or gel. Knowing that taking this simple measure can reduce the risk for patients, the nurses in these studies were not always motivated to adhere to the best practice guidelines; nor were some hospitals, in that they failed to provide the equipment and materials needed.

Becoming an ethical practitioner

Becoming an ethical practitioner requires ambition to become a good nurse and a personal investment in learning what it means to be a good nurse, the starting point for this chapter. It is based on the thinking of those who subscribe to the field of virtue ethics (Held 1990, 1993, MacIntyre 1993), which concentrates on what sort of person it is right to aspire to be, and how we behave towards one another, rather than how we decide what actions are right. Getting it right is possible only in the wider context of what sort of person it is good to be in all one's professional decisions. The view being promoted here is that a nurse who has nurtured the development of certain characteristics attributed to a good person will make a difference in terms of being sufficiently motivated towards taking the right course of action in health care practice when dealing with others. Whilst it is highly desirable that health professionals, including the professional nurse, acquire highly developed thinking and reasoning ability through the study of moral theory to defend a course of action as a morally right action, it does not necessarily guarantee that they will take that course of action in practice. You could conclude that Harold Shipman (a general practitioner, well respected in the community, who was found guilty of murdering his patients) and Beverly Allitt (a hospital nurse who was found guilty of causing the deaths of children in her care) did not need to study ethics and moral theory to know that treating patients in the way they did was morally wrong. In being cunning, dishonest and cruel they were able to commit and conceal from their colleagues their vile acts.

This chapter concentrates on the human side of ethics and what we know about human nature. We are all human beings first and foremost, which means we are fallible and vulnerable sometimes. We can have a long-lasting effect on one another's lives which can be experienced by individuals as life-enhancing or their value as persons being diminished. Health care, including nursing, is a moral endeavour as health care professionals in giving care have the potential to do much good but also to do much harm to others. Health and well-being are values we seek to maximize as part of the 'good life', so the provision of health care is a moral and cultural good (Seedhouse 1998). Health problems can leave us dependent on others to help us with our health needs. We need 'virtuous practitioners' when we are vulnerable and dependent. These virtuous practitioners are people who consistently demonstrate in their thinking, decision-making and practice a moral character and a respect for the rules and standards of professional conduct.

Nursing is a moral endeavour

Nursing as part of health care is a moral endeavour. It is not something we do in isolation from others nor is it something we do to another. It happens through relating with another person so that both parties should feel the benefit from the encounter. Caring is a key value underpinning nursing practice and has a complexity of meaning (Watson & Lea 1997). For the purposes of this chapter the dimension of caring chosen is one that captures the moral ideal of valuing all people as unique persons with basic human rights and who have similar and different needs (Sadler 1997, Watson 1997, 1999). With this in mind it might be useful for you to reflect on stories reported in the media about nurses not caring for patients but neglecting their care. For example a television drama 'Dad', shown in the UK in 2005, was based on elderly persons' experiences of abuse. Other television programmes such as 'Panorama' and 'Dispatches' also highlight instances of poor care or abuse of vulnerable patients occurring in hospitals.

Consider Case history 4.1:

- What is your immediate reaction to this?
- What individual characteristics might you assume the nurses involved failed to demonstrate and that you think are necessary to be a good nurse?

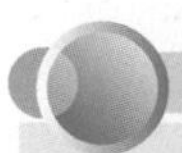

Case history 4.1

In an undercover television programme, nurses were seemingly indifferent to the visible distress of elderly patients in their care, ignoring their reports of discomfort and calls for help. Patients who were unable to help themselves were left lying in bed in their own excrement, unwashed and ignored by the nurses. The programme makers and viewers were outraged by what they described as bad care and the neglect of vulnerable persons by these nurses.

- What do you think might have influenced how these nurses were behaving towards patients, assuming that when they entered the profession they were deemed to demonstrate the profession's values of caring and ethics?
- What are the essential personal qualities all new entrants to initial programmes of preparation for nursing need to demonstrate?
- How do you think these qualities could be assessed by those selecting entrants to nursing programmes?

The standard of conduct expected of professionals when caring for patients and carers is laid down in the 'Nursing and Midwifery Council Code of professional conduct'. You might well think that in the case described in Case history 4.1 you don't need a code of ethics to know that treating patients in this neglectful and cruel way is wrong. Those nurses were removed from the register of qualified nurses and midwives maintained by the NMC and, in order to protect the public, are no longer allowed to practise. Becoming a health care professional such as a nurse is about becoming a certain kind of person and nurturing the development of those characteristics associated with being a good nurse. It is about questioning what kind of person you are, what you are trying to achieve as a health care professional and how you are relating to patients/clients and colleagues. It is about trying to better understand the potential that you as a person bring with you either for doing a great deal of good or for doing a great deal of harm. In identifying the characteristics you consider essential for becoming a good nurse you might have included in your list qualities such as honesty, kindness, generosity, justice and fairness, tolerance, compassion and respect for basic human rights in one's dealings with one another.

Virtue ethics

A virtue is a trait of character that is manifested in habitual actions. Actions spring from a firm and unchangeable virtuous character. For example, an honest person is truthful as a matter of principle, not just occasionally or when it is to their advantage. MacIntyre (1993) and Rachels (1998) argue that in today's society more emphasis needs to be placed on character building and the virtues associated with a virtuous character of someone who is motivated to take the right action in practice. Their argument in support of the revival of virtue ethics is that notions of moral duty and obligation are no longer compatible with today's world views. It is felt that modern societies have inherited fragments of conflicting ethical traditions and that people are feeling confused. A claim for a return to virtue ethics is that these virtues are needed to conduct our lives well. We are rational social beings who need and want the company of others. We live in communities, amongst friends, family and fellow citizens. Such virtues as courage, loyalty, generosity and honesty are needed for living with all of these people successfully, whatever their culture or race. These virtues all have the same sort of general value as they are qualities needed for successful living. The traditional moral philosophers would argue that it is not possible for an ethical theory that is based entirely on a virtuous character to do all the work of ethics. The idea of a core of all virtues suggests there is only one good way to live and one good way for society to develop, whereas there are many different ways to live and many possible different worlds. In the future, each world will require different systems and practices, and people with different kinds of virtue, for its development. Whilst this may be true in part, another view is that despite our differences we all have a great deal more in common. Everyone needs courage and generosity because in all situations there will be property to be managed, goods to be distributed, and some people will be worse off than others. Honesty is needed because no society can exist without communication between its members. Loyalty is needed because everyone needs friends, and to have friends one must be a friend, so everyone needs loyalty. As a framework to guide ethical nursing practice attention is paid to the major areas of life that form moral character. What are the character traits of the virtuous and the non-virtuous nurse? Virtue ethics is appealing because it provides a natural and attractive account of moral motivation. Virtue ethics makes the question of moral character its main concern. Whilst it provides understanding about moral character, moral education and motivation to act morally well, it does not necessarily provide a sufficient guide to deciding right action.

Caring: a central value for ethical practice

The concept of caring as a guide to ethical nursing practice occupied a prominent position in the nursing literature in the 1980s and 1990s with authors such as Benner & Wrubel (1989), Gilligan (1982), Leininger (1981, 1984, 1998), Noddings (1984), Tschudin (1992) and Watson (1997). Inherent in nursing practice is the moral sense of caring. Caring is a central value that underpins a special way of being and doing within the nurse–patient relationship that can promote good and enhance patients' and nurses' lives. The moral sense of caring is a universal value that guides practice. Feminist moral philosophers such as Held (1990, 1993) argue that theories of ethics that emphasize right action will never satisfactorily provide an account of what is actually done in practice. It is one thing to contemplate through reason the weighting of moral principles and to undertake rational calculation when deciding what is the right thing to do. Knowing the right thing to do does not necessarily mean that the nurse is motivated to take what is judged to be right action. The taking of action will depend on the particular qualities, virtues and vices of the nurse's character. To understand nursing ethics we must try to understand what makes a good nurse, one who is motivated to act ethically. A survey of over 200 nurses, conducted in the USA by Plunkett (1999), found that the most disturbing ethical dilemma reported by these nurses was having to work with colleagues they described as being unethical and impaired. They described their colleagues as lacking in motivation to enhance the health and well-being of their patients and clients. They were seen to condone unethical practice through their inaction; that is, they stood back and did nothing to challenge their colleagues.

The writers from the caring movement highlight particular features of the caring relationship, including ways of relating, the existence of particular conditions within the relationship, specific aims for interacting and the presence of particular caring qualities or characteristics of the caregiver. Virtuous caring qualities and characteristics highlighted include: empathy and concern for others (Gilligan 1982); being non-judgemental and accepting of others, tolerance (Noddings 1984); compassion, competence, confidence, conscience, commitment, nurturance, presence, being supportive, trustworthiness, patience, honesty, humility, courage (Leininger 1981). Through self-actualization and the development of these qualities and characteristics, the nurse will strive for the good of self and the good of others (i.e. for the good in general) (Wagner 2002). Character is the source of ethical nursing practice. Actions spring from a firm and unchangeable virtuous character. For example, the kind nurse will habitually think and act in kind ways as a matter of principle, not just occasionally or when it is to her advantage. A virtue is a trait of character that is manifest in habitual actions that is good for a person to have. In contrast, we tend to avoid people with vices such as those who have no regard for the truth, lack compassion, are cruel, disloyal and intolerant of others who have different values and beliefs.

Sadly, patients and their carers find they cannot always avoid those they would prefer not to have giving them care. An elderly relative, recently hospitalized with a fractured femur, reported to the author that he was full of praise for the care he had received. The one exception was a night nurse who he said had terrified him. He recalled she was cruel with him and seemed to go out of her way to be mean and unhelpful, removing an extra blanket from his bed given to him by another nurse, despite being told he was cold. She had not returned as promised with his drink and medication on two separate occasions despite giving him reassurance that she would. He had spent the next three nights cold in bed, in pain and too frightened to speak out. The other nurses did not challenge the nurse about how she was behaving nor did they care to bring him a blanket, a drink or medication despite knowing his situation. They said they feared her retaliation! Was this cowardice on their part? Did they lack the courage to deal with the situation? What was the nature of their responsibility for the poor standard of care he had received? What was difficult for the elderly relative to understand was that he had witnessed this same nurse being very 'kind' to some of the other patients. Whilst he could accept that nurses are human and will not necessarily like all the patients they meet, he could not accept this as sufficient reason for a nurse being so cruel and uncaring and providing poor standards of care. More importantly, he could not understand why the other nurses did not tell the 'modern matron' or support him in telling her about this nurse's behaviour. Surely they knew that what the nurse did was wrong so why were they not motivated to do something to prevent any further abuse? The two Nursing and Midwifery Council guidelines 'Reporting unfitness to practise: a guide for employers and managers' (NMC 2004a) and 'Reporting lack of competence: a guide for employers and managers' (NMC 2004b) are to support employers and managers in dealing with such incidents reported to them. Your university will also have procedures in place so that students are able to report incidences of unprofessional practice and obtain support in acting morally well in their responses.

The 'NMC Code of professional conduct'

As a student learning to engage with the process of ethical enquiry and as a guide to your ethical decision-making in practice, it is essential that you understand the shared values of the health care regulatory bodies and the nursing profession. The 'NMC Code of professional conduct' states the obligations of every registered practitioner in their everyday practice when caring for patients/clients. Before you proceed further with this chapter, we recommend that you visit the NMC website and explore the various web pages and information posted there.

Publication of the 2008 Nursing and Midwifery Council Code of Conduct: professional standards for nurses and midwives (NMC 2008) was the result of a two-year process that involved consultation with thousands of people. The 2008 code, informed by the same professional and moral values as the 2004 code, is written in everyday language, easier to understand and gives clearer guidance for responding to practice dilemmas and public protection concerns of today.

Some of the issues that were debated by nurses and midwives with the NMC for inclusion in the 2008 Code and with a request for clearer guidance included:

- Whether nurses and midwives could ever accept gifts or cash from patients.
- The need to introduce clauses on when nurses and midwives could use their profession to promote political causes (this question was triggered when a nurse appeared in uniform in a magazine promoting fox hunting).
- Accountability of nurses when off duty needed greater clarification (this could help clarify cases such as when a nurse took part in the UK *Big Brother* television programme and claimed to have had unprotected sex in the swimming pool – many nurses called for her to be removed from the register for bringing nursing into disrepute).
- Ethical dilemmas for nurses resulting from the increased use of sponsorship as a result of changing employment practices in health services provider organisations (e.g. those nurses whose salaries are paid for by companies who supply products they use in their practice may be seen to be using their professional status to endorse these products).

You can access the 2008 NMC code for reference during the ethics class at the NMC website (www.nmc-uk.org).

The Nursing and Midwifery Council

The Nursing and Midwifery Council (NMC), an organization set up by parliament to protect the public, is the professional regulatory body for the nursing and midwifery professions of the UK. The NMC maintains a register of around 682 000 qualified nurses, midwives and specialist community public health nurses. The role of the NMC is to protect the public by ensuring that nurses and midwives provide high standards of care to their patients and clients. These standards are set out in the 'NMC Code of professional conduct'. The standards already apply to you as a student. To achieve its aims, the core responsibilities of the NMC are to:

- Maintain a register of qualified nurses, midwives and specialist community public health nurses.
- Set and improve standards for education, practice performance, conduct and ethics.
- Provide advice and guidance to help nurses, midwives and specialist community public health nurses raise professional standards of care.
- Deal with allegations of misconduct, lack of competence or unfitness to practise due to ill health in the interests of public protection.
- Quality-assure education for nurses, midwives and specialist community public health nurses.

The student and the professional regulatory body

You might rightly be wondering what the professional regulatory body has to do with you, a nursing student and not yet registered with the NMC as a nurse. The NMC is highly relevant. It is responsible for setting the standards for your educational programme that leads to initial registration, including the level of entry to the programme. This includes ensuring you can provide evidence that you are of good health and character; this will be continuously monitored by your university throughout your educational programme (NMC 2004c).

Rehabilitation of Offenders Act 1974

Prior to acceptance as a suitable candidate for nursing you will have been required to apply for a Criminal Records Bureau (CRB) check. The university is entitled to ask exempted questions under the Exceptions Order to the Rehabilitation of Offenders Act (1974). As the exceptions relate to working with children, the elderly or sick people, anyone applying for nursing is required by law to reveal all convictions both spent and unspent. The Standard Enclosure check will reveal these. The role of CRB, an executive agency of the Home Office, is to assist organizations to make safer recruitment decisions and reduce the risk of abuse by ensuring that those who are unsuitable are not able to work with children and vulnerable adults. If a post involves working with children or vulnerable adults then the Protection of Children Act (POCA) list, the Protection of Vulnerable Adults (POVA) list and information held under section 142 of the Education Act (2002) will also be searched. Enhanced disclosure is the highest level of check available to anyone involved in regularly caring, training, supervising or being in sole charge of children or vulnerable adults and your details will be subjected to this scrutiny. Take some time to read the useful information on the CRB disclosure website (www.crb.gov.uk).

Competence in practice

As a nursing student it is of great significance that you will spend up to 50% of your programme learning in the practice setting, assisting in providing care for patients and their carers under the supervision of a registered nurse. The standard of competence you are expected to demonstrate in your practice as a student is clearly outlined in the 'NMC Code of professional conduct'; you should read this very carefully. In addition, the 'Guide for students of nursing and midwifery' (NMC 2002a) provides some guidance for the clinical experience you will undertake as a student; it is available at the NMC website (www.nmc-uk.org).

At different stages in your programme you will be required to demonstrate an appropriate level of competence. Before you are eligible to become a registered nurse you will be required to meet the level of proficiency described by the NMC. Lack of competence or proficiency is defined as 'a lack of knowledge, skill or judgement of such a nature that you are unfit to practise safely and effectively in any field you seek to practise'. The standard against which an individual's lack of competence will be assessed is clearly stated in the Code of professional conduct, and the same standard equally applies to the student in practice. As a learner, you need to be aware of your limitations in carrying out procedures or giving information. Lack of competence in either of these areas could put your patient in great danger.

Part of knowing one's limitations is having self-awareness, and possessing the qualities of integrity, honesty and humility to the right degree. A key component in your nursing programme is your ambition in developing these and learning skills for effective continuing personal/professional development planning.

Fitness to practise

In undertaking its role to protect the public, the NMC sets and improves standards for education, training and conduct of those of the Professional Register. It provides advice to registrants and considers allegations of misconduct, lack of competence or unfitness to practise due to ill-health. The NMC publishes Fitness to practise annual reports, which provide important detail about the nature of allegations of misconduct, unfitness to practise and lack of competence that are brought to its attention and how it has dealt with these.

NMC 'Fitness to practise annual report'

Each year the NMC publishes a report on its work in each of its areas of responsibility over the previous year. The 'Fitness to practise annual report 2003–2004' (NMC 2004d) described an increase in allegations of misconduct from 1301 in 2002–2003 to 1460 in 2003–2004. The 'Fitness to practise annual report 2004–2005' (NMC 2005a) records a slight fall in the figures to 1389 for the period of this report. Under the 1993 NMC 'Fitness to practise rules', anyone can make a complaint, but the largest number of complaints are made by employers, usually following disciplinary proceedings at the workplace. The police are also obliged to inform the professional regulatory body of any criminal conviction received by a practitioner on the NMC register. This means that, should you be found guilty of an offence, such as driving while under the influence of drugs or alcohol, in possession of drugs, etc., they will automatically notify the professional statutory body (the NMC); they will also investigate the matter, to decide whether further action needs to be taken.

The NMC also receives notice of complaints directly from patients, members of the public, colleagues, National Care Standards Commission and others. Complaints received before 1 August 2004 (the period of the 2003–2004 and 2004–2005 reports) have been dealt with under the 1993 'Fitness to practise' rules. The procedure would be as follows. A panel of the Preliminary Proceedings Committee would conduct a preliminary inquiry to decide whether or not there was a case to answer, or whether the complaint was sufficiently serious to warrant further investigation. Where there is an allegation that a registered nurse or a midwife or a specialist community public health nurse is unfit to practise for reasons of ill-health, the Preliminary Proceedings Committee then refers it to the Health Committee. During the period of the 2003–2004 report they found that the main reasons for people being referred were associated with alcohol or drug dependence, mental health problems and a smaller number of physical health problems. The Professional Conduct Committee receives referrals that are considered serious and likely to lead to removal from the professional register based on the strength of the evidence available to support the charges. In such cases, the criminal standard of proof is applied. The NMC holds its Professional Conduct Committee hearings in public and in different locations across the country.

The NMC 'Fitness to practise annual report 2003–2004' and the NMC 'Fitness to practise annual report 2004–2005' both highlight that the greatest single area of complaint is poor practice, with a total of 39% of all charges in 2004–2005. This is a slight increase on a total of 35% of all charges for the period of the 2003–2004 report. These complaints included failure to attend to patients' basic needs, inappropriate drug administration and unsafe clinical practice. Other poor practice charges were concerned with poor record-keeping and abuse of patients and clients, including theft, physical abuse, verbal abuse and sexual abuse.

The magnitude of these complaints indicates that there is an apparent gap between the shared values of the health care regulatory bodies and the registered practitioners who have been referred to the investigatory committees. What is the cause of these differences in conduct, and how may they be explained? Could it be that these nurses and midwives were lacking in competence, were unfit to practise due to ill-health or simply that they did not accept the responsibility for acting morally well?

In the first part of this chapter we provided examples of nurses who seemingly condoned unethical practice by standing back and doing nothing when they witnessed it. There is also a growing concern amongst the profession and the public about what is being perceived as a lack of competence of some nurses, including those completing the initial preparation programme and who are registering to become a qualified nurse.

New rules and competence

The current NMC, established under the Nursing and Midwifery Order 2001 (SI 2002/253), came into being in April 2002. The Order required the NMC to make new rules regarding various aspects of its functions, including the 'Fitness to practise rules' in April 2004 (NMC 2004e). All complaints received since 1 August 2004 are now dealt with under the NMC 'Fitness to practise 2004' rules.

The importance of competence features more centrally in the NMC 'Fitness to practise rules'. The NMC sees the purpose of modern regulation as being to enable practitioners rather than to police them. This includes enabling employers to engage in NMC policy development, setting standards, and to make appropriate referrals for fitness to practise investigations. It also includes enabling and supporting registrants to meet their continuing professional development (CPD) standards. Under the new 'Fitness to practise rules 2004', the NMC Investigating Committee will refer complaints to the Conduct and Competence Committee or the Health Committee. As a result, cases against practitioners who face lack of competence allegations are now separated from misconduct investigations, and there is a clear set of criteria to be met prior to referral to the Conduct and Competence Committee. New sanctions for lack of competence have been introduced. Any cases brought since August 2004 are dealt with under the 2004 rules. Charges considered by the Conduct and Competencies Committee include neglect of basic care, patient abuse (physical sexual verbal), drug maladministration, poor record-keeping, abuse of colleagues, unsafe clinical practice, drug misappropriation, failure to take action in an emergency. Allegations received after 1 August 2004 and dealt with under the new rules are reported in the NMC 'Fitness to practise annual report 2004–2005. It is important that you read this report, which is available on the NMC website and which contains some case studies.

Understanding the role of the NMC and its different committees is an important aspect of learning to become a professional.

Current work of the NMC in improving standards for practice performance

The NMC has recently reported the outcome of a number of reviews for improving standards for education and practice performance (see Activity 4.1). These include issues relating to the recruitment and selection of students for entry to pre-registration nursing and midwifery programmes and the quality of mentorship supervision and assessment of student competence in practice. The NMC considers that this work is vital to ensure public protection and that the right people are recruited into nursing programmes and nursing roles.

Other activities commissioned by the NMC are concerned with:

- Describing a level of registration for nurses working at an advanced or higher level.
- Regulating programmes for nurses from overseas countries wishing to work in the UK.
- Reviewing continuing professional development for nurses and current post-registration education and practice (PREP) requirements.
- Reviewing the 'NMC Code of professional conduct' and working with other health care regulators to share good practice, including consideration of a common code for all health professions.

Activity 4.1

Take some time to visit the NMC website at www.nmc-uk.org, where you will find hyperlinks to all the NMC reports and investigations.

The law and the NMC

Because the NMC is the professional statutory regulatory body set up by an Act of Parliament (originally through the Nurses, Midwives and Health Visitors Act 1979 and later amended by the Nurses, Midwives and Health Visitors Acts of 1992 and 1997), it has the responsibility of acting as parliament's representative in regulating the profession. This means that the NMC has a legal duty to hold professional conduct hearings into allegations of improper conduct by a nurse, a midwife or a specialist community public health nurse. The rules that govern the hearing itself are provided in a legal document approved by parliament and known as a statutory instrument (before 1 August 2004: Nurses, Midwives and Health Visitors rules 1993; after August 2004: NMC rules 2004). This statutory instrument obliges the NMC to follow a certain procedure in its investigation and hearings of these matters as referred to earlier in this section. The 'NMC Code of professional conduct' sets out the extent of the professional duty required of a nurse, a midwife, or a specialist community public health nurse. It sets out the standard of professional conduct in the practice setting, and it is important to realize that the 'NMC Code of professional conduct' carries the legal backing of parliament. As a result, the 'NMC Code of professional conduct' can be used to judge the conduct of any nurse who may have fallen below the standards demanded by the profession. It is a requirement of the NMC that registered practitioners (nurse, midwife or specialist community public health nurse) adhere to the 'NMC Code of professional conduct'; if they fail to do so, this will potentially lead to their being disciplined or even removed from the Professional Register.

The NMC determines professional duty, which may differ from the registered practitioner's legal duty. However, the NMC will not require nurses to behave in a manner that is unlawful. Each section of the 'NMC Code of professional conduct' is based on common law. A nurse who appears in court for any reason may be found liable of negligence or be guilty of a criminal offence and whilst courts have the power to order the nurse to pay compensation or to impose a criminal sentence they do not have the power to order that a nurse be prohibited from working as a nurse. This can only be determined by the NMC through its committees.

In summary, the nurse has a professional duty to the NMC which may be different from the legal duty owed to patients, clients, colleagues and employers. You can probably recognize the importance of developing your knowledge and understanding of the law as it applies to you whether you are preparing to become a registered nurse, midwife or specialist community public health nurse.

The legal basis of practice

The majority of health care situations that incur legal involvement will be civil matters. The courts of law deal with criminal offences and it is more likely that a nurse, midwife or specialist community public health nurse will be affected by civil law than by criminal court decisions. In a climate of increasing litigation, it is vital that you have the necessary knowledge and understanding of the law and how it relates to your nursing practice. The four key areas in which the law interacts with professional practice are nursing legislation, employment legislation, criminal law and civil law.

Nursing legislation

As regards nursing legislation, already discussed earlier, acts of parliament relate specifically to nursing. Much of the law controlling nursing is drawn up by the NMC from these acts.

Employment legislation

Employment legislation is concerned with protection of the individual employee and the negotiation of industrial relations between employers and unions. Matters of alleged misconduct, redundancy and dismissal are handled with reference to employment regulations.

Criminal law

Criminal law is breached when a crime is committed. For example, if a nurse or student steals medicines, bed sheets or food from a place of work, which could be a patient's home, then a criminal charge will normally be brought against the nurse. The wrongful use of drugs is also a criminal offence. Criminal charges are always brought against an individual by the Crown Prosecution Service. The NMC will automatically be informed and they decide, rather than the courts, whether or not the nurse will be permitted to continue to practise, regardless of the outcome of the charges decided by the courts.

Civil law

Civil law involves the rights and duties that individuals have towards each other. Under civil law, legal action is taken by a private individual against another individual or organization. A successful civil action results in the award of monetary compensation to the wronged individual. The part of civil law that is concerned with wrongful acts against the individual is known as the 'law of torts'. The word tort comes from the Latin meaning to injure or twist; tort allows someone to acquire the right of action or damages as a result of a breech of duty identified in law. The areas covered by torts are relevant to any nurse and student in practice. They include:

- *The tort of trespass to the person.* This is known as 'assault and battery' and is relevant to any nurse who has ever restrained a patient or given a patient an injection without their consent.
- *The tort of defamation.* This is known as 'libel and slander' and is relevant to nursing reports and records. Referring to a patient as a 'cantankerous old faggot' could result in the tort of defamation being used.
- *The tort of negligence.* This often occurs as a direct result of failure to care. The tort of negligence is of major importance for practising nurses.

Defining negligence

Negligence can be defined as the omission to do something that a reasonable person, guided by those considerations that ordinarily regulate the conduct of human affairs, would do, or to do something that a prudent and reasonable man would not do. When a patient or client feels there has been a lack of sufficient care resulting in some direct harm, then the tort of negligence can be used.

Negligence is a very difficult action to prove against a defendant because there has to be a demonstrable link between three key factors in the caring process. These are that: a duty of care has been established between the defendant and plaintiff (the person bringing the action); the plaintiff must prove that there has been a breach of that duty; as a result the plaintiff suffered consequential damage. The burden of proof rests with the plaintiff. Not all allegations of negligence are made out of a genuine concern, so it is vital that the nurse maintains accurate and comprehensive patient records in the anticipation that they will be used as evidence of what actually took place. This evidence may be called upon by the defendants several years after the alleged event and/or omission. The 'NMC Code of professional conduct' outlines the nurse's obligation in maintaining health care records. The NMC 'Guidelines for records and record keeping' (NMC 2002b) is an extremely important document; you can read it and download it from the NMC website (www.nmc-uk.org).

The duty of care

When people are in the care of any professional, including health professionals such as nurses, then a particular set of rights and duties come into action. You need to remember that people have the same rights as citizens when they come into contact with the health services as patients and clients. These rights include the duty of care. Patients rights are detailed in health service charters and include:

- The right to receive a high-level quality of care that takes account of their individual circumstances.
- To have their preferences and choices respected.
- To receive care that pays respect to their religious, spiritual and other beliefs.
- To be given full and accurate information about the care they are receiving.
- To have their dignity maintained at all times.
- To have their privacy respected.
- To be involved in making decisions about the care they receive.
- To have the right to say 'no' (to refuse care or a particular form of care).

A right can only be said to have meaning if it is seen to create an equal and opposite duty or obligation on another. The nurse–patient/client relationship establishes a duty of care from the nurse to the patient. On one level this is a moral duty. The professional nurse is expected to make a moral commitment to uphold the values and special moral obligations, rules and duties in the 'NMC Code of professional conduct' which places the patient's rights, health and well-being at the heart of health care practice. Also the duty derives from the law of torts, which imposes a duty whenever one person can reasonably foresee that their conduct may cause harm to another. This means that we as nurses have a legal obligation to care for patients (known as a duty of care) as well as a moral one.

As a student and emerging professional, you also have a moral duty to abide by the 'NMC Code of professional conduct' as well as a moral and legal duty of care to patients. The shared values as laid down in the 'NMC Code of professional conduct' are based on the notion that people have rights. An understanding about what constitutes an individual's rights is a vital goal for health care professionals and students. The 'NMC Code of professional conduct' also provides guidance for professionals and students for all their nursing activities. These should uphold and promote the rights of those the 'NMC Code of professional conduct' is aimed towards. Violation of a patient's rights is a serious matter and one of the worst offences that health professionals can be found guilty of.

The student and a standard of care

As well as establishing the legal and moral nature of our duty as nurses we also need to be clear about what is an acceptable standard of care. The nurse is expected to exhibit the expertise normally demonstrated by competent nurses. A patient has the right to expect the same level of competence from a student. As a student you are expected to reach the standards that are on a level with your training and experience. Remember that you should never accept responsibility for any aspect of nursing care unless you feel comfortable that you possess the necessary skills, knowledge and expertise to be able to fulfil what is required in a safe and competent manner. If you accept responsibility, then accountability is part of the same package. You will have no defence to claim ignorance or lack of relevant experience if you make an error. What is also very important to remember is that all nurses from time to time will feel uncomfortable in that they may not possess the necessary skill, knowledge or expertise required of them. This is often because of changes in treatments and care, or because they are working in an unfamiliar setting. Integrity and having the humility to admit that you don't know and will need to learn and develop competence are characteristics of a good nurse and a good student. If you are faced with such a situation it is essential that you seek help and training from an expert colleague or mentor before you accept responsibility for that particular aspect of nursing care.

Fair and anti-discriminatory practice

Fair and anti-discriminatory nursing practice, recognizing and respecting alternative cultures and beliefs, is constructed around the valuing of the individual as a person with rights, a key value in the 'NMC Code of professional conduct'. The moral principle of justice as fairness, together with the moral principle of autonomy, are pivotal to current health care practice and central to many of the arguments within medical and nursing ethics. Both these moral principles will provide the 'anchors' for you to understand the source of the rules or duties laid down in the 'NMC Code of professional conduct'. When you are faced with situations in practice and feel confused or lost, then it is a good idea to return to these two principles and to consider how you are applying them in the situation you are facing. It may help you to get back on track if you ask yourself how you respect and recognize an individual's autonomy. In addition, it is important to reflect and question whether you can demonstrate that you are being just and fair in the way you relate to your patient. If you find yourself treating a patient differently (or unfavourably) compared with your conduct towards other patients, you need to ask yourself what the reason is. Is it a good reason or is it due to some prejudice about age, race, gender, culture? Valuing an individual as a person with rights includes a positive acceptance of difference, arising, for example, from ethnic origin, cultural beliefs, personal attributes, social status, property, birth, health problems, political and personal opinions. An important piece of research conducted by Stockwell in 1972 and republished in 1984 demonstrated that these nurses discriminated negatively against patients who are less able to comply or who require additional care, such as people who have a sight or hearing deficit.

What are rights?

Organizations such as the United Nations (UN) try to determine through universal agreement what human rights are and how they can be upheld in countries throughout the world. The Universal Declaration of Human Rights (UN 1948) states that:

> *Everyone is entitled to all rights and freedoms within the declaration without distinction of any kind such as race, colour, language, religion, political/other opinion, natural or social origin, property, birth or other status.*

The Universal Declaration of Human Rights has 30 articles; some of the most important are listed in Box 4.1.

You will recognize that these articles are reflected in various citizens' charters and in the 'NMC Code of professional conduct'. Note the importance of consent in relation to personal rights

Box 4.1

Some of the most important articles of the Universal Declaration of Human Rights

- All human beings are born free and equal in rights.
- Everyone is entitled to all rights and freedoms set forth in the declaration without distinction of any kind, such as race, colour, sex, language, religion, political or other opinion, national or social origin, property, birth or other status.
- Everyone has the right to life, liberty and security of person.
- No-one shall be held in slavery or servitude.
- No-one shall be subjected to torture or to cruelty, inhumane or degrading treatment or punishment.
- Everyone has the right to recognition everywhere as a person before the law.
- No-one shall be subjected to arbitrary arrest, detention or exile.
- Everyone charged with a penal offence has the right to be presumed innocent until proved guilty according to the law in a public trial at which he has had all the guarantees necessary for his defence.
- No-one shall be subjected to arbitrary interference with his privacy, family, home or correspondence, or attacks upon his honour and reputation.
- Everyone has the right to seek and to enjoy in other countries asylum from persecution.

to freedom from interference, coercion, restraint, detention. Note the importance of valuing all persons equally. This means valuing their personhood. This is different from being required to like all people equally or that you will agree with what they say and do.

There may be times when you do not value what some people do, and this may create a personal conflict for you when delivering care to that person. For example, health professionals in Western culture may find it difficult to accept some cultural practices such as female circumcision, and want to work to eradicate such practices in the West (Wallis 2005). Female genital mutilation has been illegal in Britain since 1985 following the introduction of the Female Circumcision Act (Amended 2003) which made it illegal for parents to travel abroad to have the practice carried out. Other UN declarations include the UN Convention on the Rights of the Child (begun 1978), UN Declaration on Rights of Disabled People 1975 and UN Declaration on Rights of Mentally Retarded Persons 1971. As you can see, the UN clearly identifies that in trying to uphold human rights special attention has to be paid to the most vulnerable groups in societies who are most at risk of having their rights violated and experiencing unjust discrimination. These groups include those with mental health problems, disability, learning difficulties, children and elderly persons.

Upholding rights

In trying to uphold rights for all people, special attention has to be paid to those groups who are at most risk of having their rights violated. Think about the human rights abuses throughout the world today and you will find there are many examples of people oppressed, dispossessed and culturally and geographically dislocated. You will increasingly find yourself giving care to these people and it may present a challenge to understand what it means to the patient to have experienced oppression in their own country, to be dispossessed and to be living in another country that has a culture and value systems that are very different from their own.

In essence, a rights view of justice implies that someone has a duty or obligation to the person exercising his right. Different sorts of rights are talked about, including natural rights, legal rights and moral rights. Clearly a patient has legal rights not to suffer harm as a result of negligence on the part of any health care professional or student in practice. The 'NMC Code of professional conduct' is based on common law. It sets out the extent of the professional duty required of a nurse, midwife and specialist community public health nurse. As you will have read earlier, failure to adhere to the 'NMC Code of professional conduct' can potentially lead to a nurse, midwife or specialist community public health nurse being disciplined or even removed from the professional register. If your employer, or a patient or client brings an allegation against you of negligence or criminal activity, this will be dealt with through the courts.

Looking back over the period of the introduction of rights legislation in the UK, which aims to protect human rights, one is struck by its short history of less than 100 years. A useful source of information of all of the acts that aim to protect human rights in law is the Office of Public Sector Information (www.opsi.gov.uk). Important acts include the Disability Discrimination Act 2005, the Mental Capacity Act 2005, the Children Act 2004, the Mental Health Act 1983.

The Ethics Class

In this part of this chapter you will read the discussions of a group of first-year pre-registration students about their practice placement experiences. As the reader, we invite you to participate as a member of this 'virtual' ethics class. Through telling their personal stories about practice, the students are learning to engage in the complex process of ethical enquiry and we hope that you will be able to learn these skills as well. These students are beginning to use different sources of knowledge to make sense of some of the ethical issues and dilemmas they are meeting in practice. They are keen to improve their understanding about how arguments can be constructed to support a claim that one course of action will bring about a greater degree of morality compared to others from a range of possible options.

The students are examining their own values and the profession's values, together with the application of the 'NMC Code of professional conduct' (which will be referred to as the Code in this section) in practice. The students are keen to assess the usefulness of the Code in guiding right action and to understand themselves better with regard to the kind of person they are and the kind of health care professional that they aspire to become. In addition, they are learning to understand each other and what impact their own values and beliefs may have for making morally good judgements in practice.

As you read through the different stories presented by the members you may want to have a copy of the Code close by. The key question these students are asking is: How does the Code relate to my own values and beliefs concerning this situation that I am facing? You can access the code from the NMC website at www.nmc-uk.org.

Azad's story

The first story to be presented is Azad's story (see Case history 4.2). Read Azad's story and reflect on the issues before proceeding any further:

- Which parts of the Code give Azad advice about how the situation should be handled?
- What action should Azad take and why?

The Code applies to students as well as to qualified nurses. Azad is at a very early stage in his educational programme and is being asked to provide care to a patient who is aggressive and threatening violence. He is also feeling left alone to deal with the situation and he feels out of his depth. The Code places an obligation on all nurses to

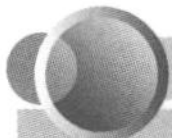

Case history 4.2

Azad's story

Azad is reaching the end of the first foundation year of the pre-registration nursing programme mental health branch. He has worked in several placement settings and is concerned about a situation he now finds himself in at his current placement. Azad is placed in an acute hospital environment and has been asked by the staff nurse, Cheryl, to stay very close to a patient who has been sectioned by the psychiatrist. The patient's name is Alan and he is very unhappy about Azad's continued presence and sees it as a gross invasion of his privacy. At the end of the second day, yesterday, Alan tells Azad that he is no longer willing to put up with his continuing presence and threatens to attack him if he doesn't remove himself out of his proximity. Azad feels threatened, frightened and unsure how to handle the situation. He is also unsure about the nature of his responsibilities in this situation and who he is accountable to for his actions.

provide a high standard of practice and care at all times. This requires the nurse or midwife to have the knowledge, skills and abilities required for lawful, safe and effective practice when working without direct supervision. It requires the nurse or midwife to acknowledge the limits of their professional competence and only to undertake practice and accept responsibilities for those activities in which they are competent. It also means the nurse or midwife is required to take part continually in appropriate learning and practice activities that maintain and develop their performance in practice.

The Ethics Class agrees the Code gives clear guidance for Azad, who should not be expected to provide close supervision, alone, to a potentially violent client. As a student in his first year, he does not have the experience and level of competence required, at this stage of his education and training, to provide the standard of care that is required. The Ethics Class discusses what it means to be accountable in the practice setting and to whom the nurse is answerable.

Accountability in practice

A major theme of accountability is the duty to answer for one's actions, to give a reasoned explanation for doing what you did. Every nurse is answerable to his employer. The employer has the ultimate responsibility for the nurse's actions. This line of accountability extends beyond the employer to the NMC itself. A professional nurse must follow the guidelines, rules and the Code of professional conduct laid down by the NMC and is therefore accountable to the NMC for her practice as a professional. As a pre-registration student, Azad is not professionally accountable to the NMC in the way he will be on qualification and registration with the NMC. He cannot be called to account for his actions or omissions as a student by the NMC. It is the qualified practitioners with whom Azad is working who are responsible for Azad's actions and omissions as far as the NMC is concerned. Students must always work under the direct supervision of a registered nurse or midwife. A student will, however, be called to account by their university or by the law for the consequences of his actions or omissions as a pre-registration student. A student can be removed from practice during a practice placement allocation by the university if their conduct is considered significantly unsafe or unsatisfactory. Normally their conduct is then subject to a full investigation to assess their fitness to continue on the programme. The NMC sets out the requirements for evidence of good health and character for becoming registered and for renewing registration (NMC 2004c). These requirements strengthen the spirit of the Code and apply to students on programmes leading to first registration, not just on entry but throughout the programme. Universities are required to set up monitoring procedures to monitor good health and character throughout the programme. These procedures will require a student to make a written declaration at specific stages of their programme that they are of good health and character.

Nurses are also accountable to their patients and clients. This is the most important line of accountability as it is the nurse's duty of care towards these people that underpins all their actions. Nurses must be in a position to explain and defend their actions either to the patient or to organizations that protect patients.

Responsibility in practice

The Ethics Class discussed the concept of accountability and how it differs from responsibility. Responsibility includes both the duty of care owed towards others that we accept as nurses and students and the personal skills, knowledge and attitudes that we apply as we carry out our duties. Responsibility, although given by a higher authority, such as our employers or supervisor, is all about our individual approaches and decisions in practice. Accountability is part of being responsible, but expresses the duty we accept to answer to other people. Thus, when we agree to undertake a given aspect of practice, such as making an assessment of a patient's blood pressure, then we take personal responsibility for it. This means we are responsible for implementing and completing the task. We also become accountable to other people for fulfilling the task, including accurate documentation and reporting.

When he accepted responsibility for the particular aspect of care of providing close supervision of the patient named Alan, Azad was by implication agreeing he had the knowledge and skills needed to perform it well, and that he had undertaken this aspect of care with the appropriate supervision and guidance and that he had been assessed as competent to do so. Professional accountability implies that Azad can give a supporting rationale to explain his actions in practice. As he is a student, the NMC would call to account the qualified registered nurse acting as his supervisor or mentor in practice. That person would have to demonstrate that she delegated the task to Azad having first satisfied herself that he was sufficiently competent to carry it out. As the student is subject to the regulations of the university, it would first investigate the student's conduct and may then refer the case to the law. Alternatively, if the police are asked to investigate the case first, the university would follow up with its own investigation to decide on the student's future.

Azad's story and the lessons learned

In Azad's story it is clear that he is out of his depth, and Cheryl, the staff nurse, should certainly have her attention drawn to the Code, which places an obligation on all nurses regarding their responsibilities towards appropriate delegation of care delivery. Specifically, the Code states nurses and midwives remain accountable for the appropriateness of the delegation, for ensuring that the person who does the work is able to do it and that adequate supervision or support is provided.

In addition, the Ethics Class suggests that Cheryl, Azad's supervising staff nurse, needs to be reminded about her obligations to act to identify and minimise any risk to patients and clients.

By asking Azad to provide close supervision to Alan who is aggressive and threatening violence, Cheryl compromised the position of a student in a way that could have led to great harm to both student and patient. The Ethics Class advises Azad he must tell Cheryl he does not yet have the experience and competence to deal alone with this situation. Azad readily admits that he had already come to this conclusion himself but that it had been extremely useful to relate his story to the group and to share their reflections. He has taken a long hard look at himself and realizes that he finds it difficult as a mature student who is used to taking risks. In his past jobs he always managed to bluff his way through difficult situations, especially in his former job as a manager in a fast food outlet. He recognizes that it is not in his character to be honest with himself when it comes to facing up to his limitations. He feels he has to work harder at being himself and being honest. He vows that in future he will seek help from his support network at the university and in practice. He now realizes that the real failure would be if he continued to attempt to do something that he is not yet fully competent to achieve and that it is potentially dangerous to try to do so. To pretend that he can manage would put his patient, himself and possibly others at risk of harm. Azad states that he now feels more confident to address this issue with Cheryl. He anticipates that she will respect his student status and value his taking responsibility for not trying to be something he is not (a qualified registered nurse), and for identifying his learning needs as a student.

Ann's story

The second story presented to the Ethics Class is Ann's story. Ann, like Azad, is sharing with the group a situation she has found quite challenging and that has made her realize the enormity of the responsibility placed on qualified practitioners to account for their professional practice. Read Ann's story (Case history 4.3) and reflect on the issues before proceeding any further:

- What traits of character do you think Brenda has that you would attribute to a good person and a good nurse?
- Which parts of the Code do you think guided Brenda's practice in relation to her care for Bill and give an example of how she demonstrated this.
- Were there any conflicts for Brenda in applying the different guiding principles from the different parts of the Code to inform her decision about how to manage Bill's care?

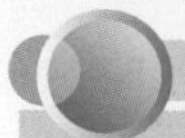

Case history 4.3

Ann's story

Ann is also reaching the end of the first foundation year of the pre-registration nursing programme adult branch. Ann has worked in several placement settings and is currently placed in a medical assessment unit. Ann tells the group that it is the best placement she has experienced. Her mentor, Brenda, is an extremely competent practitioner and always generous, giving her time and demonstrating respect for both patients and students. Brenda has given Ann a lot of encouragement and she has never felt so confident in practice before, neither has she ever been so motivated towards her studies as she is now. Ann recalls a recent incident that has shaken her confidence and shares her thoughts and feelings with the group.

The incident occurred when three nurses and an assistant practitioner had gone for the morning coffee break leaving Ann, Brenda and Graham, the unit manager, alone in the unit. Brenda had spent a great deal of time with Bill, a 70-year-old man, who was undergoing various investigations and who was most anxious about the potential outcome. Brenda had given him the time and opportunity to raise his concerns with her, to ask questions, and had provided him with information, explanations and general reassurance. Because of his anxiety, Bill was unable to relax and insisted on wandering around the unit. He had had a previous stroke and although unsteady on his feet was managing to cope by himself at home. Brenda had discussed with Bill that he should not walk about so much unaided. She also tried to interest him in other activities, acquiring his newspaper, bringing him coffee and ensuring he was comfortable in the patient lounge area with the means of summoning help when ready to move.

Ann and Brenda are dealing with a number of patients, getting them ready for various investigations, while Graham, the unit manager, is accessing electronically various patient data. Suddenly there is a call from the entrance to the unit. Bill has tried to walk from the lounge area unaided, taken the wrong turning and fallen at the entrance. He has a large cut on his nose which is bleeding and is complaining that his elbow is hurting. Graham rushes out of the office and shouts at Brenda that she should have been more vigilant. Brenda is visibly upset and says she feels responsible for Bill's injury.

- Could Brenda be considered to be negligent as seems to be implied by Graham's outburst?
- To what extent could a student be responsible in a situation where another nurse may potentially put a patient at risk?

The Ethics Class discusses at length how good it is to work in placements where there is a democratic approach to management and the standard of care is so high. Staff respect each other, whoever they may be, including the students, and they recognize that this indicates that patients are respected and well cared for. Sometimes this is difficult to achieve because of the pressures on busy NHS staff which can lead to tension.

The Ethics Class is unanimous in its praise for mentors such as Brenda, a competent nurse and a mentor who is familiar with the students' programme, learning outcomes and assessment documents. Brenda spends significant time with students and includes them in all her activities. Ann tells the Ethics Class she has always felt well supported. Brenda habitually demonstrates traits of character usually associated with a good or virtuous person and a good nurse.

The Ethics Class draws up a list of these virtues, which include compassion, competence, commitment, patience, honesty, trustworthiness, fairness, tolerance, altruism, generosity, loyalty, caring, genuineness, empathy, courage, and integrity.

Brenda demonstrates a thoughtful and questioning approach to practice, and it would appear she is clearly in touch with the personal and professional value basis for her practice. Through her practice, Brenda reflects a valuing of people as persons with different needs and this is experienced by patients, colleagues and students in their relationships with her.

Valuing of people as persons and partners in care

The Ethics Class highlighted a key principle of the Code as significant to discuss in relation to the parts of the Code guiding Brenda's practice. The Code places an obligation on all nurses 'to make the care of people their first concern, to treat them as individuals and respect their dignity'.

The Ethics Class focused their discussion on the moral principle of justice and in particular a rights view of justice and the moral duty or obligation to the person exercising their rights. The Code is informed by this moral principle, with emphasis on professionals working collaboratively with patients, clients and carers as partners in their care, to include listening and responding to their concerns, preferences and recognizing and respecting the role of patients and clients as partners in their care and the contribution they can make to it. This involves sharing with people, in a way they can understand, the information they want or need to know about their health.

The Ethics Class discussed how important it is not to lose sight of the patient as a citizen with the same rights when engaging with health services. They recognized how easy it is for hard-pressed health professionals to start making decisions on the patient's behalf. Of course, this may be acceptable if the patient has negotiated for this with the health professionals concerned.

The Ethics Class were struck by the level of respect shown to patients and reflected in Brenda's approach to their care. Brenda consistently demonstrates a valuing of patients as persons in giving time to hear their concerns, providing explanations and involving them in their care. Arising out of a valuing of the individual as a person with human and civil rights is the positive acceptance of difference. This means you must not discriminate in any way against those in your care.

The Ethics Class discussed how hard this could be for nurses who are fallible as human beings and who can make mistakes sometimes. They recognized that personal bias and prejudices can sometimes get in the way and adversely affect the care we provide if we are not consciously aware of them. As nurses it is important to be in touch with our own personal values, such as knowing who and what we represent, and understanding our relationships with others. Through reflecting on what we do in work, recreation and hobbies, we can discover meaning about ourselves, our purpose, our aims and what we seek to accomplish. Our values and meaning in life come out of what we do in our lives (Tschudin 1992). Engaging in reflective practice, we can learn about ourselves through our nursing practice, find out about the kind of person we are, our likes and dislikes, personality, temperament, whether we are thinking or feeling people.

One of the members of the Ethics Class is Frances, who is in her foundation year of the pre-registration nursing programme child branch. She readily admits that she is finding it easier to relate with children than with adults. Frances enjoys being with children and gets on well with them, but has had a few clashes with some of her lecturers for not keeping her appointments. Frances has realized she needs to work with this, to understand herself better, as she has also felt awkward when caring for children when their relatives, usually parents, are present. On one occasion a parent asked if she was always so quiet as she didn't speak very much. Frances accepts she needs to develop her skills of self-awareness and communication with help from peers and mentors. The Code places an obligation on all nurses 'to act to identify and minimize the risk to patients and clients'.

The Ethics Class discussed the moral principles of beneficence (to do good) and non-maleficence (to do no harm) which have been the traditional basis of the nurse–patient, doctor–patient relationship over many years. The professional's duty as a competent practitioner is to act in the best interests of the patient. This might give the impression that the professional knows best, placing the patient in a more passive role.

Respect for patient/client autonomy and duty of care

More recently, respect for the individual, including respect for autonomy, means a more equal doctor–patient, nurse–patient relationship in health care. The conflict arising for Brenda was that clearly she was being guided by the Code in demonstrating her respect for the patient's right to be a partner in his own care and to contribute to decisions made. This reflected a respect for patient autonomy. Brenda was guided by the moral principles of beneficence and non-maleficence which underpin the nurse's duty of care to the patient.

In Ann's story, Bill was exercising his autonomy in choosing to walk unaided despite Brenda's advice. She had undertaken several actions out of her 'duty of care' owed to Bill, the patient. These had been to respect his rights to exercise his autonomy and pointing out that he could be placing himself at risk of harm whilst at the same time negotiating parameters in order to reduce the risk of his falling. Brenda's conflict is that to override a patient's autonomy is a very serious thing to do and would have to be justified and documented clearly in his records. On the other hand, as his nurse, she owes him a duty of care. In this case, it involves managing the potential risk. If Bill suffers harm then she may face an inquiry and be investigated in the judicial courts of law for a breach of the duty of care. This could take place many months, if not years, after the incident (long after the details have been forgotten), and so accurate documentation is vital.

The Ethics Class reviewed the tort of negligence under civil law and they were in no doubt that a duty of care existed and that Brenda had a duty of care to Bill. The Ethics Class believed that Brenda did not breach her duty of care. Brenda had spent a great deal of time appealing to Bill not to walk about without assistance and had tried to help him relax so that he did not feel compelled to walk around so much due to his anxiety. In undertaking this kind of caring activity, Brenda was exercising her duty of care as she was acting in Bill's best interests by trying to minimize any risk of his falling. Despite her appeals, Bill had chosen not to take Brenda's advice. This was Bill's choice and Brenda could not be held responsible for the results of his actions. Bill was exercising his rights in deciding not to summon help when he moved from the patient lounge area.

Bill's fall and lessons learned

If Bill had fallen and his fall did not result from any hazard in the environment (such as a slippery floor, or an obstacle in his way), then this was an accident. Judgements about the standard of care would be judged against what a competent nurse would be expected to do in such a situation. The Bolam test would be applied. As we have discussed, Brenda is clearly not incompetent. For negligence to be proved there would need to be a link proved demonstrating that there had been a breach of duty or a lapse in the standard of care and that the patient suffered damage as a result. Bill had injured himself but not as a result of a breach of duty or standard of care on Brenda's part.

The Ethics Class also reflected on the comment made by Graham to Brenda at the time of the incident. This had greatly upset both Ann and Brenda, as well as other patients who had heard the comment, which Graham delivered in a loud voice. All had felt that it was undeserved and counterproductive to team harmony. The Ethics Class raised the importance of team leader character traits, including genuine concern, loyalty, trust and fairness as important to nurture team harmony. The Code clearly states the obligations of the nurse 'to co-operate with others in the team'. The team includes the patient or client, their families and carers, and the wider community and nurses are obliged to work with others to protect and promote the health and well being of those in their care.

The Ethics Class concluded that Graham had contravened the Code by responding as he did, suggesting in a loud voice, to be overheard by other patients, relatives and staff, that Brenda's practice had not been of the standard it should have been. It was agreed that Graham needed to be reminded of his obligations outlined in the Code.

Gordon's story

Gordon is a pre-registration nursing student near the end of his first year in the branch programme and has been invited to attend the Ethics Class to present his story, which is concerned with an issue of informed consent while working in a primary care setting. Ann has invited Gordon because she has got to know him through sharing some of the same placements over the last 12 months, and is enthusiastic for Gordon to share his story with the group to help them start thinking about their roles and responsibilities relating to patients' consent to health care treatment or care.

Read Gordon's story (Case history 4.4) and consider how the Code is relevant. Reflect on the

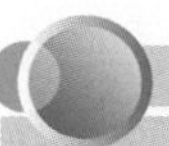

Case history 4.4

Gordon's story

Gordon is a mature student and, prior to commencing the programme, had worked in his family butcher's business. He is very enthusiastic about his future career and intends eventually to work in the community setting as a specialist community public health nurse. He is dedicated to promoting men's health and to undertaking research to inform the development of future local services and service delivery. Gordon's story unfolds from the time he was attending a community placement in primary care and had met Donald, who was attending for a prostate-specific antigen (PSA) blood test at the health centre.

Donald had told Gordon how he had found himself on the screening programme. It was nearly 2 years since he had originally consulted his doctor about a painful knee. He was prescribed medication and advised to rest the joint. During the consultation the doctor suggested that he would do a health check which included blood pressure reading and taking a sample of blood to check his blood chemistry. This seemed a good thing to do at the time and Donald had cooperated fully in allowing the doctor to proceed. Several weeks later Donald received a letter from his doctor asking him to make an urgent appointment to discuss his blood test results. He was told that the blood test to screen for prostate cancer had shown abnormally high levels of PSA; this was highly significant and indicated the need for urgent treatment. Donald was shocked and a prostate biopsy was undertaken. Donald didn't speak about this to anyone in his family, not even his wife and close friends. He was convinced he had cancer and there was no cure, and he felt at the time it was best nobody should know. For 12 months Donald bottled up his feelings and this had put a strain on his marriage as his wife had asked him why he seemed so distant and didn't talk to her very much. The biopsy had come back inconclusive and he was advised to have another biopsy which was clear. Donald attended regularly for the blood test which remained abnormally high. He also began to search the Internet to learn about prostate cancer and the validity and reliability of the screening test. Eventually, Donald had felt able to question his doctor about the controversy surrounding the usefulness of the screening test and treatments. Donald's doctor agreed with his decision to do nothing further on the basis of the blood test findings and that he would attend for the next screening test after 1 year.

Donald had told Gordon that, if he had known what he knows now about the test, including research findings that indicate levels can fluctuate and come down from high levels, the prognosis, treatment options and complications, he would never have cooperated and agreed to a test in the first place. It was just presented as a good idea to do a health check and PSA test and prostate cancer was never mentioned. He had been naïve and ill-informed at the time. No matter the outcome of the test, based on his own study of the topic and others' experience and the treatment options available, he would never consent to medical invasive intervention. What then is the point of the test?

Although in this case the doctor was responsible for obtaining consent, Gordon is in no doubt that in Donald's case consent to the test was not based on understanding and therefore was not a valid consent. Nurses are often best placed to know about the emotions, concerns and views of patients and clients and may be best able to judge what information is needed so that it is understood.

issues before proceeding any further with this section:

- Reflect on what you think happened in this case and how the Code might help you identify what is good practice in obtaining informed consent prior to medical and/or nursing procedures.
- The Code is also based in law. What does the law say about valid consent?

After hearing Gordon's presentation about Donald, the Ethics Class highlights several issues for discussion as described in the sections following.

Doctor–patient relationship

What was the nature of the doctor–patient relationship when the test was first done? Was this a traditional doctor–patient relationship in the sense that the doctor sees himself as the expert, knows what is needed and will do what is best for the patient? (In such a relationship the doctor will usually be making the decisions whereas the patient/client adopts the passive patient role placing all his trust in the doctor). This kind of relationship would seem to be out of step with current thinking in today's health care service which is about promoting patient autonomy and respecting the individual's right to be involved in decisions about their own care.

Did the nature of the relationship change over time? The Ethics Class thought there was evidence of significant change. Donald is now, after 2 years, directing his own care from a position of 'being informed' and it seems the doctor now values and respects Donald's right to contribute to directing his own care.

The right to withhold or withdraw consent

The Code gives some clear guidance based on respect for autonomy about a person's right to decide whether or not to undergo any health care intervention – even where a refusal may result in harm or death to themselves or a foetus, unless a court of law orders to the contrary.

The right to withhold or withdraw consent is protected in law and a doctor or health professional may face an action for damages if a patient is examined, provided treatment or care without consent. Consent may be linked to the tort of trespass to the person known as 'assault and battery'. Assault is described in law as 'an act which causes in the person subjected to it an apprehension of the immediate infliction of battery'. Battery is physical contact with another person. The Ethics Class considered whether or not valid consent had been obtained in this case. Donald had implied consent in that he had cooperated and complied with the doctor's wishes. However, his consent was not based on any understanding of the relevant information as none was presented or discussed at the time. In law, consent that is not based on sufficient understanding of the relevant information is not valid consent. It makes no difference whether consent is expressed verbally or in writing. The Ethics Class concluded that, in this case, the doctor had obtained consent in that it had been given by Donald through his compliant response and actions. However, the doctor had not obtained informed consent, which is the standard required in law and the standard required of health professionals in practice. The Code gives clear guidance on this and you should read the relevant section outlining the key principles and expectations of the profession.

The Ethics Class then went on to discuss the complexities involved when obtaining consent:

- What kind of information and how much information is sufficient?
- What happens when patients and clients cannot assimilate information and/or understand the information, whatever the reason?
- What about the patient or client who doesn't want the responsibility of selecting for him/herself a course of action from several options and asks the health professional to decide?
- What about the patient or client who decides not to undergo treatment or care, even when a refusal will result in harm or death to him/herself?

Valid informed consent

In law, valid consent is that which is based on information which:

- Is given in a form that the patient can understand.
- Involves explanation of the nature of the examination, treatment or care procedures.
- Mentions the existence of any alternatives.
- Mentions substantial risks.
- Mentions the consequences for life, including medical adverse effects, but a patient may be advised on the prescribed course of action, together with reasons.

The Ethics Class tried to consider the issue of informed consent from Donald's viewpoint. Reconsidering the situation, what information and explanation would Donald have expected and needed at the time in order to provide valid informed consent? It was agreed that, for his consent to be valid, the doctor would need to discuss with Donald and check his understanding about: the nature of the test; the purpose of the test and why he is recommending the test; how it is carried out and by whom; what is known about the validity and reliability of the test; predictive ability and margin for error; the different viewpoints about the usefulness of the test (it is not known if the test will save lives by detecting cancers at an earlier stage or prolong patients' survival). Some argue the test may be detecting cancers that will never cause symptoms as they are so slow-growing (Concato et al 2006). What might be the consequences for Donald if the test is positive? What options will Donald have to choose from when making decisions about the course of treatment to take? What is known about each option (for example, treating prostate cancers can cause adverse effects such as impotence and incontinence)? Knowing what he knows now, Donald is withholding any consent to any further biopsy or treatment, even if his PSA should remain high. Donald is exercising his right to decide in the light of uncertainty about the evidential base and potential risk of adverse effects. Living a life being impotent and incontinent is not what he would value for himself and he is not willing to take that risk. Donald has the right to change his mind and may well do so in the future if the research programme provides more compelling evidence of the benefits of having the test and treatment options are developed without such adverse effects.

The Ethics Class raised the question about whether or not Donald would have wanted the test in the first place, knowing what he does now. What is the point of knowing he has a high PSA if, in light of all of the evidence, he would not consent to treatment anyway? At least, by him not knowing, he might have avoided the emotional and psychological trauma caused both to himself, his wife, family and friends.

Gordon's story and the lessons learned about informed consent

The Ethics Class summarized their discussion and concluded that informed consent means that the person obtaining consent has explained to the patient, in language the patient can understand, about what is happening to him and for what the consent is being sought. Informed consent means the patient can make a decision about what is to happen to him as a result of having all the information he needs to really understand the impact of his decision on his health and well-being.

Ann had pointed out to the group that it was not always so straightforward and that she had experienced patients who preferred not to be given information about what was happening to them. They had asked that the doctor and nurse do whatever was necessary. In fact, some patients had become unnecessarily distressed when given information about adverse effects, complications, probability of success and failure of procedure. The Ethics Class questioned the competence of some health care professionals in communicating with patients. The professional practitioner working with the principle of autonomy would demonstrate their respect for the patient's rights. They would sensitively explore with the patient and discover what and how much information they want to know at any one time, how they want to be given the information and how they wish to contribute to the decision-making. The group concluded that, if patients are being expected to direct their own care, then provision is needed that ensures equity of access for all patients to information resources and provides help in preparing patients to undertake such an active role in directing their own care.

Complexities of informed consent

Frances and Azad reminded the group there are situations in which people are not able to give informed consent for a number of reasons. They talked about examples they had encountered in relation to children and some patients with mental health problems.

Informed consent in relation to children – Frances' story

Frances recalled a situation in which a child had been knocked down in the street by a car and had suffered severe injuries requiring emergency surgery. The mother's partner accompanied the child to hospital as the mother had gone shopping and could not be contacted. There is no authority in law, apart from that given to a parent of a minor under 18 years of age, where a relative can give valid consent for a patient. The mother's partner was not the biological father and could not give valid informed consent for the emergency surgical procedures. Further attempts to contact the mother failed. The child's condition was life-threatening and the decision was made by the surgeon to proceed with surgery without obtaining consent from a biological parent. The law accommodates particular situations like these for life-saving procedures where any patient is unconscious and/or unable to give valid consent.

The Ethics Class noted the following points about the law and consent of children and young people. The consent of a child under the age of 16 years is fully acceptable if a child fully understands. If the child doesn't fully understand, then parental consent should be sought, except in an emergency where there is not time to obtain it. It was also noted that, for a young person over 16 years, parental consent is not necessary unless the person is not competent to give valid consent, when consent of a parent or guardian will be sought. However, such authority only extends until the child is 18 years of age.

The group also noted that they had read examples in other nursing texts and articles about situations arising in which parents do sometimes refuse to give consent for life-saving treatment. An example would be parents who are Jehovah's witnesses refusing to consent for a child to undergo surgical interventions and blood transfusion. Nobody in the group had experienced this in practice but realized that in such cases, time permitting, court action may be taken so that consent may be obtained from a judge. However, this could have serious implications for the child and the family if they objected so strongly to the decision because it violated their beliefs. The result might be that the child is ostracized by the family. It was also understood that cases like this would be considered individually and might lead to different courses of action in relation to the medical and legal decisions.

The group agreed there is a lot more to be considered by health care professionals when taking such decisions, including potential harm for the child due to disharmony in future family relationships. The students agreed ethics is a complex process and realized they have yet much to learn. However, they felt that, in view of such uncertainty, when in doubt it is useful for students to refer and stick to the rules provided by the Code.

Informed consent in relation to patients with mental health problems – Azad's story

Azad discussed with the group occasions in the mental health setting when obtaining consent from a patient was not feasible. He recalled the case of a mentally ill person who was perfectly rational before the onset of her illness and whose severe depression impaired her rationality but not completely. The difficulty for the health care professionals is being able to assess the patient's degree of autonomy. Does the patient understand what is happening to her, have the will to assert autonomy and take action? In addition, how does the health care professional know what the patient would want for herself rather than what the decision-maker would want for himself? These are very difficult situations and involve health professionals and carers in complex and difficult decision-making.

In the case recalled by Azad, the patient called Margaret had refused treatment and had not been eating or drinking for several days. If a patient refuses to allow treatment, then, apart from the very special circumstances of being detained under the appropriate section of the Mental Health Act (1983), which permits treatment, no treatment can occur. Margaret had been admitted as an emergency admission for 72 hours; this permits assessment, not treatment. The mental health team and Margaret's relatives had all been involved in trying to decide what was right to do and whether or not, out of the professionals' duty of care for Margaret, it would be defensible to override Margaret's autonomy. The doctors were not yet willing to place Margaret under a different section which permits treatment as they felt she was competent to give informed consent. Azad had brought a copy of the Mental Capacity Act 2005 to the group, which he had downloaded from the Office of Public Sector information at http://www.opsi.gov.uk. The legislation aims to protect those who lack capacity to give informed consent. The relatives and staff did not agree with the doctors' view and felt Margaret lacked the capacity (as defined in the Act) to give consent. It had been a difficult and complex case that had made Azad realize there is much more to ethical decision-making in the area of consent than just following the rules, looking for guidance in law and being of good character as a health professional.

The Ethics Class identified that there are situations when patients are subjected to examination, treatment and care in the absence of consent. These include: for life-saving procedures, by order of statutory power; in certain cases where a minor is a ward of court and the court decides that a specific treatment is in the child's best interest; treatment for a physical disorder where the patient is incapable of giving consent by reason of a mental disorder and the treatment is in the patient's best interest.

Consent and the nurse

In all of the situations recalled from practice at the Ethics Class, doctors had been responsible and accountable for obtaining informed consent for medical treatments. The nurses and the students had been very closely involved as members of the multidisciplinary team providing care for the patients, supporting their relatives and carers. The nurses contributed to the discussions and decision-making. If a nurse does not feel that sufficient information has been given in terms that are readily understandable to the patient, taking account of such things as language, ethnicity, culture, it is for her to state this opinion and get the situation remedied. The nurse is often best placed to know about the patient's circumstances, feelings, concerns and views, and it is important to inform the members of the care team what information is needed by the adult or child so that it is understood.

The Ethics Class also realized that all of the principles they had discussed in relation to obtaining informed consent for medical treatment also apply to all health care interventions including nursing care. Aveyard (2005) examined the way nurses obtain informed consent prior to nursing care procedures. Analysis of the data collected from focus groups and critical incidents suggests that consent was often not obtained by those who participated in the study and that refusals of care were often ignored by the nurses in the study. The author reports that participants in the study were often uncertain what to do when the patient was unable to consent. This is never a defence or an acceptable reason for a nurse to ignore the patient's refusal of care. Demonstrating moral perception and sensitivity may well result in the student finding herself in situations where she does not know what to do or how to react morally well. In such situations, exercising the virtues of integrity, honesty and concern will lead the student to ensuring the patient has access to a competent and compassionate health care professional.

Ann recalled a patient refusing to attend to personal hygiene but who would not let the nurses help her. Several nurses wanted to coerce the patient and stated in a threatening manner that she would contract hospital infections if her hygiene wasn't attended to and might die. The sister reprimanded the nurses; this was not acceptable behaviour and they were required to apologize to the patient. The sister reminded them of the Code and the requirement to make the care of patients their first concern, treating them as individuals and respecting their dignity. She also reminded them of the need to uphold the reputation of the nursing profession at all times.

The nurses concerned were genuinely sorry for what they had done and angry at their own behaviour. At the time they were feeling the pressure of their workload and felt hindered by this patient. The sister remarked how easy it is to slip into a culture of disrespect when constantly having to cope with the pressure of workload and that nurses needed to help and rescue each other from this. The actions of the sister were exemplary and appropriate for an effective manager. She demonstrated that there was zero tolerance amongst the profession for such behaviours and that individuals would be called to account to their profession for their actions. Eventually the patient was reassured that she would be able to maintain the privacy she needed and was supported to attend to her personal hygiene in her chosen way.

Examples of registrants being removed from the professional register for the abuse of elderly persons are discussed in NMC News (see, for example, NMC 2005b). The code requires of its members to act quickly to protect patients and clients from risk if they have good reason to believe that a colleague, from their own or another profession, may not be fit to practice for reasons of conduct, health or competence.

Being fit to practise

As a nurse or a nursing student you have an obligation to be fit to practise. If you feel stressed or too ill to work it is your obligation to let someone know. Remember that part of being fit to practise is being of good character, which includes physical and emotional wellness. It is essential to uphold the trust placed in you by sometimes extremely vulnerable people. The Ethics Class discussed several incidences when they had been concerned about a practitioner's conduct in practice. One incident had involved a nurse swearing and shouting at an elderly patient. When the student involved had suggested she would help the patient, the nurse who was the student's mentor, became aggressive and accused the student of undermining her. The student spoke to the appropriate member of the academic staff as laid down in the university policy relating to students reporting incidents of unprofessional conduct observed during practice experience. This is an important stage when the student is able to discuss the observed conduct so that a judgement can be made as to whether the observed conduct constitutes a breach of professional behaviour or is a result of a misunderstanding. As a student you must familiarize yourself with your university's policies and procedures in relation to reporting incidents of unprofessional conduct. This may extend to fellow students whose conduct is deemed sufficiently unprofessional to warrant reporting to a senior member of staff either in placement or to the university.

Georgina's story

Georgina is in the foundation year of the pre-registration nursing programme child branch and has been learning a great deal about the reforms taking place through the 'Every child matters' programme, which is about making services more effective to improve health outcomes for children and young people. Georgina has been learning about how important it is that nurses, midwives and specialist community public health nurses can work effectively with other agencies, including social services and education, and contribute to the health and well-being of vulnerable children and young people. She is immensely interested in this area having brought up children of her own and being a grandparent. She has also worked in the past as a care support worker in a children's medical ward and considers she has a lot of experience helping to care for vulnerable children. Now read Georgina's story (Case history 4.5) and reflect on the issues before joining the next Ethics Class:

- Reflect on the issues and identify how the Code might help guide what Georgina should do.
- Consider the concept of duty of care in the moral, professional and legal sense and how this might apply to Georgina or any student in this situation.

The Ethics Class considered the Code in relation to guidance on what to do in such a situation. The requirement placed on nurses and midwives to provide a high standard of practice and care at all times and the need to keep their knowledge and skills up to date throughout their working lives became the focus for their discussion. Although Georgina had felt confident that her previous experience as a health care assistant had enabled her to deal effectively with caring for children, she was now having to face up to the fact she is a student and has much to learn. Her placements are intended to help her learn and achieve practice competencies under the supervision of a registered practitioner. The Ethics Class pointed out to Georgina that, as she is a student, and although she might have a lot of experience caring for children and adolescents, she needed to accept the limitations of her role and realize why she was undertaking the pre-registration education programme. It was obvious that, despite her previous experience, Georgina

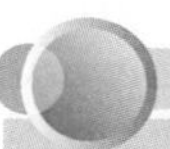

Case history 4.5

Georgina's story

Maxine, aged 14 years, lives on a small housing estate with her mother and two brothers. Her mother has multiple partners and Maxine has never known her own father. Georgina has been visiting the house while on placement with the paediatric outreach nurse, Carol, to provide care and support for Maxine's brother who has diabetes and is having difficulty complying with his treatment. He has been found unconscious on several occasions recently as a result of skipping meals to stay out with friends.

During these visits, Maxine is always at the house and states she has 'bunked off' school. During a visit, Georgina is left alone with Maxine as Carol and Maxine's brother wish to talk in private. Maxine is very talkative and asks Georgina if she can keep a secret. She tells Georgina the reason she is not attending school is that she keeps feeling sick and has vomited on several occasions. She is sure that she is pregnant as she obtained a test kit and it shows positive. She instructs Georgina that she must not tell anyone as she thinks the father is her mother's current boyfriend. He has told her that she has not to tell anybody about their affair and she still sleeps with him when her mother is not around. She fears that if her mother finds out she will throw her out and have nothing to do with her again. Her mother's boyfriend has told her he believes this will happen and that when she is a little older they will go away together. Maxine reminds Georgina that she has told her this in strictest confidence and it is her duty not to divulge this information to anyone.

Georgina told the Ethics Class that she felt confused, shocked and at a loss as to what she should do. Maxine was not the patient, but in a way Georgina had established a relationship with Maxine giving her time and listening. She had been identified as a nurse by Maxine, someone with the knowledge and skills to help. Georgina had not made it clear to Maxine that she was a student not a nurse. Georgina had at this point become acutely aware of the limitations of her role as a student.

lacked the knowledge skills and abilities required for lawful safe and effective practice without direct supervision. As a student, Georgina has an obligation to uphold the 'NMC Code of professional conduct' and not to act in a way that could bring discredit to nursing as a profession. The Ethics Class suggested to Georgina that her actions in not informing Maxine that she was a student nurse had led them to believe that she was unclear about the appropriate and lawful boundaries of her role and responsibility as a student nurse. They felt it was Georgina's responsibility not to take on the persona of a nurse and attempt to practise beyond the scope of her role as a student. They agreed that supervisors need to be confident that students are trustworthy and will adhere to the agreed plan of work. This is of particular importance in situations where the student is working under their supervisor's distant supervision and their attention is with the patient.

Georgina at first was resentful and told the group she had decided to undertake the pre-registration nursing programme merely to obtain the qualification of registered nurse. She had felt, on entry to the programme, that she had already learned a great deal in her role as a health care assistant. In her view, she knew just as much and was able to do the same things in practice as some of the qualified nurses she had worked with. She questioned what was wrong with seeking formal recognition from within the profession and the multidisciplinary team for what she was already doing. Georgina did eventually admit she had felt challenged by this situation and this had led her to reconsider her attitude and personal beliefs. Georgina had reflected on the incident with the Ethics Class and now realized that, although she had some strengths, she also had significant gaps in the level of her knowledge, understanding and her self-awareness. She acknowledged that her previous experience had not prepared her to deal with this kind of situation and that her skills and competence were inadequate.

Working with confidentiality in practice

The Ethics Class then considered what they should do as students if they were ever asked to keep a secret. Although Maxine was not the patient in this case it is highly likely she had not made any distinction in her own mind that she wasn't talking to a nurse with the knowledge and experience to help. Even if Georgina had initially failed to make it clear she was a student and not a nurse and to explain the difference, she should have been alerted by Maxine's question 'Could she keep a secret?' As a nursing student, her correct response would have been to make it absolutely clear that she was not a nurse. In addition, she should have explained the difference between a nurse and a nursing student and that as a student she would be obliged to share with her mentor any information Maxine should wish to divulge to her. If Maxine had then decided not to disclose her secret, Georgina would have been obliged to inform her mentor about what had happened. Where there is an issue of child protection and/or a vulnerable adult, the nurse must act always in accordance with national and local policies and within the law.

The mentor in this situation did take Maxine's revelation extremely seriously and used her skills to explore this sensitively with Maxine and Georgina. Every organization has a local child protection person and clear policy that reflects the national policy and guidelines to be followed in such situations. In terms of confidentiality, there are clear directives and procedures to follow when health professionals believe that disclosure of information is justified to protect children from abuse and neglect. Considerations will include decisions about how such sensitive information is recorded, what is written, where it is written and who to tell, including other agencies to be involved. What is paramount is the health, well-being and safety of the child. In this particular case, the Ethics Class realized that if proven guilty the mother's boyfriend may well be facing a criminal conviction for having sexual relations with a child. This is an extremely serious offence.

You can find out more about the 'Every child matters' programme and the Department for Education and Skills document 'Cross government guidance: sharing information on children and young people' at www.ecm.gov.uk. The document proposes changes of practice for health professionals and to clarify what weight should be given to public interest in protecting children from abuse and neglect. This follows some high-profile and tragic cases and in particular the Lord Laming enquiry into the death of Victoria Climbie. In this report, serious concerns were raised that information about vulnerable children was not recorded properly and communication between professionals from different agencies was poor with fatal consequences for the child. The outcome is to make it easier for health professionals to share crucial information when there are concerns by access to an online child protection database.

The Ethics Class went on to consider the issue of confidentiality and the guidance available in the Code. It is clear that breaches of confidentiality are viewed very seriously and improper disclosure of information is a serious breach of the Code. Confidentiality forms the basis of the professional–patient relationship and involves trust on the part of both the patient and the health care professional. The patient is required to give honest information and the health professional is required to keep secret the patient's disclosure. Respect for a person's autonomy underpins the principle of confidentiality, and to override autonomy by breaking a confidence always needs to be taken extremely seriously and must be justified. Sharing of information is justified only with the permission and consent of the patient. It is important always to make clear to patients that you need to share information with other members of the team involved in the delivery of their care.

The Code states the nurse's obligation if she is required to disclose information outside the team and if the patient's consent cannot be obtained, for whatever reason.

Disclosures may be made only where: they can be justified in the public interest (usually where disclosure is essential to protect the patient or client or someone else from the risk of significant harm); they are required by law or by order of the court.

By breaking confidence, the health professional may cause some degree of harm to the patient. They will be faced with making a difficult and complex ethical decision weighting the moral principles of autonomy and non-maleficence, to guide right action with no clear moral rights or wrongs to choose between. What would seem to be important is the honesty of the professional in not misleading the patient and in ensuring that the patient or client understands the parameters within which information may be disclosed.

Breaching patient/client confidentiality

The Ethics Class recalled that on several occasions they had observed breaches of patient confidentiality. Some of these included nurses being overheard discussing patients in public places such as hospital dining rooms, in lifts and on public transport, and discussing and sharing information about patients and families they know as friends or neighbours with others in their circle. The group recalled the university policy and guidelines for students in relation to patient confidentiality and privacy and any written assignment using patient information. The obligations of the student are clearly outlined, and include procedures to follow in obtaining the patient's permission to use the information and maintaining anonymity of information so that nobody can identify the patient or place of care. The Data Protection Act (1998) applies here in stating the rights of the individual: that no person can share information about someone without his permission and that information obtained has to be used in accordance with the reason someone gave it to that person in the first place.

Ann raised with the group that, on occasions, when patients' relatives and friends made enquiries about a patient, she had found it difficult telling them that she could not give them information. Some relatives did not seem to understand when it was explained to them the reason why and could get angry and upset. It was difficult to communicate over the phone with somebody who is angry and upset. However, she did her best to be helpful and always offered to pass on messages to the patient or to ensure the enquiry was given to the qualified nurse.

Gordon raised with the group his concerns about the reflective diary he was keeping and as encouraged by the course leader. This contains patient and staff information, although private to himself. The Ethics Class agreed the principles for maintaining anonymity should apply equally to the reflective diary. It also should be kept securely and should not be left in any place where it might be discovered and read by others.

Sabina's story

Sabina's story (Case history 4.6) is the last story to be presented to the Ethics Class before the students move into the branch programmes. They will then continue these sessions during their first branch year while undertaking an ethics module to examine moral theory. The focus will be on the use of reason and logic, to identify and analyse moral dilemmas and evaluate the usefulness of moral theory as ethical frameworks for providing justification for the courses of action taken as right action. Sabina is in the foundation year of the pre-registration nursing programme learning disability branch and has been concentrating on the issues surrounding patient/client rights. Sabina is keeping a reflective diary and is thinking a great deal about health work and how what you do in practice situations can contribute to health and well-being.

Sabina asked the Ethics Class to reflect on the case of Mary and to suggest a course of action that they considered would best contribute to Mary's health and well-being. Reflect on Sabina's story about Mary and ask yourself the following:

- Why do you think health and social care practice, including nursing, has an ethical dimension?
- Reflect on the issues and consider which parts of the Code give guidance to the team about what action they should take.
- Does the Code provide nurses with all of the answers? Is there anything else needed to guide health professionals in deciding on the right course of action to take?

The Ethics Class discussed the story about Mary's situation and was immediately struck by the nature of the health professional's work and in particular the importance of maintaining good relationships with patients/clients and others in the team. They discussed what working towards the aim of creating better health might mean in terms of intervening in another person's life and that it may not always be welcomed by that person. Everyone in the Ethics Class agreed that health and well-being is a 'good' that they themselves value and pursue in their own lives. They acknowledged that this judgement is based on their own combined

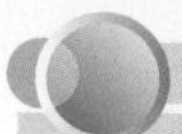

Case history 4.6

Sabina's story

Sabina presents her story about Mary to the Ethics Class. Mary is 51 years of age and lives in a supported tenancy scheme. She has a learning disability and a diagnosis of schizophrenia. Mary has been involved with mental health and social services for most of her adult life. There have been some long-standing issues regarding her financial vulnerability, particularly with regard to her boyfriend Isaac.

Sabina has been on placement with the learning disability team for only 2 weeks and tells the Ethics Class she is getting to know Mary quite well. She has learned that Mary is very independent and, prior to the tenancy scheme, lived by herself for a period of 9 months with outreach support as required. Isaac, her boyfriend, visited and stayed over frequently when she was on her own but, as the house has become fully occupied and fully staffed, these visits have 'dropped off'. Mary now only sees Isaac at his house. This has been entirely their decision and has not been influenced by staff or other tenants.

Several months ago staff noticed bruising to Mary's arms following an overnight visit to her boyfriend. Mary had told some of the tenants that she had banged herself, while telling others the bruises had appeared by themselves. Mary was vague when, due to this contradiction, she was asked if she could clarify the situation. When asked directly if she had been abused in any way, Mary categorically denied this.

Mary had agreed to attend her general practitioner to rule out any physical cause for the bruising as this was one of the explanations Mary had offered. The tests were negative and the matter wasn't pursued any further by the learning disability team.

Only last week, more severe bruising was observed and it had been explained to Mary that staff had a duty to take action because of the possible implications of this. Mary had hinted at her boyfriend being responsible and that he had been hitting her because he wanted more money despite her having none left as he had already taken it from her. However Mary would not cooperate with the team's suggestion that the police should become involved and again was adamant that she was not being abused in any way.

The team had begun to question what they should do and there were different views being expressed about the right course of action to take.

personal values about the perceived quality, cost and consequences of health and well-being, and that not all individuals will necessarily share the same values, beliefs and judgements about health, what it means as a 'good' to be pursued and the ways in which to achieve it, assuming that we know its meaning. The students discussed the various theories of health they were learning about.

The importance of personal values and the dilemmas created in practice

Azad told the Ethics Class that he felt he was learning a great deal about what 'working for health' means in terms of working to remove obstacles in the way of patients/clients achieving their full potential for health and well-being and what this might mean in practice (Seedhouse 1998). In addition, he had learned that, whilst there are many similarities shared by individuals, there are differences between individuals in their values, beliefs, desires and aspirations. He had experienced situations in which patients and clients, given the opportunity, had constructed very different lifestyles for themselves compared with his own and those of the health care professionals caring for them. Whilst Azad shared the profession's valuing of the desirability of individual freedom to make personal value choices as a benchmark of a fair and just society, sometimes, in his view, patient/client choices had resulted in a lessening of their health and well-being. He believed it was sometimes very difficult for health professionals to stand back and to respect patient choices, especially when, in the professional's opinion, the patient had refused to consider what might appear to be better options for creating their own health and well-being. In Mary's situation, some members of the team had felt that they should not stand back but must report the matter to the police. They had argued this would be best for Mary because they were of the opinion that she was not making the best choice in selecting a partner for herself. Isaac should be dealt with in order to reduce the risk and remove the danger of further abuse which might escalate.

The Ethics Class agreed that, because of the very nature of the work health professions do, health work does have an ethical dimension. Whatever the health professional does will have the potential to affect another person for better or worse. His actions can contribute to creating health and well-being, leaving the patient/client feeling enhanced as a person, or causing great harm and suffering. The Ethics Class had also begun to recognize the potential for a conflict of values between professionals themselves, between professionals and their patients/clients and between their relatives as well as between different groups in society. The story of Mary had clearly illustrated these conflicts and they were beginning to realize this reflected the complexity of health care ethics. The challenge is in deciding between different courses of action and what interventions in other people's lives will produce the greater degree of morality. They recognized that this requires careful thought and deliberation and honest reasoned judgements. Codes of professional conduct and the law can clearly state the health professional's obligations towards patients/clients but they do not always provide a means for deciding between different options. Mary's situation raised the question as to which course of action would bring about the greatest degree of morality. The dilemma the team faced was whether to take the course of action that respects Mary's autonomy and right to make decisions about her own life or to take the course of action based on acting in her best interests that protects Mary but which overrides her autonomy. Gordon and Ann were very keen to point out that Mary as a citizen has rights and the right course of action is that she should be able to make her own decisions and choices about how she lives her life from the options available to her.

The Ethics Class discussed what they consider is important in their own lives, and members of the group spoke about how they valued their own relationships, which they believed made their lives worth living. However, they did not think they would knowingly choose a relationship where they were bullied for money and/or were a victim of physical violence. Sabina told the Ethics Class that on several occasions Mary had spoken to other tenants about Isaac, saying he was the most important person in her life. Ann and Gordon again referred to the Code. Particular sections of the Code outline the nurse's obligations in relation to respect of the patient/client as an individual with rights, including the right to refuse any health care intervention and the right to confidentiality of information.

Working with the complexities of autonomy in practice

Hilary is another student undertaking the pre-registration nursing programme and who is about to enter the mental health branch. Her module assignment has led her to study the moral principle 'autonomy'. This is a complex principle to understand and to apply to real-life situations. Hilary, like her fellow students Ann and Gordon, felt that Mary's right to make decisions about her own life and relationships was underpinned by a respect for patient autonomy. Hilary felt that she would base her judgement about the right course of action out of a felt obligation to respect this moral principle and to respect Mary's decisions as an autonomous person. In addition, Hilary pointed out that the Code clearly states the obligation of the nurse.

In most ethics literature an autonomous person is said to be in control of their own destiny. They can decide what they want and do what they want without interference from anyone else. This view, that autonomy is a right, is a simplified version of what is indeed a complex principle, one that is not easy to understand when applied in practice. Autonomy is also thought of as a personal quality, with a person having different degrees of autonomy in different aspects of their life. The higher the degree of autonomy, the more a person is able to do. Georgina described the times when she visits her dentist as times when she is less in control. On one occasion she was so frightened that she could not understand simple directions and had bitten the dentist by clenching her teeth when he had instructed her to open her mouth wide.

Sabina described how she had felt during a recent episode when her grandmother was in hospital after sustaining a broken hip during a fall. The patient in the next bed had told her that her grandmother was not eating or drinking and the meals delivered by support workers were always removed untouched. Sabina had subsequently discovered that her grandmother, who could not feed herself without assistance due to Parkinson's disease, was frightened she might make a mess if she tried to help herself. She had taken the decision not to try, but to wait until she got home when she would have the support needed. Sabina had been extremely angry and upset about this and subsequently visited at every mealtime to help her grandmother eat her meals and drink.

Both the above examples demonstrate that there are ways in which the degree of autonomy can be reduced. Feeling anxious and distressed, as in the dentist's chair, can affect thought processes and the capacity and ability to process simple information effectively. Patients talk about being anxious when accessing health services and this may affect their ability to process the information that is given to them. The second example illustrates how a physical disability can be a serious obstacle to doing even the most natural thing that we want to do, when we want to do it. This makes us vulnerable and dependent on others for our needs. Not having food and drink is serious and will have detrimental effects on a person's health and well-being. Neglecting a patient's nutritional and hydration needs in this way is not an acceptable standard of practice and must be met with zero tolerance by the profession.

The Ethics Class identified how the health professionals might work with Mary to help enhance her autonomy in her relationship with Isaac. One strategy might be to spend time with Mary to encourage her to talk about her relationship with Isaac and so better understand its importance to her. They would want to ensure Mary had access to essential information and services that can help with difficult relationships such as one that is abusive and to ensure that she does understand what her options might be. In addition, measures could be taken to afford Mary and Isaac some privacy so that they are able to spend more time together at Mary's house with access to support from the team.

Georgina reminded the Ethics Class that Mary had a learning disability and that some members of the team had wanted to inform the police against Mary's wishes. They had argued this was the right course of action to take, that it was in Mary's best interests to do this. Sabina referred to the plight of her grandmother who had not been assessed appropriately or consulted about her care needs by the nurses and in particular how she would meet her nutritional needs. Was this because she was elderly and had Parkinson's disease and therefore considered less competent as a person who therefore had less of a right to respect for autonomy? Could it also be the case that having a learning disability might mean others assume a person is less competent and so not able to make their own choices about how to conduct their own lives and choose the relationships they wish to make? It could be that well-meaning health professionals feel it is their moral, professional and legal duty to protect patients/clients like Mary from making choices they consider are harmful to the patient's/client's health and well-being. After all, the health professional has a moral and legal duty to promote good and prevent harm. Legally, the health professional could face a claim of negligence under the Law of Tort if they do not intervene and it is subsequently proved that the patient/client suffered harm as a result of their non-intervention. The Ethics Class discussed risk assessment and wondered how the measure of potential risk can be made with any confidence by the professionals.

Lessons learned about intervening in patients'/clients' lives

Azad told the Ethics Class how in some situations health professionals had questioned whether their true motive for overriding a patient's right to respect for autonomy was always out of concern and acting in the best interests of the patient/client. They acknowledged that perhaps their decisions were sometimes more about their own self-interests. Within contemporary nursing practice, individual accountability is paramount and health professionals are feeling challenged to balance limited resources with their desire to achieve high standards of nursing practice. This is at a time when both the public and policy-makers have growing expectations and are increasingly demanding.

The Ethics Class concluded that ethics in health care is a complex process and there is not always a clear answer as to the best course of action to take to achieve the greatest degree of morality. The Ethics Class considered they had utilized a range of sources of knowledge and had brought together all of the different discourses to make some sense of what was going on in Mary's case. They had raised questions about the facts of the case, research base for care, the law, moral principles, the Code of professional conduct and professional values, client's own and others' personal values and beliefs and the measurement of risk. In particular, Azad had been learning about the evidence base for risk-assessment tools used in the field of mental health. Some staff had raised their concerns about the validity and reliability of these tools and that they were sometimes used to assess the threat of danger to the general public. Should patients/clients be denied their freedoms just in case they are a threat to others? How can a prediction of threat be quantified, assuming it can be qualified and at what level of threat is the client's freedom curtailed?

The Ethics Class recognized that working for health and well-being in health care practice is ethical practice and this necessarily requires the health care professional to engage in careful deliberation about what kinds of interventions in other people's lives will produce the greater degree of morality.

Ethics and what is required of health professionals

In this chapter it has been argued that health professionals require certain character traits that are compatible with good moral character, the good nurse and good nurse–patient/client relationships. Some of these traits or virtues, such as kindness, honesty, compassion and concern, you may have already nurtured before deciding to join a health care profession. They may have influenced your decision to join the profession in the first place. Here we are arguing that moral virtues can be developed with the right sort of professional education. This requires commitment, courage and motivation on your part as a nursing student, to learn and develop moral perception, moral sensitivity and to act morally well. The stories that we have shared demonstrate how in some situations, when a bad outcome occurs in practice, the health care professional, whilst admitting to unkindness, dishonesty or cowardice, might choose to shrug it off as being the result of a situation not in her control. Remember Ann's story (Case history 4.3) about the way in which a patient was being threatened by the nurses to comply with attending to personal hygiene and how the sister had intervened? How the nurses had gone on to defend their action claiming it was the result of pressures of workload which was out of their control? The sister was acknowledging that, despite the pressures of the workload, it was unacceptable to act in a manner that was ethically wrong. This kind of integrity is necessary of both the health care professional and students and indicates acceptance of responsibility in some meaningful way, even in situations when outcomes are not necessarily within their control. In this particular difficult and typical situation of today's busy and demanding health service environment the sister demonstrated integrity in accepting responsibility and acting morally well. The outcome was good as a result of her action and as a manager she had already presented a written report and begun negotiations to secure funding to appoint an additional staff member to the team.

Balancing the responsibility in practice to achieve the economic targets of the health service with a commitment to act morally well in practice, the health professional is vulnerable and fallible. However, health care professionals and students can achieve a greater degree of control over the kind of person they become through cultivating certain virtues such as integrity, honesty, courage and compassion. Even in the face of difficulty beyond their control, the good nurse remains steadfast in exercising the virtues and endeavouring to act well. In Ann's story, the sister was honest in accepting the situation as it was and displayed courage in facing up to her responsibility for ensuring the standard of care provided to patients even in the face of adversity. The sister demonstrated a genuine valuing and respect for the patient as an individual and for her staff nurses and acted morally well in aiming to maximize the patient's and the nurses' autonomy.

Reflection and discussion

Although this chapter has focused on what sort of person it is good to be as a health care professional, the health care practitioner nevertheless has a duty of care towards each individual patient and towards each group of patients. This can involve making difficult ethical decisions, having to choose between different courses of action, none of which is satisfactory in a moral sense. Remember Ann's story of her mentor Brenda, and how on the one hand she was motivated to respect Bill's autonomy and right to choose how he would manage his anxiety, whilst at the same time she was acutely aware of her obligation to do good and not harm, that she owed Bill a duty of care in both the moral and the legal sense. The 'NMC Code of professional conduct' clearly outlines that you must respect patients' and clients' autonomy and that you have a duty of care to your patients. Brenda had to choose between overriding Bill's choice, not respecting his autonomy in order to prevent potential harm befalling Bill or respecting his autonomy, taking the risk he might fall and be harmed. To override patient autonomy and choice is an extremely serious thing to do and needs to be thought about carefully with a strong argument to justify such a course of action. On the other hand, a decision to stand back and do nothing could result in great harm to the patient and a claim of negligence against the health care professional.

You will have learned, through reading this chapter, of the importance of knowing the 'NMC Code of professional conduct' as a first guide to decision-making in your practice. You may be perplexed at times, perhaps not always knowing what the moral dilemma is that is facing you in practice. Your moral perception and sensitivity will lead you to want to work it out and to reach a level of understanding so that you can act well. Use the 'NMC Code of professional conduct' as an anchor to return to for help and to identify the ethical issues.

You may feel tempted to try to hide behind the 'NMC Code of professional conduct', or to hide behind those you might blame for a situation in which you may find yourself. The Ethics Class quickly realized that the health professional's responsibility in ethical decision-making in practice is to choose the course of action that will result in the greatest degree of morality. This requires further study of ethics, including consideration of moral theories and moral principles that focus on acquiring the right answer about what is the right course of action to take in a given situation. It involves you in developing your ability to analyse and construct complex arguments using knowledge from a range of subject disciplines and sources. We anticipate that you have already reached this stage of your journey in your ambition towards becoming a competent health care professional, a good nurse. The next stage of your journey is to learn to construct your arguments so that you can give informed views and contribute in a meaningful way to ethical decisions made within the multidisciplinary team. You will need the necessary philosophical knowledge and ability to apply logic and reasoning in constructing convincing arguments to support what you believe to be true as justification for what you do in practice.

References

Aveyard H 2005 Informed consent prior to nurse care procedures. Nursing Ethics 12(1):19–29

Benner P, Wrubel J 1989 The primacy of caring: stress and coping in health and disease. Addison Wesley, California

Boyle CA, Henly SJ, Duckett LJ 2001 Nurse's motivation to wash their hands: a standardised measurement approach. Applied Nursing Research 14(3):136–145

Concato J, Wells CK, Horwitz RI et al 2006 The effectiveness of screening for prostate cancer: a nested case–control study. Archives of Internal Medicine 166:38–43. Online. Available: http://archinte.ama-assn.org 1 Feb 2006

Department for Education and Skills 2005 Cross government guidance: sharing information on children and young people. Online. Available: www.dfes.gov.uk Dec 2005

Gilligan C 1982 In a different voice: psychological theory and women's development. Harvard University Press, Cambridge, MA

Gould D 2004 Systematic observation of hand decontamination. Nursing Standard 18(47):39–44

Held V 1990 Feminist transformations of moral theory. Philosophy and Phenomenological Research 50:321–344

Held V 1993 Feminist morality: transforming culture, society and politics. Chicago, University of Chicago Press

Leininger M (ed) 1981 Caring: an essential human need. Proceedings of three national conferences. Charles Slack, New Jersey

Leininger M 1984 Care: the essence of nursing and health. Charles Slack, New Jersey

Leininger M 1998 Caring: a central focus of nursing and health care services. In: Leininger M (ed) Care: the essence of nursing and health. University Press, New York, p 45–59

MacIntyre A 1993 After virtue: a study in moral theory. Duckworth, London

Noddings N 1984 Caring: a feminine approach to ethics and moral education. University of California Press, London

Nursing and Midwifery Council 2002a Guide for students of nursing and midwifery. NMC, London

Nursing and Midwifery Council 2002b Guidelines for records and record keeping. NMC, London. Online. Available: www.nmc-uk.org

Nursing and Midwifery Council 2004a Reporting unfitness to practise: a guide for employers and managers. NMC, London

Nursing and Midwifery Council 2004b Reporting lack of competence: a guide for employees and managers. NMC, London

Nursing and Midwifery Council 2004c Requirements for evidence of good health and good character. NMC, London

Nursing and Midwifery Council 2004d Fitness to practise annual report 2003–2004. NMC, London

Nursing and Midwifery Council 2004e Fitness to practise rules 2004. SI 2004/1761. NMC, London

Nursing and Midwifery Council 2005a Fitness to practise annual report 2004–2005. NMC, London

Nursing and Midwifery Council 2005b The NMC tackles elder abuse. NMC News 13:6

Nursing and Midwifery Council 2008 Code of Conduct: professional standards for nurses and midwives. Online. Available: www.nmc-uk.org

Plunkett P 1999 New Hampshire nurses: what are our concerns, resources and education in ethics? Nursing News 49(3):3

Rachels J 1998 The ethics of virtue and the ethics of right action. In: Cahn SM, Marki P (eds) Ethics: history, theory and contemporary issues. Oxford University Press, New York, p 669–681

Rowson RH 1999 An introduction to ethics for nurses. Scutari Press, London

Sadler J 1997 Defining professional nurse caring: a triangulation study. International Journal of Human Caring 1(3):12–21

Seedhouse D 1998 Ethics: the heart of health care, 2nd edn. Wiley, Chichester

Stockwell F 1972 The unpopular patient (Study of nursing care project reports, series 1 no. 2). Royal College of Nursing, London

Stockwell F 1984 The unpopular patient. Croom Helm, London

Tschudin V 1992 Values: a primer for nurses. Baillière Tindall, London

Wagner AL 2002 Nursing student's development of caring self through creative reflective practice. In: Freshwater D (ed) Therapeutic nursing: improving patient care through self awareness and reflection. Sage, London, p 121–144

Wallis L 2005 When rites are wrong. Nursing Standard 20(4):24–26

Watson J 1997 The theory of human caring: retrospective and prospective. Nursing Science Quarterly 10(1):49–52

Watson J 1999 Postmodern nursing and beyond. Churchill Livingstone, Edinburgh

Watson R, Lea A 1997 The caring dimensions inventory (CDI) content validity, reliability and scaling. Journal of Advanced Nursing 25:87–94

Further reading

Creel RE 2001 Thinking philosophically. Blackwell, Oxford, p 112–125

Dimond B 2005 Legal aspects of nursing, 4th edn. Pearson Longman, Harlow

Mason T, Whitehead E 2003 Thinking nursing. Open University Press, Buckingham

Chapter Five

5

Learning and working as a nursing student in a multicultural world

Alison Spires

Key topics

- Multicultural society
- Supporting diversity employment policy
- Quality issues relating to diversity
- Gender differences
- Transcultural care

Introduction

This chapter is about learning and working as a nursing student in a multicultural world. It focuses on the importance of diversity in the modern health service in the 21st century, both from the perspective of the nurse as care-giver and the perspective of the patient or client as a recipient of care. Throughout the chapter the importance of cultural issues in nursing practice are addressed.

The diversity of the population in northern Europe has increased dramatically over recent decades. This has both enriched our societies and also caused us to reconsider many practices that have been taken for granted. An example is given in Case history 5.1.

From this case history it becomes clear that the students' wishes were being respected, but within the constraints of current knowledge about infection control and the need for patients to feel secure in the knowledge that the person caring for them was a legitimate practitioner. So let us consider how such radical changes have developed and impacted on everyday nursing practice.

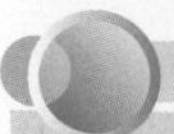

Case history 5.1

Religious dress and social norms in nursing

Increasingly the nursing profession in the UK is attracting students from a wide variety of religious faiths. This brings with it issues to do with dress as an expression of faith and cultural identity. A group of female Muslim health care students at a large university felt that the uniform regulations of the university did not allow them to express their faith fully, as it expected all students to conform to the standard policy of wearing a semi-fitted short-sleeved tunic-type jacket and trousers. Many of the students were wearing a variation of their religious dress as uniform. The students made representation to the senior level of management within their university to try and obtain some guidance about what they could wear that would allow them to express their faith and care for patients at the same time. The university authorities sought a compromise between the students who wished to wear their traditional dress and the university and partner hospital trusts who their dress to be more in keeping with a nursing uniform. A decision was made that enabled the students to wear looser trousers, a longer tunic with long sleeves, which could be rolled up when giving care, and a hijab (headscarf), providing it was clean and laundered daily and tucked into the tunic. This compromise was acceptable to the students.

Comments and discussion

There are health and safety implications for health professional staff when they wear their own clothes as uniform. Uniform is manufactured to be washed at a high temperature to ensure destruction of micro-organisms and ensure stain removal. Personal clothing may not stand high-temperature washes, and additionally it is not acceptable to allow one's own clothing to be soiled by patients' body fluids. A flowing dress of any kind, religious or not, may interfere with manual handling operations and long skirts may sweep the floor if a nurse bends down, for example, to empty a catheter bag. This has implications for cross-infection from micro-organisms in floor dust. Long sleeves are in danger of being contaminated by patients' body fluids, so it is essential that sleeves can be rolled up when performing nursing care.

In instances where uniform is a problem, both sides should continue their endeavours to seek a negotiated solution and should not walk away from the issue.

Historical background to the concept of diversity

It is clear that, since the formation of the National Health Service (NHS) in 1948, there have been changing needs in the health care requirements of the population of the UK. Prior to the formation of the NHS, provision of health care was from a mixture of local authority, charity and government sources – an eclectic mix of services which left many people lacking in provision and some with none at all. The National Health Service Act in 1946 effectively nationalized health care provision and brought the majority of services under the control of the Ministry of Health, with some under the control of local authorities. A reorganization of services in the early 1970s saw all services united under government control. The formation of the NHS was predicated upon a comprehensive service, free at the point of delivery to all. Very quickly it became clear that there were neither the monetary nor staff resources to meet the demand, and some staff shortages were met by recruiting heavily from Commonwealth countries in the 1950s and 1960s (Webster 2002).

Along with those recruited into the NHS from Commonwealth countries such as the West Indies, people, including health care workers, have come to the UK from many other countries since the inception of the NHS – for economic reasons, as invited workers, as political refugees, or to escape persecution because of their beliefs. From the 1960s, immigration into the UK increased, with people arriving from India, Pakistan, Bangladesh, Hong Kong and more recently from African and eastern European countries. The formation of the European Union (EU) further opened up opportunities for workers from EU countries to seek employment in the UK. Thus, in the early 2000s, the sociocultural make-up of the UK is such that the black and minority ethnic population of the UK constitutes 7.6% of the total population, up from 1% in 1950. The Department of Health (2003) stated that the Greater London area contains half of all people from the black and minority ethnic population of the UK, with the totals in individual London boroughs ranging from 5% to

50%. The West Midlands, Greater Manchester and West Yorkshire also have black and minority ethnic residents, with 84% of the total black and minority ethnic population of the UK living in the four areas mentioned. Leicester and Birmingham are predicted to increase their black and minority ethnic populations to a majority by 2010 (Department of Health 2003). This has important implications for health care provision in these areas and for nursing. But we must be in no doubt that, in this third millennium, the UK is a multicultural society and part of a multicultural world.

With increasing international travel and migration since the end of World War II, the majority of the world's countries now contain more than one cultural or ethnic group. But multiculturalism is not just about different races and different colour of skin, it is also about the traditionally distinctive and diverse cultures of all countries of the world including the UK. Indeed, the islands that make up the UK have within their borders groups of people who each see themselves as culturally distinct from their neighbours. People are proud of their Scottish, Irish, Welsh or English ancestry, and of the cultural dimension of that ancestry. They are also as proud of the fact that they may be highland or lowland Scot, mountain or valley Welsh, Londoner, Liverpudlian or Bristolian English, rural or urban dweller. History tells us that over the years the UK has become a host country to many groups of immigrants. Even within one single society it can be argued that it contains many different cultures. Men and women and boys and girls, old and young, ill or healthy, all these groups in any society are expected to behave in ways that their culture determines is appropriate for them.

Multiculturalism in health care provision

Cultures are also divided into subcultures. For example, the NHS can be said to be a subculture of British society, and, within the NHS, nursing, medicine and physiotherapy, for example, can be identified as further subcultures. Each subculture has its own clear and distinctive set of implicit guidelines for behaviour. New entrants to health care professions are often referred to as needing to be 'socialized' into their professions. It is clear that health professionals do form a separate cultural group within society, but can the same be said for patients? Is there a 'patient' culture? Helman (1994) states that society divides up its members according to their health status as 'healthy' or 'ill'. However, this may be a label applied by a health professional to a person rather than by the person themself.

There are also other ways of dividing society up into categories of subcultures. The 1991 census was the first to elicit information about ethnic origins of the population of the UK, and the 2001 census added to this with questions about disability and religious affiliation. The percentage of black and minority ethnic groups is not currently high, but according to James (1995) this is likely to double over the next 40–50 years. Without doubt, each different cultural and minority ethnic group adds value to the diversity and complexity of UK society. Valuing the cultural background of each and every client and patient is crucial in the provision of culturally aware, culturally sensitive and culturally competent nursing care. Valuing diversity in caring is an important and fundamental issue for health care provision and for nursing in the UK.

Cultural perspectives of health and illness

Cultural determinants of health and illness and of life and death and the understanding of such perspectives is important in contemporary society where diverse communities of people hold differing beliefs and values. The knowledge and explanations of their health and illness that indigenous British people use is based upon a Western tradition of medicine. This has its roots in ancient Greek scientific thought together with an understanding of the nature and causation of disease brought about changing knowledge since the middle ages. Immigrant peoples bring with them their own explanatory models of health and illness which may stem from different beliefs about health and disease. Understanding the differences between these assumptions and beliefs about health and illness provides a basis for healing. With such a diverse population, learning about each individual religious or ethnic grouping within the UK is no mean task for you to undertake, and it may not actually be necessary. Looking at your own culture and/or religion and working out how to explain this to someone from another cultural or religious group may be a useful first step in recognizing and valuing diversity. Read the two case histories of people from very different cultural backgrounds and think how their views reflect your own beliefs. The first (Case history 5.2) is of Jack who is a native of Newcastle; the second (Case history 5.3) is of Chooi, a woman of Chinese-Malay origins.

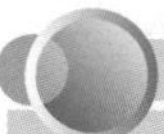

Case history 5.2

Jack's view of his diet and his health

Well, I was brought up on chips and peanut butties (sandwiches) for breakfast and lunch. We used to have potato scallops for tea with some gravy on them and then at about 10 at night me Dad would go down to the chippie for a round of fish and chips. On Sundays we'd have a proper meal of roast chicken. This was pretty much like what all my mates would have. Now I has me lunch at the pub, a couple of rounds of beer and a bag of crisps and go home to a fry up that me wife does for me. My health? Well the doctor says I've got to lose weight on account of my blood pressure being that high, stop smoking and take some exercise. I guess the pills he's given me will do all that for me.

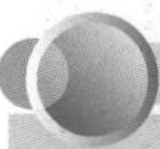

Case history 5.3

Chooi's beliefs about diet and health

My family are quite strict Buddhist and so we are vegetarians, but that means we eat a lot of fruit and vegetables as well as rice at every meal. We see food as being strongly linked to health; it is like a medicine and at different seasons of the year if we are ill we eat different kinds of food to make us strong and healthy. We see health as a balance between the different elements in the body and we eat foods to keep those elements in balance.

What is culture?

In order to explore the concept of diversity in caring, we first need to define what we mean by culture. Culture has many meanings. When some people talk of culture they are referring to art, opera and music; to others, culture can mean the distinguishing characteristics of a workplace. For example, we often talk of the culture of the NHS, the culture of the armed forces or of the civil service. From an anthropological perspective culture is taken as meaning the set of guidelines that individuals use and which tells them how to behave in their own particular part of society. We can tell from this definition that anthropology is the study of people and their relationships within their social setting. Helman (1994) uses the analogy of a 'lens' through which an individual perceives and understands his or her own world. Anthropology theory suggests that people's behaviour is partly governed by the specific society in which they grow up and in which they live. Culture provides the guide for determining values, practices and beliefs within any given society. It determines how people accommodate themselves within their own culture because it is related to the way that people live. Culture relates to morality, beliefs, social norms and accepted behaviour. Individuals in any culture are expected to adopt and comply with that culture's rules. What is acceptable in one culture may not be acceptable in another culture. For example, female circumcision (also known as female genital mutilation and normally abbreviated to FGM) is an accepted and deep-rooted practice in a number of African countries. Ng (2000) stated that, in the 1990s, some 50% of Kenyan girls were still being circumcised, and it was estimated in 1994 that this procedure had been performed on over 100 million girls and women worldwide (Henley & Schott 1999). In the UK, there is legislation in place (Prohibition of Circumcision Act 1985) which prohibits the practice, and the World Health Organization does not support it. However, it is important that nurses understand why such practices are still carried out and to know what practical help and advice they can provide to women and girls on whom this procedure has been performed; see Henley &

Schott (1999), or read Waris Dirie's (1998) personal account of female circumcision in her biography 'Desert Flower'.

Culture determines how nurses and patients react and respond to the actions of nursing interventions. 'Transcultural' nursing, as the term implies, means that the provision of nursing care is to do with a meeting of two or more cultures: the culture of the nursing profession, the nurse's own cultural background and the cultural background of the patient, and maybe even male/female culture and age/youth culture. Transcultural care thus focuses on issues to do with the way each cultural group understands what health is and the causes of illness, what treatment is intended to achieve and what contribution nursing care makes to the total picture. Our behaviours as people in all our roles in life are learned from observing others in our immediate society, and, in comparing what we do with what others do, we alter our own behaviour to fit in. This is a useful way of describing culture from a health care point of view since it allows us to look at our own nursing culture, and also be concerned with the cultural background of the individuals who become patients and clients of the health care services.

Culture and health care

The NHS was set up in 1948 to cater for the needs of a fairly homogeneous 'British' culture. Mares et al, writing in 1985, felt that the NHS had not really begun to take into account the composition of the population in the provision of care. They felt that NHS service provision and staff training were still geared to the way of life, family patterns, dietary norms, religious beliefs, attitudes, priorities and expectations of the majority population. In 1994, Thomas and Dines felt that initiatives by the NHS to meet the health care needs of minority ethnic groups appeared inadequate, and that there was little evidence of what might constitute good practice in this area. Papadopoulos, writing in 1999 about Greek Cypriots living in London, felt that their health care needs had not yet been fully recognized. Vydelingum's research (2000) indicated that patients of South Asian origin felt a general dissatisfaction with their health care in hospital settings. Despite a number of reports from the Department of Health in the 1990s (e.g. Department of Health 1992) which highlighted the particular needs of minority ethnic groups, it seems that such ideas have not yet been translated fully into action in the NHS, although there is now considerable thought and action in this area.

Whatever we might like to think, there are examples of racism and prejudice to be found within the NHS; some might term this 'institutional racism'. These examples range from not providing interpreter services and using patients' own young children as interpreters, not providing appropriate food or calling it 'special' food, failing to provide services for particular medical conditions common in specific ethnic groups, and failing to adapt patient records to reflect particular naming systems. Yet numerous examples of good practice can also be found. These include health promotion literature in different languages (see Figure 5.1), the provision in some areas of interpreter services for patients, the provision of education for health professionals in the areas of culture and race and the provision of literature for health professionals to consult (e.g. UK Transplant Coordinators Association, undated).

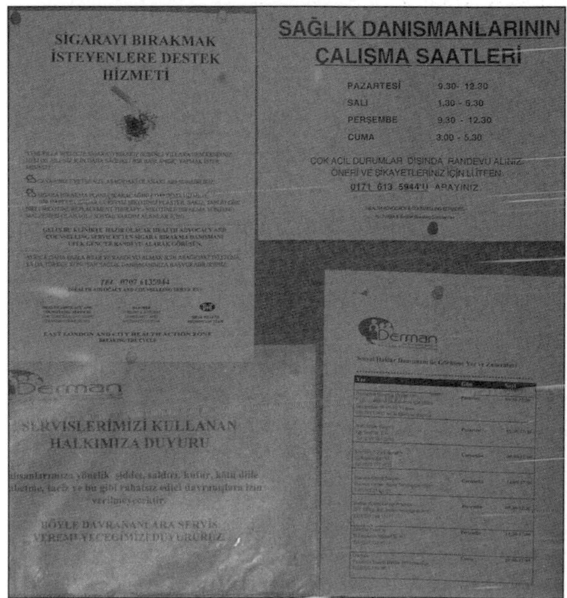

Figure 5.1 • Health promotion literature in different languages.

However, James (1995) spells out the health disadvantages that continue to encumber the black and minority ethnic population of the UK. The rates of ill-health and mortality in minority ethnic groups differ from those of the white population and differ between minority ethnic groups themselves. Black and minority ethnic communities face additional disadvantages to those of the indigenous white population in that they are more likely to be concentrated in lower-paid occupations, are more likely to be unemployed, are more likely to live in poor housing and have access only to schools that are poorly equipped. Box 5.1 lists disadvantages that have been identified in terms of health.

James (1995) and Nazroo & Smith (in Macbeth & Shetty 2001) identified some major influences on health and illness in these particular cultural groups. We need better understanding of the aetiology of illness in these groups and among all minority ethnic populations within the UK. It is not enough to say 'it is cultural differences'. This is a view echoed by Macbeth & Shetty (2001) in the introduction to their book 'Health and Ethnicity'. This book aims to 'explain the diversity in "biomedically" measurable health conditions due to determinants and factors that can be called ethnic', and acknowledges that, although we explain ideas of illness and health within a Western biomedical model, 'this in itself is a cultural phenomenon'.

Box 5.1

Health disadvantages of black and minority ethnic populations in the UK

- *Perinatal mortality*: higher among babies born to African-Caribbean-born and Pakistani-born women (Balajajan 1993, Department of Health 2003).
- *Congenital abnormality*: higher rates among Asian infants (Balajajan & Raleigh 1993).
- *Coronary heart disease*: higher mortality in people from the Indian subcontinent than other racial/ ethnic groups (Balajajan & Raleigh 1993, Department of Health 2003).
- *Hypertension, cerebrovascular accident*: higher prevalence among people from the Caribbean, Asia and African countries (Balajajan & Raleigh 1993, Department of Health 2003).
- *Diabetes*: the incidence among people from the Indian subcontinent can be four times higher than among the UK white population (Department of Health 2003).
- *Mental health*: suicide rates among young Asian women and diagnosis of schizophrenia in men of African-Caribbean origin are higher than the national average (Balajajan & Raleigh 1993, Department of Health 2003).
- *Cancer and palliative care*: services are accessed less frequently by minority ethnic groups (Department of Health 2003).
- *Dental health*: children in all minority ethnic groups, especially Pakistani and Bangladeshi children, are less likely to have visited a dentist (Department of Health 2003).
- *Smoking*: rates are higher among minority ethnic men, including black and Irish, and especially Bangladeshi men (Department of Health 2003).

Defining health

Lewis in Macbeth & Shetty (2001) discusses the meaning of health in a cultural context and makes the important point that in some cultures it is not possible to find a word that means the same as health. If the word 'health' is not translatable into another culture's language, then this has crucial implications for that culture's understanding of what health means to them in the context of the UK health care system. Indeed, even in English, there is confusion about the term health. As Lewis points out, it can include illness, and it is said that the NHS is a misnomer since it is mainly about the treatment of illness and disease.

When it was founded in 1948, the World Health Organization took its definition of health to be 'a state of complete physical, mental and social well-being, and not merely the absence of disease or infirmity'. This is such a lofty ideal and is probably unattainable, representing a wish rather a reality. The ancient Greeks defined health as the four body humours (blood, yellow bile, black bile and phlegm) in balance; a biomedical definition would centre around the concept of perfect homeostasis.

It is clear, however, that health means many different things to people of the same and different cultures, and this causes problems when trying to define and provide interventions for illness and disease, as well as health promotion initiatives. Defining illness and disease is problematical too. If someone has diabetes, there is a lack of the glucose-controlling hormone insulin. Diabetes can thus be recognized as a hormone-deficiency disease, but does this make that person ill or unhealthy? Disease can be diagnosed by examining the results of minute changes in body biochemistry, yet that person may show no signs of illness and indeed will not feel 'ill'.

A couple longing for a child may need to embark on lengthy and expensive medical interventions to help them conceive. Are they ill? This question needs to be asked because it is only the NHS or a private health service that can provide the intervention necessary to assist conception.

The impact of Western beliefs on other cultures

The global spread of the Western biomedical view of health may have radically altered the perception of health and illness in other countries. As part of a medical team working for an international expedition in a jungle village in Peru in the 1980s, my medical colleague and I were able to persuade a family that saving up their hard earned cash to take their child to the USA for treatment would be to no avail, since even the advanced medical systems of the USA had no cure for microcephaly (congenitally small brain). This family had the view that Western medicine could provide a cure for literally everything, and this view was further supported by our presence in their village with our antibiotics, de-worming medicines, iron tablets and injections and powdered baby milk. Our primary aim and purpose was to provide medical care for expedition members, and I wonder now about the ethics of providing the indigenous population with a very limited amount of help for their acute problems. We were there for 6 months. Did we have a right to impose our health system on theirs, even if they did see it as superior and cure-all, and when we departed to leave them with nothing? Yet would we have accepted their health system had anything gone wrong with any of us? Probably not. The point is that there are so many different explanatory models worldwide for health and the causes of illness that the health care system in any one country cannot possibly encompass them all. Any system has to follow the prevailing medical culture, which in the UK NHS is the Western biomedical model. UK doctors and nurses will explain disease and illness and treatment and nursing care in predominantly biomedical terms. UK-educated nurses and doctors will not find this problematical, yet they may have to adapt their explanations for people from different cultures who have not been exposed to the UK health care system. However, Helman (1976), in 'Feed a cold and starve a fever', found that even the predominantly middle-class patients from outer London used in his research still explained their illnesses with reference to ancient Greek theories of hot and cold and the four humours (blood, black bile, yellow bile and phlegm).

Alternative beliefs about health care in the UK

The last 20 years or so have seen a significant growth in the UK of complementary and alternative approaches to medicine and health care. Complementary and alternatives are defined in the sense of their relationship to biomedicine. Thus, every town now appears to have its alternative health practice, such as homeopathy, osteopathy and chiropractic as alternatives to biomedical medical treatments, orthopaedics and physiotherapy. A complementary health practice may offer aromatherapy, reflexology and a massage as complementary to biomedicine, working alongside it to assist the healing process. Health systems from other countries are also in operation in the UK, such as Chinese herbal medicine and Ayurvedic approaches to health and illness care which originate from the Indian subcontinent. Although some alternative medicine may be available on the NHS (e.g. osteopathy), such approaches are characterized by their cost to the client at the point of delivery, in contrast to the NHS which is mainly free at the point of delivery. Although this situation is changing gradually, the problems of their acceptance in the UK are the continuing general antipathy of the health professions towards them and the fact that most (apart from osteopathy and chiropractic) are not currently regulated in the same way that the traditional biomedical professions are. However, this is changing and in a few years all the major therapies will only be practised legally by registered practitioners.

Why do people brought up in the Western culture of health and illness consult alternative and complementary practitioners and other sources of help? The answer has to be that for many people, especially those with long-term health problems, Western biomedicine does not meet their needs.

With these issues in mind there is much that nursing can do to acquire the knowledge and understanding to be culturally aware and to provide culturally sensitive and culturally competent care, as well as to acknowledge cultural diversity in health care.

Diversity and health care: empowering the NHS

Recognizing diversity

With the growth of the black and minority ethnic population in the UK and the understanding that the UK's indigenous population is culturally diverse, there has been a clear move in recent years to attempt to understand the cultural dimension of health and disease as well as an attempt to understand those issues to do with race and ethnic origin that impact upon a person's health. Thus government policy has moved towards creating a strong strategy to focus on equality and diversity within the NHS plan, both in terms of employment and in care delivery (Department of Health 2003). The NHS plan, which was published in 2000, deliberately set out to put patients and people at the core of the health service, and recognized the need to empower people to work differently to deliver services which the diverse community of the UK requires. Whilst much has been done to acknowledge equality and diversity issues in the NHS, the Department of Health concedes that there is still much that needs doing in this area. The Department of Health (2003) in defining equality and diversity states that equality is 'essentially about creating a fairer society where everyone can participate and has the opportunity to fulfil their potential'. Diversity is seen as the 'recognition and valuing of difference' where people are expected to participate in 'creating a working culture and practices that recognize, respect, value and harness difference for the benefit of the organization and the individual'. There is an emphasis on the valuing of difference that has not been stated in previous policy documents. It suggests recognition that differences make people unique and that commonalities 'connect us all for the benefit of the organization and the individual'. To reflect the changing mood towards equality and diversity in the UK, the government is seeking to merge a number of organizations – the Commission for Racial Equality (CRE, http://www.cre.gov.uk), the Equal Opportunities Commission (EOC) and the Disability Rights Commission (DRC) – into one body.

Quality aspects of supporting diversity

The NHS plan in terms of providing a quality service and promoting equality charges health and social care providers to make sure that:

- Public services are accessible and responsive to the needs of all users.
- All public sector bodies work to promote equality and work to eliminate discrimination, and that the public sector leadership implements such requirements.
- Employment strategies in the public sector promote equality and diversity.

To ensure there is a direct impact on improving patient care, the NHS is expected to invest in the training and development of its workforce in order to eliminate discrimination and harassment, to improve diversity and to improve the working lives of its employees. It is the job of local health service managers at the strategic level to ensure that these government imperatives are acted upon and that such ideas become translated into reality for patients and all workers in the health and social care sectors.

The NHS employs over 1.2 million people in its workforce (September 2002). Within such a large workforce we could expect to see a wide and representative distribution of the population as a whole with representation from across the full age range, equal distribution of both genders at all levels of the organization, a meaningful representation of workers from black and minority ethnic groups, workers who are disabled, workers from a number of different religious orientations, workers of various sexual orientations and workers from all kinds of families (Figure 5.2). The NHS plan states that, as an employer, the NHS is committed to equality and positive recognition of diversity, and seeks to attract people from a wide range of backgrounds and communities to work for it. It would seem unwise to establish 'quotas' for people of differing backgrounds to work for the NHS, but perusal of the statistics makes it clear that there is still much work to be done in the area of equality of opportunity. The employment statistics for the NHS workforce in 2002 indicates the following:

- 103 350 doctors.
- 367 520 qualified nursing and midwifery staff.
- 116 598 qualified scientific, therapeutic and technical staff.
- 15 609 qualified ambulance staff.

These people were supported by a further 689 364 staff working in support and other roles such as porters, cleaners, secretaries, managers, drivers.

The proportion of female medical staff working as consultants has grown in recent years from 17% in 1992 to 24% in 2002. The male/female ratio of medical students has changed over time so that now medical school intakes comprise about 51% women (see Activity 5.1). This increase in female doctors is an important factor in terms of choice for clients in the NHS. With policies that value diversity and insist on it being respected, the NHS should increasingly be able to accommodate such requests and requirements. Consider Case history 5.4, for example; how do you think Amina was able to cope with these two experiences of the health service? Or consider the case of John (Case history 5.5).

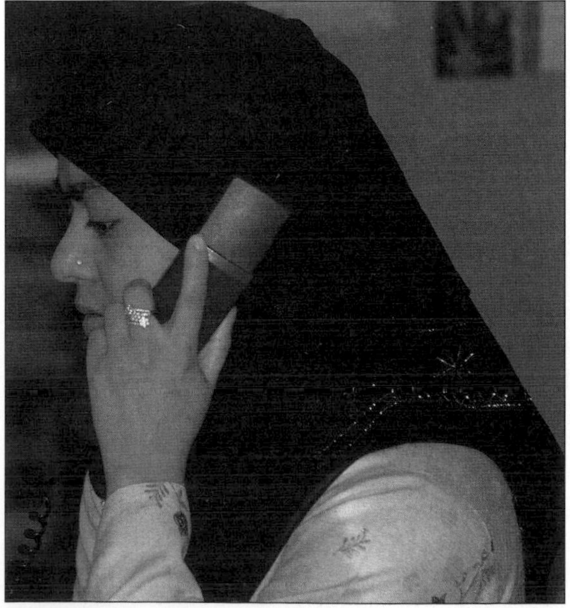

Figure 5.2 • A member of the health care team.

Activity 5.1

Think of the potential implications the changing ratio of female to male medical and nursing staff could have for health care service provision and the kinds of facilities that might need to be developed.

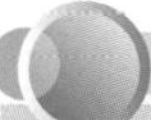

Case history 5.4

Amina

Amina is an 18-year-old Muslim woman who is expecting her first child. Her religion forbids her to be seen by any man other than her husband. During her antenatal care she is attended by a female midwife and her general practitioner (GP), who is male, but there is a female GP available. When Amina was admitted to hospital she was seen by a male obstetrician because there were no female obstetricians.

Later she was admitted for a surgical procedure and was seen by a female gynaecologist.

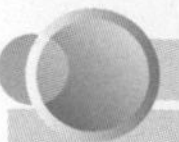

Case history 5.5

John

John is a 75-year-old who is having trouble passing urine. He has lived on his own since his wife died nearly 20 years ago. He is attended by a female nurse in the accident and emergency department, which he finds intensely embarrassing and asks if he can be attended by a male nurse.

Attitudes towards personal preferences and cultural expectations are gradually becoming recognized and are influencing how health care is delivered. Many people in the West who do not have religious grounds for seeking same-sex care are benefiting from the cultural understanding that is arising from our increasingly multicultural society.

Another approach to ensuring that policies relating to promoting diversity and equality are being respected is through collection of data about the ethnic origin of NHS staff by the government. Since 2001, staff appointed to the NHS have been asked to categorize themselves against a new list which for the first time includes those of mixed race background. The 2002 data indicate that 63% of newly employed NHS workers were white, 4% black, 22% Asian, 8% other ethnic groups, with 3% not stated.

Promoting diversity in nursing

Nursing is often seen as not being a suitable occupation by some minority ethnic groups. This has significant implications for the ability of the NHS to provide a service that supports such populations. The reasons for this attitude may go back to traditionally held values in a number of societies where nursing is considered as being 'dirty' work, and not having the same 'kudos' or status as medicine. Sadler (1999) reported on a project in a city in the north of England that looked at the reasons why specific minority ethnic groups did not apply for nursing training and sought to encourage applications from these groups so that the workforce could become more representative of the local population. Interviews with sixth formers, health care students, parents and careers advisers indicated that there were a number of negative attitudes held about nursing, including subservience to doctors, low pay, hard work but mentally unstimulating, the 'bedpan' image. For some they saw a conflict between the requirement of wearing uniforms and religious requirements, such as wearing the hijab to cover hair, and the issue of nursing men. Measures were put into place to increase knowledge and awareness among the target population and to help people gain the relevant qualifications for entry to nurse training. These initiatives met with success in increasing the number of Asian school leavers coming forward for nurse training. The local NHS trust and the local community hopefully will now benefit in the future from a workforce that is more representative of the local population.

Quality and professional implications of gender preference

Nursing has traditionally attracted more women than men, and the number of men in training has not varied much over time. The traditional Western view is that nursing is 'women's work', and it is sad to report that common stereotypes of men in nursing are still popularly held. Research carried out in Canada (Evans 2002) indicated that prevailing gender stereotypes of men as aggressively sexual, or gay, 'negatively influence the ability of male nurses to develop comfortable and trusting relationships with their patients'. Clearly this has not deterred men seeking to train for the nursing profession, yet there is still much work to be done in challenging such prevailing stereotypes. Chur-Hansen (2002), in her research in Australia, looked at patient preferences for female and male nurses, and concluded that situations in which patients prefer a male or female nurse are not clear, and that the degree of intimacy in a clinical situation was found to be predictive of same-gender preferences. This is where both male and female nurses find themselves in a dilemma. If a female nurse senses that a male patient is uncomfortable with her care, is the answer to ask a male colleague to take over? If a male nurse senses a female patient's discomfort, should he ask a female colleague? This is where a balance between meeting a patient's needs and acknowledging one's own sensitivities is important. If nurses aspire to ensuring that patients have choice, then there should be no hesitation in asking a nurse of the patient's gender to take over. The 'Nursing and Midwifery Council Code of professional conduct' says that you must recognize and respect the role of patients and clients as partners in their care and the contribution they can make to it.

> *This involves their preferences regarding care, and respecting these within the limits of professional practice, existing legislation, resources and the goals of the therapeutic relationship.*

This can be interpreted that a request or implied preference for a same-sex nurse should be acted upon, but only insofar as professional practice or resources will allow. Any patient has the right to refuse care and the Code of professional conduct, Clause 3, makes it clear that consent must be obtained (including consent by cooperation) before a nurse gives any treatment or care. Nurses should always seek advice from others if they find themselves in delicate situations where a patient refuses care from them because of their gender. It can be argued that the provision of gender-sensitive care is about the provision of culturally sensitive care as well. Culture in this instance is seen in the sense of the differing worlds of men and women, as well as in the more traditional sense.

In terms of gender, it is crucial that we seek to treat men and women as equal in the provision of health care. One area where this aspect is acknowledged as being unmet is in the 'gendering of coronary heart disease'. Lockyer & Bury (2002), in a literature review, suggest that, for various reasons, less attention has been paid to women's risk and occurrence of coronary heart disease (CHD) than to men's risk and occurrence. This has implications for nurses and other health professionals who may view women as lower risk, and it has also influenced such things as the provision of coronary rehabilitation programmes which are predicated upon male needs. When research done on men is applied to women, it may ignore specific needs related to being female and experiencing CHD. Lockyer & Bury stress that women are less likely to be referred for investigative tests, are diagnosed later and are less likely to be recommended for surgery. The idea of 'gender-neutral' care put forward by Lockyer & Bury means that nurses make decisions about caring for women with CHD based on their knowledge and experience of caring for men with CHD. Women's needs are therefore not being met.

Quality and ethnicity in patient care

The government's diversity agenda seeks to improve patient care, citing its own report 'Study of black, Asian and ethnic minority issues'. This report indicated clearly that inequalities in health and social care in terms of access, treatment and outcomes were due in no small part to the persistence of discrimination and harassment in the NHS. The NHS is therefore seeking to make a clear link between performance in delivering high standards of care and in supporting diversity. A study cited by the Department of Health ('The business of diversity') indicated that 80% of organizations that had made significant progress in delivering equality and diversity were also high performers. They had systematically integrated equality and diversity values into their business cultures, with success identified as being due to good leadership, the existence of corporate values, identifying people with responsibility for diversity, supporting and training staff and ensuring that diversity is a thread running through all corporate activity. The NHS aspires to this high performance, but a huge organization of such complexity and diversity will inevitably experience problems in reaching such a goal. It is incumbent on each individual worker in any health care organization, from the most experienced and senior of consultants, nurse managers or chief executives to the newest student nurse or medical records clerk, to work towards the promotion of equality and diversity. For nurses, much of this lies in the provision of excellent quality nursing care based upon the principles enshrined in the 'NMC Code of professional conduct', which says that:

you are personally accountable for ensuring that you promote and protect the interests and dignity of patients and clients, irrespective of gender, age, race, ability, sexuality, economic status, lifestyle, culture and religious or political beliefs.

This can be seen as the provision of culturally competent care. Consider Case history 5.6, which illustrates the importance of every member of our health care society having a good understanding of people's values and beliefs. The rest of this chapter will explore the issue of culturally competent care, and conclude with some ideas for good nursing practice in the area of transcultural care.

Culture and nursing care

McGee (1992) tells us that it was Florence Nightingale who first articulated the need for nursing care to take into account the cultural dimension of a society. Nightingale asserted that women who chose to work in India must know the language, religions, superstitions and customs of the women they cared for. However, it is only in the last few years that this cultural dimension to nursing care has begun to be addressed in nursing textbooks and in nurse education programmes. For many practitioners, this still represents a gap in their knowledge, and unfortunately many nurses continue to think that it is enough to provide care that

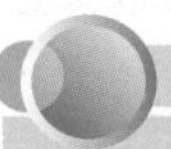

Case history 5.6

Symbols of faith

In the operating theatre it is the responsibility of the whole operating team to ensure that the privacy and dignity of patients are maintained while they are anaesthetized, during surgery and in recovery afterwards. Jay Singh was a Sikh gentleman in his thirties who underwent surgery to his knee following a sports injury. A devout observer of his faith, he was wearing his kacchera (undershorts) and kara (steel bangle) when he arrived in the anaesthetic room. The other symbols of his faith he had allowed to be removed and placed in the care of his relatives before he left the orthopaedic ward.

The theatre staff were uncertain about the procedures to follow in respect of these religious symbols of faith. Should they tape the kara as would be done for a wedding ring or should they remove it after the anaesthetic had been given? It is certainly permissible in operating theatre practice to tape the bangle to the wrist, although care should be taken not to damage it or apply tape directly to hirsute skin. There was no necessity in this instance to remove the bangle. If the patient was having major surgery involving the insertion of intravenous lines or if the wrist was swollen or injured it would be permissible to remove it, but the patient's consent should always be obtained in advance where possible.

Comments and discussion

After Jay was moved onto the operating table, a member of the theatre staff started to remove the kacchera. Is removal of this garment appropriate in these circumstances?

It would be wrong to remove the garment fully, and the theatre team should ensure it is wrapped loosely around the ankle of the non-operated leg. The whole theatre team are responsible in that each should be aware of the patient's cultural background. Problems may arise in situations where Sikh patients are incontinent as their garments will clearly become soiled. It is always best to ask the patient directly in these circumstances what they would like to happen. If the patient is unable to decide for any reason, the nurse can approach the relatives.

It is important to maintain a patient's dignity in respect of his religious belief when he is unconscious and not aware of what is happening. Religious expression is a fundamental aspect of culture and a person is religious even if they are unconscious. If health care students and professionals do not attempt to assist patients to adhere to their own beliefs and expression of faith when unconscious, then they are only paying lip-service to good practice in transcultural care.

is 'individualized'. By declaring that 'I treat everyone equally' or 'I treat everyone as an individual' might imply that I have not thought through the special needs of that person in relation to their cultural background. It is worth considering how your own beliefs and values could differ from those of someone from a different culture. Consider the questions posed in Box 5.2; then consider Amina's response to these questions.

Box 5.2

Differences in beliefs and values across cultures

Consider your response to the following questions

- How do your beliefs about *hygiene* influence your approach to washing and eating?
- How do your beliefs about *fasting* influence your approach to someone who prefers not to eat during daylight?
- How do your beliefs about *death* and the *care of the body and soul* influence how you care for a dying or a dead person?

Amina's response to these questions

As a Muslim we have very strict rules about hygiene and hand-washing before eating as well as before praying. We use running water to wash with and so in our homes we do not have sinks with a plug. Bathing is not part of my culture; we prefer to take a shower as we believe it to be more hygienic. We use the left hand for cleaning activities, including using toilet paper. The right hand is only used for clean activities, such as eating, so it is important that the right hand is always free to do this otherwise it will feel horrid if I have to use my left hand.

Every year at the time of Ramadan we fast during daylight hours. This means nothing to eat or drink. Of course, the elderly, weak and sick people are exempt as well as women who are pregnant or who are menstruating. But many people prefer to fast. We make sure that we eat at dusk. We believe that this form of self-discipline is good for the body as well as the soul. I am teaching my children to get into the habit of fasting during Ramadan. At the end of Ramadan we have a big celebration with our family and friends and lots of different foods to eat.

The International Council of Nurses' 'Code for Nurses' (ICN 1974) states that the need for nursing is universal. Inherent in nursing is respect for life, dignity and the rights of man. It is unrestricted by considerations of nationality, race, creed, colour, age, sex, politics or social status. It was Leininger (1991) who first put forward a model for cultural aspects of caring. She coined the phrases 'transcultural' and 'cross-cultural' in referring to the fusion of nursing and anthropology. She felt that anthropology had a significant contribution to make to modern nursing. She argued that, just as a patient's culture influences their own beliefs about health and illness, so a health professional's cultural background will influence his or her own beliefs and values about illness states and how they are managed, and about health and how it is maintained. Transcultural care has been in existence for as long as nursing has. Anyone who gives care to another person does so in the context of the cultures from which they both come. Sometimes that may be the same culture; sometimes it may be different cultures. In any nurse–patient interaction there can be misunderstanding as well as understanding; some misunderstandings may be based on cultural issues. What has happened in recent years is that cultural issues in health care have become more clearly articulated. The need for increased cultural awareness and understanding, awareness of racial and ethnic group issues, and race discrimination have become important items on the modern health care agenda.

Transcultural care

Andrews & Boyle (1995) represent transcultural care as a synthesis of nursing concepts and other borrowed concepts, suggesting the following:

- Caring exists in all cultures.
- The way in which caring is carried out is culture-specific.
- The meaning of caring varies cross-culturally.
- What constitutes care varies cross-culturally.
- Where care matches client expectations, the more accepted it will be.

They suggest that caring in a transcultural sense is concerned with shared meanings and the degree to which carer and client agree or disagree on the cultural symbols of health, illness, disease and caring. These meanings are said to influence all carer–client interactions.

For effective transcultural care, a nurse needs basic knowledge of how different cultural groups define and treat illness, promote and maintain health, prevent illness and structure their health care systems (see, for example, Henley & Schott 1999). Many authors have articulated their own beliefs about what constitutes transcultural care. Andrews & Boyle (1995) see transcultural care as a fundamental element of all care, not just care given to minority ethnic groups and foreign populations. The nurse skilled in transcultural care techniques will possess sophisticated assessment and analytical skills, will plan care with sensitivity to an individual's culture and will implement interventions that are culturally relevant and acceptable. In fact, all nurses and health professionals should aspire to be culturally aware and seek to become skilled in delivering culture-sensitive care. Such a person as a 'transcultural nurse' should not exist, because this emphasizes difference and suggests that the transcultural nurse should be 'consulted' when a patient from a different cultural group to that of the health professional is being cared for. So transcultural and culturally competent care must not be just about how white people look after black people, and it is not just about the care of minority ethnic groups. Leininger's (1991) view that 'every nurse comes from a particular group . . . and we cannot come to a care situation free from our religious, social and cultural influences' is important in understanding our own communication processes in a health care context. People are not always aware of the extent to which these influences operate in their daily lives, and see themselves as possessing 'normal' thoughts and behaviours. This can lead to the 'pathologizing of culture', which is when cultural expression itself is seen as abnormal in a health context.

Abdullah (1995) agrees with this view, stating that caring involves the intellectual analytical ability of the nurse to relate relevant and culturally appropriate knowledge in the delivery of effective care. Providing quality individualized patient care cannot be achieved without considering the context of the client as a whole person and factors associated with their personal being such as culture, belief and tradition. This means that each nurse has to think about his or her interactions with patients from all kinds of cultures and backgrounds, and has a responsibility to learn about a patient's culture.

Herberg (1995) states that transcultural care is concerned with the provision of care in a manner that is sensitive to the needs of individuals, families and groups who represent diverse cultural populations within a society. Developing cultural sensitivity is something that comes with the experience of meeting people from diverse backgrounds and acknowledging that there is a need to learn, and then to use that learning in an appropriate way. Nurses and other health professionals therefore need to understand the variables in people's behaviours, such as differences in values, religion, dietary belief and practices, social hierarchical structure, family patterns, and beliefs and practices related to health and illness, if they are to begin the process of offering culturally sensitive care. DeSantis (1994) goes further and suggests that nurses need more than cultural sensitivity. They need competence in the use of culture.

Koskinen & Tossavainen (2004) reported on a programme to learn intercultural competence by a period of study abroad. Such 'elective' placements have been used by many nursing schools in the UK to give students insight into other cultures, and many medical students undertake a period of clinical placement overseas or in another part of the UK. The effectiveness of such placements as a way of gaining intercultural competence has not been evaluated extensively. British-born nurses are often hampered by the fact that they are not fluent in the language of the country they choose to go to, and rely on the ability of the local nurses and patients to speak to them in English, which for someone who is ill seems hardly fair. Koskinen & Tossavainen reported on the experiences of Finnish students coming to the UK. These students found the experience to be a major culture shock, citing language problems, loneliness, isolation and homesickness as serious difficulties. They needed much 'emotional resilience to respond effectively to the shock of intercultural immersion'. My own experiences of supporting students involved in an exchange programme with Swedish students echo Koskinen's & Tossavainen's findings. Additionally, it would be impossible for *all* students to undertake such programmes because of availability, cost or family and personal ties, and the profession needs to seek alternative ways to develop intercultural competence.

It is also important for the NHS and the nursing profession to consider how to support nurses from other countries who come to the UK to work. Staff shortages in the NHS have encouraged many trusts to recruit from overseas, and while for some adaptation may be relatively simple, for others it is not. Gerrish & Griffith (2004) stated that industrialized nations, including our own, who recruit from the global health market need to invest in providing support to enable overseas nurses to adapt to working in a different health care system and social and cultural context. Between the years 2000 and 2002, over 14000 overseas-trained nurses entered the register in the UK. Whilst many were from developed nations, it could be considered unethical to recruit from the less well-developed nations as it deprives them of their trained nursing workforce. It is important to note that differences in the role of the nurse were potent factors in determining how successful overseas nurses were at adapting to UK culture. Technical procedures were likely to be less stressful for these nurses than, for example, managing a patient's discharge home. Transcultural care has thus taken on an additional dimension since the growth of overseas nurses entering the register.

Providing transcultural care

Transcultural care is the integration of the concept of culture into all aspects of nursing and the provision of health care. In terms of nursing care it is the ability to step out of or suspend one's own cultural traditions (values, beliefs and practices) in order to try and perceive the situation as others do. DeSantis suggests that transcultural care includes several components; these are discussed below.

Nurse–patient negotiation

If a nurse makes all the decisions about the care to be provided for individual patients this inevitably means that the patient's needs are viewed from the nurse's own cultural perspective. This may not be appropriate for that patient's care. Many patients may be content for the nurse to make a large number of decisions about care on their behalf. If this is the case, the nurse and patient should first agree that this is acceptable to the patient.

Simultaneous dual ethnocentrism

What do we understand by the term 'dual ethnocentrism' and why is it important? Culture always operates, is always present and always influences what patients and nurses do in any health care encounter. We all make judgements according to our own belief systems, which in turn are culturally determined. The concept of dual ethnocentrism makes nurses aware that everybody operates under the influence of their own specific culture. Nurses can then begin to appreciate the culture of the 'other', and can then attempt to use aspects of the patients belief system in mutually acceptable care interventions.

Multiple cultural contexts and clinical realities exist in the nurse–patient encounter.

Each nursing care encounter is the interaction of three cultures:

- The nurse's professional culture.
- The patient's interpretation of the health care system based upon their culture.
- The context in which the nurse–patient encounter takes place (institution, home, surgery).

If we accept the above premise, then it allows us to understand that there are multiple realities operating simultaneously in all health care situations.

Patients are cultural informants

The nurse can help the patient to explore their own meaning of the health care situation during, for example, the assessment process. Part of this is for the health professional to assess matters such as a patient's beliefs and understanding about health and sickness. These personal explanatory models will influence how each patient may hold different explanations about the same signs and symptoms, as each culture puts its own meaning on health and illness events. The patient is the authority on their own culture, and the nurse must take what the patient says about this culture as correct for that patient. By acknowledging that each individual is a unique product of their own culture, with a unique perception of their own health and illness experiences, their uniqueness can be incorporated into the health care encounter.

The cultural dimension is fundamental to the nature of nursing

When culture is seen as something separate to be assessed, the cultural dimension of care can be incorporated into the nursing process in a more routine way. But using a separate cultural assessment tool only when there are distinct ethnic/racial/cultural/religious aspects of an individual may make culture a distinctive factor rather than something that affects every individual in everything that they do.

To become competent in acknowledging and drawing on cultural factors, nurses need to be able to:

- Recognize the limitations that their own cultural values, beliefs and practices can impose upon them.
- Be open to cultural differences.
- Have a patient/client-oriented focus.
- Use cultural knowledge and resources to address health care problems.

Recognizing your own cultural perspective, especially if you are part of a dominant or majority culture, is important. Realizing that life may be different for others may be hard to acknowledge for some nurses. It may be that the nurse working with a transcultural perspective is one who has studied other cultures in depth and understands their differences and the specific needs of people using health care services. Nurses may function as 'cultural brokers', who strive to perceive the situation from the patient's perspective, compare it to their own and mediate between the two cultures to produce interventions that are mutually agreed and appropriate to the care situation. Nurses must always scrutinize their own beliefs and practices in relation to those of their patient. In this way nurses' own cultural beliefs are brought further into their consciousness. Consider Case history 5.7.

Making transcultural care a reality

Tripp-Reimer & Brink (1984) suggest that 'cultural brokerage' provides the way for nurses and other health professionals to carry out transcultural care. This includes the ideas described below, and could form the basis of a cultural dimension to the assessment and planning stages of the nursing process.

- An assessment should be carried out of how the patient and family understand the current health care problem and intended treatment.
- There should be a comparison of the nurse's and patient's perspectives.

The nurse can explain and interpret medical and nursing care for the patient, and is able to take into account the patient's own explanatory model. The result of this is an effective working partnership, with both the nurse and the patient understanding each other's perspective. There may be occasions when nurse and patient cannot find mutually acceptable understanding, and nursing interventions are not possible. If neither is able to find solutions the nurse has the responsibility to compromise, but such problems should be referred to appropriate sources of help. No nurse need feel that he or she is without peer or manager support in difficult situations. Each party must abide by the solutions and monitor progress. If no compromise is possible, the patient has the absolute right to decide on what health care measures to take, although there may be legal and ethical reasons why this may not be appropriate in specific incidences.

Onward referral must be used when no compromise is possible or when the nurse feels unable to accept the patient's decision. This is the nurse's

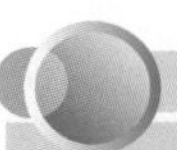

Case history 5.7

A child in pain

A situation occurred on a children's ward in a large inner-city hospital where a student nurse and a staff nurse were caring for a small boy of Afro-Caribbean origin. Jackson Browne, aged 5 years, had been admitted with a sickle cell crisis precipitated by a high temperature during a viral infection. The student nurse observed that Jackson seemed to be in severe pain and was visibly distressed, and approached her mentor to administer the prescribed analgesia. When the mentor and student returned to the child, his parents had arrived. When discovering the student and mentor were about to administer analgesia, the boy's parents refused to allow them to do so, indicating vociferously that it was not part of their beliefs to allow this, as children in their family had to learn how to bear pain. An altercation ensued between the staff nurse and parents, and Jackson became further distressed. The student made valiant efforts to soothe Jackson who was crying with pain and the distress at seeing his parents angry. The ward manager was forced to intervene and eventually Jackson received the analgesic and calm was restored to the parents, nurses and the child.

Comments and discussion

Sickle cell anaemia affects people of West African, Afro-Caribbean, Cypriot, South Asian and Middle Eastern origin, among others, and is caused by an abnormality in the structure of the red blood cells. This abnormality means that the cells can change shape from round to sickle-shaped. When sickle-shaped, the red cells block the peripheral venous system, causing occlusion and often very severe pain. Such a sickle cell crisis, when many of the red blood cells change shape, can be precipitated by any number of reasons, including infection, dehydration and sudden stress, both physical and psychological.

This situation raises many issues to do with ethics, consent to treatment, management of pain, perceptions of suffering and intercultural communication. Often, the opposite of this situation is found, with patients in sickle cell crisis often undermedicated in terms of analgesia. Many studies have found that people suffering from sickle cell crises are thought to be exaggerating their pain and so receive a lesser amount of pain medication. Underusage of pain medication causes distrust, anxiety, fear and resentment in affected patients and this is not exclusive to any particular cultural or ethnic group.

In Jackson Browne's situation, the family culture, in which a stoical response to pain was valued by the parents, clashed with the institutional culture of the hospital and the children's ward philosophy of care. It is important for families to be involved in care decisions about their children and good communication is essential when dealing with families in such instances. A children's nurse sometimes needs to be an advocate for the child, even when advocating for the child against its parents. Whilst we acknowledge that parents most often know what is best for their child, in this situation the nurses felt that they could not leave the child to suffer.

There are support organizations for people and families with sickle cell disease and a similar related condition known as thalassaemia, and it is often helpful to put families in touch with these organizations. You can find the addresses of two organizations at the end of the chapter. Many hospitals located in areas of the UK where sickle cell disease and thalassaemia are common, employ specialist nurses to advise and counsel patients and their families.

responsibility. The patient also has the right to seek assistance elsewhere.

Some dilemmas in respecting cultural perspectives and values

Practising with this kind of open, non-judgmental approach to care can be challenging for a nurse. This often has to do with ethical issues. For example, some religions such as Jehovah's Witnesses, may object to a blood transfusion, and it is hard for nurses to see a patient exsanguinate before their eyes when a blood transfusion would save that life. If that patient is a child, it is harder still. However, for the family of the child, it could be so shocking that blood had been given that they can no longer accept the child as part of their family, and the child faces social death as a result of the decision to give a blood transfusion. Much transcultural care literature seems to imply that nursing and caring must be value-free and non-judgemental, but this dehumanizes nurses and other health professionals as no one individual can be forced to be all-accepting. In such cases, nurses and doctors may feel more comfortable with the decisions about care and treatment being taken by a court of law. However, nurses can allow themselves to intervene directly in other situations. For example, if a parent hits a child in hospital (even if physical chastisement is part of the family or group culture), a nurse can remonstrate with the parent. Also, in the UK, nurses can register a conscientious objection to abortion and not take part in such a procedure, even though it may be allowed legally.

Mediating care delivery

DeSantis (1994) suggests that brokerage has three forms:

- It focuses on patients to help them cope with the health care situation.
- It focuses on practitioners to assist them to provide care in a culturally acceptable and appropriate way.
- It provides for a mediation between patients and practitioners who have different health care orientations.

The end-point of brokerage may be simply an understanding of another person's point of view.

Nursing therefore needs to incorporate cultural assessment devices into nursing assessment. There are some examples of specific cultural assessment devices around, but these are often unwieldy and, although being comprehensive, are perhaps of little value clinically. They also tend to be separate from other assessment tools and may just be providing one more form to be filed away in a patient's notes.

Nursing also needs theory and concepts related to the issue of culture and care. No longer is it enough merely to exhort nurses to be culturally aware and give culturally sensitive care, or to present inventories of cultural practices, as this promotes a recipe approach to care. Such theories and concepts include understanding of the differences between culture and ethnicity. Culture is the observable factors such as food, dress, language, values and beliefs. Ethnicity refers to a subjective perspective of one's own heritage and to a sense of belonging to a group that identifies itself and is identified by others as distinguishable from other groups. Culture therefore includes those things about the ethnicity of the person. There needs to be a balance between knowledge that is ethno-specific, and the introduction of concepts, which are useful in an understanding of people across cultures. There is a need to have an understanding of how cultural bias may make interventions less effective as well as an understanding of approaches that can be used to make health care interventions more effective. A goal for transcultural nursing care could thus be described: 'To provide care that is relevant and culturally acceptable to patients'. However, it is important that care is culturally acceptable to the nurse as well as to the client.

Care within a nursing framework

Most nursing models and theories mention the importance of understanding a patient's social background; we could take this to mean their cultural background. The model of Roper, Logan and Tierney (see Roper et al 1996) – a model of nursing based on a model of living – recognizes that there is a social element to each of the activities of living. The activities that are socially based (working and communication, for example) have more overt emphasis, but it is nevertheless important to recognize that physiological activities of living such as breathing, eliminating and eating and drinking also have clear-cut sociocultural elements. This approach however, makes it easy to slip into a reductionist approach, whereby we ask questions such as 'What do different cultures eat?' We may end up, therefore, with statements such as 'Jews don't eat pork', and hold this as an uncontested belief. This could lead the nurse into difficult situations such as that described by Henley & Schott (1999), who cite a Jewish patient who recalled being 'told off' by a nurse for eating ham; in fact, he chose not to be an observant Jew, and he was stunned at the nurse's comment. This kind of stereotyping means that descriptions of cultural norms are not always helpful when it comes to offering culturally sensitive care. On the other hand, ignorance of dietary rules can also cause difficult situations. A nurse who opened the packaging on a Kosher meal for an observant Jewish patient did not understand that she had acted inappropriately and did not appreciate the patient's annoyance at having to wait for another meal to be delivered to the ward.

Leininger's 'sunrise' model (Figure 5.3) attempts to depict her theory of cultural care universality and diversity, and offers perhaps a wider perspective than models such as that of Roper et al. However, models such as this look very complex, so we may tend to lose sight of their intention and may have difficulty in understanding exactly what it is they are meant to depict and convey.

It may be a useful exercise for you to look at a number of different nursing models and try to tease out the cultural element in each of them. Most have something to say about 'social' influences. Human societies are clearly complex structures, but we need a simple model that puts culture into an appropriate context and to see how it affects the nurse–patient relationship.

A simple model (Figure 5.4) for examining culture and its relationship to nursing care takes on board all the necessary factors. This model offers a concept of transcultural care in which it can be seen that the nurse–patient relationship is at the core of nursing care. The assessment component of the nursing process is a key factor, and both patient and nurse bring their own personal cultural experiences to the encounter. This model can be applied to any 'health' or 'illness' event.

Littlewood (1989), in discussing the link between nursing and anthropology, said that anthropology might be more useful in terms of nurses' understanding of patients' subjective worlds than, for example, knowing about physiology. Western systems of healing place primacy on a biological understanding of disorders. Nursing could be a very powerful force and try to supplement this understanding by seeing things more from the patient's viewpoint, recognizing that illness is both physically and socially disruptive. This suggests that nurses could begin to incorporate the patient's own explanatory models of illness into their own assessment of the patient. Rather than just ask the patient for their understanding (which may or may not fit into the nurse's preconceived notions) the nurse could ask the patient, for example, 'How will you know when you are healed (or better)?' Models of illness (even simple things such as coughs and colds) are in general culturally determined.

Is there a problem with transcultural care?

There is a real danger that ethnospecific or culture-specific care can lead to over-generalization and making assumptions about individuals' health practices that can result in cultural stereotyping. There is some fear, therefore, that transcultural care may reinforce the very problem of paternalism and ethnocentric care that it seeks to address. Some nurses may feel that, if they offer 'individualized' care, they offer 'culture-sensitive' care. These 'transcultural nurses' may be so bound up with their own beliefs and values in offering such care that they cease to be sensitive to anything other than their own belief and value system. Some nurses may project their own cultural expectations as they attempt to offer culture-sensitive care, making it difficult, if not impossible, for the patient to express their own ways of thinking and behave as they would do normally.

Culture is not static; it is a dynamic process and within any one culture the experience of the individual varies and changes with time. There may be a danger in providing culture-specific care as it may divert attention away from the uniqueness of the individual.

Mason, in her 1990 research, compared mothers in Jamaica and Northern Ireland and found no causal relationship between cultural background and maternal behaviour. Differences between women's experiences of motherhood within the two cultures were just as great as those between the two cultures. There is an argument, therefore, that to draw up a list of culture-specific practices is not appropriate because of the huge variation within a culture as well as between cultures. There may actually be very little that we can recognize as culture-specific.

Mason (1990) warns us that we should not make gross generalizations about people based on

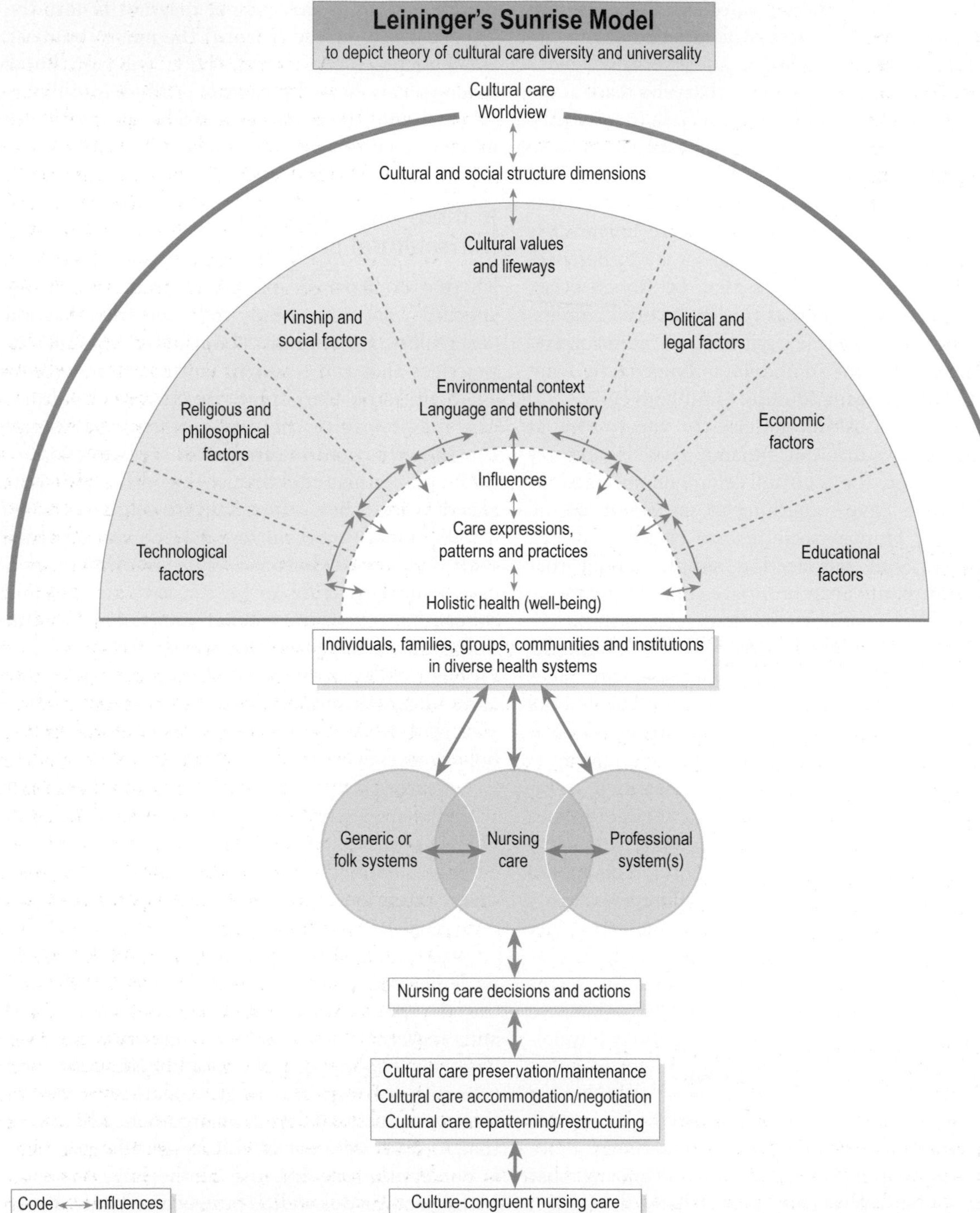

Figure 5.3 • Leininger's 'sunrise' model of transcultural care. (Reproduced with permission from Leininger 1991.)

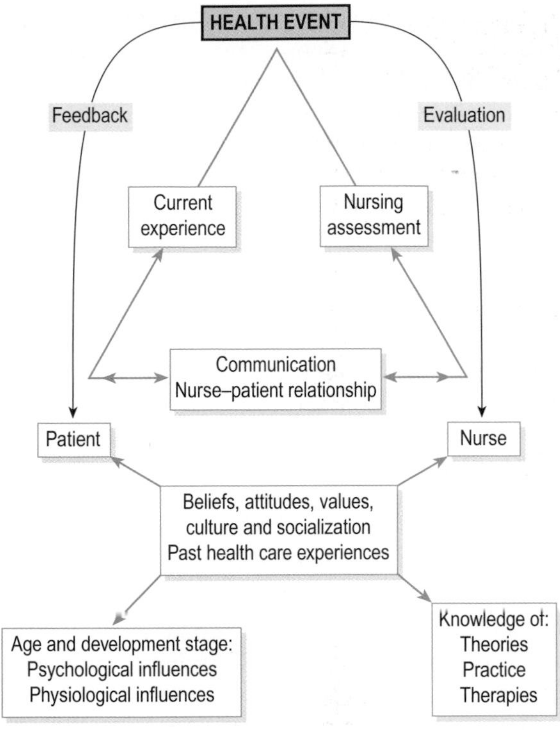

Figure 5.4 • A simple model to depict the influence of culture on the nurse–patient relationship.

our preconceived notions of their 'culture'. If we do this we may be guilty of stereotyping and ignoring individual specific needs. Nurses may then run into the trap of further dividing cultures, and the usefulness of this is questionable. People are certainly 'cultural' beings, but it is not helpful always to view patients in this way; for example, a person in pain may simply need their pain relieved rather than have their pain behaviour interpreted as culturally determined.

Providing culture-sensitive care: an example from nursing practice (pain)

Pain is the most commonly occurring universal symptom of disease, illness and injury, and is the most frequent and compelling reason for seeking health care. Pain as a problem has exercised the minds of philosophers and medical men down the centuries, and still poses a problem for modern health care. It is a primary danger signal that all is not well with the body, and is a central perception not merely a primary sensory modality; that is, pain is felt with the whole being, and affects the way a person thinks, feels and behaves. It forces individuals to take note that something is amiss. From what we know of pain, the physiological mechanism does not vary widely from person to person or from culture to culture. What does vary considerably is the psychocultural component of pain, and this gives rise to many different pain behaviours across cultures. This makes pain a very difficult symptom for heath professionals to deal with.

Definitions of pain are culturally influenced, and its expectation, manifestations and management are all embedded in cultural contexts. So, not only should health professionals consider how they might conceptualize the importance of pain relief (based on physiology), they might also consider how they might understand the whole meaning of the pain experience for an individual based on that individual's psychosocial make-up.

Pain behaviour is the result of a complex physiological, psychological, social and cultural interaction, a concept put forward by Melzack & Wall (1988) as the 'gate control theory of pain'. In building upon Melzack and Wall's work, Bates (1987) suggests that pain behaviours are learned though two powerful psychosocial processes: that of social learning (Bandura 1977, cited in Bates 1987) and that of social comparison (Festinger 1954, cited in Bates 1987).

Social learning theory suggests that our behaviours in relation to entities such as pain are learned as we grow up in the social world by imitating the behaviours of others and by appropriate reinforcement of behaviour. For example, it is common in the UK for families to reinforce 'brave' pain behaviours in children, and this is likely to lead to stoic 'stiff upper lip' responses as adults.

Social comparison theory suggests that people are continually evaluating themselves and try to present themselves to others in the best way that they can. Thus, when a person is in pain, he or she will wish to behave in a way that is congruent with the rest of the social group. Thus, the behaviours related to pain in any one cultural group become the socially desirable behaviours (see Figure 5.5).

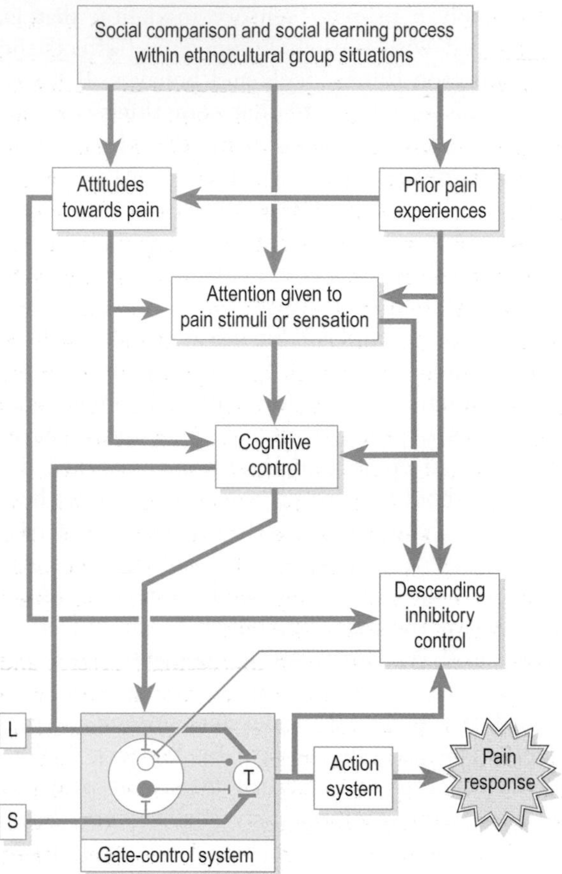

Figure 5.5 • A biocultural model of pain perception. L, large-diameter fibres; S, small-diameter fibres; T, transmission. (Reproduced with kind permission from Bates 1987.)

These biocultural theories lend support to the notion that we learn our pain behaviour as part of social learning, beginning in very early childhood, and by mechanisms of social comparison. That is, we continually compare our own behaviours in all sorts of situations to the behaviour that we observe in others; thus our pain behaviours will become the socially desired behaviours of our specific cultural group. Bates suggests that it is likely that the cultural group experience influences the psychophysiological processes responsible for pain thresholds (when a stimulus is reported as causing a pain sensation), perception of pain severity and pain response.

There have been numerous studies on pain behaviours and responses in different cultural groups over the last 50 years, but such studies are only of value if we use the results to make a difference in the understanding and management of pain. Knowledge of cross-cultural variations in pain behaviours only helps if such knowledge is used by health professionals in their assessment and treatment of pain. This kind of knowledge can be dangerous: it can lead to the stereotyping of people and their response to pain, and this in turn can detract us from an individualized plan of care for the person in pain. We must learn to accept intracultural variation as well as intercultural variation in all behaviours related to health and illness.

Some of the first cross-cultural research into pain was conducted by Zborowski in 1952. He looked at Americans of differing cultural backgrounds who were in hospital for a variety of health problems (herniated intravertebral discs, neurological disorders and other disorders). He found differences in pain behaviours between the cultural groups, but also similarities. Where there were similarities there were often different meanings ascribed to pain by the differing cultures. Two important features arise from Zborowski's study. First, those patients who made more complaints about their pain were often labelled as problem patients (Jewish and Italian people); second, those who tended to express their pain with minimal expression and were withdrawn were often labelled as 'model' patients (people of Irish, Anglo-Saxon and German origin). This demonstrates how culture can be damaging if nurses stereotype patients.

Just as patients have their own culturally determined pain behaviours, so too will nurses come to a patient encounter with their own culturally determined attitudes to people in pain. There is vast potential for culture clash here, with the result that pain can go unrelieved because the pain behaviour of a person from one culture is not recognized as such by the carer from another culture. Other cross-cultural research into pain has looked into this concept. Davitz et al (1976) conducted research on 554 nurses in six different countries to test their attitudes towards pain and suffering. They demonstrated that there were marked cross-cultural differences in the way nurses from different countries rated pain and distress, based on patient case studies. For example, Japanese and Korean nurses indicated that they believed the patients in the case studies suffered higher degrees of pain than did American and Puerto Rican nurses. American nurses scored the lowest ratings of patients' pain. Clearly, the implication here for nursing practice is that pain may go unrecognized and therefore unrelieved. The report of the Royal College of Surgeons (1990) on pain after surgery states that for pain to be unrelieved is bordering on professional negligence. We need, therefore, to construct pain assessment tools that can somehow take the cultural-behavioural element of pain into account, and make the nurse's assessment more objective and free from his or her own cultural influences. This is not likely to be an easy task. Henley & Schott (1999) indicate that a number of studies have shown that people experiencing pain from sickle cell crises are often thought to be exaggerating and so are given lower levels of pain relief than is required. It is important that, in those areas where the cultural make-up of the population would indicate a high likelihood of admission for sickle cell crises, there are protocols in place for the assessment and management of pain in this specific condition.

Other studies have found similar situations where there were differing perceptions of pain on part of the nurse and patient. Calvillo & Flaskerud (1993) compared Mexican and Anglo-Saxon American women's responses to cholecystectomy pain, and found that there was a huge gap between what patients said about their pain and what their nurses said. Nurses evaluated *all* pain as being less than the patients' evaluations of their own pain. This presents a powerful argument for changing current pain management regimes to put pain control into patients' hands. Pain is an intensely personal experience and it is simply not possible to experience another person's pain. Pain assessment is therefore very difficult.

Differing cultural backgrounds are therefore likely to produce differing pain behaviours; however, there is as much intracultural variation as there is intercultural variation. The cultural background of carers is an important determinant of inferences of pain and distress, and this in turn suggests that there is a need to assess pain and evaluate responses to pain therapies in relation to the ethnic and cultural background of the patient. There is a need to address methods of pain management for different cultural and ethnic groups, and nurses need to understand that differing cultures attach very different meanings to pain. In recent years, much work has gone on in trying to derive different methods of pain relief and some of this can be based on cross-cultural research. For example, acupuncture, a traditional Chinese approach to pain management, was for many years considered 'fringe' medicine. Since the 1970s, there has been a gradual acceptance of the efficacy of pain relief from acupuncture and it has now become a popular and effective method in the mainstream of modern medicine. Other methods from other cultures may well become accepted into Western medical thought.

With society becoming increasingly diverse and multicultural and with people from a wide range of ethnic origins, it is important that we understand how cultural factors influence pain experiences. Bates (1987) argues that we must pay attention to how people learn to think about pain, which she suggests is culturally determined. Bates also suggests that we need to pay attention to a whole host of other variables which will vary cross-culturally, such as attitudes, values and experiences, and look at how these influence psychological, verbal and behavioural responses to pain.

In terms of pain relief, Henley & Schott (1999) indicate that none of the major world religions forbids the use of analgesics, and this includes analgesics of the opiate group. In general, it seems that people in all religious groups agree that pain should be controlled or eliminated wherever possible. However, within any religion, members may feel that pain should be borne without complaint as it is sent from their God, or that the suffering of pain will offer atonement from sin. It can be difficult for nurses to 'stand by' and accept that the patient's choice may be to suffer pain.

Culture would appear to be inextricably intertwined with all aspects of an individual, including the suffering of and response to pain, and it cannot be ignored in the assessment and management of

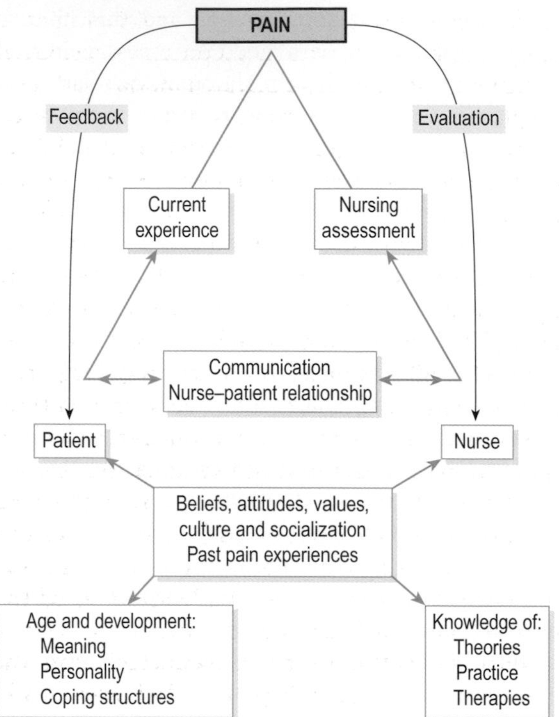

Figure 5.6 • Adaptation of Figure 5.4 to depict the influence of culture on the nurse–patient relationship when the patient is in pain.

pain. The model depicted in Figure 5.4 can also be adapted to represent a model for understanding the cultural influence in pain (Figure 5.6); this simple model can also hold true for many other health and illness events.

Good practice in transcultural care

It must be possible to determine what good practice in transcultural care should be. It should be based upon the key elements of knowing and understanding each patient's cultural background, the nurse's understanding of his or her own background, effective patient assessment, appropriate evaluation of care, the patient's own experience and good communication within an effective nurse–patient relationship.

This section is not intended to be an all-encompassing summary of what differing minority ethnic and cultural groups do in their everyday lives, nor will it provide all the answers for the nurse. There are many other texts that can do that. It is merely intended to give some examples of where the nurse can make a difference in the provision of care that is culturally sensitive.

Patient assessment

Nursing care plans will usually contain some kind of assessment tool which helps the nurse take a nursing history from the patient and identify problems that can be managed by nursing intervention. Such assessment tools could incorporate a cultural element, but the nurse has to be careful not make the questions asked seem unusual in any way. Cultural enquiry perhaps should become part of the norm for assessment. It is usual practice for a patient to be asked his or her religion; this may open the way for a nurse to enquire if that means anything specific in terms of, for example, food preferences and personal hygiene practices. Once the information is obtained it must be used. Vydelingum (2000) quotes South Asian patients in his study who felt that questions were asked only for the sake of the form being completed rather than seeking real information that could be used in the construction of a care plan.

Patients' explanatory models

Each person views their health situation from their own cultural background and experience. Nurses are uniquely placed to bridge the gap between the medical viewpoint and that of the patient. By placing emphasis on the patient's understanding of the illness, anxieties and possible misunderstandings can be minimized. Patients are usually asked their personal understanding of their medical condition or for their explanation of the operation they are having, and this will be faithfully documented. Littlewood (1989) suggests that it is the nurse more than most health professionals who has the possibility of exploring the person's understanding of illness, and can negotiate between the goals of the doctor and the goals of the patient. Herberg (1995) suggests that nurses' attitudes are influenced by a value system of rational, analytical and biomedical practices. Therefore nurses must be careful not to allow their own attitudes to stand in the way of accepting ideas, beliefs and practices about health care that are incongruent with their own. Put simply, the nurse must believe in the patient's viewpoint. In addition, the 'NMC Code of professional conduct' states that nurses must respect the patient's autonomy.

Spiritual needs and transcultural care

As mentioned above, patients normally will be asked their religious belief as part of the admission/assessment procedure. It is important to be aware that a professed religion does not necessarily mean that a person is active in that religion, or that agnostic, atheist or humanist perspectives mean that a patient does not have any kind of spiritual life. A nurse should be willing to engage in communication with a patient about their spirituality, and indeed he or she can do so without necessarily sharing the same belief system. Religious belief should be documented carefully. Terms like Christian, Hindu, Moslem, Jew all need further definition, as the person the nurse identifies to help the patient spiritually may be inappropriate and this may cause great offence. Cortis (2004) and Maclaren (2004) both suggest that it is not at all realistic to expect nurses to give religious 'care' as such to all their patients. Even if a nurse shares the faith of the patient he or she is nursing, it would be inappropriate for that nurse to make assumptions about the way that patient expresses their faith. Gone are the days when the ward sister conducted prayers on her ward every morning, or a children's nurse baptized a very ill baby without permission from the parents. Such practices persisted in some areas of the NHS well into the 1960s and 1970s. Now they would be rightly considered as patronizing and culturally insensitive.

Neuberger (2004) suggests that religious labels are partly anthropological: they provide guidelines for the way people live, group themselves in particular communities, mark life-cycle events and keep distance from other groups. Eisenbruch (1984), for example, argued that, although death itself is universal, the response to death is not and each cultural group will have its own appropriate responses. In the UK, the most generally acknowledged way of dealing with loss, as with pain, is the 'stiff upper lip', a response of stoicism that is alleged to have its roots in Victorian values. Grief is viewed as essentially a private emotion and great emphasis is put on a rapid return to normality. However, the changing response from the public to deaths and disasters over recent years, perhaps starting with the death of the Princess of Wales in 1997, has demonstrated that such stoic values in UK society may be changing, with people more open to showing their emotions. Murray-Parkes et al (1997) noted that there have been few cross-cultural studies on grief and mourning, suggesting that one reason for this is the reluctance of anthropological researchers to interpret their observations of grief and mourning in other cultures. A series of articles in the nursing press (Nursing Times 1992) and books by authors such as Green (1991) and Neuberger (2004) have gone a long way in assisting nurses in their understanding of the customs and rituals associated with death and dying in different cultural groups. Neuberger gives the example of how Jewish people deal with death. She asserts that Jews are very much in the 'here and now', with a deep and strong hold on life, and a belief in an afterlife and a physical resurrection. Such an emphasis on life, Neuberger argues, makes Jews 'less than good' at dealing with a dying family member and this may be interpreted by nurses as callousness. A body is not left alone after death, and the custom of having 'watchers' who stay with the body day and night after death and recite psalms is still continued by many Jews. Clearly this may pose a problem for nurses, so the provision of a side room may be helpful to both the family and to nurses in dealing with the numbers of people involved.

It is important to acknowledge that it may be difficult for a patient to adhere to the traditions and rituals of their religion while in hospital. At the very least, privacy can be offered, and maybe each nurse has an obligation to know and understand something of the patient's belief system if they are to offer appropriate care.

Communication and interpretation

Chevannes (2002) is clear that health professionals must meet the health needs of the whole population, and that lack of skill to communicate interculturally is evident among nurses. Language is often an issue in this respect. When interpreters are used to assist patients to communicate with health care professionals, it should be appropriate for the situation. Many women would not want a male interpreter, especially if problems of a highly intimate nature are being discussed, and indeed vice versa. Richardson (1994) suggests that interpreters must understand the issues involved and be able to help the patient (and family) understand. It is preferable to use professional interpreters; many hospitals keep a register of interpreters and also provide posters and leaflets for patients informing them how to access the service as part of their diversity agenda. However, an English-speaking friend or relative may still be required to make the initial approach to the hospital. Professional services are preferable to the use of family members or volunteers from hospital staff because a professional interpreter will ensure that he or she presents information as given and will not edit information which may render it inaccurate. This will also help to ensure that the patient and health carer talk to each other and not to the interpreter. Members of staff are often used as volunteers to interpret for patients, but such use can take them away from their own jobs. Extreme caution should be taken if children are to be used as interpreters for family members. They may speak English well, but will have a very limited medical vocabulary, are not able to grasp the concepts involved, and certainly should not be expected to cope with the responsibility. It would be wholly unacceptable, for example, if a child were asked to interpret news of cancer or other serious illness.

It is not only people who *speak* a different language who require assistance with communication. The deaf population may also require the presence of a sign language interpreter to assist them in understanding what is being said, and for the interpreter to present the patient's view. It has often been suggested that nurses should learn a language additional to their own; this could be British Sign Language. Many people will have observed that health professionals make poor attempts to communicate with deaf people, often making the error of shouting, and of standing too far away, or covering the mouth, for the patient to lip-read successfully. Parts of the deaf community in the UK form a highly distinctive cultural group, and all deaf or hard of hearing people should have their needs for good communication recognized in the same way as people from other cultural groups.

One issue that is often encountered with Asian women centres around the fact that, as well as experiencing difficulty with speaking and reading English, they may not be able to read their own language. This poses problems for health professionals in the provision of information about such things as cervical smears and breast self-examination. Watts et al (2004) suggest that videos in different languages may be successful in assisting women to access health care in these areas, as conventional approaches with written information have excluded groups of people from access.

Eating and drinking

Eating and drinking are part of what we all do every single day of our lives. The more common dietary preferences are generally catered for in the provision of food and fluids in hospital. Most hospital menus will give a choice so that people who are vegetarian, or wish to eat, for example, a low-fat diet, or a high-fibre diet, can eat their preferred food. Many people do not mind what sort of food they eat or how it is prepared. However, for some people such aspects of eating and drinking are very important manifestations of their religion or culture. Although all cultures have a shared need of food, ethnocentric thoughtlessness can result (Gerrish et al 1996). People should not be expected to suspend their beliefs or their food preferences because they are ill. Families may wish to overcome deficiencies in hospital catering by bringing in food prepared at home but while this may solve a problem for one individual, it does nothing to address the issue in general terms. However, nurses should be able to advise relatives on what foods are appropriate to bring in for such patients, and be knowledgeable about their own hospital policy and protocols in this respect.

The South Asian community continues to have a much higher than average risk of coronary heart disease and diabetes. For various reasons Asian families may be unaware of current Department of Health guidelines on healthy eating. Local health promotion initiatives on food preparation can assist women from minority ethnic groups in this respect. Asian cookery clubs set up in South Bedfordshire helped women to adapt their traditional cooking in line with dietary recommendations. Evaluation of these clubs demonstrated that this model of helping individuals to follow healthier diets was effective in facilitating dietary change (Snowden 1999).

In the 1970s it was unusual for a hospital to provide Asian menus. Today, hospitals should provide menus to cater for a wide variety of different food preferences. The nurse has a responsibility to make such menus available for all patients who need them, and to assist each patient to make appropriate choices from that menu. However, Vydelingum (2000) cites a number of authors who have found that there is still poor provision of nutritional services to meet religious needs. Thomas & Dines (1994) have suggested that, where Asian meals are provided, they are rather limited, usually being vegetarian, and that provision for Afro-Caribbean meals is virtually non-existent. Information files on wards and departments could indicate what nurses and others need to know concerning the provision and serving of food to different cultural groups. It is also necessary to understand that different cultures have different beliefs concerning food eaten during illness. Helman (1976) found in his research among white English patients in a GP practice that people believed that, if they were suffering from a fever, they should not eat, but if suffering from a cold, they should 'feed the cold'.

Fasting is important in many religious groups; for example, Muslims may choose to fast during Ramadan between sunrise and sunset (see Box 5.2). Muslim patients are often permitted not to observe such a fasting requirement when they are ill, but may still choose to do so. The nurse must ensure that the patient has his or her need for food and drink met, and will need to discuss with the patient how this can be accommodated.

Personal hygiene and washing

Attention to these aspects of personal care occupies much nursing time, and ensuring the comfort and cleanliness of patients is a core activity of nursing. A patient of white, British origin may be entirely happy to wash either in the bath or under a shower or from a bowl of water put by the bed. He or she may not like removing underwear for surgical procedures, but will comply with such a request from a nurse. However, a patient of Asian origin (e.g. a Hindu) may find such practices as washing from a bowl of water unacceptable because running water is considered essential for cleanliness. Nurses must learn to adapt their practices in this respect to allow the patient to feel clean and comfortable. Patients of Muslim origin distinguish between the 'clean' right hand and the 'dirty' left hand. The siting of intravenous infusions is therefore important.

Sikhs wear five identifying symbols, including the kara (a steel bangle which should never be removed) and kacchera (undershorts, which are intended to reinforce notions of sexual morality and modesty). Kacchera are never removed totally; the wearer changes kacchera by removing one leg from the old pair and putting it into the leg of a new pair before removing the old pair from the other leg. This garment is also worn when showering. See Case history 5.6 for further discussion.

Summary

It can be argued that a transcultural view of caring will assist the nursing profession to see all patients as empowered human-beings. To move nurses into culturally informed clinical practice, and to embrace diversity, the concept of culture must be viewed as basic to the nature of caring, and responsible for shaping human responses to health, illness and other life situations.

Modern nurses in the 21st century must attempt to provide health care within the context of understanding the effects of culture on patients and on themselves. In a multicultural and multiracial world this simply cannot be ignored. Nurses and other health professionals must seek to develop competence in culture care and begin to operate from a transcultural position.

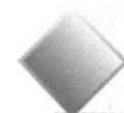

References

Abdullah SN 1995 Towards an individualised client's care: implications for education. The transcultural approach. Journal of Advanced Nursing 22:715–720

Andrews MM, Boyle JS 1995 Transcultural concepts in nursing care. Lippincott, Philadelphia

Balarjajan R, Raleigh VS 1993 The health of the nation: ethnicity and health. A guide for the NHS. Department of Health, London

Bates M 1987 Ethnicity and pain: a biocultural model. Social Science & Medicine 24(1):47–50

Calvillo ER, Flaskerud JH 1993 Evaluation of the pain response by Mexican American women and their nurses. Journal of Advanced Nursing 18:451–459

Chevannes M 2002 Issues in educating health professionals to meet the diverse needs of patients and other service users from ethnic minority groups. Journal of Advanced Nursing 39(3):290–298

Chur-Hansen A 2002 Preferences for female and male nurses. The role of age, gender and previous experience: year 2000 compared with 1984. Journal of Advanced Nursing 37(2):192–198

Cortis JD 2004 Meeting the needs of minority ethnic patients. Journal of Advanced Nursing 48(1):51–58

Davitz LL, Sameshima Y, Davitz JR 1976 Suffering as viewed in six different countries. American Journal of Nursing 76:1296–1297

Department of Health 1992 Health of the nation: a strategy for health in England. HMSO, London

Department of Health 2003 Equalities and diversity strategy and delivery plan to support the NHS. HMSO, London

DeSantis L 1994 Making anthropology clinically relevant to nursing care. Journal of Advanced Nursing 20:707–715

Dirie W 1998 Desert flower. Virago Press, London

Eisenbruch M 1984 Cross-cultural aspects of bereavement. 1: A conceptual framework for comparative analysis. Culture, Medicine and Psychiatry 8:283–309

Evans JA 2002 Cautious caregivers: gender stereotypes and the sexualization of men nurses' touch. Journal of Advanced Nursing 40(4):441–448

Gerrish K, Griffith V 2004 Integration of overseas registered nurses: evaluation of an adaptation programme. Journal of Advanced Nursing 45(6):579–587

Gerrish K, Husband C, MacKenzie J 1996 Nursing for a multi-ethnic society. Open University Press, Buckingham

Green J 1991 Death with dignity: meeting the needs of patients in a multi-cultural society. Nursing Times Book Service, London

Helman C 1978 'Feed a cold and starve a fever'. Folk models of infection in an English suburban community and their relation to medical treatment. Culture, Medicine and Psychiatry 2:107–137

Helman C 1994 Culture, health and illness, 3rd edn. Butterworth-Heinemann, Oxford

Henley A, Schott J 1999 Culture, religion and patient care in a multi-ethnic society: a handbook for professionals. Age Concern, London

Herberg P 1995 Theoretical foundations of transcultural nursing. In: Andrews M, Boyle J (eds) Transcultural concepts in nursing Care, 2nd edn. Lippincott, Philadelphia

ICN 1974 Code for nurses: ethical concepts applied to nursing. International Nursing Review 21(3–4):103–104

James J 1995 Ethnicity and transcultural care. In: Basford L, Slevin O (eds) Theory and practice of nursing. Camion Press, London

Koskinen L, Tossavainen K 2004 Study abroad as a process of learning intercultural competence in nursing. International Journal of Nursing Practice 10:111–120

Leininger MM (ed) 1991 Culture care, diversity and universality: a theory of nursing. National League for Nursing Press, New York

Littlewood J 1989 A model for nursing using anthropological literature. International Journal of Nursing Studies. 26(3):221–229

Lockyer L, Bury M 2002 The construction of a modern epidemic: the implications for women of the gendering of coronary heart disease. Journal of Advanced Nursing 39(5):432–440

Macbeth H, Shetty P 2001 Health and ethnicity. Taylor and Francis, London

Maclaren J 2004 A kaleidoscope of understanding: spiritual nursing in a multi-faith society. Journal of Advanced Nursing 45(5):457–464

Mares P, Henley A, Baxter C 1985 Health care in multiracial Britain. Health Education Council/ National Extension College, Cambridge

Mason C 1990 Women as mothers in Northern Ireland and Jamaica: a critique of the transcultural nursing movement. International Journal of Nursing Studies 27(4):367–374

McGee P 1992 Teaching transcultural care. A guide for teachers of nursing and health care. Chapman & Hall, London

Melzack R, Wall PD 1988 The challenge of pain. Penguin Books, Harmondsworth

Murray-Parkes C, Laungani P, Young B 1997 (eds) Death and bereavement across cultures. Routledge, London

Neuberger J 2004 Caring for dying people of different faiths, 3rd edn. Radcliffe Medical Press, Oxford

Ng F 2000 Female genital mutilation: its implications for reproductive health. An overview. British Journal of Family Planning 26(1):47–51

Nursing and Midwifery Council 2008 Code of professional conduct. NMC, London

Papadopoulos I 1999 Health and illness beliefs of Greek Cypriots living in London. Journal of Advanced Nursing 29(5):1097–1104

Richardson J 1994 Cultural issues in critical care nursing. In: Millar B, Burnard P (eds) Critical care nursing: caring for the critically ill adult. Baillière Tindall, London

Roper N, Logan W, Tierney A 1996 The Elements of Nursing: a model for nursing based on a model for living, 4th end. Churchill Livingstone, London

Royal College of Surgeons 1990 Report of the working party on pain after surgery. RCS, London

Sadler C 1999 Promoting diversity. Nursing Standard 13(39):14–16

Snowden WD 1999 Asian cookery clubs: a community health promotion intervention. International Journal of Health Promotion and Education 37(4):135–136

Thomas VJ, Dines A 1994 The health care needs of ethnic minority groups: are nurses playing their part? Journal of Advanced Nursing 20:802–808

Tripp-Reimer T, Brink PJ 1984 Cultural brokerage. In: Bulechek GM, McCloskey J (eds) Nursing Interventions. Saunders, Philadelphia

UK Transplant Co-ordinators Association (undated) Organ donation: religious and cultural issues. UK Transplant Co-ordinators Association, London

Vydelingum V 2000 South Asian patients' lived experience of acute care in an English hospital: a phenomenological study. Journal of Advanced Nursing 32(1):100–107

Watts T, Merrell J, Murphy F, Williams A 2004 Breast information needs of women from minority ethnic groups. Journal of Advanced Nursing 47(5):526–535

Webster C 2002 The National Health Service: a political history, 2nd edn. Oxford University Press, USA

Zborowski M 1952 Cultural components in responses to pain. In: Conrad P, Kerns R (eds) The sociology of health and illness. St Martin's Press, New York

Chapter Six

6

Using a 'toolkit' of activities in your placement

Jenny Spouse

Key topics

- Making the most of the activities in the 'toolkit'
- Being a nurse and doing nursing
- Finding out about your placement setting
- Planning your nursing experience
- Learning from practice
- Developing your professional self
- How am I doing?

Introduction

This chapter will guide you through a series of activities designed to help you develop professional knowledge and expertise and meet the Nursing and Midwifery Council (NMC) outcomes for entry to your chosen branch of the professional register. If you choose to do the activities on a regular basis during your placement, you will develop your knowledge and understanding and so be in a strong position to complete your course assignments. Even more importantly, you will be learning how to learn in and from your practice as you progress through your placement and so improve your practice and patient care.

The 'toolkit' described in this chapter was designed to help you develop the independent learning skills that you need for the whole of your programme and your future career as a health care professional.

Making the most of the 'toolkit': what is it? and why?

You may be asking yourself various questions such as 'What is this toolkit all about?', 'Do I have to use it?' or 'How is this going to help me with all the other work I have to do for my assignments and my practice placements?'

The toolkit provides activities designed to alert you to the educational opportunities in your placement. It also guides you through activities that are concerned with your practice placement. We suggest various activities for you to do while in practice which you can tailor to reflect your placement experiences and your assignments. The following is a summary of what the toolkit is designed to do for you:

- Help you recognize educational or learning opportunities in your placement.
- Prepare you for your written assignments.
- Alert you to the kinds of knowledge you need to develop throughout your first year.
- Encourage you to investigate your practice and use relevant knowledge from a range of sources.
- Develop your ability to apply to your practice the concepts, values and approaches that you learned in the classroom and from your reading.
- Help you to develop your practice as a first-year nursing student.
- Help you to demonstrate achievement of the outcomes for entry to the branch programme that have been specified by the professional statutory body.

Throughout this chapter you will find activities designed to help you use your course theoretical material and to relate it to your practice when giving care. Of course, your learning should not stop there and we hope you will want to do some extra reading and develop a broader and deeper understanding about how to care for your patients/clients.

The activities will take you through the steps of planning your learning and your practice development while helping you to consider how you can demonstrate your progress. Depending on how much you already know before you start the placement, some activities will take approximately 10–20 minutes, whereas others can be done over a period of days. The activities will encourage you to work rather like a detective investigating a case, looking for clues and then finding supporting evidence to support your arguments.

Working like a detective

Before you start on your detective work, you will need to keep a small notebook in your uniform pocket so that you can make notes and review them when you have some free time both on your placement and when you are off duty. You will have the opportunity to write a report on your observations (see below). If you want, you could transfer your notes to an electronic file or database so you can use the information later when writing up your practice-based assignment or your portfolio. The kinds of things you might want to include are:

- The title of the investigation.
- The dates.
- The placement name and your name.
- An introduction to the activity.
- The NMC outcome(s) it relates to.
- A description of what took place (the event/s).
- Your discussion of the event, drawing on relevant course material and additional material from your reading.
- Your conclusions.
- What you have learned and how you will use this learning when giving care and working with practice colleagues.

Figure 6.1(a) shows a form that can be used to report a practice experience; Figure 6.1(b) is an example report of a typical practice experience.

You will need to keep your reports in a safe place, so you may find it helpful to store them in a ring file, or write them up electronically and put them on a memory stick so you can use the information for your assignments.

If you choose to do these learning activities during each of your first-year foundation programme placements, you will develop your writing skills and assignments will become much easier to complete. Your knowledge and enjoyment will also increase as you become confident about what you are learning. This will be reflected in your placement and development of your practice skills. So, even though it may seem quite daunting at this

Figure 6.1 • (a) A form that can be used to report a practice experience; (b) an example report of a typical practice experience.

(a)

Investigation:	**Date:** **Placement:**	**Relevant NMC outcomes:**

The activity:

What took place (the event):

Reflections on the event:

Action and references for further reading:

(b)

Investigation: *care of patient receiving a blood transfusion*	**Date:** *June 1st 2007* **Placement:** *Beckton Ward*	**Relevant NMC outcomes:** *Care delivery: 2.1, 2.2, 2.3, 2.4*

The activity:

Setting up an IVI and administration of a unit of blood

What took place (the event): *I observed my mentor assist the doctor to set up an IVI and to monitor the patient. He was an elderly gentleman (85 years old) who had been admitted with iron deficiency anaemia caused by malnutrition. I then assisted her in checking the blood when it arrived and she taught me the different observations that need to be made to ensure the patient does not have an adverse reaction.*

I was impressed by the way the nurse talked to the patient (who had a hearing aid) and checked that he understood what was going to take place and why. She spent some time ensuring he understood how to care for his arm once the infusion was in place. She also discussed the procedure that would take place when the blood transfusion started.

My mentor showed me how to record the different observations and told me what I should look out for, such as an increasing pulse rate, or the patient becoming sweaty or breathless, or a rash appearing. She also explained what these different symptoms could mean.

Reflections on the event: *I had not realized what a potentially dangerous procedure a blood transfusion could be and felt quite nervous about doing the observations in case I missed anything. Fortunately my mentor was helpful and told me to go to her if I had any worries at all.*

I must read up about blood groups and how a blood transfusion helps with anaemia.

I need to think about how this patient is going to manage his own care if he cannot use his left arm (he is right-handed so at least he can do some things himself).

Action and references for further reading: *read up my nursing textbook and physiology.*

point, working through the activities in the toolkit has lots of advantages.

When you start on a placement you will find it helpful to talk to your mentor about the kinds of patients you want to study and the related social and biological sciences and so benefit from your mentor's experience of the placement and knowledge of the patients. This can save you a lot of time.

Preparing for your assignments and examinations

All your theoretical and practice-based assignments are designed to support your professional development. By using the toolkit you will be able to accumulate evidence for your assignments, including your practice-based assignments, and to develop the essential skills for your skills schedule.

So, in preparation for working through the toolkit, you will need copies of any related course/programme documents, such as:

- Learning outcomes for each placement experience.
- Skills schedule.
- Placement details.
- Assignment information.
- The welcome pack for your placement and any information about the learning opportunities available.

Meeting professional standards

NMC outcomes for entry to the branch programme

The Nursing and Midwifery Council of the United Kingdom (NMC) sets standards that all nursing and midwifery students must achieve before they progress from their foundation programme to the branch programme and from the branch programme to become a registered nurse or midwife. As a nursing student, you must demonstrate that you have achieved the outcomes for entry to the branch programme. All your assignments (including the practice-based assignment) and the skills schedule are designed to help you meet these requirements. For simplicity's sake and because these requirements have been set by the NMC, we will call them either 'NMC outcomes for entry to the branch' or 'NMC proficiencies for registration'.

The NMC outcomes for entry to the branch programme are set out in the Appendix at the end of the book (an electronic version of the NMC outcomes can be obtained from the NMC website at www.nmc-uk.org). They are described under four headings (domains), all concerned with helping you develop your professional knowledge in preparation for your branch programme and promoting high standards of professional practice and good quality of patient care. It is essential that, by the end of your foundation course programme, you can demonstrate both in writing and in your nursing practice that you understand and use these attributes.

By reading through the information for your foundation course, you will find a list of the NMC outcomes that you have to achieve in order to successfully complete the foundation course programme and progress to your chosen branch programme. If you check the foundation course assignments against each NMC outcome, you will see that they are all based on these NMC outcomes.

As you read the various activities in the chapter, you will see specific NMC outcomes mentioned. Activities 6.1–6.4 will help you gather evidence and increase your knowledge and understanding of the outcomes as they relate to your specific placement and NMC domains 2 and 3, and relate to care delivery and care management for individualized patient care. For activities 6.11–6.13, rather than provide an activity for each outcome, you are invited to map your work against a number of NMC outcomes, which are all concerned with those in domain 1.

Developing your portfolio of evidence

NMC outcome 4.1 (under the domain of personal and professional development) requires you to demonstrate responsibility for your own learning through the development of a portfolio of practice

and to recognize when further learning may be required. You can accumulate different pieces of evidence for your portfolio by doing all the various activities and keeping your work in a folder.

The section titled 'Learning from practice' later in this chapter provides some advice on how to develop your portfolio and helps you to assess your development by giving you some questions to ask yourself and other people about your performance (such as colleagues including your mentor and even your patients). Many students have difficulty writing in an academic style, so this section also provides guidance about how to write a good assignment.

Reusing the activities in the toolkit

You can 'recycle' the toolkit for each of your placements as the activities have relevance throughout your course/programme and any placement in your foundation programme. You might therefore want to make copies of some of the pages so you can save them for your next placement. How extensively you use the toolkit is entirely up to you, but the work you do will help you with your revision and your assignments. Box 6.1 lists the learning outcomes you might be expected to achieve.

Please note: You will find blank copies of Figure 6.1(a) and the templates in Activities 6.1–6.3, 6.11–6.15, 6.19, 6.20 at http://evolve.elsevier.com/Spouse/commonfoundation.

Box 6.1

Learning outcomes you could achieve by using the activities in the 'toolkit'

- Develop a clear understanding of your beliefs and values about being a nurse and giving nursing care.
- Plan your placement experience according to your learning needs and in collaboration with your mentor.
- Demonstrate skills of self-management.
- Demonstrate knowledge and behaviour that reflect understanding of professional and ethical practice.
- Demonstrate the ability to take responsibility for your own learning.
- Seek and utilize supervision to support your professional development.
- Create an action plan for your development, based on self-assessment of competence and collaboration with your mentor and other clinical staff.
- Increase your capability in patient care delivery and management.
- Demonstrate integration and progression of knowledge concerned with different aspects of patient care and professional practice.
- Develop your skills and expertise as a reflective practitioner.
- Create a portfolio of evidence.
- Develop expertise as an action inquirer into your own professional practice.
- Demonstrate acquisition of essential nursing skills.
- Operate within the principles of confidentiality and professional practice.
- Develop your writing skills and skills of literature searching.

Being a nurse and doing nursing

- What kind of nurse do you want to be?
- What are the attributes of a good nurse?
- Why is teamwork important for patient care?
- How does the 'NMC Code of professional conduct' protect patients?

These are the questions that you will address in this section. They are designed to raise your awareness of what is meant by good nursing practice and the kinds of help you may need to achieve your goals. Being able to recognize and talk about your vision of good nursing practice may also help you decide on what you want to achieve in your career, perhaps even whether nursing is the right choice.

Ensuring that patients receive high-quality care is the responsibility not only of the individual

Activity 6.1

What makes a good nurse?

Allow 20 minutes for this activity

This activity relates to NMC outcomes in all the domains.

Make some notes in response to these questions (you may want to come back to these questions as you go through the activities in the toolkit and to add your ideas as you see other nurses giving care).

Spend a few minutes thinking about why you want to become a registered nurse.

What do you want to be like as a person and as a practitioner?

How do you see yourself caring for patients?

What do you think are the most important features of a good nurse?

Comment

Views of some first-year nursing students (from: Spouse J 2003 Professional learning in nursing. Blackwell Science, Oxford)

Nicola. Perhaps my view of general nursing, there's some stereotyping I'm sure, there's just as much basic chores in what there might be aspects of nursing as general – part of the job really. When I got back last week [from observation on a psychiatric ward], it made me think: 'Yes I think this is what I want to do'. Sort of made it clear in my mind but I think that I do want to do it even more perhaps. . . . That scares me more than anything else, the actual physical, injecting, taking blood pressure, rather than like sitting down and talking to people. I'm sure you can do damage talking to people but it's not like doing physical damage. I think it's horrendous. . . . My mother, she was always the one who nursed me, when I had been ill at home, so I do think we do, carry on that sort of, 'play the role-model'. I don't know how I'd nurse actually, if it was me. I think sitting down and talking about it. You can't talk about someone being sick; obviously you've got to do some practical.

Ruth. If you realize what makes you feel nice, if you were in a strange bed and things like that. Then that would help you to appreciate the little touches for a person, coming into a ward, so there is value in all those sort of reminders. I've always just thought a loving attitude, really, to actually like want to hold people's hands and I think you need an element of toughness in you too, not to be pushed around by people . . . and in yourself. Well I think you need to know the workings of the body. You can learn all the theory in the world but really you've just gotta, to get on with people. They're the main things.

Jack. But somehow this idea of sitting down talking to patients, getting to know them as individuals, not treating them as the appendix in bed 6. Not doing the back round at 3.00 p.m. Actually giving them the tablets when perhaps they want the tablets and not at 6.00 p.m. when perhaps they don't need them. Giving them at 4.00 p.m. when they've got a pain. It just seemed so sensible to me then.

nurse; there are several different teams of people who work with nurses to ensure that the health care system delivers effective care. In preparation for each placement it is worth identifying what these teams are, whether they are the same for each placement, who makes up these different teams, how each team contributes to patient care and how they are all coordinated. An important influence on everyone's work is that of the professional statutory organizations, which define standards designed to protect the public. In this section you will begin to explore what this means for nurses. The activities in this section are related to NMC outcomes 1.2, 1.5, 2.2, 2.11, 3.1 and 4.1 (see the Appendix at the end of the book).

Your vision of being a nurse and doing nursing

Understanding your own motivations for becoming a nurse is an important aspect of being a nurse. This is fundamentally different from doing nursing. Being a nurse reflects your attitudes and beliefs about working with people and caring for other people. You may anticipate having close physical contact with people as being part of nursing, or spending a lot of time listening, teaching and talking to people; alternatively, you may see yourself mothering tiny children and working alongside their parents as they struggle to come to terms with their child's illness. Doing nursing is about the kinds of

Activity 6.2

Working together

Allow 10 minutes now and more time on your placement visit

Role	Contribution to patient care
Cleaner	
Porter	
Physiotherapist	
Occupational therapist	
Ward clerk	
Pharmacist	
Radiographer	
Consultant	
Registrar	
House officer	
Bereavement officer	
Catering officer	
Social worker	

Comment

You might discover that your placement setting is supported by only some of the people listed here, or you might find that several are missing from the list. Make a separate list in your notebook and find out about the roles of the people not identified here and then consider why there may be differences. Check your speculations with your mentor and see if you can get any further information.

As you work through this exercise you may wonder how the work of all these different teams of people is coordinated. This is a question you can work on during your placement by taking on your detective role, asking questions and more usefully observing what people are doing at different times during the 24-hour cycle of care. Don't forget to make notes in your notebook as these will help you to formulate your questions.

tasks and activities you envisage undertaking when delivering care. Some of these tasks are often glamorized by television programmes that misrepresent the true nature of nursing and hide the essential caring activities that nurses undertake every day.

The first-year students talking in Activity 6.1 are describing some of their beliefs about how patients should be cared for. How do their views match with yours? Knowing how you feel and think patients should be cared for and then being able to describe these beliefs makes it easier for you to talk about your practice. By writing about them you are on the way to meeting NMC outcome 2.2 (see the Appendix at the end of the book).

Working together

Being an effective nurse also means being an effective team member. You will notice that placement settings are staffed and visited by a wide range of people who all contribute to ensuring that the delivery of health care is smooth and effective. Some of these people will have professional qualifications, whereas others are working for national vocational awards and others are receiving on-site training for their job. Activity 6.2 is designed to help you understand the roles of these various team members and to see how to work with them.

The 'NMC Code of professional conduct'

You should have a copy of the 'NMC Code of professional conduct'; make sure you take the opportunity to examine its implications for you as a student. Then try working through Activity 6.3. You might also spare a moment to consider whether other professions have a similar code or how such codes are developed. (Try looking on the worldwide web for some codes; Chapter 2 gives advice on how to do this.)

Finding out about your placement setting

- What do I need to know?
- Why do I need to know it before I go there?

Activity 6.3

Patient care and the 'NMC Code of professional conduct'

Referring to the 'NMC Code of professional conduct', write short notes against each of the following areas of practice as to how the Code influences patient care.

Allow 20 minutes for this activity

Using your copy of the 'NMC Code of professional conduct' write short notes against each area of practice on how the Code influences patient care regarding:

Technical procedures

Care delivery

Care management

Physical, emotional and spiritual needs of patients

Comment

You will see that the 'NMC Code of professional conduct' is very comprehensive and is designed to make sure that patients receive care only from practitioners who are capable of delivering it at a safe and competent level. This means that practitioners have the responsibility for ensuring that patient care is only delegated to people who are capable of delivering it. Thus they need to assess students before they delegate patient care responsibilities to them. Managers have the responsibility of ensuring that the skill-mix of staff on duty will allow this to be possible.

- What do I do with my findings?

This section will help you make the most of your various placements, to identify what you need to know before you arrive and how to develop your learning agreement. As nursing is a practice-based profession, it means that you must view each placement as an important opportunity to learn not only clinical skills but also the related knowledge that supports your clinical judgement and the care that you give. Finding out about your placement in advance is a useful way of preparing. It means you can decide what preparatory revision you need to do, the kinds of journal articles you should be reading and the skills that you need to refine. Each of these preparatory activities helps you to make the most of your placement as well as to put you in a good position to be successful.

Being informed

The information you need about your placement is of two types: social and professional.

Social information is concerned with:

- Is there an induction programme to the organization (NHS trust/independent or voluntary organization)?
- Is there a welcome letter and pack for the placement?
- How do I get there (what is the best transport to take)?
- What are the duty times the staff are expecting to see me?
- What are the meal break times and where do I go?
- What is the name of my mentor and the names of the other staff working in the placement?
- Are there any ground rules staff have about attendance or anything else (such as clothing/uniform)?

You have the above checklist for the social information you might need. Now use Activity 6.4 to help in making a list of the *professional information* you want.

During your first week in a placement you will work with your mentor or another member of the

Activity 6.4

Professional information you might require to prepare for placement experiences

Allow 5 minutes for this activity

The areas you may be interested in are:

- Student support available.
- Patient care.
- Clinical speciality.
- Patient-centred learning opportunities on and away from the placement.
- What I need to revise in preparation for the placement.
- What I need to do for my assignments.

Comment

Abraham developed the following list of questions when asking 'What do I need to know about my placement?'

- How many patients are cared for in this setting?
- What is wrong with the patients nursed in this placement (kinds of diseases/ conditions)?
- How is nursing care organized (team, primary nursing or task allocation)?
- What special information do I need to have before I arrive?
- Is there a recommended reading list to help me get started?
- Where can I find a copy of the menu of learning opportunities (visits, investigations, etc. to see and so on)?
- Which of my learning outcomes can I achieve here?
- Which skills can I develop here?.
- What would be good subjects for my practice-based assignment?
- What learning resources are available close by (e.g. library, computer, reading materials)?
- What is the name of the link lecturer, the times she/he comes to the placement and how can I contact her/him?

staff. (If this does not happen you need to alert the nurse in charge and the practice experience manager/practice experience facilitator.) This gives both of you the opportunity to assess your learning needs and your level of capability, and helps your mentor decide on the kinds of patients you can care for safely.

Your revision in preparation for the placement will help you to plan what you want to achieve with your mentor. This is a very difficult thing to get completely right so don't be upset if your mentor feels you are being overly ambitious or that you could do more. Having a preliminary assessment of your practice helps your mentor fulfil their professional responsibility of ensuring patients receive high-quality care and do not come to harm.

Planning your learning experience

- Being self-directed.
- Identifying your learning needs.
- Writing a learning agreement.
- Begin to address NMC outcomes of domain 4 (personal and professional development).

In this section you will explore how to use your preparatory work from the previous section to develop a learning agreement for your placement. This includes identifying your learning needs and the help you will need, and negotiating that help. In undertaking this work you will demonstrate your achievement of NMC domain 4 relating to personal and professional development. Important elements of undertaking this work are the opportunities to:

- Gain an increased understanding of the importance of self-directed inquiry.
- Develop your self-awareness.
- Review your current abilities and focus on your strengths and limitations.
- Identify your professional development needs.
- Draw up a list of qualities and attributes that you wish to develop.
- Create a timetable for meeting the requirements of your placement.
- Identify the resources that you can use to help you achieve your learning outcomes.

A learning agreement

Why use a learning agreement?

Learning agreements (or learning contracts) provide a way of planning your learning experiences with the support of an experienced practitioner or teacher and for getting the help you need to be successful. By planning your own learning, you will have greater control over your studies and the process of learning. As a result, you will probably feel that you own the plan and therefore can be more committed to the learning. This is supported by research that shows that when adults plan their learning for their own personal development they are likely to be more successful. One condition of this is when personal development is associated with a course to improve competence. This is when learners must seek the guidance and support of a more experienced practitioner. The structure (or the organization) of the learning to be achieved needs to be more explicit. So a learning agreement provides this kind of structure on a day-by-day basis.

Eight steps of a learning agreement

A learning agreement can be thought of as having eight stages (Anderson et al 1996).

1. *Learning needs*. The learning needs are the gap between where you are now and where you need, or want, to be. You need to be clear about what these are for you. (Your placement learning outcomes will help you identify the knowledge you need to develop.)
2. *Learning outcomes*. These are specifications of exactly what you need to learn in order to fill the learning gap. This involves describing what will be learned, not the strategies adopted.
3. *Learning resources and strategy*. These are the materials that you will need and who might be involved to help you meet each of these objectives.
4. *Evidence of accomplishment*. Your successful completion of your placement learning outcomes, assignments and skills schedule. As mentioned earlier, you may find it helpful to keep a small notebook in which you can keep track of what you have achieved by the end of each shift. You can use this record as a basis for discussion with your mentor and make a report of your meetings to go into your portfolio.
5. *Evidence for validation*. This involves deciding how you and your mentor will recognize your progress: for example, deciding what skills you can practise and become good at during the placement and so having a list of them on your learning agreement; getting your skills schedule signed off regularly throughout your placement rather than leaving it to the last minute. Other criteria you may choose could be concerned with how you use your interpersonal skills when caring for patients, their relatives and working with other members of the clinical team. When you and your mentor assess your development of knowledge, you may be looking for your ability to describe accurately the patient's condition and the treatments they are receiving, or your ability to explain the actions, dosage and adverse effects of some of the commonly used drugs.
6. *Review*. Review the agreement with your mentor, or another member of staff, as you progress through the placement to check your progress and whether you can add any new learning targets.
7. *Carry out the agreement*. This means undertaking the learning steps specified.
8. *Evaluate the learning*. This will come from how you are feeling about your progress and the feedback you ask for from your mentor and any of the other placement staff. It is also the role of your mentor to write an accurate record of your progress.

You can see that a learning agreement provides a means for you and your mentor to assess your learning needs, to make plans to have these met and to evaluate your progress against your targets and thus identify future learning needs. If you choose to use this approach you will be taking a valuable step towards managing your own learning and thus meeting the relevant NMC outcomes for entry to the branch programme (see Box 6.2) and your learning outcomes for completing the foundation programme.

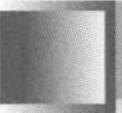

Box 6.2

NMC outcomes for entry to the branch programme: personal and professional development

Student can demonstrate responsibility for own learning through the development of a portfolio of practice and recognize when further learning is required. That is, can:

- Identify specific learning needs and objectives.
- Begin to engage with, and interpret, the evidence base that underpins nursing practice.
- Demonstrate awareness of own personal responses to unfamiliar situations and be able to discuss them coherently with a trusted colleague.
- Where necessary, seek and make use of appropriate help from relevant sources.
- Recognize learning need by articulating confusion, misunderstanding or ignorance to mentor or other appropriate person and is able to provide evidence of documenting practice experiences in learning log.
- Identify and plan to meet learning needs based on assessment of performance and feedback from mentor or appropriate colleague.

Student can acknowledge the importance of seeking supervision to develop safe nursing practice by:

- Recognizing own limitations and strengths and understanding of implications of acting without appropriate supervision and guidance.
- Demonstrating awareness of difference between role as a health care assistant and role of nursing student and is successful in adjusting performance.

Creating your learning agreement

You have already begun to think about what a learning agreement is and will have some ideas about what you *must* learn and what you *would like to* learn during a placement. Now you need to plan how you can bring all these together so that when you work with your mentor you will have a draft of your own learning agreement that you can discuss together (Activity 6.5). This will help you get the best benefit from the placement and prepare for your assignments.

Activity 6.5

Creating a learning agreement

Make a list of the skills and knowledge you are bringing to your placement (these can be what you have learned on the programme so far as well as the life skills you have accumulated from being who you are and the kind of life you have led so far).

Read through the learning outcomes for your placement and write three lists:

List 1: what I bring to the placement.
List 2: what I must learn on this placement.
List 3: what other things I would like to learn.

Using a (highlighter) pen check the learning outcomes on list 2 that you are most worried about as these are the ones you need to get the most help with from your mentor and other clinical staff.

Below is an example of how Grace (a first-year ward student) made her lists. You will see that she has listed what she wants to learn against the NMC outcomes.

(Cont'd)

Activity 6.5

Creating a learning agreement *Continued*

List 1: What I bring to the placement	List 2: What I must learn from my first placement (NMC outcomes in brackets)	List 3: What I would like to learn
Mother of three children (8, 12, 15 years of age)	The purpose of professional regulation and the function of the Nursing and Midwifery Council (1.1, 1.2)	How to be a member of the team
Managing finances of the home	Identify personal responsibilities under the Health and Safety at Work Act and legislation relating to moving and handling (2.8, 3.1)	To work like the other nurses
Running my home and making sure the family are clothed and fed and get off to school every day	Explain the measures required to maintain the security and confidentiality of client records in all formats (1.3)	To understand what is wrong with the patients
Handling my 15-year-old and her friends so she feels valued and respected as an adult (even though she gives me grief with her tantrums)	Reflect on how personal and professional values and attitudes have potential to influence the care given (2.1, 2.2)	To be able to give good-quality care to the patients
Caring for my children and showing them how much I care for them even when I am very tired	Demonstrate social skills of warmth, respect and basic empathy, including verbal and non-verbal communication (2.1, 2.2)	To develop my technical skills and knowledge that ensures I do a good job
Make sure my kids do their homework	Describe the rationale for using a systematic approach in relation to the assessment of patients (2.4, 2.9)	How to make patients comfortable
Worked as a care assistant for 3 years before starting the programme, so know the basic skills and how wards are run and no longer feel embarrassed with some of the nursing work	Discuss planning care with a registered nurse (2.5, 2.10)	How to ensure I do not cause patients any harm
	Demonstrate core essential caring skills, including first aid and basic life support to the required standard within the school and clinical environment (2.6, 2.7, 2.8, 4.2)	How to survive a shift
	Identify factors that promote effective teamwork (3.2)	How to talk to patients without sounding silly or unoriginal
	Identify and use appropriately the commonly used SI and non-SI units for measurement of weight, length, volume, time, temperature, pressure, etc. (3.3)	

SI (Système Internationale), the international system of units.

Comment

By the time Grace had completed her different lists she was quite surprised by what she had learned about herself. She had not realized how valuable much of her past life she was bringing into her nursing. She realized that she had developed good time-management skills and was able to organize her work to meet deadlines. She knew she was good at dealing with children who were tired and temperamental, and understood that some of these skills of patience, listening and paraphrasing would be helpful when working with confused or distressed people.

Preparing and drafting an action plan

As you work through each of your placements you will find it gets easier to plan your learning and take more control over it. Now try Activity 6.6.

When you meet with your mentor discuss your list and what help you can receive to achieve your learning outcomes. This could include:

- Working alongside your mentor and assisting with giving care;
- Giving care to specific patients either under the close or distant supervision of your mentor or another member of staff;
- Keeping a detailed record of the care you have given and then finding more about it by reading texts and journal articles in quiet times.

Activity 6.6

Preparing and drafting an action plan

Allow 45 minutes for this activity

- Before you meet with your mentor look at the assignments that you need to do for your course and think about how you can go about managing all of them before their submission dates.
- You should also have some ideas about the practical skills you want to develop and what you want to write about in your practice-based assignment. This will give you the focus for your meeting with your mentor.
- On a piece of paper plan what sort of evidence you will need and how you are going to document it in preparation for your next meeting with your mentor for your portfolio.
- When you meet your mentor ask for advice about who can help you and especially when they are not on duty with you.
- Using your *duty schedule* agree some dates when you are both on duty at the same time to arrange times to work together and to discuss your progress.

Comment

This is your first step in learning to become an action inquirer. The planning stage is vital to give you some sense of how much time you will need. Here is an example of how Savoula mapped out her placement.

	Week 1	Weeks 2–4	After week 5
Skills schedule	Work alongside mentor and co-mentor until I feel confident about working on my own and staff are confident about patient safety and my skills. Discuss my performance with one of these people at the end of the week and agree an action plan for the next week. Write up notes from reading three patient care plans and notes. Check notes of unfamiliar terms. Keep a drug diary to enter the names of any drugs I don't know and check their actions and side-effects.	Review how I feel about my skills and what others I need to practice. What help do I need? Carry on with keeping notes in my drug book. Watch two or more different nurses assess a patient and discuss the nursing care plan. Work through a nursing assessment form and negotiate to conduct an assessment on my own with a follow up review with the patient's nurse. Check my skills schedule and arrange to have those I feel confident about supervised and signed off.	Begin to review notes and evidence. Discuss with mentor. Check my skills schedule and arrange to practise those outstanding skills, and, when OK, have them supervised and signed off.

(Cont'd)

Activity 6.6

Preparing and drafting an action plan *Continued*

	Week 1	Weeks 2–4	After week 5
Practice-related assignments	Think about the patients I want to talk to about being a patient and in hospital. How will this help with my practice-related assignment? Make a plan of the kinds of questions I might ask Do I need to ask the patient's consent and how do I do that? (Ethics)	Talk to three patients and relatives to find out about their experiences of being ill, what caused them to see the doctor, the investigations they had before their diagnosis was confirmed and what happened before they came in for treatment. Find out how they manage being in hospital. Find out how they feel about going home and what help they will need and get. Make notes of these findings.	Find and read assignment topics and write some preparatory notes and do some reading around it.
Exams/assignments	What anatomy and physiology can I learn about whilst on this placement? What are the most common diseases and what is the related anatomy and physiology? What kinds of investigations and treatments do patients have? Can I watch any of them? What preparation do I need to do? What preparation do patients have before they go for their investigation? Can I attend the outpatient clinic for this placement and meet patients coming for their first visit and patients attending for their follow-up visit after discharge?	Read patients' nursing and medical notes, especially those of several patients with the same diagnosis. What are the common themes? What parts of the body are affected; what is the anatomy and physiology? What is causing the problem? How is the diagnosis made? What everyday nursing care do these patients need? What special nursing care do they need? Make notes of my answers to these questions and keep them in a file for this placement.	Go through my files of information and write summaries of what I have learned. Make a list of things I still do not understand and check them out with my mentor or another member of staff. Can I write a care plan for one of these patients?

Comment

As you can imagine, Savoula took quite a long time at different moments to plan this. As she settled into the task she became more aware of what she wanted to achieve and what help she would need. It gave her a good starting point to write up her first learning agreement. When she finished it she discussed it with her mentor and saved it in her portfolio file for future review.

Writing a learning agreement

Activity 6.7 is designed to help you with the final stage of writing your own learning agreement.

Learning from practice

- What are the skills I am going to learn?
- How do I learn to bring theory into my practice?
- How can I provide good nursing care?
- Will this help me with my assignments?

This section offers an opportunity to connect your classroom learning with your clinical practice experiences and so create your evidence to demonstrate achievement of the NMC outcomes in domains 2 and 3 (see the Appendix at the end of the book).

In the classroom and through your reading, you will have been introduced to some important but

Activity 6.7

Writing a learning agreement

Allow about 30 minutes for this activity

- It is important to remember that learning agreements are intended to be a creative framework for learning rather than a new kind of restriction.
- Remembering what you need to think about in your learning agreements from your reading in Activity 6.1, you are now ready to plan what you want to achieve. This should be stated in terms that allow the reader to know what the outcome will look like (rather as in patients' care plans).
- Write target dates for all things you want help with. This includes: getting feedback from your mentor or another named member of the team; having your skills schedule signed off (preferably in at least three stages); preparing for your assignments such as dates by which you will have a first draft completed for sharing with a friend or your mentor; the date by which you want feedback; the last date by which you must have finished your final and corrected version.
- Make a list of the resources that you will need and what you need to do in preparation.

Comment

You have now drawn up a learning agreement for yourself. This may involve negotiating specific learning agreements with your mentor and your link lecturer. As with all learning agreements, you are the person managing your own learning and you will need to consider how and when you review and evaluate this. A professional practitioner looks to the future, seeing continuous development as a way of life that is satisfying, challenging and enjoyable. How you maintain your learning agreement is very important, as it relies on good planning and assertiveness as well as insight into the demands and pressures your mentor is working with.

If you can successfully negotiate your learning needs as a result of planning, working alongside your mentor or another practitioner and receiving coaching, you will have made a great deal of progress towards meeting the NMC outcomes for professional development.

generalized principles concerned with your role as a nursing student, caring for people who are experiencing ill-health and factors that may contribute to ill-health and to wellness. You will also have been introduced to a range of caring skills. As you will know, while you are on placement, you will be confronted with people who are ill. Most students respond to this by immediately forgetting all they learned in class and trying to start learning completely anew.

Using the activities in this chapter will help teach you how to relate your generalized classroom learning to specific patients. With practice at using the activities, you will learn how to recognize common or general characteristics of some patient problems. By doing so you will be able to complete the circle of going from the general to the specific and back to the general, only you will have used theory to inform your practice and your practice to inform your theory.

The suggested activities are designed to:

- Help you believe in your own abilities.
- Value your everyday practice and to recognize its importance.

Rather than identify specific outcomes for you to address with one activity, you will undertake a patient-focused activity and use it to show achievement of your several NMC outcomes (see the Appendix at the end of the book).

This section will help you to be able to:

- Identify key aspects of patient care that you need to practise.
- Develop your knowledge about specific skills and practices.
- Relate course-related principles and knowledge to your everyday practice.
- Develop a repertoire of language and knowledge that helps you to describe your practice in a professional manner.

- Develop knowledge and understanding of the needs of patients nursed in your placement appropriate to your stage in the programme.
- Participate in clinical work as a team member who is supernumerary to the workforce but who contributes to patient care.
- Undertake work that prepares you for your assignments and examinations.
- Understand what it means to be an empowered learner.
- Further develop your capabilities for lifelong learning and problem-solving.
- Recognize the value of reflective practice.

Developing your practical and experiential knowledge

Learning in practice is possibly different from learning in the classroom or from texts, although we are only recently beginning to recognize this. As a student, the important thing for you to learn is how to learn and to recognize learning opportunities. At the beginning, everything is new and this can feel overwhelming as there seems to be so much that is unfamiliar. Expertise in practice requires an alert mind and a sensitive ear for what patients experience and yet sometimes have difficulty in describing. This level of expertise is developed through thoughtful analysis of personal practice. Rather in the same manner that barristers document their cases and study exceptions to normal experiences, so health care practitioners develop their expertise through careful documentation and review of both familiar and unusual outcomes of care. Both groups of professionals study such examples with the intention of finding relationships, and thus patterns of behaviour or experiences, that can lead them to effective solutions to problematic encounters. This approach of action inquiry makes learning evolve from practice that is more satisfying for everyone involved. The skills that the National Committee of Inquiry into Higher Education (1997) believed to be necessary were those of critical thinking and being able to:

- Analyse a situation.
- Problematize aspects that are either unfamiliar or confusing.
- Find resources such as journal articles or knowledgeable colleagues.
- Learn from these sources.
- Apply the information wisely and critically, or testing whether the information has relevance to the specific, problematic case.
- Evaluate and record the results (in your pocket notebook).

Through such inquiry, practice can become stimulating and satisfying. Everyday care is regarded as dynamic and challenging, with opportunities to test intuitive hunches that have been informed and developed from reading and internalizing associated literature.

Seeing and understanding

Being a professional includes being able to notice what is taking place, what is the ordinary and the extraordinary and knowing how to respond appropriately to it and having the language to describe it. All the unfamiliar words and phrases or the jargon that practitioners use often overwhelm newcomers. So as a newcomer wanting to feel part of the team, you need to familiarize yourself with these phrases and words as well as to learn how to see and understand what you are looking at. With practice and persistence you will find it becomes easier as you accumulate experience and learn about your placement and the care people need. Try Activities 6.8–6.10.

Activities 6.9 and 6.10 can both be completed several times for different patients. In fact, you are likely to learn a great deal if you do repeat these activities. You are more likely to be able to remember theory when you can associate it with individual patients, and by following these activities you will develop a portfolio of mini-case studies.

If you are on your second or third placement, you will find it helpful to write a case study of a patient. This means you analyse all the different aspects of your patient's nursing and health care needs and the role of the various practitioners (physiotherapist, pharmacist, doctor, nurse and so on) in helping your patient recover. When you

Activity 6.8

Seeing in practice

Allow 10 minutes' observation in total

- Negotiate with the nurse in charge a time when you can observe the ward in action for 10 minutes and to discuss your observations afterwards.
- Find a quiet place in your placement/ward, clinic, etc. and watch what is taking place.
- Make notes in your notebook of all the significant things you see happening.
- Write a summary of what you noticed over that time and include a list of the key points, personnel or events that you want to discuss with the charge nurse, giving each a priority rating (say, 10 being the highest, and 1 the lowest).
- When you meet with the charge nurse (or it could be another student), see whether you have captured all that took place and given each event the same level of importance.
- Consider how much you noticed and how much you missed.
- Try using this activity again at the end of your placement and notice if there is any difference in what you see and prioritize.

Comment

One of the most important skills to learn in your first year is to recognize what you are looking at. This may appear nonsensical, but if you think back to the first few days of the programme you might remember how unfamiliar everything looked. As a result, you probably didn't notice many things that you now take for granted. The same principle applies whenever you go into an unfamiliar (placement) setting. The accuracy with which you are able to record events and prioritize them is an indication of your progress. You may be surprised by how much you have learned from this simple activity.

Activity 6.9

Learning in practice: attending to physical needs

This activity can help you develop the knowledge and skills to meet the NMC outcomes. Your learning agreement specifies the areas of practice that you want to understand and develop further and these should be the focus of this activity.

During the second week of your placement, negotiate with your mentor to care for one particular patient for the duration of their hospitalization or your placement. The aim is to learn as much as you can about their experience of being a patient and their needs for nursing care.

- With your mentor's support and supervision negotiate with the patient to provide their care and discuss their illness and treatment.
- Read their nursing care plan and make notes about the essential care they are receiving.
- Read your patient's medical notes to discover the history of their illness and the signs and symptoms that led them to seeking medical help (you may need to use your nursing dictionary to understand some of the terms).
- If there is anything in these notes that you don't understand, make a note and use your nursing textbooks to find out as much as you can. If you get stuck, seek the advice of your mentor or another nurse or your link lecturer.
- Choose one or two elements of your patient's care to study in great depth (your choice may depend on what you would like to understand better or what will help you with your assignment).
- Your studies should include the following:

  A description of the care/task.

  A labelled diagram of the anatomical area (a cross-section of the skin if it is prevention of pressure sores, or the mouth if it is mouth hygiene; or, if you want to study nutrition or hydration, a labelled map of the path of different nutrients/fluid after it has been swallowed). You can probably use the study guides you had from your course to do this.

  Review the normal function of the anatomical area; so if, for example, you are studying mouth care, you need to think about the work of the salivary glands, the tongue and the teeth in maintaining the mouth in a healthy condition.

  A discussion of the potential problems that can occur to that part of the body as a result of inadequate care or damage (e.g. from infection).

  The symptoms of inadequate care.

  A description of good care, preferably using one or two articles on the subject to support your arguments.

Comment

You can use the above steps to guide you through writing about patient care as often as you feel able. You can write about specific skills or tasks (such as mouth care).

Activity 6.10

Learning in practice: attending to emotional, social and cultural needs

Another approach is to explore your patient's emotional, social and cultural needs. Your aim is again to learn as much about their experience of being a patient and their needs for nursing care.

- With your mentor's support and supervision, negotiate with the patient to provide their care and discuss their illness and treatment.
- Read their nursing care plan and make notes about the essential care they are receiving.
- Talk to your patient about how she/he is feeling about:

  Being in hospital.

  Being ill.

  Being away from home and friends and/or pets.

  The other people in the ward.

  Sleeping in a hospital.

  The hospital food.
- Try to find out if the person has visitors, how she/he feels about having visitors, how far they need to travel to come for the visit and so on. What you want to discover is how it feels to be a patient in a strange environment. (You may notice some similar experiences to your own if this is your first placement.)
- Make some notes about your conversation and the conclusions you have arrived at.
- If it is appropriate and your patient is willing to share their feelings with you, try to find out whether this person has any cultural or religious needs regarding:

  Their diet.

  Hygiene.

  Being cared for by people of a different sex or faith.
- Are this person's needs being met? If they are being met, how is that being achieved? Has a nurse documented these needs in the nursing care plan? Check the care plan.
- Does your placement have any special arrangements for people whose first language is not English? Try to find out what these arrangements are and whether you can find out more about them.
- Write a summary of your findings, drawing on information from your course or after searching out a journal article that can advance your understanding.
- Discuss your findings with your mentor or another member of the nursing team.

---

complete your case study you can map it against the NMC outcomes concerned with care delivery and care management (see the Appendix at the end of the book, or the NMC website at www.nmc-uk.org).

Developing your professional self

This section of the chapter is organized in a slightly different way than the earlier sections. It is designed to help you demonstrate achievement in domain 1 of the NMC outcomes (professional and ethical practice). Reading through this section you will notice several activities that invite you to gather information from a range of sources, to think about your reading and explore examples in your practice setting. You can then write a short report about your findings. Remember that writing up your findings is as important as doing the detective work. Writing helps you to recognize what you understand and what is challenging your thinking, so writing can be used to help your learning. You may also find it helpful to plot your learning on a spidergram or mind map, or to chart it in some way so that you can summarize everything on one sheet of paper. As an example, Figure 6.2 (p 177) shows a mind map developed by Savoula. You can find out more about mind maps on the website of Tony Buzan (www.buzanworld.com).

Each of the activities in this section (Activities 6.11–6.14) is related to one of the NMC outcomes in domain 1 regarding professional and ethical practice (see the Appendix at the end of the book). Each outcome has been subdivided into smaller specific standards for you to meet, with a corresponding activity for you to undertake that will help you gather evidence and thus develop your understanding and produce evidence of achievement for your portfolio.

Activity 6.11

Discuss in an informed manner the implications of professional regulation for nursing practice

Outcome and activity	Activity notes
Student demonstrates awareness of the role of the professional statutory body and its role in protecting the public. **Activity** Read the 'NMC Code of professional conduct' and drawing on your work for Activity 6.3 discuss how public protection is ensured.	
Student demonstrates awareness of the 'NMC Code of professional conduct': standards for conduct, performance and ethics, in everyday behaviour while on and off duty. **Activity** If a student was persistently late for duty or failed to notify the staff that they were having difficulties attending how might this contravene the 'NMC Code of professional conduct'?	
Student demonstrates an awareness of, and can apply ethical principles to nursing practice. **Activity** Consider your responsibilities and actions if you discovered a member of your placement team was verbally and physically abusing a patient/client.	
Student demonstrates awareness of legislation relevant to nursing practice. **Activity** Describe what you would do if a patient/client told you they were using hard drugs and had some in their bedside locker. Drawing on your course materials and any further reading give an explanation for your proposed actions.	
Student demonstrates the importance of promoting equity in patient/client care by contributing to nursing care in a fair and anti-discriminatory way. **Activity** Describe your actions if your elderly and blind patient/client is incontinent because she has been unable to receive the necessary assistance to get to the toilet in time.	

Activity 6.12

Demonstration an awareness of the 'NMC Code of professional conduct'

Outcome and activity	Activity notes
Student demonstrates awareness of the ëNMC Code of professional conduct' whilst engaged in patient care and interactions with patients, their carers and colleagues. **Activity** Read the ëNMC Code of professional conduct' and using two examples from your practice discuss how to try to adhere to it.	
Student demonstrates understanding of professional responsibilities to protect and serve society by acting in a thoughtful and considerate manner towards patients, their carers and colleagues. **Activity** Describe one situation from your recent experience where you feel you have worked in a thoughtful and considerate manner towards: (a) a patient and their carer (b) your colleagues in practice.	
Student demonstrates willingness to accept responsibility for personal actions and decisions, by ensuring that appropriate guidance and supervision have been sought and utilized. **Activity** Describe how you felt about the feedback you have received during this placement either if you sought feedback on your performance or where you have sought guidance on patient care.	

Activity 6.13

Demonstrate an awareness of, and apply ethical principles to, nursing practice

Outcome and activity	Activity notes
Student demonstrates awareness of responsibility to behave with integrity, honesty and in the best interests of patients, their carers and colleagues. **Activity** Describe one situation from your recent practice where you can demonstrate that you have met this outcome.	
Student's actions and speech demonstrate respect for patients, their carers and colleagues, and understanding of the importance of confidentiallty when discussing or documenting aspects of patient care or practice. **Activity** Drawing on relevant programme material describe one situation where you gave care to a patient that demonstrates that you understand this outcome in your daily relationships with patients and colleagues.	
Student demonstrates willingness to consider ethical issues that challenge personal beliefs and values and to explore reasonable explanations whilst acting in the best interests of patients, their carers and colleagues. **Activity** Describe how Activity 6.1 has influenced your approach to patient care giving an example from your recent practice.	

Activity 6.14

Demonstrate an awareness of legislation relevant to nursing practice

Outcome and activity	Activity notes
Student demonstrates observation and utlilzation of health and safety regulations in practice activities and general conduct and has attended relevant mandatory training days (please include list of dates). **Activity** Make list of the health and safety regulations that relate to your practice. Against each regulation write a short paragraph describing how the regulation influences each of the following. • your nursing care (e.g. moving and handling) • your own health and safety (i.e. what could happen to you if you did not follow the regulation) • your patients and their carers • your colleagues.	
Student demonstrates observation and utilization of employers' policies in everyday practice. **Activity** Make a list of placement and school policies that affect you in the clinical placement and check that you have identified ones with your mentor. Discuss the relevance of the school and placement policies for your everyday behaviour in your placement. Drawing on two placement policies and examples from your own placement experiences, discuss how they influence your nursing care and membership of the clinical team.	
Student demonstrates observation and awareness of relevant legislation relating to mental health, children, data protection etc. in everyday practice. **Activity** Choosing a patient in your placement, identify two pieces of relevant legislation and explore how they influence health care provision.	

How am I doing?

- Reviewing your personal development.
- Planning your assignments.
- Reviewing your portfolio.

As you work through the activities in this chapter, you might find it helpful to check your progress by self-evaluation in preparation, say, for meetings with your mentor and with your personal tutor as well as with your link lecturer. An important step to reviewing your progress is to develop your self-awareness; a self-awareness checklist (see Activity 6.15) will help you to keep track of your plans so that, if you choose, you can review your learning agreement. The checklist has a number of statements that are extremes of awareness. It is unlikely that you fit neatly into either extreme, but by working through the list you can begin to think about your attitudes and feelings about receiving advice and guidance.

You will have planned your learning as a result of carefully checking your assignments for this placement, and you will have developed a list of the kinds of knowledge and skills you wanted to learn when you wrote your learning agreement.

Activity 6.15

Self-awareness checklist

Allow 20 minutes for this activity

The checklist is made up four different types of abilities or attributes. Consider each pair of statements, decide where you fit between them and circle the appropriate number.

Circle the number that reflects your strengths and weaknesses 1 = I need help, 5 = I feel strong about this						
Self-management						
I am poorly organized	1	2	3	4	5	I am well organized
I rarely feel good about myself	1	2	3	4	5	I feel good about myself most of the time
I rarely get the most out of new situations	1	2	3	4	5	I get the most out of new situations
I am poor at coping with stress	1	2	3	4	5	I am good at coping with stress
I find it difficult to describe what I feel	1	2	3	4	5	I am good at describing what I feel
I am not clear about what is important	1	2	3	4	5	I am clear about what is important
Confidence						
I find it difficult to identify my own professional needs and development	1	2	3	4	5	I feel confident about looking at my professional needs and development
I find it difficult to take responsibility for my own learning	1	2	3	4	5	I am committed to my own empowerment and learning
I am not very good at seeking help from others	1	2	3	4	5	I feel comfortable seeking help to develop
I feel self-conscious when I work with colleagues in one-to-one situations	1	2	3	4	5	I enjoy working with colleagues in one-to-one situations
Skills						
I am not confident about (skill)	1	2	3	4	5	I am reasonably confident about this skill
I am finding it difficult to study while I am on duty	1	2	3	4	5	I can negotiate time to study while on duty
I find it difficult to talk about my own experience as a student	1	2	3	4	5	I am able to talk about my own experiences as a student
I am not good at problem-solving	1	2	3	4	5	I am good at problem-solving
Support						
I don't feel confident to talk to my mentor about my professional development	1	2	3	4	5	I have support from my mentor about my own professional development
I don't know who to go to for support	1	2	3	4	5	I know who to go to for help if I have a problem outside my scope

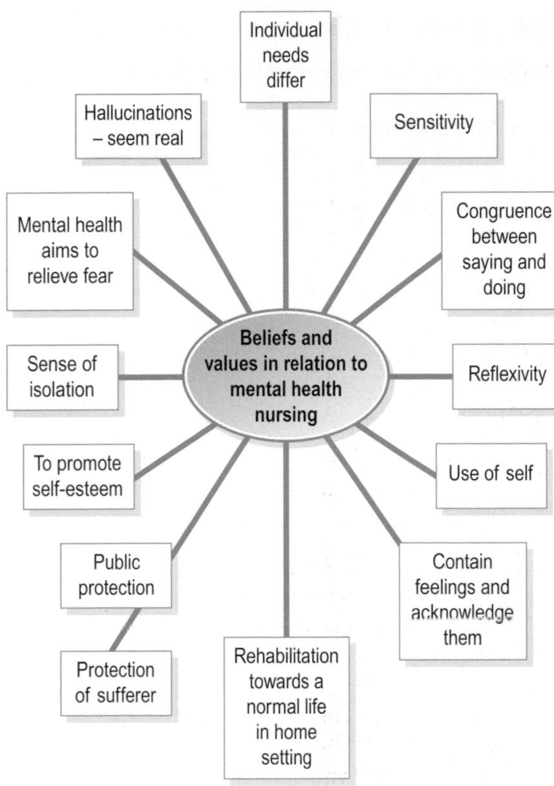

Figure 6.2 • Savoula's spidergram of her beliefs about mental health care.

Perhaps you used these strategies to plan what you wanted to achieve with your assignments. This section helps you to monitor your progress and plan for the future. By accepting responsibility for your own learning, and using some simple activities, you can monitor your progress and plan to have your future learning needs met by using a framework of questions to:

- Review your progress to date.
- Check your development of professional skills and knowledge.
- Begin to learn how to take criticism as being concerned with what you do rather than who you are (see Activity 6.15).
- Review and plan how to meet your future learning needs.
- Plan your learning and your assignments.
- Consider using reflective practice.

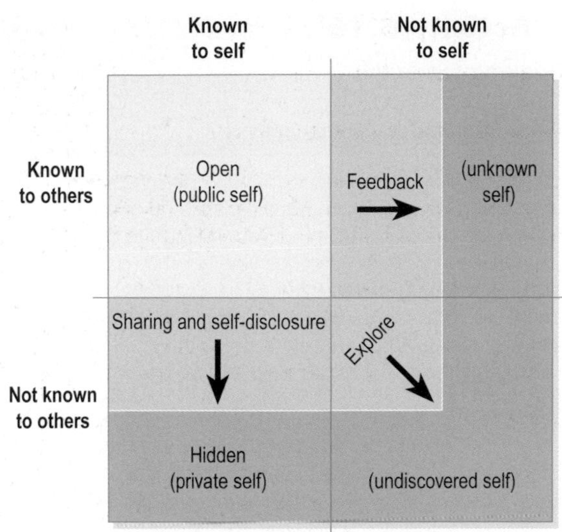

Figure 6.3 • The Johari window. (Adapted from Luft 1969.)

Learning from others

If you have asked your colleague(s) for feedback (Activity 6.16, p 178), they may have provided some unexpected insights. Quite often we have areas of ourselves that we are unaware of. Two researchers developed a way of describing this using a diagram they called the Johari window (Figure 6.3). This is a useful tool to think about your practice when you want feedback on your performance.

Think of the Johari diagram as being a window through which you can view yourself. The *open* area shows things that are known to you and to others. The top left section is open and represents the part of yourself that you consciously present to others. The *hidden* part represents things about yourself that are known to you but not to others. Some things may best remain hidden, but trust and teamwork are easier if you can open up and share this part of yourself. The *unknown* part of you is known to others but unseen to you. By receiving feedback in a positive way you can become more self-aware. The *undiscovered* part of you consists of feelings, abilities and so on that you are not aware of and which others have not yet seen, but which one day may come to the surface. Revelation in this area is usually spontaneous and cannot be planned, although exploratory processes such as counselling or psychotherapy can facilitate its

Activity 6.16

Seeking feedback

Allow 30 minutes for this activity

When you have gone over the list and decided where your strengths and weaknesses lie, ask one of your colleagues (another student or your mentor) to go over your checklist with you and see whether they hold the same view of you. Listen carefully to what they say, especially when they support your strengths. By doing this you can develop a sense of how others see you and so gain a stronger understanding of your learning needs.

Comment

Over a period of time you can build up your stock of information from colleagues and this will enable you to develop a realistic profile of your strengths and weaknesses. It is worth noting that in some cultures there is a tendency to underestimate strengths and to concentrate too much on weaknesses, so take care to maintain your own levels of self-esteem.

emergence. The easiest way of discovering some of the hidden parts of ourselves is to find out and reflect on how others see us (Activity 6.17).

Some examples

> *I find it very difficult to ask my mentor to do this activity as I feel very vulnerable and insecure in this placement. Because of this, I don't want to burden him with any more of my needs.*
>
> *(First-year student)*

This student is expressing a feeling that many people feel but don't talk about when they are going to discuss their performance. It takes a lot of maturity to separate out the act from the person. As a learner it would be remarkable if you or I were right first time when we are learning a new skill or profession. Most practical activities take a great deal of practice to get right. Nursing is very complex, but most of the practitioners take their skill and expertise for granted and some may forget the struggle most newcomers and novices experience. Learning new skills and behaviours in an unfamiliar setting with people who are busy and worrying about caring for very ill people makes learning even more challenging.

Activity 6.17

How others see us: reflective practice

Allow 30 minutes for this activity

Make a note of comments and reactions you received from meeting with your mentor when you discussed your values and beliefs, and reflect on how you have responded.

- Make a mental note of what you were saying and doing.
- Observe other people's reactions to what you were saying or doing.
- Note your own feelings about their reactions.

Comment

The effect of this exercise is to raise your awareness rather than your self-consciousness, as the latter can block your rapport with your colleagues. One way to think about reflective practice is to use the character Zaphod Beeblebrox that science-fiction writer Douglas Adams (1979) developed in his book 'The hitchhiker's guide to the galaxy'. Beeblebrox had two heads, one of which viewed the world differently from the other. Reflection is rather like using each of the heads in different ways but at the same time, perhaps using 'one head' to think about your practice and the other to recognize how you are feeling. If you can learn to do this, it will support your learning and increase your reflective skills.

Case history 6.1 is a scenario between a mentor and a student who has just received some honest comments about her performance.

- What parts of the 'NMC Code of professional conduct' is Phil is bound by?
- What do you think are his responsibilities towards his patients?
- What do you think are his responsibilities towards Janice?

Phil has a duty of care towards his patients by making sure that Janice is giving high standards of care. If he discovers that the quality of care the patients receive from Janice is unsatisfactory or that she is potentially putting his patients at risk then he must tell her. Janice also has a responsibility to learn how to develop her practice. By resisting Phil's comments she is making a difficult job for her mentor even more challenging. She is also failing to demonstrate that she is willing to take

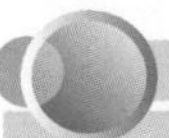

Case history 6.1

How Phil views Janice's performance

Phil: *Janice, how do you feel you're getting on now you've reached the end of your third week on the ward?*

Janice: *I'm doing fine.*

Phil: *There are some areas where the staff are pleased with your performance, but we have concerns about some other areas.*

Janice: *You don't like me; perhaps I should have a new mentor.*

Phil: *I do like you; you are a very nice person. But I have spoken to several colleagues who share my concerns. The feedback related to this aims to be constructive and it aims to help you identify areas for your future learning needs. We are here to help you so you can achieve your learning outcomes.*

responsibility for her own learning *and* failing to acknowledge the importance of seeking (and using) supervision to develop safe nursing practice.

- So how do you think Phil feels about sharing his concerns of Janice's performance after this experience?
- What do you think Janice must do to ensure she develops the necessary professional skills to become a registered nurse?
- Do you think Janice's performance is demonstrating the necessary knowledge to meet the NMC outcomes in domain 4?

Self-review

You can also use the Johari window (Figure 6.3) to think about your learning needs. You started this chapter with an activity that encouraged you to identify your learning needs based on your analysis of your placement requirements (your assignments and so on). When you worked with your mentor and planned your placement experiences, there were probably some differences between what they thought you needed to learn and your own thoughts. Your own thoughts match what might be known to you and known to others, whereas your mentor, because of their professional experience may have insights that you are not aware of and this matches 'Known to others' but not 'Known to self' in the Johari window. As a result, a blind spot surfaces as you work together throughout the placement and the programme. The important thing is to try to keep learning about yourself and being open to commentaries from others. The more you know about yourself and how you behave in different circumstances, the more adaptable you can be when you are helping others. Being conscious about your actions and knowing why you are using them in every context may seem excessive. By increasing your self-awareness, you gain freedom of choice and understanding that can inform your practice that cannot be achieved otherwise. Try Activity 6.18.

In order to help you practise the process of reflecting on your learning, you will find it helpful to undertake a self-review at the end of each section of this chapter. The self-review template is a series of questions to help you think about and consolidate what you have learned from working through a section of the chapter (see Activity 6.19). You may well find it helpful to discuss the questions with your tutor or mentor or with a colleague. In your portfolio you may have created

Activity 6.18

Self-review

Reflecting on your learning

- Reflect on your development as a practitioner: what have you achieved so far?
- Reflect on your personal development: has there been any increase in your self-confidence or improvement in your core skills?

Identifying the next steps for your learning

- What further preparation do you now need to do before completing your next assignment?
- Which skills do you need to develop? (You may find it helpful to refer to your responses to the various activities as well as to your learning agreement).

Application to your practice

- Think about the changes that have affected or may affect your work situation:

  What changes do you now plan to make in the way that you work?

  What other steps do you propose to take?

Activity 6.19

Self-review template

Chapter section title or activity numbers: ____________________ **Date of completion:** ____________________
Now that I have completed this section of the chapter, what have I learned and what do I want to record?
What have I learned about myself?
What have I learned about my strengths and shortcomings?
What information do I have that could be used for my portfolio?
Identifying the next steps of my learning
As a result of working through this section of the chapter, is there anything further I would like to find out about:
1. My practice? 2. Knowledge related to my specialist practice?
Have I checked through the placement learning outcomes and the NMC outcomes for entry to the branch?
Have I reviewed each section of the chapter and identified what help I might need to develop my skills further?
What skills and knowledge do I want to concentrate on next?
What help do I need?
How am I going to record this information in my portfolio?

a personal record section. If you have not, use the template to help you to complete a self-review sheet which can then be added to your portfolio.

Getting started

Getting started with my assignments

Before you begin to put pen to paper, you should carry out some initial planning so that you can explore the help available to you and work within realistic time-scales. You might like to draw up a personal action plan like the one shown in Activity 6.20 to help you choose your assignments, focus on who can help you, and set target dates for starting and completing them. Although there is no compulsion for you to complete the activities in this chapter, you are strongly advised to do so as they will help you complete your assignments.

Preparing for my assignments

In this part you will be learning how to read a text analytically and to take notes that will help you to use relevant and essential information in your assignment (Activity 6.21).

Activity 6.20

Getting started with my assignments

Comment

Setting dates to complete different parts of your assignments makes it easier to manage all of them. It also gives other people a better opportunity to support you and to play their part, such as reading material for you, watching you in practice and so on. It should also save a great deal of anxiety and stress towards the time that your assignments are due to be completed and so help you to enjoy your programme much more.

Assignment	Who can offer me help and advice?	Who else needs to be involved?	Which patients or relatives?	Target dates to start/complete
Skills schedule				
Practice-related assignment				
Exams/ assignments				

Activity 6.21

Preparing for my assignments: what am I looking for in my reading and writing?

Allow 20 minutes for this activity

- Spend a few minutes thinking about a recent journal article or book that you have read. List the factors that tell you that this is a good article.
- Read through an earlier assignment that you have done and compare it with your list.
- Identify the differences between the two pieces of work.
- Compare your list with the following one that Chooi made when she did this exercise.

Chooi's list

- Structure

Readability. The language used was simple and easy to understand. The grammar, spelling and vocabulary were correct.

Presentation. The paragraphs were complete and long enough to deal with the one idea being discussed. The pages were numbered and the work looked orderly, as if the writer cared about its appearance.

Content. This was referenced to current and relevant journals and texts.

(Cont'd)

Activity 6.21

Preparing for my assignments: what am I looking for in my reading and writing? *Continued*

- Process

  Writing. This was fluent and described the issue before proceeding to discussing the pros and cons of the argument.

  Arguments. Included supporting references from the literature.

  References. These were summaries of what the author had said rather than quotations, and their relevance to the writer's arguments were spelt out.

  Subsections. These were summarized and the relevance of the section to the overall argument of the paper was made clear.

  Conclusions and recommendations. These brought together all the earlier discussions and arguments.

- Outcome

  The paper gave me a very clear understanding of the topic and I could follow the arguments fairly easily without having to back-track; they were logical, and good explanations were given all the way through. I felt as if the writer was speaking to me.

  Because the writer was discussing her personal experiences, she used the first person. Using 'I did this' or 'I felt' made her writing feel much more realistic and appealing. I could sense that she had worked out what she was going to say and had ordered her thoughts quite well.

  References. When I wanted to read one of the articles she mentioned, I found that my local library did not have the journal, but I was able to give the interlibrary loans section all the information that they needed to get a copy. I found it was possible to locate all the references that she gave.

Comment

Chooi has given a very good description of the quality of essay that everyone hopes to achieve. See how her findings compare with your own and make some comments on the differences.

Looking at the care plans of several patients should allow you to gain a broader understanding of aspects of their care needs and to recognize patterns in their experiences and management of their symptoms and care. In the same manner, reading widely, using journal articles and textbooks, provides a broader understanding of theory and how it relates to your everyday practice. This is a good strategy to help you get started writing and can be used for any assignment. Another vital strategy is to check the question and make sure you understand what you must do. If your university provides a copy of the marking criteria for course work, you will see where you can gain most marks and what aspects you must address.

Good marks are awarded for demonstration of understanding of the key elements of the subject. You can demonstrate this by discussing the topic in relation to your own experiences in practice (keeping names of patients confidential of course) and the relevant literature. Try to think of the process as having a discussion with a friend who holds a different view and you are trying to persuade your friend to take on your perspective because of the strength of evidence you are bringing into your argument.

Getting writing started

- Identify an issue of interest and gather all the information that you can to inform your understanding and planning.
- Create a spidergram of the main points of the reading.
- Use the spidergram to write notes summarizing each piece of reading you do. Don't forget to get all the reference details such as the name of the authors, the date of the publication, the title and the location of the publisher and the publisher's name.
- Develop an action plan that allows you to explore all aspects of the problem and to investigate it effectively.
- Implement and monitor the plan for its effectiveness and the results.

- Collect the findings from your results and review them in the light of your reading. This may mean that you have to go back to your reading for more information.
- Write a report of your findings and conclusions and making your recommendations as a result.

A few tips

- Use a friend to help you plan your work and to discuss your reading. Students who work in this way do better in their assignments.
- Write anything you can think of the first time you face the blank page. It doesn't matter if it isn't coherent. The aim is to get going. You can always correct it afterwards.
- If you are using a word processor to write your assignment, use the spell-check and the grammar-check carefully (sometimes what you are trying to spell/say is misunderstood if you get it wrong).
- Professional writers leave enough time to review their paper after they have written it. Usually you need 2 or 3 days to 'forget' what you have written and can thus go back to it with fresh eyes.
- Ask a friend to read through your assignment to spot any mistakes or parts that don't make sense.

Writing essays is hard work and is a skill that takes time to develop. Indeed, it is probably the most challenging part of being a student. Having feedback on written work from trusted friends is valuable, especially if they know nothing about the subject. It is also helpful to exchange your work with another student, as this helps you to see how someone else approaches the same problems as well as getting further feedback. If you would like to follow these ideas up further you will find several books that are aimed at helping students develop their writing skills. One of them is the Open University publication 'The good study guide'. Chapter 2 also provides some helpful advice.

A word of warning about PLAGIARISM

You must only submit work that is entirely yours. Your lecturers and your course handbooks will have explained what is meant by plagiarism, so you will know that you must always reference any work that is not your own. Normally, this relates to quotations or material that you have used to explore a topic for an assignment. Working in collaboration with a friend to learn about your coursework and prepare for your assignments is not plagiarism. What is considered as plagiarism is when you share/copy the writing of a friend's assignment and then give the impression that your assignment is all your own work. If you have any doubts, consult your course handbooks or talk to your link lecturer/personal tutor.

Another, similar, form of plagiarism is to download prepared essays from the worldwide web and submit them as your own. This is often easy for the markers to recognize as plagiarism, and universities now use sophisticated software to scan students' assignments. Students who plagiarize the work of others and present it as their own are severely penalized by the university and this can lead to expulsion. It also contravenes the 'NMC Code of professional conduct'.

Writing a reflective account

One way to write up reflections is to focus on examples of care you have been involved in with patients/clients. You should reflect upon care situations and consider your role in these. What did you do? What did you learn from the situation? You are asked to relate theory to these examples so consider what is relevant. Depending on the examples of patient care you choose to include, you might want to discuss the patient's/client's problems and the related physiology. It would be good if you also describe any psychological issues, such as the patient feeling depressed about their diagnosis and so on. As you describe each issue you must relate it to relevant theory. So, for example, describing your patient's experience of depression means that you must relate it to your reading and learning about depression. Writing about other aspects of care may mean you need to discuss your patient's care and the rationale for their care. When you discuss all these aspects you are also analysing what happened and using theory to explain your discussions and justify the position you are taking. Don't forget that you must always protect your patients' right to confidentiality. Chapter 4 will give help with this.

Another important part of your reflections is to discuss the factors that have helped you learn. For example, you may feel that your mentor and your practice were particularly important, or the seminars, or the enquiry-based learning (EBL) activities, or sharing experiences with your peers. Having summarized what you have learned and what helped you, the next stage is to identify what you need to learn in the future. This process of reflection, self-analysis and planning should prepare you for your next placement and your next learning agreement and thus help you to progress through the course.

In conclusion

Having worked through the activities in this chapter once, you will have developed a range of important skills and knowledge that will help you throughout the rest of your programme and in the future. You can see how you can use the same activities in different placement settings to develop your professional knowledge and skills as they relate to the special needs of patients. It is hoped that you will continue to develop your knowledge this way and accumulate a sound base of professional (craft) knowledge to inform your practice and make it stimulating and enjoyable.

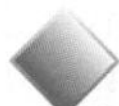

References

Adams D 1979 The hitchhiker's guide to the galaxy. Pan Books, London

Anderson G, Boud D, Sampson J 1996 Learning contracts: a practical guide. Kogan Page, London

Luft J 1969 Of human interaction. Mayfield Publishing, Palo Alto, CA

Section Two

Essentials of care delivery

Carol Cox

CHAPTERS

Introduction

Learning how to provide nursing care that reflects the highest standards must be the aspiration of all nursing students. Being able to demonstrate that you have the knowledge and skills to deliver care of a uniformly high standard is an essential requirement of both the professional statutory organization (the Nursing and Midwifery Council, NMC) and your programme provider. Naturally, the level of expectation will differ according to your stage in your pre-registration programme. Nevertheless, your readiness to progress from the common foundation programme to your branch programme will be assessed as to your ability to deliver professional nursing care, and that you have the underlying knowledge to do so. This section focuses on some of the core attributes and knowledge that you require to deliver such care.

Frameworks for describing high-quality care have been developed by different professional and government organizations within the UK. One of these was a 'toolkit' for benchmarking the fundamentals of care (Department of Health 2001). The intention of developing a toolkit was so that health and social care personnel would use the benchmarking document to address issues of concern within their areas of work in order to improve services already provided as well as to monitor existing practices. The Department of Health (2003) noted that: 'the benchmarks are relevant to all health and social care settings . . . and can be used in primary, secondary and tertiary' care settings.

They are applicable to all patient/client/carer groups. What is of primary concern is that all health care practitioners engaged in benchmarking, including patients and carers, where involved, should agree the indicators that demonstrate best practice within their area of care. The importance of getting these fundamental aspects of care right is essential if patient/client/carer care is to improve. Getting the fundamentals right was reinforced in 'The NHS plan' (Department of Health 2000) to improve the patient experience. It is so important that, since the introduction of 'The NHS plan' and the 'Essence of care' (Department of Health 2001, 2003), many health care organizations have begun special programmes designed to ensure staff have the necessary skills and knowledge to guarantee high standards of care.

The 'Essence of care' toolkit (Department of Health 2001, 2003) is one strategy introduced throughout England to provide health care practitioners with a framework to take a patient-focused structured approach to sharing and comparing practice. It enables health care practitioners to identify best practice and to develop action plans that can improve care. We have used this framework as a structure for this second section of the book. The benchmarks that were developed by the Department of Health (2001) covered eight essential areas of patient care:

- Continence and bladder and bowel care.
- Personal and oral hygiene.
- Food and nutrition.
- Pressure ulcers.
- Privacy and dignity.
- Record-keeping.
- Safety of clients with mental health needs in acute mental health and general hospital settings.
- Principles of self-care.

Since then, other benchmark standards have been added; for example, in 2003, a benchmark relating to communication between patients, carers and health care professionals was added.

Professional knowledge for the benchmark statements

In the three chapters of this section, we explore issues associated with the art and science of nursing. Within each chapter we provide examples of how the art of nursing and caring is manifest within the applied science of nursing. This is evident in the way in which care is delivered and the way in which practitioners communicate with their patients, their carers and with other health care professionals. Hand-in-hand with the idea of nursing being an art is the importance of nursing being a science. We will be exploring the science of nursing within the context of food and nutrition, personal and oral hygiene as well as in communication skills. These chapters provide the theoretical underpinnings that are so important for effective, professional nursing care delivery. In the narrative that follows, you will be introduced to the sources of knowledge that may be used to inform practice, caring relationships and caring behaviours.

In 1978, Carper's seminal research was published in a research article titled 'Fundamental patterns of knowing in nursing'. Carper's four fundamental patterns of knowing are empirical (scientific) knowledge, aesthetic (art) knowledge, personal knowledge and ethical knowledge. The combination of these ways of knowing provides nurses with a sound basis for nursing practice.

Empirical knowledge is synonymous with science, which in nursing is scientific knowledge associated with evidenced-based practice. Empirical knowledge may be equated with formal research-based knowledge that describes, explains or predicts natural and social phenomena. Empirical knowledge is related to factual evidence that can be used to inform clinical decision-making. It is objective, obtained through the senses, can be verified and quantified. Inductive and deductive reasoning are logical thought processes involved in the discernment of empirical knowledge.

Aesthetic knowledge is associated with the art of nursing. Aesthetic knowledge contributes to our understanding of how nursing is undertaken. It involves an expression of skill and the personal qualities of caring that lead to a difference in the patient's health. According to Carper (1978), the art of nursing is based on actual experience. Carper (1978, p 16) indicates that aesthetic knowledge begins with the 'singular, particular, subjective expression of imagined possibilities'. Therefore, the art of nursing is expressed through creativity and style in planning and providing care that is both effective and satisfying to the patient and nurse alike. The nurse's skilful delivery of care is provided in partnership with the patient and reflects a holistic and problem-solving nursing process.

Personal knowledge involves a 'knowing, encountering and actualizing of the concrete individual self' (Carper 1978, p 18). Through the discovery of self, reflection and synthesis of perceptions of what the nurse knows from life experience, a nurse can establish a satisfactory nurse–patient relationship. Personal knowing is associated with the inner experience of becoming an aware being. In the process of establishing the nurse–patient relationship, efforts of authenticity, rather than detachment in interpersonal relations, occur on the part of the nurse, resulting in an experience of interconnectedness between the nurse and patient. Personal knowing allows the nurse to be able to see the patient holistically; subsequently, the relationship with the patient becomes therapeutic.

Ethical knowledge involves the moral component of knowing. Ethics maintains a focus on 'matters of obligation or what ought to be done' (Carper 1978, p 20). It involves 'all voluntary actions that are deliberate and subject to the judgment of right and wrong' (Carper 1978, p 20). In relation to nursing, ethical knowing involves making moral choices even when value judgements may conflict. Cultural and spiritual/religious beliefs that confront the nurse in day-to-day practice within a multicultural society may challenge the nurse's assumptions about moral and ethical behaviour. Therefore, it is important to recognize that ethical knowing is subject to personal knowing as well as empirical evidence. Ethical knowledge influences the way we live in the world and nurses are responsible for the choices they have made.

Carper's four fundamental patterns of knowing are woven into the narrative of the chapters that follow. As you consider the empirical, aesthetic, personal and ethical knowledge conveyed in this section, you will gain a sound foundation upon which to base your nursing practice.

Communication between patients, carers and health care professionals

In Chapter 7, Shuling Breckenridge and William Blows provide the basis for understanding how to communicate with patients, carers and health care professionals on a daily basis. Having a good understanding of the nature of communication as well as the importance of communication is essential for building trust within the nurse–patient relationship. By drawing on the 'Essence of care' framework for communication skills (Department of Health 2003), they provide a guide to explore the nature of communication in the context of nursing and health care. The related anatomy and physiology of hearing, sight and speech and the psychosocial importance of communication are explored in detail. Illustrative points for consideration are provided throughout the text to help you to develop your skills of critical appraisal when communicating with patients/clients, carers and health care professionals.

Food and nutrition in health care delivery

In Chapter 8, Hannele Weir and Alison Coutts discuss some of the complexities associated with the process of creating our meals. They indicate that the process involves, first, production of food and the policies that underpin the selling and consumption of food – who consumes what and where they consume it – and the factors that impinge on what people eat. Through their discussion you will realize how important it is to understand and acknowledge that food choices are heavily dependent on the socioeconomic circumstances of people and their countries, and that accessing 'good' food for a healthy life is more complex than simply following health education messages.

Chapter 8 is organized according to the structure of the 'Essence of care' food and nutrition benchmarks (Department of Health 2003). You can find these benchmarks, which is our framework, on the Department of Health website (www.publications.doh.gov.uk). This framework is focused on three levels: individual patients, communal/community and government activity/action. These levels provide the necessary wider context for understanding the social meaning (non-nutritional significance) of food, political and fashion trends in food production, purchasing, preparation and consumption.

Promoting hygiene in health care delivery

In Chapter 9, Maria Dingle, Carol Cox and Alex Grayson consider essential issues related to personal and oral hygiene. We have used the

Department of Health (2003) 'Essence of care' definition of personal hygiene to discuss this important aspect of care delivery: 'The physical act of cleansing the body to ensure that the skin, hair and nails are maintained in an optimum condition'. Oral hygiene is described as the 'effective removal of plaque and debris to ensure the structures and tissues of the mouth are kept in a healthy condition' ('Essence of care' benchmarks on personal and oral hygiene; Department of Health 2003). You cannot learn the artistry of delivering care to meet this standard without working alongside an experienced practitioner on many occasions and for practising your skills of observation and critical thinking when delivering care. However, this chapter will contribute to your understanding of the related science and we hope you will be able to recognize its salience when giving hygiene care to your patients. First, the anatomy and physiology of the integumentary system are described, followed by the skin appendages, including the hair, glands and nails. The functions of the skin are presented, including thermoregulation, and protection from infection, including a discussion related to methicillin-resistant *Staphylococcus aureus* (MRSA). We discuss the structure of the mouth in relation to personal and oral hygiene. You may meet patients who are suffering from infestations of parasites, such as worms, fleas and so on, and we shall discuss why this happens and how to provide the necessary nursing care to reduce the symptoms. Practical methods of providing personal and oral hygiene care are detailed.

With such a diverse range of people living in the UK and with nurses travelling and working across the world, it is important that you begin to consider the special observations and needs of your clients, especially in such a sensitive area of personal hygiene, so we discuss some of the special needs associated with specific populations, different religious and cultural attitudes to personal hygiene and the significance of touch when giving care. We conclude with an examination of how your nursing role relates to hygiene and the promotion of safety, comfort, privacy and dignity.

Conclusion

This section of the book provides an introduction to the fundamental, essential aspects of nursing care and how to deliver care that is sensitive to personal needs whilst understanding the related scientific knowledge. The core message of the chapters in this section is the importance of delivering care that is focused on the needs of your patients and their best interests.

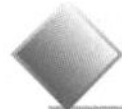

References

Carper B 1978 Fundamental patterns of knowing in nursing. Advances in Nursing Science 1(10):13–23

Department of Health 2000 The NHS plan: a plan for investment, a plan for reform. Department of Health, The Stationery Office, London

Department of Health 2001 Essence of care. The Stationery Office, London

Department of Health 2003 Essence of care. Department of Health, NHS Modernisation Agency, London

Chapter Seven

7

Communication between patients, carers and health care professionals

Shuling Breckenridge, William Blows

Key topics

- Importance of communication in nursing
- What communication is
- Anatomy and physiology of speech, hearing and vision
- The nurse–patient relationship
- The complexity of communication and potential for misunderstanding
- Self and communication
- Matching communication to different contexts
- Transcultural communication
- Communication strategies with different patient/client groups
- Record-keeping and using information technology

Introduction

Nurses must be able to communicate with patients, carers and health care professionals on a daily basis. Therefore, having a good understanding of the nature of communication as well as the importance of communication is essential for building trust within the nurse–patient relationship. In discussing the nature of communication, we have used the benchmark standards from the UK Department of Health 'Essence of care' (Department of Health 2003) framework within the context of nursing and health care. To help you develop the necessary knowledge you will have an introduction to the related physiology of hearing, sight and speech along with an exploration of the psychosocial importance of communication. Communication in nursing practice can be complex and challenging to the novice and we shall be discussing some strategies that you may like to develop and use with different patient/client groups. Keeping accurate records is essential to ensure continuity in care delivery and so we shall discuss record-keeping as well as the use of information technology and its importance in communication.

What is communication?

Communication has three fundamental components, all of which are necessary for it to live up to its name: these are the sender, the receiver and the message (Figure 7.1). This diagram does not fully represent the complexity of interactions in that it depicts communication as a one-way process (Bradley & Edinberg 1990) because the reality is that messages are simultaneously going back and forth between both parties, but it does enable a reasonably simple analysis. The message is encoded into a symbolic representation of the thoughts and feelings of the sender and then, in turn, decoded and interpreted by the receiver. Communication is judged as successful when the received message is close enough to that of the sender. The potential for things going wrong at any of these stages is considerable. The coding of the message is achieved through a number of channels.

Channels of communication

Because of the power of human language, it is easy to equate the message with words and overlook other ways in which we communicate, such as with our bodies, with posture, with gestures, and with tone of voice and intonation. Non-verbal communication consists of all forms of human communication apart from the purely verbal message (Wainwright 2003). While verbal communication is perceived mainly through the ears, non-verbal communication is perceived mainly through the eyes, although it is occasionally supplemented by other senses.

Humans are the only species to have developed elaborate systematic language and we tend to concentrate on verbal messages. Other species use sound, colour, smell, ritualistic movements, chemical markers and other means to transfer information from one member to another. Scientists are constantly discovering how complex and subtle communication systems are, even in the lowliest of species, and how necessary these systems are for survival. Non-verbal communication is often of a more primitive and unconscious kind than is verbal communication, and powerfully modifies the meaning of words.

In face-to-face communication, verbal and non-verbal channels are open and carrying information. When they give a consistent message (congruence), the receiver is likely to receive the message at face value as being sincere. When there are inconsistencies, non-verbal communication is normally taken to be more reliable than the words spoken (see the example in Case history 7.1). This is summed up in the cliché 'Actions speak louder than words'. We commonly hear people say 'It's not so much *what* he said, it's *how* he said it', or 'Even though she's tough with you, you know she really cares'. The subtlety of human communication arises from the interplay of these various channels. The capacity to be ironic or sarcastic, or to mean the opposite of what is said, depends on the exploitation of this rich resource in human communication.

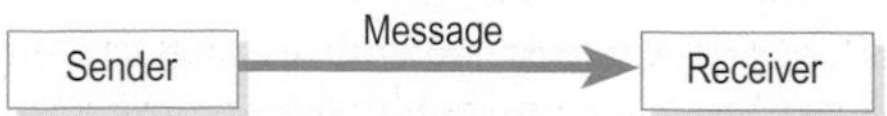

Figure 7.1 • The three components of communication.

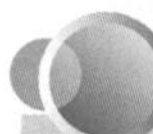

Case history 7.1

Incongruence in communication

As David prepared to leave the acute psychiatric ward where he had spent the past 3 weeks, everything that he said to the nurse suggested that he was confident about managing his own life after his discharge home. Despite David's words, the nurse sensed that, far from being confident, David was actually apprehensive about leaving the ward. At first, the nurse was unsure of the basis for this interpretation, but when asked to justify the assessment by a colleague, realized what had been observed. David had avoided eye contact by looking down at the floor, he was hesitant in packing his belongings and, as he turned to leave, his shoulders dropped slightly and he adopted a heavy posture as he walked away. It was the non-verbal communication that reflected his true feelings, and David was given the opportunity to talk about his fears and address the issues involved before being discharged.

Modes of communication

Not all communication is face-to-face with all channels open. Consider the variety of communication modes that a nurse might use in the course of a day's work:

- Rules and procedures.
- Memos.
- Reports.
- Letters.
- Information technology (e-mail, discussion forums, Internet sites).
- Telephone/mobile calls.
- Face-to-face contact.

Written rules of procedure or safety regulations may be referred to as impersonal and faceless, because they are sent from 'the authorities' to a generalized person of no particular identity. A memo can have personal or impersonal qualities, depending on whether it is sent from one person to another or is of a general nature. A report is a more formalized method of information-sharing and may be written to selected individuals or for general access. A letter is more commonly a communication between two individuals, the writer having in mind a particular person when it is written, although it can, of course, also be generalized and public.

Information technology is increasingly being used as a method of communication in all walks of life. It may take the form of direct messages, such as electronic mailing systems, or data files that are accessible to others. There are an increasing number of nurse discussion forums which offer topical debate and information on contemporary issues. A telephone call allows for the immediate interaction that is missing from the written word, so that the message is not only in *what* is being said but also in *how* it is said. If a telephone message is written down, it is reduced to the written channel only. Only in face-to-face contact are all channels open. That is why, when important matters are being discussed, there is no substitute for face-to-face meetings. Lovers have always known this!

Different modes for different uses

Everyday experience shows that we gradually learn the subtleties of each mode of communication and use them to suit our purposes. Making a complaint about an aspect of one's health care, for example, is most easily done for some people by writing a letter, so that the complainer is in sole charge of the language used. Another person might prefer the fuller contact of a telephone call but avoid face-to-face encounter. All of this points to the complexity of human communication.

Channels of non-verbal communication

Use of touch

Touch has been said to:

- Connect people.
- Provide affirmation.
- Be reassuring.
- Decrease loneliness.
- Share warmth.
- Provide stimulation.
- Improve self-esteem.

On the other hand, not all touch is interpreted positively, even when so intended by the nurse (Davidhizar & Newman 1997). Because of these potential positive or negative effects, nurses need both to understand touch and to value the ability to use it therapeutically. Touch, in a nursing context, may be either instrumental (which includes all functional touch necessary to carry out physical procedures such as wound dressing or taking a pulse) or expressive (used to convey feelings). Nurses are unusual in that they are 'licensed touchers' of relative strangers. This legitimized transgression of the normal social code requires that nurses are sensitive to the reactions of patients.

Cultural uses of touch vary from country to country. Murray & Huelskoetter (1991) noted that cultures such as Italian, Spanish, Jewish, Latin American, Arabian and some South American countries typically have relationships that are more tactile. Watson (1980) identified England, Canada

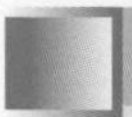

Box 7.1

Points to consider in relation to touch

- Reflect on any recent experiences that involved you touching patients.
- Determine if your touch was instrumental or expressive.
- How sensitive were you to how the patient interpreted your touch?
- Consider the respective age, gender, ethnic background and social class of the patient and yourself.
- How appropriate was your touch?

and Germany as countries where touch is more taboo. These cultural differences in social codes heighten further the need for sensitivity when judging if touch is appropriate (see Box 7.1). Whitcher & Fisher (1979) found that the use of therapeutic (expressive) touch by nurses pre-operatively produced a positive response to surgery among female patients, but not male patients. There is some evidence that males may perceive touch differently to females in relation to aspects of status or dominance (Henley 1977).

Proxemics

Proxemics refers to the spatial position of people in relation to others, such as respective height, distance and interpersonal space. Hall (1966) originally identified four different interactive zones for face-to-face contact and considered anything less than 4 feet as intrusive of interpersonal space in most relationships other than intimate ones. The four zones are used differently according to the topic of conversation and the relationships of the participants. Patients in hospital settings may not perceive that they have any real personal space. French (1983) suggested that an area of 2 feet around a patient's bed and locker could be viewed as personal space. One's spatial orientation and respective height to the other person are also significant and should be considered when engaging with others.

Posture

Posture conveys information about attitudes, emotions and status. For example, Harrigan et al (2004) suggested that depressed and anxious patients can be identified purely by non-verbal communication. A person who is depressed is more likely to be looking down and avoiding eye contact, with a down-turned mouth and an absence of hand movements. An anxious person may use more self-stroking with twitching and tremor in hands, less eye contact and fewer smiles. Of course, the nurse's posture carries just as many social messages. The ideal attending posture to convey that one is listening has been variously described in the literature (Egan 1998).

Kinesics

This includes all body movements and mannerisms. Gestures are commonly used to send various intentional messages, particularly for emphasis or to represent shapes, size or movement, or may be less consciously self-directed and sometimes distracting to others. Head and shoulder movements are used to convey interest, level of agreement, defiance, submission or ignorance.

Facial expression

Facial expressions provide a running commentary on emotional states according to Argyle (1996), and Ekman & Friesen (1987) identified six standard emotions that are universally recognizable across all cultures by consistent movement of combinations of facial muscles, namely happiness, surprise, anger, fear, disgust and sadness.

Gaze

Eye contact is a universal requirement for engagement and interaction. In Western society listeners look at speakers about twice as much as speakers look at listeners (Argyle 1996), although there are cultural variations to this. When people are dominant or aggressive they tend to look more when they are speaking. The absence of eye contact may indicate embarrassment, disinterest or deception.

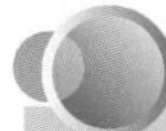

Appearance

Our self-presentation makes statements about our social status, occupation, sexuality and personality. Some aspects of appearance can be easily manipulated, such as our dress and hairstyle, but other features are beyond our control, such as height. Both types of presentation communicate messages about who we are. Nurses have often discussed the merits and disadvantages of wearing a uniform. Uniforms and other forms of regalia make nurses easily identifiable to others and provide additional information about seniority and qualifications. In some contexts, uniforms may be seen to present a barrier to establishing therapeutic relationships by reinforcing the power of the professional in the relationship. Try Activity 7.1.

Paralanguage

Paralinguistics includes those phenomena that appear alongside language, such as accent, tone, volume, pitch, emphasis and speed. It is these refinements of the lexical content that provide meaning to spoken communication. It is possible to use the same actual words but with contrasting paralanguage and convey an entirely different meaning. After reading Case history 7.2, which concerns communication with an unconscious patient, try Activity 7.2.

Physical environment

The nature and organization of the physical environment in which any communication takes place will have significant impact on the interaction. In Case history 7.2, the patient is completely at the mercy and compassion of her nurses. Fortunately, Deana is blessed by having nurses who are sensitive to her need for sensory stimulation and companionship, even though they are not getting an obvious response from Deana. She may have different nurses who are less aware of the importance of communication, both through touch and through sound, to help her remain orientated, even though she is unable to communicate her level of consciousness. Less skilful or less insightful nurses might treat her as an object that needs specific tasks to be done, so Deana might be treated as a work object rather than a human being, and simply a bed number that needs attention.

Activity 7.1

Think about your chosen branch of nursing and the different contexts in which it takes place.

- How does the wearing of a uniform affect relationships with others?
- What are the advantages and disadvantages of wearing a uniform in these different settings?

Case history 7.2

An unconscious patient and communication

Deana is a 48-year-old woman who is in an acute medical ward following a cerebrovascular accident. She has been unconscious for 2 days since she first experienced a bad headache and then gradually became unconscious. Deana's chances of surviving depend upon how much intracranial bleeding has taken place and whether it has been stopped. All of her physical care is undertaken by the nursing staff. She is entirely reliant on the actions of others for her survival. The nurses are by necessity in total control. Even though she is unconscious, each of the nurses who attend to her physical needs converse with Deanna as they go about their work, either giving information to explain their actions or just chatting to pass the time of day.

Activity 7.2

Reflect on these questions, which relate to Case history 7.2.

- How might you feel about talking to someone like Deana who is unconscious and unable to respond or indicate whether she is hearing or understanding what is being said?
- What other methods of communication might you use with Deana?
- Why do you think the nurses are taking the trouble to talk to Deana?

You might like to discuss your answers with a colleague and then perhaps with your mentor and compare their responses to yours.

Another clear example is the difference between visiting patients in their homes and nursing them in a hospital ward. Being a visitor in a patient's or client's home significantly alters the power relationship and thus the locus of control. The nurse has less control over the environment in the patient's home setting and is a guest. Hospital buildings are unusual settings for most patients and provide consistent reminders that the health care professionals are in control of the environment to a large extent. Wilkinson (1992, 1999) recognized that nursing environments were often not conducive to open communication, even if the nurses were highly skilled in it. Making the most strategic use of facilities available according to the nature and purpose of the exchange is an important aspect of nursing communication.

The functions of non-verbal communication

All of the channels of non-verbal communication described above are extremely important and may constitute up to 90% of the communication taking place. They do of course occur in various combinations with each other, not separately as above. The various functions of non-verbal communication are summarized in Box 7.2.

Observation of channels of communication

So how are humans able to develop all these subtleties in their everyday speech and language use? Why is it important to understand the physiological processes? With these questions in mind, complete Activities 7.3 and 7.4.

Speech, hearing and vision: anatomy and physiology

Understanding how we are able to hear, speak and see is important to help you support people who have a deficiency in one or more of these senses. It is useful to remember that normal communication involves all three senses, although we may believe it is our hearing that provides all the information.

Box 7.2

The functions of non-verbal communication

- *To replace speech*. A meaningful glance, a caring touch, a deliberate silence. Also, specific symbolic codes such as Makaton (if you are interested, information about Makaton is readily available on the Internet).
- *To complement the verbal message*. The main function, and used to add meaning to speech. If we say we are happy we are expected to look happy. We use gestures to provide clarification and emphasis.
- *To regulate and control the flow of communication*. We generally take turns in conversation by prompts indicating 'I am finishing, you can take over'. Some may use non-verbal communication to dominate.
- *To provide feedback*. We monitor others' non-verbal communication to interpret their reactions; for example, are they listening, worried? Have they understood? There is evidence that patients place great emphasis on non-verbal communication because of the technical nature of some verbal messages given by health carers (Ambady et al 2002, Friedman 1982).
- *To help define relationships between people*. An example is the wearing of a uniform in the hospital setting to indicate role, function and status.
- *To convey emotional states*. Emotions and attitudes are recognized primarily on the basis of non-verbal communication.
- *To engage and sustain rituals*. Argyle (1996) identified an additional function, namely ritualistic. Certain meaningful behaviours are expected at ceremonies such as weddings and graduations.

Activity 7.3

Next time you are in a public area, take time to observe the non-verbal messages that are being used. Identify the channels and functions of the messages that are exchanged.

Activity 7.4

If you have access to recording equipment, arrange to both audiotape and videotape a short conversation with a fellow student. Replay the interaction in the following order:

- Audiotape (alternatively you could listen to the videotape, facing away from the TV).
- Videotape with the sound turned right down.
- Videotape with the sound.

Make notes as you replay each stage. In particular, contrast the different stages, noting limitations of the first two playbacks. Identify how meaning is changed by additional data.

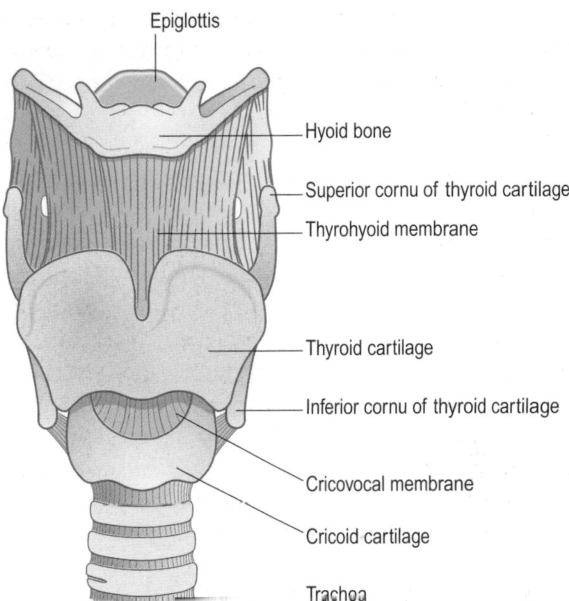

Figure 7.2 • Anatomy of the larynx. (Reproduced with kind permission from Waugh & Grant 2006.)

If you worked through Activities 7.3 and 7.4 you might have discovered some interesting attributes of speech; for example, that using verbal and the non-verbal forms of communication is important when we are talking with other people. So we communicate with each other through our ears, through our eyes and through our body posture or body language. So an understanding of the anatomy and physiology of speech, hearing and vision will help you to appreciate why some people can't speak, hear or see.

Speech and language

Although language is not unique to humans, the use of speech to convey concepts seems to be. So how do we manage to create sounds that are shaped into words to convey concepts such as mathematics, music, history, love and so on?

The physiology of speech can be divided into two distinct entities:

- The mechanics of speech, which involves manipulating air to create vibrations (sounds).
- The neurophysiology of speech, which helps us to create sentences (language construction), to understand what is being said (perception) and which helps us use and control the various muscles involved in speech.

The mechanics of speech

Air is supplied from the lungs by carefully controlling breathing to allow regulated volumes of air to pass through the upper airway passages. The muscles involved are those of normal breathing (i.e. the diaphragm and the intercostal muscles between the ribs). At the top end of the trachea is the larynx (or voice box), which is a hollow structure made mostly from tough cartilage and lined with mucous membrane (Figure 7.2). The narrowest point of the air passage inside the larynx is called the glottis, and across this point are stretched the vocal cords. These vibrate in the air passing across them creating sound. Variations in the pitch of this sound are achieved by changing the tension on the cords; volume is changed by varying the force of air released from the lung across the vocal cords. Some muscles of the larynx attach to the corniculate cartilages (which are mounted on the aretinoid cartilages).

The corniculate and aretinoid cartilages are involved with opening and closing the glottis, and the production of sound. The muscles attached to these cartilages adjust the tension on the cords, changing the vibration frequency, and thus the sound produced. These sounds are not yet words. To achieve this we need the help of the tongue, jaw, lips and mouth. Precise muscle movements of the tongue, throat and lips allow for the shaping of the laryngeal sounds into recognizable words. Figure 7.3 shows in diagrammatic form the various anatomical features involved in vocalizing sounds (Seeley et al 2006).

Some people who have suffered from a traumatic injury to the neck or have developed cancer of the larynx, have had their larynx removed surgically. This is known as laryngectomy ('ectomy' means removal). Without the two cartilages opening and closing the glottis, air cannot vibrate as it passes up the throat, leaving the patient without a voice. This represents a major change in 'body image' and a huge challenge for the patient, who must learn to speak through other means. Some patients were given a speaking tube that fitted through the neck and allowed air to pass through, thus mimicking the larynx. With modern technology, patients can learn to produce artificial speech from a synthesizer (Blows 2005).

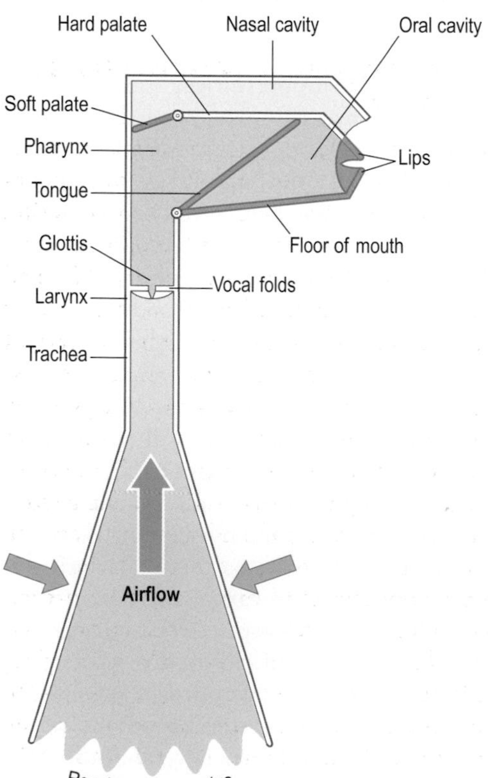

Figure 7.3 • The anatomy involved in speech production. (Reproduced with kind permission from Kindlen 2003.)

The neurophysiology of speech

In the part of the brain called the motor cortex, there is an area, known as Broca's area, which has specific control over the muscles of speech. However, the complexity of speech requires several different groups of muscles to work together, and so neuromuscular control of speech is far more sophisticated than that for other muscles. The brain shows lateralization for speech; that is, only one side of the brain carries out the function of controlling speech muscles. More than 95% of right-handed people have their Broca's area on the left side of the brain for speech, whereas in left-handed people the figure is about 70%. So, for the majority of people, speech is a left-sided brain function.

Broca's area is a region in the frontal lobe of the left cerebral cortex located below the primary motor cortex (see Figure 7.4). It appears to be a major site for the coordination of the muscles of speech (i.e. muscles of the tongue, lips and jaws). There may be muscle motor memory stored here that assigns specific muscle movements that will be required for the pronunciation of words.

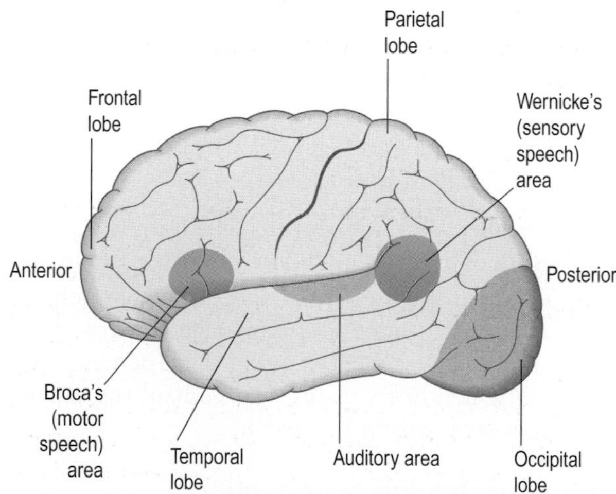

Figure 7.4 • The location of Broca's area and Wernicke's area in the cerebral cortex. (Reproduced with kind permission from Waugh & Grant 2006.)

Creating speech is so sophisticated that it requires several related areas in the brain to work together, so near to Broca's area are deeper structures in the brain tissues that are also involved. These include an area known as the caudate nucleus (part of the basal ganglia), parts of the insular (a region of cortex hidden behind the temporal lobe), the peri-aqueductal grey matter (within the brain-stem) and the cerebellum. Studies of people who are mute, or people who cannot make sounds, found that they have damage or lesions in one or other of these areas. It has not yet been possible to determine the exact relationship of these structures or their specific contribution to making speech.

Speech and language

Being able to make and shape sounds into speech is only part of the process. Another important aspect is how we create words and sentences and language that is grammatically correct. Learning to shape sounds takes practice as well as the ability to recognize sounds as having specific meanings. We achieve this through another part of the brain, thought to be Wernicke's area. This seems to be the major site for recognizing and understanding words and producing meaningful speech. Wernicke's area is located in the posterior part of the auditory association cortex within the left temporal lobe (Figure 7.4). The auditory association area lies next to the main auditory cortex, the area that deals with hearing.

Generating language for speech

Language is either spoken or written, and the pathways connecting the various areas of the brain are different for spoken words than for written words. Spoken language involves hearing words (i.e. input to the auditory cortex); vocal responses involve Wernicke's area, followed by Broca's area and the main motor cortex to operate the muscles of speech. Written language first involves seeing words written down (i.e. input to the visual cortex); verbalizing those words again involves Wernicke's area, linked to Broca's area and the main motor cortex.

Aphasia

Aphasia means the inability to speak, but there are many types of aphasia depending on which part of the brain is involved in the problem. A simple division is to classify aphasia into the two main centres primarily involved: Broca's aphasia (lesions of Broca's area) and Wernicke's aphasia (lesions of Wernicke's area). In Broca's aphasia, the patient understands spoken and written words; they know what they want to say, but they have significant difficulty in trying to say it (this is known as 'expressive aphasia'). In Wernicke's aphasia the opposite is true; the patient has the ability to speak but lacks the comprehension and understanding of what is said to them or what they want to say (this is known as 'receptive aphasia') (Carlson 2004). Stroke, or cerebrovascular accident, occurs when the blood supply to a part of the brain is interrupted, resulting in the death of the brain cells in this part of the brain and thereby affecting the person's speech or language, or both.

Communicating with people who have speech deficits

As indicated above, aphasia is an impairment of language affecting the production or comprehension of speech and the ability to read or write. Aphasia is caused by injury to the brain, most commonly from a stroke (see Case history 7.3) and particularly in older adults. The aphasia can be so severe as to make communication with the patient almost impossible, or it can be very mild. Expressive aphasics are able to understand what you say, receptive aphasics are not. Some victims may have a bit of both kinds of the impediment. For expressive aphasics, trying to speak is like having a word 'on the tip of your tongue' and not being able to call it forth. When communicating with individuals who have aphasia, it is important to be patient and allow plenty of time to communicate and allow the aphasic to try to complete their thoughts, to struggle with words. Avoid being too quick to guess what the person is trying to express. Ask the person how best to communicate and what techniques or devices can be used to aid communication. A pictogram grid can be used as these are useful to 'fill in' answers to requests such as 'I

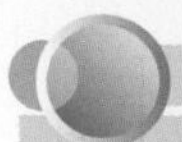

Case history 7.3

Communicating with people who have speech deficit as the result of stroke

Mrs Smith, a 65-year-old woman, is in a rehabilitation ward. She was left non-responsive after a massive stroke a year ago. She has been receiving extensive speech and physiotherapy and making slow progress. Mark, a student nurse, is on placement on this ward and finds it is very difficult to communicate with Mrs Smith. He tries to apply the communication skills learned in class but it doesn't seem to work. Mrs Smith either hardly responds to him or seems to be frustrated when he doesn't understand what she is trying to say. However, Mark observes his mentor, an experienced nurse who handles the situation very well. Mrs Smith seems to be a different person when she sees the nurse coming to give her care. Mark notices that the nurse shows genuine interest in Mrs Smith's well-being and speaks to her in simple and caring language. The nurse is very patient with Mrs Smith by being a very good listener with appropriate non-verbal behaviour. Mark can tell that Mrs Smith trusts the nurse and is very relaxed in the nurse's presence.

After further reading, Mark gained a better understanding of stroke from both biomedical and biopsychosocial perspectives and realized that stroke can affect human lives in a most abrupt manner. He discusses his learning with his mentor, who points out that caring and communicating with people who suffer stroke involves multiple skills and comes with much practice. When oral communication is not possible or minimal, non-verbal cues such as spending time with patients can convey a nurse's commitment and caring, and furthermore gain the patient's trust and foster a therapeutic nurse–patient relationship. Mark also learned that each patient is different and should be treated as an individual. Gaining an understanding of stroke and the patient's experience of living with stroke is imperative in the process of delivering care to and communicating with stroke patients.

need' or 'I want'. The person merely points to the appropriate picture.

Hearing

The receiving and understanding of sound is a vital means of human communication. Contrary to how things appear, we do not 'hear' with our ears. The ear is actually a structure designed to convert sound waves into nerve impulses. It is not until these nerve impulses arrive at the conscious brain, the cerebral cortex, do we become conscious of the sound. The part of the cerebral cortex that allows us conscious appreciation of sound is a part of the temporal lobe called the auditory cortex.

Anatomy of the ear (Figure 7.5)

The outer ear

The external ear consists of the auricle (that part seen on the side of the head) and the external auditory meatus (the auditory or ear canal). The ear canal is about 2.5 cm long, but much shorter in children, and is lubricated by a wax-like secretion called cerumen. Blockage of this canal, by a foreign body in children, or by cerumen in adults, can result in significant loss of hearing until the blockage is cleared. At the end of the canal is a delicate membrane called the tympanic membrane (or ear drum).

The middle ear

The other side of the membrane is an air-filled cavity called the middle ear. This is connected to the pharynx via a canal called the auditory or eustachian tube. Air can pass up or down this tube as necessary in order to equalize the air pressure on the two sides of the tympanic membrane. This is required to prevent any unequal pressure that would cause the membrane to bulge and perhaps become damaged. The lower end of the eustachian opens into the throat via a valve-like flap which opens on swallowing or chewing. Tympanic damage caused by unequal air pressure changes is called barotrauma and if severe enough can result in complete rupture of the tympanic membrane, causing loss of hearing.

Connecting the tympanic membrane with the inner ear are three tiny bones, the ossicles. They are linked together by joints allowing them to move in relation to vibrations of the membrane. The first bone, attached to the inner surface of the tympanic membrane is the malleus (or hammer). The second bone is the incus (anvil) and the third is the stapes (stirrup). This last bone is anchored to a membranous 'window' (called the oval

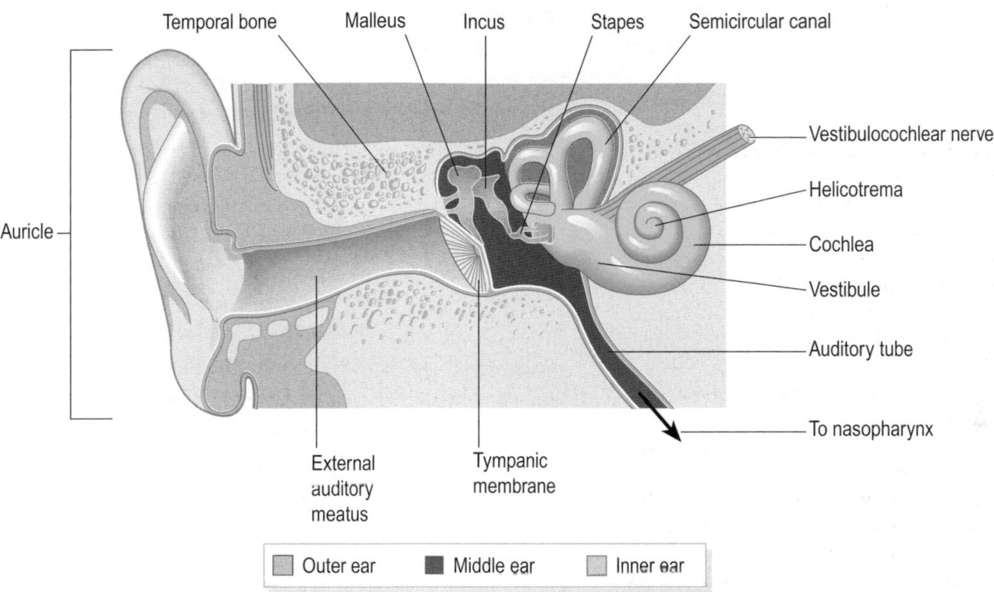

Figure 7.5 • Anatomy of the ear. (Reproduced with kind permission from Waugh & Grant 2006.)

window, or fenestrae ovalis) in the bony cavity that forms the inner ear.

The inner ear

The inner ear consists of a cavity (the bony, or osseous, labyrinth) in the temporal bone of the skull, and a membrane enclosing a space, the membranous cavity, within the bony labyrinth. The membranous cavity is filled with a fluid called endolymph, whilst a slightly different fluid, the perilymph, surrounds the membranous labyrinth and separates it from the bony labyrinth.

The inner ear cavity consists of three main parts. The vestibule is the main central compartment to which the stapes attaches (via the oval window). Extending from the vestibule are two main structures, the cochlear (the organ of hearing) and the semicircular canals (the organ for monitoring balance). The cochlear is subdivided into three compartments by the manner in which the membranous labyrinth is attached to the bony labyrinth. The upper compartment (the scala vestibuli) and the lower compartment (the scala tympani) are outside the membranous labyrinth and therefore contain perilymph. The middle compartment (the cochlear duct) is inside the membranous labyrinth and therefore contains endolymph. Sitting on the lower membrane (the basilar membrane), inside the cochlear duct, is a vibration-sensitive structure, the organ of Corti, the function of which is to convert waveform vibrations into nerve impulses (Figure 7.6). The cochlear is curled, like a snail shell, with the wide end merging with the vestibule, and the narrow end terminating with the helicotrema. The organ of Corti extends the full length of the cochlear and tapers in width, the widest end being close to the vestibule and the narrowest end being at the helicotrema.

The organ of Corti contains about 1600 epithelial receptor cells, also called hair cells because of their tiny hair-like extensions (called stereocilia). These hair cells are bathed by endolymph and are covered by another membrane, the tectorial membrane, which is attached along one edge to the bony labyrinth of the cochlear. The tips of the stereocilia are embedded in the tectorial membrane, which acts like a roof over the hair cells (Figure 7.7). There are four parallel rows of hair cells along the length of the organ of Corti: three rows together, and a fourth row offset from the

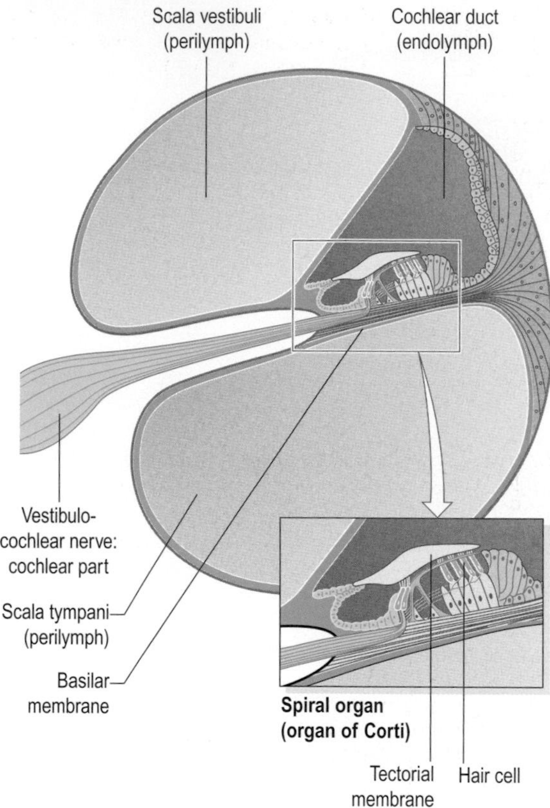

Figure 7.6 • The organ of Corti. (Reproduced with kind permission from Waugh & Grant 2006.)

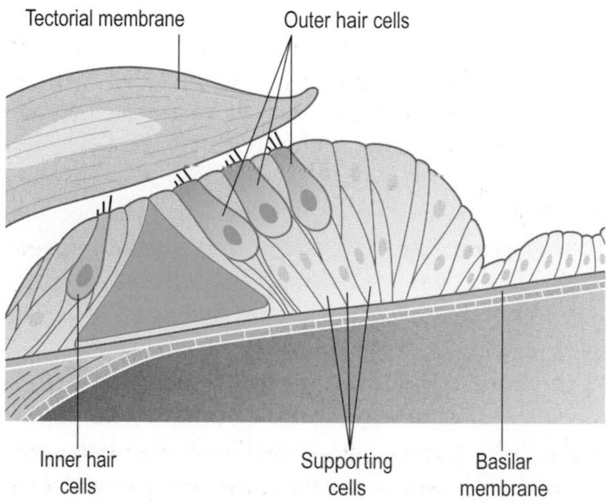

Figure 7.7 • The hair cells of the cochlea. (Reproduced with kind permission from Kindlen 2003.)

others and angled slightly towards them (Shier et al 2004).

Physiology of hearing

The whole hearing system is sensitive to vibrations. The source of the sound causes vibrations to occur in the air, and these move outwards like ripples on a pond. Such vibrations are funnelled down the auditory canal to the tympanic membrane, which then also vibrates. Tympanic membrane vibrations are transmitted through movements of the ossicles to the oval window, resulting in vibrations occurring in the membrane covering the oval window (Figure 7.8). The purpose of the ossicles is both to amplify the vibrations and to concentrate them onto the oval window. This amplification/concentration effect results in vibrations of the oval window being about 22 times greater than the vibrations of the tympanic membrane. The oval window vibrations cause ripple-like waves in the perilymph of the vestibule. These waves pass down the cochlear in the upper chamber, the scala vestibuli, and are transmitted across the upper membrane to the endolymph within the cochlear duct below. This in turn vibrates the basilar membrane and the organ of Corti on that membrane.

Different sound frequencies cause vibrations in different parts of the organ of Corti; this is why humans are able to appreciate different sounds. The brain recognizes which hair cells on the organ of Corti are affected by vibrations and which are not. It is then possible for the brain to interpret this as specific sounds. Part of this achievement is due to the differing abilities of the basilar membrane to vibrate throughout its length. At the oval window end, the basilar membrane is stiff and narrow (despite the cochlear being widest at this point) and it vibrates here at a frequency of about 20 000 Hz. At the helicotrema, the basilar membrane is at its widest (although the cochlear is narrow) and more flexible. Here it vibrates at about 20 Hz frequency of sound. Between these two points the basilar membrane varies gradually in width, stiffness and flexibility, allowing for a wide spectrum of sound appreciation.

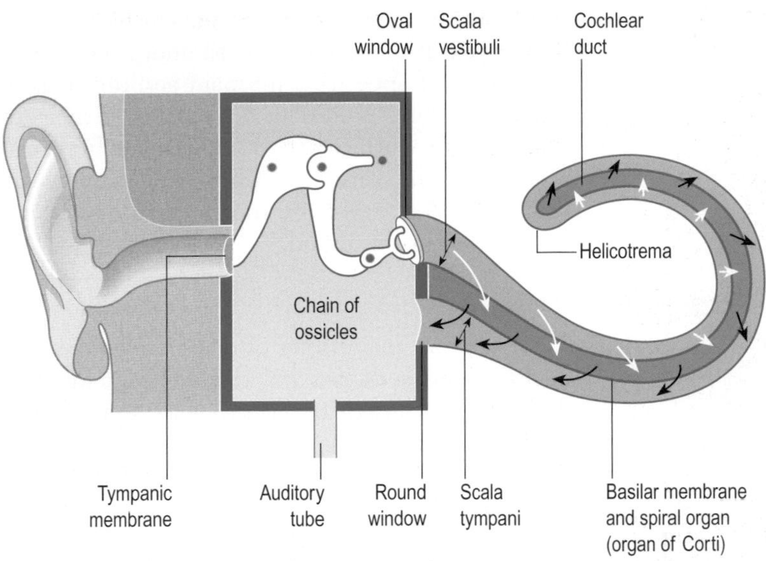

Figure 7.8 • The physiology of hearing. (Reproduced with kind permission from Waugh & Grant 2006.)

The neurophysiology of hearing

At rest, the stereocilia on the hair cells are upright and potassium channels in these structures are partly open, allowing small quantities of potassium to enter the hair cells. As a result, the hair cells release low levels of neurotransmitter into the synapse between the hair cell and the neuron below. This neuron then sends low-frequency impulses (also called action potentials) along the nerve to the brain. Endolymph and tectorial membrane vibrations created by incoming sounds cause the stereocilia of the hair cells to bend one way or the other. If they bend towards the longer stereocilia a greater increase in potassium (and calcium) into the hair cell occurs. This causes more neurotransmitter to be released and therefore greater intensity of action potentials sent to the brain. If the stereocilia are bent towards the shorter ones, the potassium input to the hair cells is cut off and no neurotransmitter is released. This results in no action potentials being sent to the brain (Shier et al 2004).

Impulses from the organ of Corti pass along three orders of neurons (Figure 7.9), the first being those of the cochlear nerve. Hair cells are connected to nerve endings that are terminations of the cochlear nerve. This nerve is one branch of the vestibulocochlear nerve, the eighth cranial nerve that passes to the cochlear nuclei of the brainstem. From here, second-order neurons partly cross to the opposite side (known as decussation) to another medullary centre, the superior olivary

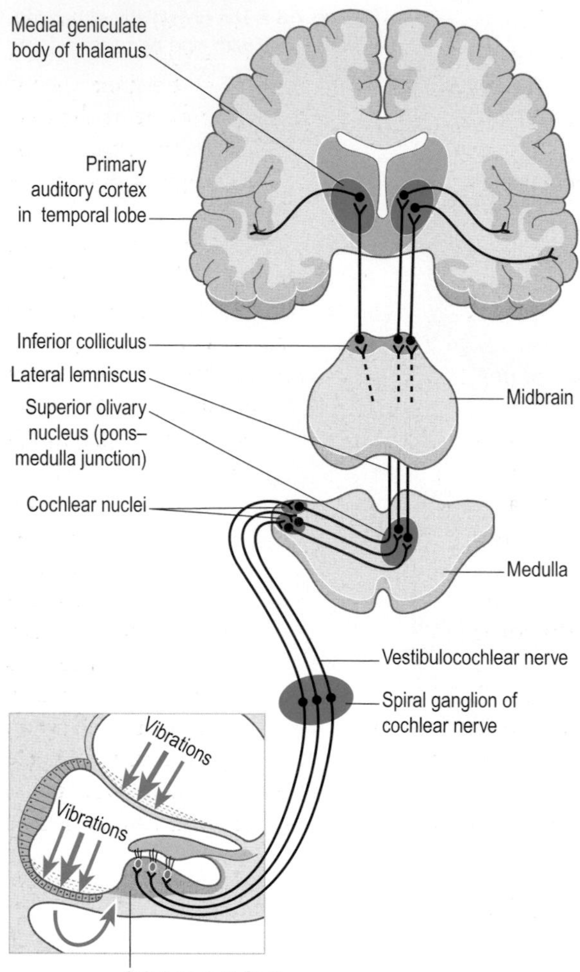

Figure 7.9 • The neurophysiology of hearing.

nucleus. Others pass to the superior olivary nucleus on the same side as their origin. From these nuclei, ascending neurons course through the pons and midbrain and terminate in the medial geniculate nucleus of the thalamus. The third-order pathway is to the conscious brain, the auditory cortex of the temporal lobe, which is part of the cerebral cortex.

The brain has the ability to sort out the many thousands of different impulses sent from the different parts of the organ of Corti, and to interpret these as specific sounds. Part of the brain's role is to store all previous auditory information in an area called the auditory association area, which surrounds the auditory cortex and acts like a sound library (see also Wernicke's area under the neurophysiology of speech). The main auditory cortex can access this stored data to assist in the correct analysis and identification of sounds. The brain can also judge the direction from which sound is coming, its distance from the ear, and detect any movements in the sound.

Deafness

There are two main types of deafness: conductive deafness and sensorineural deafness. Conductive deafness is caused by a problem that occurs somewhere along the mechanical pathway that conducts vibrations through the ear. This would mean any disruption of the anatomy or function of the tympanic membrane, the ossicles, and so on. Treatment can be as simple as unblocking the external canal to more complicated surgery. Sensorineural deafness is caused by any problem occurring in the neurological pathways that convey impulses from the organ of Corti to the brain. Treatment usually involves the use of a hearing aid to boost stimulation of the organ of Corti.

Communicating with people who have hearing deficits

Hearing-impaired people need to supplement hearing with lip-reading. It is important, therefore, to provide a conducive environment with reduced background noise and proper lighting to allow patients/clients to lip-read. There are a few things you can do to make it easier for the patient/client to lip-read: for example, face the patient when speaking, keep your hands away from your mouth while speaking and do not exaggerate lip movements when speaking. Gestures and visual aids can also be very helpful. If the person wears a hearing aid and still has difficulty hearing, check to see if the hearing aid is in the person's ear. Also check to see that it is turned on, adjusted and has a working battery. If these things are fine and the person still has difficulty hearing, find out when they last had a hearing evaluation. Keep in mind that people with hearing deficit hear and understand less well when they are tired or ill. If the person has difficulty understanding something, find a different way of saying the same thing, rather than repeating the original words over and over. Write messages if the person can read and be concise with your statements and questions.

Vision

Analogous to what was stated about the ear, we do not actually 'see' with the eye. The eye is a mechanism for converting light intensity into nerve impulses. We only see the world around us when those impulses arrive at the conscious brain, the cerebral cortex.

Anatomy of the eye

The eye is mounted inside a bony socket called the orbit. Each eye is moved around in the orbit by six muscles controlled by three cranial nerves from the brainstem (Blows 2001). The internal structure divides the eye into two main compartments: the anterior and posterior cavities (Figure 7.10). These are fluid-filled compartments; the anterior cavity contains aqueous (water-like) humour, the posterior cavity contains vitreous (jelly-like) humour. Both fluids are crystal clear to allow for the passage of light.

The wall of the eye is composed of three layers: the outer sclera (the white of the eye), the middle choroid coat (a vascular layer) and the inner retina (the light-sensitive layer). At the front of the eye, the sclera becomes a round clear patch (the cornea), which bulges forwards slightly due to the pressure of the aqueous humour of the anterior cavity. Also towards the front, the choroid layer becomes the ciliary body, the base to which suspensory ligaments attach for holding the lens. Suspensory ligaments play a vital role in changing the shape of the lens for the purpose of accommodation, which is the ability to focus on objects at different distances. Accommodation is automatic, governed by the brainstem via the third cranial nerve. Problems with accommodation are not uncommon. Myopia is near-sightedness (i.e. the ability to see close up but distance vision is blurred). The opposite is hypermetropia (hyperopia; i.e. far-sightedness, where close objects are seen as blurred but distance vision is clear). Presbyopia is a natural age-related change in the lens resulting in a gradual loss of normal accommodation. Like all ageing processes it is not preventable. The 'near-point' is the closest an object can get to the eye and remain in focus.

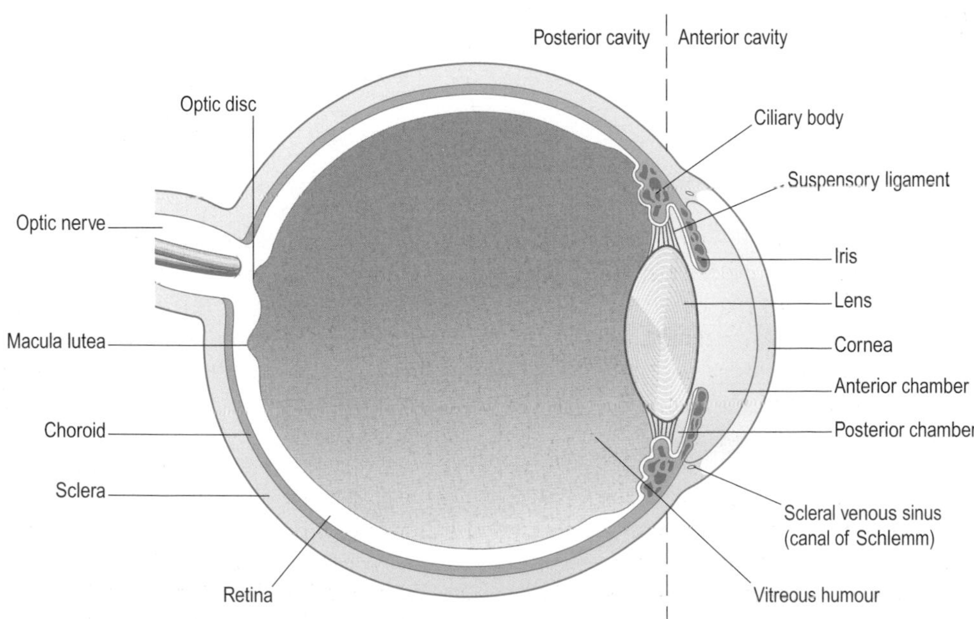

Figure 7.10 • Section through the eye. (Reproduced with kind permission from Waugh & Grant 2006.)

In presbyopia, the near-point extends gradually further away, from a normal 23 cm to sometimes an arm's length or more. Fortunately, accommodation errors can be corrected with suitable glasses (Seeley et al 2006).

Extending forwards from the ciliary body is the iris, which divides the anterior cavity into an anterior chamber and a posterior chamber. The aqueous humour that fills both is produced from the ciliary body and flows forwards through the pupil, the opening at the centre of the iris, and is reabsorbed by a canal (the canal of Schlemm) in the anterior chamber. In this way, the aqueous humour is constantly being renewed, being derived from blood plasma and returning to blood plasma. The iris can close the pupil (in bright light) or open the pupil (in dull light) in order to regulate the amount of light falling on the retina. Like accommodation, this action is automatic, being controlled by the third cranial nerve.

The retina is unique in one respect: it is the only part of the nervous system that is visible from the outside world. It is formed during embryological life as a forward growth from the brain, and can be viewed using an ophthalmoscope. It is the light-sensitive layer that converts light into nerve impulses. These travel to the brain via the optic nerve (the second cranial nerve).

Physiology of vision

Light passes through the cornea and the pupil, and is concentrated and focused on the retina by the lens. The retina has two main cell types: rods and cones (Figure 7.11).

The rods are specialized retinal cells for responding to black and white and to night (low-light) conditions; cones are similar cells for responding to colour and to day (bright-light) conditions. Rods have a high sensitivity to light (this is needed in low-light situations) and there are many of them (100 000 000, or 10^8, per retina). Compare this to the cones, which have low sensitivity to light (suitable for bright light) and are fewer in number (3 000 000, or 10^6, per retina); cones do not respond at all well in low-light situations. There are three types of cones (red, green and blue), providing a full spectral colour range; they are more concentrated at the fovea (Figure 7.11). Both rods and cones carry out phototransduction, which is the conversion of light energy to nerve impulses. This involves complex chemical changes starting with a light-sensitive pigment called rhodopsin (or visual purple) which is partly produced from vitamin A.

Rods and cones are attached to a second layer of cells (the bipolar cells), which in turn are connected to ganglion cells leading to the optic nerve.

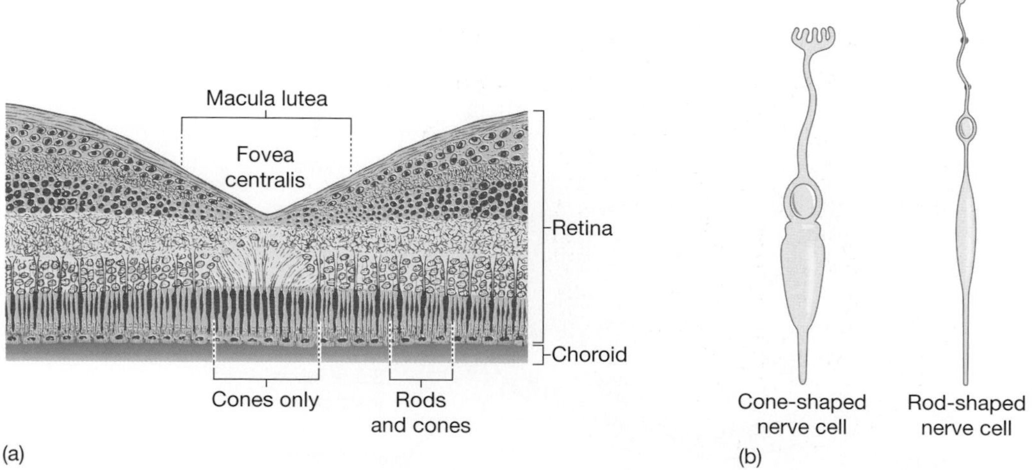

Figure 7.11 • The cellular structure of the retina (b) The light-sensitive cells of the retina. (Reproduced with kind permission from Waugh & Grant 2006.)

The surprising aspect is the manner in which these layers occur in the retina. The rods and cones are the innermost layer (towards the choroid), and the ganglion cells are the outermost layer (nearer to the vitreous humour) (Figure 7.11). This means that light striking the retina must first pass the ganglion and bipolar cells before reaching the rods and cones. Convergence (i.e. several rods linked to a single bipolar cell) occurs across the retina; this also applies to cones but to a lesser extent.

Another surprise is that light deactivates the rods and cones; that is, light switches them 'off' not 'on'. In the dark, both rods and cones produce a neurotransmitter at the synapses between them and the bipolar cells. This chemical increases activity in the bipolar cells, which in turn affects the activity in ganglion cells. Some bipolar–ganglionic synapses are excitatory, increasing ganglionic activity; others are inhibitory, decreasing activity. In the light, the rods and cones produce far less neurotransmitter and therefore the bipolar and ganglion cells are less affected by them. In this way, variations in light or dark on the retina are communicated to the ganglion cells, and thus to the optic nerve (Shier et al 2004).

The neurophysiology of vision

Impulses generated by the retina travel along the optic nerve and arrive at the optic chiasma (Figure 7.12). Here the two optic nerves join, allowing the

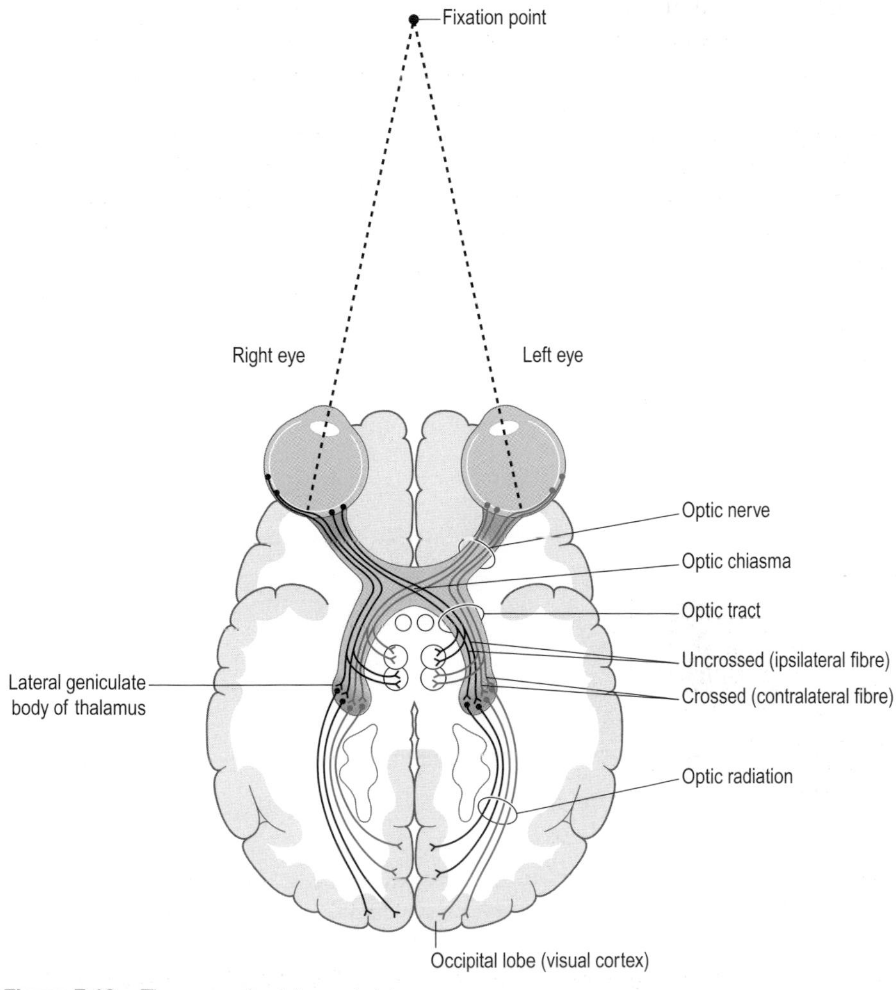

Figure 7.12 • The neurophysiology of vision.

lateral half of each retinal output to remain on the same side, while the medial halves (nearest the nose) cross to the opposite side (known as decussation). From here backwards the visual pathways (called optic tracts) are contained within the brain. The left optic tract carries impulses from the left lateral and right medial retinas; the right optic tract carries impulses from the right lateral and left medial retinas. These pass to part of the thalamus called the lateral geniculate nucleus, and from there they pass via the optic radiations to the visual cortex in the occipital lobe of the cerebrum. The impulses arrive upside down and split between the two sides, which would create a very strange view of the world.

The visual cortex reassembles the picture into the view we are familiar with. Around the visual cortex is the visual association area, which allows for the identification of visual stimuli. So, if you look at a chair, you know it is a chair because the new visual stimulus will be compared with previous stimuli stored in the visual association area.

Communicating with people who have sight deficits

Treat the visually impaired like a sighted person as much as possible. Use the word 'see' and 'look' normally. Make use of whatever vision they still have. Remember that, legally, blindness is not necessarily total blindness. Use large movements, wide gestures and contrasting colours. When you speak, let the person know whom you are addressing. Explain what you are doing as you are doing it (e.g. looking for something or putting the wheelchair away). Encourage familiarity and independence whenever possible. Leave things where they are unless the person asks you to move something.

How the body links each part of the sensory system

The brain processes all the different senses separately (e.g. vision in the occipital lobe, hearing in the temporal lobe), but when we perceive the world the different senses are all active together. Somehow, the brain must unite the senses after processing, and this is the job of the entorhinal cortex (Figure 7.13). This is part of the temporal lobe of the cerebral cortex located beneath the brain close to the hippocampus. Output from all the major sensory areas pass to the entorhinal cortex where they are integrated into a single

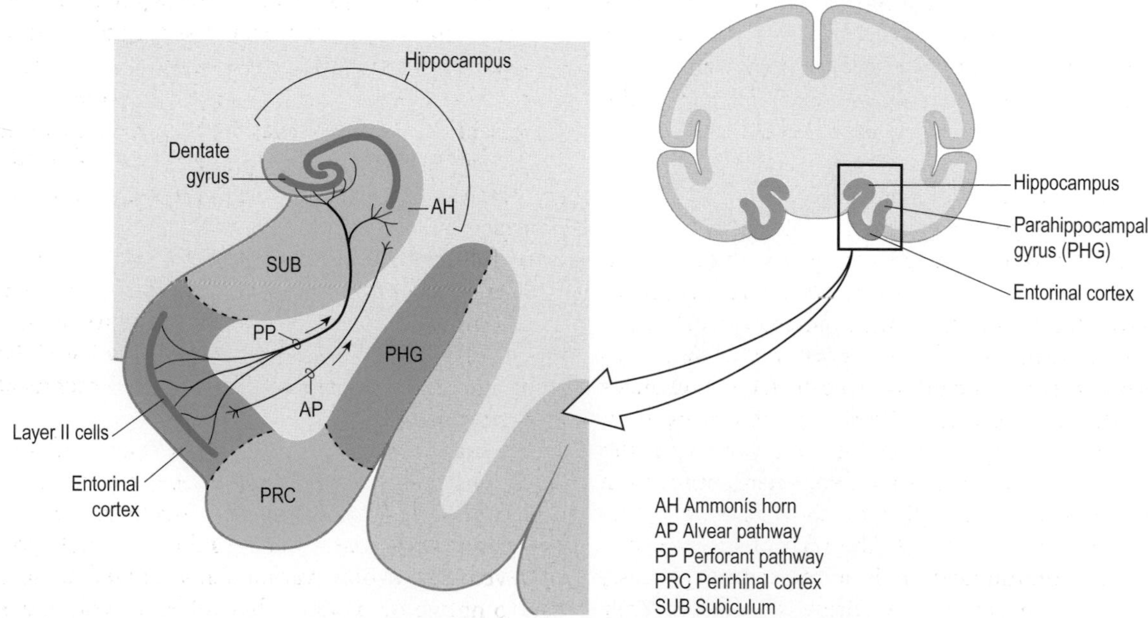

Figure 7.13 • Entorhinal cortex and hippocampus of the brain. (Adapted from Blows 2003, with permission.)

package, which is then sent to the hippocampus. The hippocampus is the part of the brain used for short-term memory, but it is also a key area for influencing thought. Thinking is a function of the frontal lobe, and much of what we think about is based on our sensory understanding of the world around us. The package of integrated senses created by the entorhinal cortex is used by the hippocampus to influence that thinking.

The devastating disorder of schizophrenia is generated by losses of some cells and disruption to others in both the entorhinal cortex and the hippocampus, creating the opportunity for serious disturbances of perception (such as hallucinations) and thought disorder. This results in withdrawal of a person from reality and creates corresponding communication problems. The cause of schizophrenia is unknown, but it is likely to have a polygenic origin (i.e. the combined effects of gene errors with, as yet unidentified, environmental factors) (Blows 2003).

The importance of communication in nursing

Nursing, by definition, takes place in the presence of others and can be viewed as essentially an interpersonal process (Peplau 1988). If one accepts this perspective, then nurses' competencies and sensitivity as communicators will largely determine the effectiveness of nursing care, wherever it takes place.

The definitions of communication have a tremendous range (Department of Health 2003). It can be described as a process that involves a meaningful exchange between at least two people to convey facts, needs, opinions, thoughts, feelings or other information through both verbal and nonverbal means, including face-to-face exchanges and the written word. We human beings are born with the ability to vocalize, but not with the knowledge and skills that define communication competence. The ability to communicate effectively is learned. In fact, the pursuit of effectiveness in communication is a frustrating process; frustrating because it is lifelong and everyday experiences that remind us of just how complex and elusive effective communication actually is; frustrating because to become more effective requires that we first realize our inadequacies. There is a risk in only perceiving communication as a repertoire of skills, so that the activity is reduced to an overly mechanistic process (Hartrick 1997).

The contents and activities of this chapter are designed to achieve a balance between the behavioural and relational aspects of nursing communication. The relational element is an acknowledgement of the phenomenological or subjective nature of human encounters. In other words, the nurse and the patient are unique individuals, with their own constructed views of the world, who bring their perceptions, values, interpretations and experiences to any interactions (Barkausmas et al 2003).

A view is sometimes expressed that communication skills are more significant in mental health nursing than in other specialities. This would seem to undervalue the significance of communication with other client groups and implies that relating to patients is not central to nursing. It is certainly the case that mental health nurses engage in complex relationships in their working lives, but communication is equally as important for all of the other care groups. Nurses working in an intensive care unit or in an operating theatre still require sophisticated communication skills, as do nurses trying to relate to an individual with severe learning disability or to families in a children's ward. Each context has its own challenges, but a consistent feature is the need for effective communication (see Case history 7.4).

It follows from these general remarks that nursing students are expected to take seriously the communication aspects of their work and to develop key professional communication skills alongside more obvious practical or technical competence.

We suggest that you keep a daily record of conversations you observe taking place, or conversations that you have conducted, while you are in your foundation year. Keeping a diary will help you to develop your observation skills, as well as help you to notice techniques that different colleagues use in different situations. After a while you will

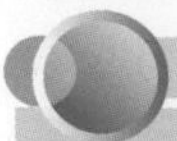

Case history 7.4

Communicating with people who have sight difficulties, hearing difficulties and with a learning disability

Richard is a 19-year-old young man in a surgical ward for acute appendicitis. Richard is autistic. He functions cognitively at about the level of a 3-year-old. He is non-verbal and communicates through gestures and a form of British Sign Language used by the developmentally disabled. He also has sight difficulties and requires spectacles to see. He lives in a residential centre for developmentally disabled people.

Being hospitalized for surgery is a stressful event for Richard. The nurse in charge realizes that Richard is a special patient and requires the nurse who looks after him to be equipped with multiple communication skills. In order to provide Richard with the most appropriate care, an emergency caring conference was held to discuss Richard's care plan. Because Richard's sight and hearing difficulties, compounded by autism, present a considerable challenge, a comprehensive care plan was laid out to address his special needs. A senior nurse who has previous experience working with patients with difficulties similar to Richard's takes on the task to look after him.

First of all the nurse obtains a very detailed social history of Richard from his mother, as this information is extremely important in understanding Richard as a person and will greatly contribute to effective communication with him. Second, the nurse prepares herself by reviewing the sign language that Richard uses. Thus when she is ready to introduce herself to Richard, she already has a very good idea about Richard and how to approach him. At the end of her shift, the nurse writes down a few key points which serve as reminders for the nurses on the next shift, who may be less experienced in looking after patients with multiple communication barriers. It is highlighted that, even though Richard is on an adult ward, his cognitive level requires nurses to use nursing skills from other branches of nursing such as children's nursing and mental health nursing.

Because the ward took a very proactive approach in caring and communicating with Richard, he has remained very calm and cooperative. Consequently, he is fit to be discharged as early as possible so that he can return to his usual living environment. Another ward conference is held after Richard has been discharged in order that the nurses may reflect on the experience gained through his care. It is identified that it is important to remember that there is no single method that suits all patients with communication or learning disabilities. Each patient should be treated as an individual. A sound understanding of issues pertaining to these difficulties and disabilities is crucial. The ability to use sign language proved to be vital in Richard's case. After the conference, the rest of the nurses on the ward, including all the nursing students, decided that they were all going to take a training course on how to use sign language.

develop a shorthand system of documenting your observations which will be speedier. Spending some time during a quiet period, either at home or while at work, considering what you have observed will help your learning and skill development. Don't forget that you need to respect the 'NMC Code of professional conduct' and maintain confidentiality, so no using real names.

Contextual and demographic changes impact on the nurse as communicator. The significant number of older people in our society means that many more older people are able to enjoy a healthy and active life. This in turn means that you are likely to meet older people requiring routine surgery at quite an advanced age. This presents a challenge for nurses. Some of the very old people and people who are physically frail often feel isolated from society because of their inability to go out and meet people or engage in many of the daily routines of shopping, going to the cinema and so on. A responsibility often lies with nurses and other health and social care professionals to assist these people to be included in society, to have a voice in a comprehensive health system and in society generally.

Shorter stays in hospitals and an emphasis on a community-based service also change the context of nursing communication. Hospital staff often complain that they have insufficient time to get to know the patients; and community staff sometimes feel they have insufficient time to meet the demands of increasing caseloads. Communication between hospital and community, and between different community agencies, largely dictates whether community care works or does not work. The increasing cultural diversity of our society creates another kind of challenge, and learning how to communicate with people who do not share a common language can be challenging for nurses working in hospitals, nursing homes or in the community.

The nurse–patient relationship

You may have read critiques in the nursing press about the loss of the artistic elements of nursing care, as practitioners become technically knowledgeable about normal and abnormal body function. This use of technical knowledge has become essential as medical care treatments have become more sophisticated and nurses have taken on more and more of the activities that doctors previously undertook. Nevertheless, the emphasis of nursing education has been to promote holistic care and to treat the person rather than the illness. The implication of this shift is that both nurse and patient are now seen as people who bring their full humanity to their relationship, the quality of which contributes significantly to the therapeutic effectiveness of any treatment the patient receives. This can be both reassuring and daunting for a nurse: reassuring, because all personal resources, and not only the competence achieved as a direct result of training, are relevant to the professional role; daunting, because there is no opting out of recognizing the relevance of the nurse's whole personality and behaviour to the treatment of a patient. However, the policy is often hard to implement when there is a high turnover of people going through bed spaces and staff work long shifts and so often only care for a group of patients once or twice during their hospital stay. Community nurses often, by contrast, are able to develop relationships with their clients that last several years. So both these experiences of health care provision create a challenge for the nurse.

The inevitability of communication

Human beings have a basic drive to relate to one another which is expressed through communication. When two or more people are together they cannot help but communicate. It is difficult to imagine strangers on a train sitting together for any length of time without some form of communication taking place between them, even if no-one speaks. Smiling is a communication, as is not smiling. One cannot *not* communicate as there is no opposite of 'behaviour'. All behaviour has message value even when this is not consciously intended, and once a message has been sent it cannot be retracted.

Relating

Babies cannot survive without someone relating to them. Their bodies are made out of the bodies of their closest relatives. Their capacity to be fully human in an emotional sense is realized through relationships with others. As children mature, this external relating gradually becomes internalized, so that the quality of their earliest relationships with others profoundly affects the way in which they relate to themselves. In turn, this inner world of relating is projected onto the outside world, affecting the way they relate to other people. It is helpful for a nurse to be aware of this basic pattern of relating and of how the present is built on the past.

The human need to relate remains fundamental and universal. It does not go away with time or maturity. Its very intensity and permanence give rise to the multifarious ways in which it is expressed – in love, in sex, in marriage, in friendship, in work, in social activities, in sport, in religion – and is the glue that holds families, communities, organizations and nations together. It can also be suppressed or hated. Nevertheless, the 'me/you' issues of life never go away; they determine our happiness and sense of fulfilment.

The complexity of communication and potential for misunderstanding

Shortcomings of both intimate and work relationships are often similar, centering around poor communication: not being listened to, not knowing what is going on, not being valued for one's individual self, not being taken into account. Statements such as 'We live in the same house but we just don't communicate' or 'No-one tells me anything around here' suggest the feelings of anger, frustration and even helplessness that are aroused by poor communication. They also show that sending a message is not, in itself, communication. The message has to be received and understood by the receiver for communication to take place. Perhaps it is not surprising that users of the National Health Service have consistently highlighted dissatisfaction with communication. Indeed, it seems there is a significant correlation between the general satisfaction of patients and their specific satisfaction with nursing communication (Ricketts 1996).

Many studies have identified communication problems in the delivery of health care (Hewison 1995, Lilly et al 2003, Wilkinson 1999). Nurse education has responded to these findings to some extent but there is no room for complacency. The reasons for the problems are complex and often specific to the area being researched, but include: lack of skills and training; lack of resources and time; emotional vulnerability; the location of power; and even some deliberately perpetuated bad practices between agencies. This has to be seen within the complicated and elaborate network of relationships with patients, colleagues, informal carers and multidisciplinary agencies.

The nurse's relationships

Figure 7.14 maps the variety of relationships that a nurse is likely to experience. Having so many relationships with such a wide range of people means that the nurse needs to be sensitive in how she uses different approaches to communicating, depending on the context, the age, the ability and the state of mental or physical health of the other

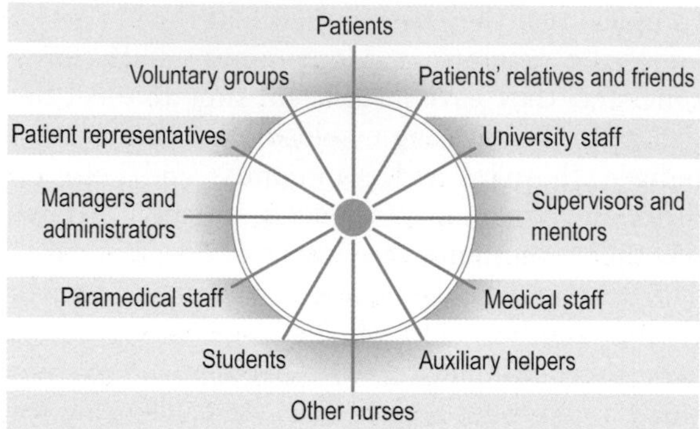

Figure 7.14 • A web of relationships.

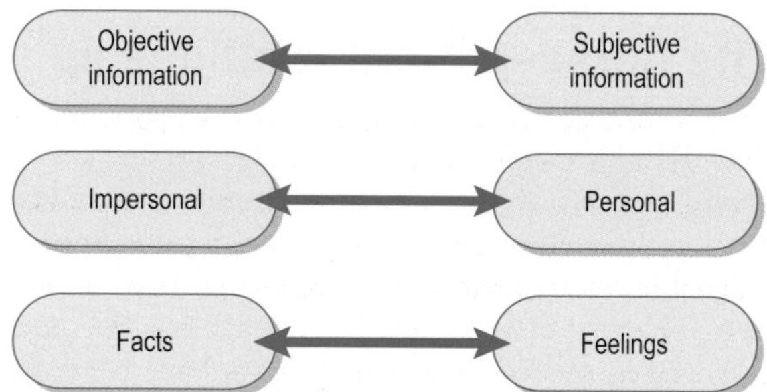

Figure 7.15 • Dimensions of communication.

person or persons involved. Most young children are still learning how to make the subtle judgements required to communicate effectively in different circumstances. Such naivety is charming in children but less so in adult professionals.

Consider the dimensions of communication identified in Figure 7.15. Any communication is likely to be biased towards one end of each dimension, depending on the context and the people involved. For example, a doctor who says 'And this patient's blood pressure?' is likely to expect an answer of objective information rather than an expression of personal feelings about the patient's treatment.

Personal flexibility

Some people are flexible in their use of different communication styles and manage to respond to different contexts in an appropriate way. Others find it difficult to adjust so that, for example, they always talk impersonally and factually even when an expression of feelings and subjective views is of pressing importance. Another person might be emotional and subjective when a cool look at the facts is what is really needed. The multifaceted role of the nurse within a complex social context necessitates the nurse to be flexible in matching the appropriate communication to the individual(s) and the set of circumstances.

The way in which we communicate can be seen as dependent on our whole personality. Certainly, what is communicated between two people is a product of the interaction of the three basic components: sender, receiver and message (see Figure 7.1). A patient who is asked the question 'How are you?' by two different nurses might pick up quite different meanings. From one, it might be an empty phrase, said perhaps while the nurse was attending to something else. From the other, it might be a genuine empathic enquiry into the patient's thoughts and feelings at the time. Which message is received will depend on the patient processing all of the information available. The judgement about the meaning of that information will depend on the patient's own expectations and personality.

Self and communication

You will have realized by now that communication is a complex process. Being able to engage in a meaningful exchange with another person, irrespective of their ability to hear, see or respond verbally, requires considerable skill. Being able to do so with children or with adults who are mentally confused or physically frail requires even greater sensitivity and skill. In this section, we explore the various factors that might influence how effectively we communicate with others, including what we bring to the conversation.

The conscious and unconscious mind

You may be aware that the conscious mind is aware that it knows; the unconscious is not aware that it knows. The Viennese father of psychoanalytical therapy, Sigmund Freud, was the first to study the unconscious mind seriously and through his written accounts of his clients he has greatly enriched our understanding of human nature. Many of his views are still considered to be controversial. Freud theorized that the common experience of not knowing why we do things, or the act of discovering that we are saying things that we didn't want to say and are contrary to our conscious wishes, suggests there is another part of our mind at work, the unconscious mind. Freud believed that we can discover our unconscious mind through our dreams.

Self-awareness

Facets of ourselves that are beyond our consciousness are also beyond our control and may adversely impact on our best of intentions. Such facets of ourselves include our attitudes, our values, our beliefs, our emotional state and feelings and influence our behaviour. If we are able to develop a high level of self-awareness and understanding of our beliefs and values, we are more likely to have more productive relationships with friends, colleagues and clients, and to have a greater sense of self-purpose. By developing an increased self-understanding we can make the best out of situations that could otherwise become unpleasant or cause unhappiness.

Having a stronger sense of self nearly always results in being able to distinguish between personal feelings and attitudes and those of other people that they are projecting. A classic example is when a patient feels he has fallen in love with his nurse, or when a relative feels very hostile and angry towards his loved ones or their nurse. Such feelings reside outside the nurse and could be the result of having to rely on the nurse for help and support. Understanding this and being clear about personal levels of responsibility helps one to cope effectively in such situations. Having an understanding that how you see yourself may be different from how others see you is important to learn and is essential to becoming an effective communicator.

We all develop and hold a personal and particular view of the world and relationships with others that is different to how others perceive it. This subjectivity, or personal world view, and its influence on how we relate to others and to the world in general, means that nurses, who are directly involved in interpersonal relationships, need to be aware of how their beliefs might be influencing, or be influenced by, external behaviours and factors. Stein-Parbury (1993, p 60) states:

> *Nurses need to develop acute self-awareness whenever they engage in interactions and relationships with patients, because the primary tool they are using in these circumstances is themselves. Without self-awareness, nurses run the risk of imposing their values and views onto patients . . . Through self-awareness, nurses remain in touch with what they are doing and how this is affecting patients for whom they care.*

Increasing self-awareness

Rogers (1974) emphasized the view that the degree to which we understand ourselves is the degree to which we are able to understand and help others. The first point to make is that this is a pursuit of the unachievable. The idea that we achieve complete self-awareness on a certain day is unrealistic. The concept of self-awareness is best thought of as a continuum. Many believe that our lifelong task is to inch our way along that continuum of self-awareness, in the understanding and acceptance that we will never reach its end. Our progress is more likely to be achieved through introspective processes such as reflection, self-exploration and self-assessment and by interactive activities such as self-disclosure, discussion and feedback (see Case history 7.5).

Burnard (2002, p 15–16) defines self-awareness as a process:

> *Self-awareness refers to the gradual and continuous process of noticing and exploring aspects of self, whether behavioural, psychological or physical, with the intention of developing personal and interpersonal understanding . . . to have a deeper understanding of ourselves is to have a sharper and clearer picture of what is happening to others. In a sense it is a process of discrimination.*

Case history 7.5

Increasing self-awareness (from Betts 1995)

Julie, a student on the learning disabilities branch, watches the replay of a video recording of herself interacting with a fellow student. She is both fascinated and disconcerted by what she observes. Seeing herself from the outside presents a contrasting image to her 'internal' view of herself. She notices repeated mannerisms which previously she had no idea she used. She is able to check out later with her peers how they had experienced these behaviours and is not too surprised to discover that others had perceived them as a distraction. As a result of this experience, Julie is aware of aspects of herself that were previously beyond her consciousness. This learning experience has increased her options and further refined her capacity to communicate effectively with others.

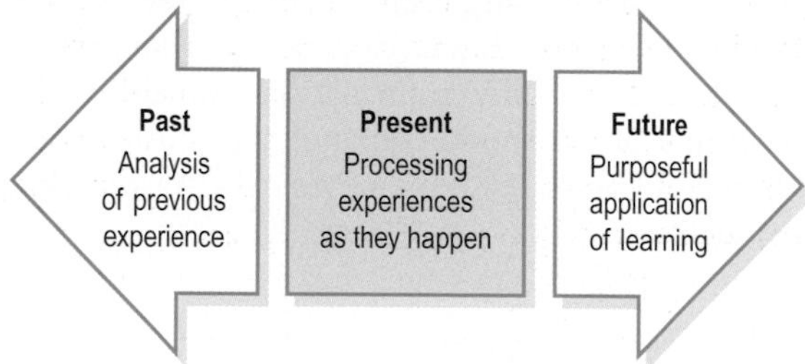

Figure 7.16 • Three dimensions of reflection. (Adapted from Betts 1995.)

Learning about self, relationships and communication through reflection

Since Schön (1983) coined the term 'reflective practitioner', it has appeared frequently within nursing literature. The suggestion is that nurses incorporate 'reflection' into their practice, but confusion exists regarding the meaning of the word. Boud et al (1985) state succinctly that 'reflection' in this context refers to 'turning experience into learning'. This is a purposeful and conscious activity requiring structured time and effort rather than an automatic process. Different methods can be used to achieve this, such as introspection, writing, discussion or clinical supervision. One common misconception of reflection is that it consists purely of historical analysis (see Figure 7.16).

Kemmis (1985) stressed that reflection is not an end in itself but that it leads to informed, committed action. Learning to become an effective and reflective communicator eventually leads to the ability to 'process', or to analyse and respond effectively to, what is happening during an interaction rather than only after it has finished. Being able to process experiences accurately allows us to choose the way in which we wish to respond. This results in our ability to have more control over our use of self, to become more intentional in our use of self. Schön (1983) referred to processing experiences as they happen as 'reflection in action', and to retrospective reflection after the event as 'reflection on action' (see Figure 7.16).

For some people, reflective writing is productive as a medium for the recording and analysis of interactions. The use of learning journals or communication diaries to record, analyse and evaluate specific experiences may suit some people. Walker (1985) suggested that writing provides an objectivity and clarity to experiences by removing elements of subjective feeling that can obscure issues. These written records also provide data for further review in tutorials, supervision sessions or with peers. Some examples of reflective questions are listed in Box 7.3.

Box 7.3

Examples of reflective questions (adapted from Betts 1995)

- What was the context of the interaction?
- What was the purpose of the interaction?
- What actually happened?
- What were my behaviours, thoughts, feelings at the time?
- What were the other(s)' behaviours?
- What do I imagine were the other(s)' thoughts and feelings at the time?
- What were my thoughts and feelings afterwards?
- What do I imagine were the other(s)' thoughts and feelings afterwards?
- How successful was the interaction?
- What skills did I use well/not so well?
- Given the opportunity, how would I do it differently?

Matching communication to different contexts

You will realize from the discussion above that we are arguing that we can consciously choose how to communicate with others, and indeed this is the essence of communication. Effective communicators are more likely to make the right or appropriate choices in the situations they face because they are clear about what they hope to achieve (Heron 2001). To be successful in making such decisions, you need to develop sensitivity and empathic understanding to read each situation accurately and to respond appropriately. The nurse's choice of intervention is determined by the needs and resources of the other person at the time. Nurses are likely to choose to use any one of the range of helping strategies (TACTICS) depicted in Figure 7.17.

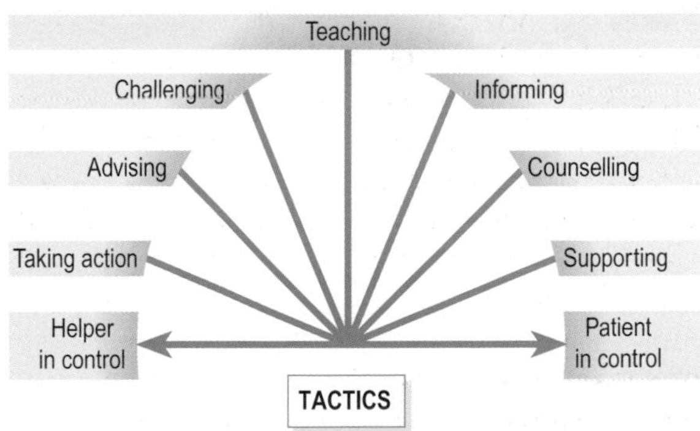

Figure 7.17 • Strategies (TACTICS) for helping. (Adapted from the National Institute for Careers Educational and Counselling model.)

Moving from one extreme strategy of 'taking action' to the other extreme of 'supporting', the basis of the helping relationship changes by degrees from 'helper in control' to 'patient in control'. The issue of where the balance of control lies between helper and patient distinguishes one strategy from another and gives each its own special characteristics. None of these TACTICS or strategies is intrinsically superior to others. The art of effective communication, in nursing, concerns diversity, and choosing the appropriate strategy according to the needs of the patient and/or carer at the time (see Case history 7.6).

Taking action

The 'taking action' strategy (Figure 7.17) implies that the nurse is working on behalf of the individual. This type of strategy is indicated when a patient is incapacitated through some aspect of ill-health or loss of function, and the type of communication is by nature directive. The rationale for such helping is founded in a judgement that patients are unable, temporarily or permanently, to perform an action or represent themselves. Consequently, nurses need either to take this responsibility themselves or to refer on to another who is more able to do so.

Consider the position of Anna in Case history 7.7:

- How do you think Anna might attempt to establish a relationship with Maria?
- How do you think Anna will be able to communicate with Maria?

The decision to take action for others (to take control) is a significant judgement that should be based on careful consideration of all the factors. As a general principle, it is preferable to negotiate and empower patients in their own decision-making, but situations arise in which a more paternalistic approach is required in the interests of the patient.

An alternative form of taking action for others involves an advocacy role for nurses. Gates (1994, p 2) defines advocacy as:

> *The process of befriending, and where necessary representing, a patient . . . in all matters where the nurse's help is needed, in order to protect the rights or promote the interests of that person.*

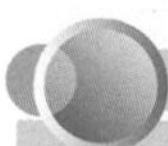

Case history 7.6

Adaptability as a prerequisite for effective communication

Simon is an experienced nurse on a children's ward. He is the supervisor of Anita, who is a common foundation programme student on placement. Anita is required to write up observations of nurse–patient interactions to meet the learning outcomes of one of her modules.

What impresses Anita about Simon is his versatility as a communicator. At one point he demonstrates a close rapport with a 6-year-old girl, and at another he listens attentively to the concerns of a worried mother. Anita notices that Simon matches his intervention to the individual in a seemingly effortless manner. He recognizes when it is appropriate to advise or give information to patients and relatives, and also when it is more appropriate to encourage self-disclosure or emotional expression through the effective use of counselling skills.

Anita reflects on the crucial importance of developing the ability to be adaptable and intentional in nursing interactions and hopes to achieve Simon's level of competence, judgement and confidence.

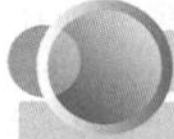

Case history 7.7

Maria

Maria has schizophrenia. She was admitted last night under an emergency section of the Mental Health Act, after being found wandering the streets, shouting at passers-by and trying to get into people's houses. She is fearful that she is being followed by two women who are out to do her harm. Her psychotic state of mind makes it difficult for her to make rational decisions or to look after herself. The nursing staff consider her to be a danger to herself and to others on the ward. A nurse (Anna) takes on the task of staying with Maria wherever she goes. This causes even more suspicion on Maria's part, but the decision is made that she needs this constant observation to protect her from harming herself or others. There is no negotiation about this care plan because it is judged that Maria is not in a position to understand the reality of her situation. The nurses are taking action on her behalf until she is able once again to make decisions for herself. Despite Maria's acute illness, Anna tries to begin to communicate with her in an attempt to establish some kind of relationship with her.

Nurses sometimes find themselves in a position to represent the patient's interests, as, for example, in a multidisciplinary team meeting. Alternatively, for some issues, it may be more appropriate to refer the patient to an 'outside' advocacy agency.

Advising

The most crucial aspect of giving advice is first to assess if advice is appropriate. Inappropriate advice-giving may have more negative consequences than doing nothing. Advice comes from the adviser's frame of reference and usually consists of what the adviser would do in the given situation. Stein-Parbury (2000) notes that offering advice and suggesting solutions is a common response to others who present problems. She warns that this response may be habitual rather than based on considered choice and that nurses may need to unlearn this customary response and refrain from their usual way of responding.

Inappropriate advice can undermine the self-determining competence of others and may also encourage dependence rather than autonomy. The other potential problem is that the advice may not work out well in practice, resulting in a loss of confidence in the nurse. As a general rule, advice is inappropriate in the case of personal issues but it is sometimes more appropriate in specialist issues. The medical model relies on the expertise of the doctor, and sometimes views the patient as a passive recipient of advice who is expected to comply with the solution that is offered. This attitude is changing, largely as a result of lobbying from patient and carer representative groups to move towards partnership and greater empowerment of patients in their treatment.

Having warned against excessive use of advice, there is clearly a need for such interventions within a nursing context. Activity 7.5 invites you to consider a number of scenarios and decide whether or not giving advice is appropriate in each case.

Activity 7.5

Respond to each of the following scenarios, indicating if advice is appropriate or not. Think carefully about why you arrive at the decision you make.

- A 21-year-old male university student has an extreme episode of anxiety that is mainly related to his impending final examinations. He asks the community psychiatric nurse if he should give up his degree studies.
- A woman, caring for her partner who is recovering from a stroke, contacts the community nurse because she is struggling to help her partner transfer from the bed to a chair.
- A 10-year-old boy wants to know when he can start playing football again following an appendicectomy.
- A female resident with a learning disability lives in a group home and asks one of the care staff for advice about a sexual relationship she is considering starting with another resident.

Principles of giving advice

When advice is indicated, there are a number of factors to consider. First, it is important to assess the person's level of knowledge and understanding of their situation along with their emotional and physical states. These will influence the starting point, the language used and the timing and amount of advice given. It is possible to prescribe advice at different levels. Heron (2001) identified 19 different types of prescription, ranging from directive approaches through to more subtle influencing. This is a question of matching the level of influence to individuals and their circumstances and resources. Finally, it is important to evaluate the response to the advice, by judging the other's level of understanding and degree of acceptance or rejection of the suggestions (try Activity 7.6 which concerns reflection on giving advice).

Activity 7.6

Think of an occasion when you were given advice. Recall the context and nature of the experience. Reflect on the following questions:

- Was the advice appropriate at the time?
- How well was it given?
- How would you have delivered such advice if roles were reversed?

Now, in the light of your reflections, list what you think are the principles of giving advice effectively.

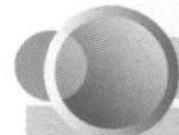

Challenging

Egan (1998) discriminates between the word 'challenge' and the term 'confrontation'. Many people construe confronting and being confronted as unpleasant experiences to be avoided. Egan (1998, p 184) defines challenge as:

> *An invitation to examine internal or external behaviour that seems to be self-defeating, harmful to others, or both and to change the behaviour if it is found to be so.*

Successful challenges increase awareness and promote insight by enabling others to come face-to-face with aspects of themselves or their behaviour. Heron (2001) emphasized that, in a helping context, challenge is a non-aggressive and non-combative intervention, unlike the meaning of the term in some other situations. Sensitive challenging is an advanced communication skill but necessary within the repertoire of strategies available to nurses. Case history 7.8 describes scenarios in which challenging is appropriate.

Principles of challenging

There is a difference between a constructive and a destructive challenge. Constructive challenges throw a searchlight on alternatives and leave the other person with something on which to build or change. Destructive challenging is delivered unskilfully and leaves the other person feeling bad or put down, with nothing to build on. The goal is to raise the consciousness of unused strengths and potential.

Another principle of the effective challenge is specificity or being unambiguous about the focus of the challenge and being clear about the message one wants to give rather than generalizing.

Empathic understanding is a crucial element of challenging. This involves listening carefully to the other's perspective and acknowledging their position while encouraging an alternative. Challenging without empathy is brutal and destructive because it invalidates the subjective reality of the other person.

Assertiveness is a feature of effective challenging. Furthermore, assertive communication is the key to communicating important messages to others. It also helps individuals to stand up for their rights and, when appropriate, the rights of others (e.g. advocacy). The message should have sufficient strength without being apologetic or overzealous. Aggression is destructive and passivity is ineffective. Non-verbal communication should be congruent with the spoken message, as suggested earlier in this chapter.

The context of the challenge is important, in terms of both timing and setting. The first scenario in Case history 7.8 demonstrates this well. The nurse did not challenge her colleague at the time of the incident but selected a strategic moment and setting with the desired result.

Case history 7.8

Challenging situations

During a particularly hectic shift on a children's ward, a nurse observes one of her colleagues expressing her frustration in an angry exchange with a 14-year-old male patient. The nurse thinks that her colleague's response is excessive and takes the opportunity at a quieter moment in the coffee room to challenge her about what happened. The firm but sensitive intervention highlights the unacceptable nature of the exchange without alienating the colleague.

Sarah, a 28-year-old woman, has been an inpatient on the mental health unit for 3 weeks. Her depression has started to lift and she is now more able to engage in therapeutic dialogue with one of the nurses. She talks about her life, in particular the things that have gone wrong. The nurse listens carefully and notices that there is a theme running through all of Sarah's life situations. She describes events as if she has no power or control over how things turn out. It is as if life is all down to fate rather than to choice. The relationships that have gone wrong and the missed opportunities she has experienced are the fault of others. She sees herself as a victim of circumstances with no resources to influence the outcomes of these situations. The nurse uses a skilful combination of empathy and challenge to bring into relief this pattern of victim that runs through Sarah's life situations. Together they explore ways in which Sarah could take more responsibility and control over life events.

Finally, Egan (1998, 2002) suggests that effective challengers are open to challenge themselves by not immediately rejecting or disputing any challenge, but, instead, clarifying and considering the alternative perspective before deciding how to respond.

Assertiveness and aggression

Assertiveness

Assertiveness is the ability to express your thoughts, your ideas and your feelings in a direct, honest and appropriate way. It means that we have respect both for ourselves and for others. We are consciously working towards a 'win–win' solution to problems. A win–win solution means that we are trying to make sure that both parties end up with their needs met to the extent possible. Assertive communication is the key to successful relationships for the client, the family, the nurse and other colleagues. An assertive communicator effectively influences, listens and negotiates so that others choose to cooperate willingly.

Bower & Bower (1991) developed a framework for developing assertive responses known as the 'DESC script'. This is a useful tool, although not all steps are used in every situation:

Describe the situation.
Express what you think and feel.
Specify your request.
Consequence.

To build your assertive skills you will need further study and application (see Box 7.4). Riley (2004) emphasized that there are three essential criteria for success: timing, content and receptivity. For example, if you need to discuss mentorship issues with your mentor, the best time would be a scheduled meeting and in a private location where there is less chance of interruption. At the end of a long shift, when both of you are tired and ready to go home, would be an inappropriate time.

Aggressiveness

People sometimes confuse assertiveness with aggressiveness (see Box 7.5). Aggressiveness involves expressing our thoughts, feelings and

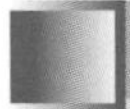

Box 7.4

Communication techniques that can help you convey a positive assertive attitude

- Use suitable facial expressions, always maintaining good eye contact.
- Keep your voice firm but pleasant.
- Pay careful attention to your posture and gestures.
- Listen and let people know you have heard what they have said.
- Ask questions for clarification.
- Have a positive attitude about communicating directly and honestly.
- Feel comfortable and in control of anxiety, tenseness, shyness, or fear.
- Feel confident that you can conduct yourself in a self-respecting way whilst still respecting others.
- Honour the fact that you and the other person both have rights.
- Look for a win–win approach to problem-solving.

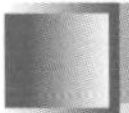

Box 7.5

A comparison between assertive and aggressive styles of communication (Phelps & Austin 2002)

Assertive

'I am OK, you are OK'.
Engage in direct, fair confrontation.
Use of clear direct statements of wants, objective words, honest statements of feelings and confident congruent messages.
Lift yourself up without putting others down.
Mutual respect.
'I win, you win' strives for 'win–win' or 'non-lose' solutions.

Aggressive

'I am OK, you are *not* OK' is an attack on the other person.
Use of loaded words, accusations, superior haughty words, labelling of the other person.
Air of superiority, flippant, sarcastic style causes hurt, defensiveness, humiliation.
'I win, you lose' beats out others at any cost.

beliefs in a way that is inappropriate and more seriously violates the rights of others. It can be active or passive, but, no matter which, it communicates an impression of disrespect. By being aggressive, we put our wants, needs and rights above those of others. We attempt to get our way by not allowing others a choice. Where assertiveness tries to find a win–win solution, aggressiveness strives for a win–lose solution: 'I'll be the winner, you will be the loser'. Communication should have positive benefits for you and for others. Aggressive behaviour is destructive as it provokes anger and may lead to retaliation.

Giving information

Many studies over the past 20 years have highlighted shortcomings of information-giving in health care settings. Perhaps in such a large and complex system it is inevitable that the exchange of information is not always as good as it could be. The potential for information to get lost or become corrupted as it passes between agencies, departments and individuals is considerable. We live in the information age in which new technologies, better education, lobbying groups and increased expectations have resulted in greater and more immediate access to all kinds of information. The health arena is no exception, and patients, carers and professionals rightly expect to receive relevant, accurate and understandable information. Information empowers patients and elevates them to partnerships in care, rather than passive recipients of treatment.

It is easy to confuse information with advice. On one level, the distinction is clear in that information is neutral and non-prescriptive, whereas advice involves suggesting or presenting solutions. On a second level, things are more complex. The informer may believe that the message is given in a non-prescriptive way but may underestimate the social influence that is inherent in the way that it is given, or the very fact that it is provided by a person who is seen as an expert.

Principles of giving information

A starting point and the first principle of giving information is to determine the other person's readiness to receive information. Benner (2001) indicates that capturing the patient's/client's readiness to learn is an advanced judgement that is characteristic of expert nursing practice. This involves picking up and determining cues from patients to judge if, when and how much information should be given. This will vary with individual patients, some of whom will be eager to gather every scrap of information about their condition whereas others would prefer not to know very much at all. These same cues give indications as to the timing of the information-giving.

Having decided that information-sharing is the appropriate intervention, it is important to clarify what the patient already knows and to assess the accuracy of their knowledge. This demonstrates that information sharing begins with open questioning rather than the imparting of facts, and allows the informer to pitch the information at the right level. Doing a preliminary assessment allows you to pitch the information at the right level and to keep it relevant. You may find that you do not have sufficient understanding or knowledge and that you need to get help from a more senior colleague.

When it comes to the actual information-giving, there is some evidence that people recall opening statements (primacy effect) and attach high significance to these messages. This is particularly likely if the opening statement is emotionally significant to the patient, such as a confirmation of a diagnosis. An example of this is the confirmation of a positive HIV (human immunodeficiency virus) test result. Staff working in this speciality have learned that the capacity to absorb information directly following the receipt of this news is poor. The need for follow-up interviews and giving out written information is helpful as it means the patient can re-read the information when they are feeling less anxious, and can also share the information with a close relative or friend.

A second principle is not to give too much information at once. Too much detail can result in confusion and misunderstanding.

A third principle is to ask the patient or carer to tell you what they have understood using their own words. Using this technique helps patients to remember more accurately what has been said and it has the advantage of letting you assess whether they have understood the important points.

Using accessible language

Health care jargon and technical language often exclude patients and carers from meaningful communication (see Case history 7.9). Throughout their education, nurses are introduced to a wide new vocabulary, and to survive and be successful they have to learn how to use it correctly (Gumperz 1968). This socialization process soon becomes forgotten as, with increasing familiarity with the vocabulary, nurses can often forget that patients and their carers are completely unfamiliar with the language. Use of nursing jargon and acronyms provides a shorthand communication system between professionals, but it is often an inappropriate style of speech with patients and carers (Kagan et al 1986).

Case history 7.9 illustrates the kind of vocabulary that is distinctive of a specific discipline in medicine and which is beyond the understanding of most people who have not studied medicine. As an example of communication it is very poor. As a means of helping someone understand what is happening it is very bad. So it is always important to spend some time with your patients, ensuring that they understand the information they have been given and to give them the chance to ask for clarification, particularly if the patient is elderly. It is also important to remember that someone may have good spoken English, or Welsh, but not be able to read it, and to be sensitive to people whose first language is not English. Most health care providers have access to interpreters and to written information in different languages.

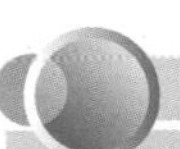

Case history 7.9

Inappropriate use of language

Information given by a psychiatrist to a patient's partner:

Your partner's symptoms are characteristic of a bipolar affective disorder. This condition is typified by fluctuating episodes of hypomania and periods of depression. Your partner's premorbid personality is cyclothymic, which is not uncommon in these cases. Symptoms are usually fairly well controlled by lithium carbonate, although neuroleptics or antidepressants may be required at certain times. Any questions?

The nurse as a teacher

The educational role that nurses should undertake is crucial to helping patients and their carers learn how to maintain and promote their own health and well-being. Being a teacher also includes supporting the professional development of colleagues. With increasing emphasis on using strategies that help people learn in their workplace, the contribution that each member of the health care team can make towards increased understanding and use of good practices is crucial to the welfare of patients. Even as a foundation course nurse you will find that you have something to teach either a colleague or a patient. Figure 7.17 locates teaching at the midpoint of a continuum of control. This is indicative of the diversity of possible approaches to helping someone learn, ranging from approaches that assume the only person with knowledge is the teacher to the opposite approach, which is facilitative and relies on trying to support the learner in learning for themselves. As you can imagine the different approaches require very different communication skills.

The educational role of the nurse with patients/clients and carers

Learning how to help patients or clients and their carers to carry out techniques and procedures is an important nursing skill. The nursing theorist Dorothea Orem (2001) believes that patients have a responsibility to maintain their own health by extending their self-care functions as necessary. She suggests that, if an individual is unable to do this, the next logical caregiver is an immediate family member or close friend. In the UK, it is estimated that there are 6 million non-professional carers (National Health Service 2000). This means that 6 million people are using everyday nursing skills to support the health and well-being of a friend or relative, and it is important that they understand how to use such skills safely and effectively. Inevitably, the nurse is the first person to provide such support, even to the point of teaching a patient how to take their drugs safely when they go home from hospital, clinic or nursing home.

There is a danger in teaching skills in isolation of the theory that informs the practice. For example, teaching a carer the practical skills of an aseptic technique with no attention to the principles of asepsis will not help the carer if, for some reason, she/he has to adapt the procedure because of a shortage of resources. Being able to teach a client/patient and their carer effectively means that you need to be able use educational psychology and the principles and practice of teaching and learning.

The helping relationship and counselling skills

Defining counselling

Counselling is a professional activity in its own right, and it may be more appropriate in the nursing context to think of nurses using counselling *skills* rather than being counsellors to their patients. Each person brings their internal world and outward behaviour into a common space in which the counselling work is carried out. This can happen only if the space is protected from intrusion or distraction and the two people are engaging with each other in a voluntary way.

The basic aim of counselling is to help individuals to help themselves. The British Association for Counselling (1992) makes the following comments on the nature of counselling:

> *The overall aim of counselling is to provide an opportunity for the client to work towards living in a more satisfying and resourceful way . . . Counselling may be concerned with developmental issues, addressing and resolving specific problems, making decisions, coping with crisis, developing personal insight and knowledge, working through feelings of inner conflict or improving relationships with others. The counsellor's role is to facilitate the client's work in ways which respect the client's values, personal resources and capacity for self-determination.*
>
> *The goal of counselling is to enable people to be in closer touch with their own resources so that they can move towards greater freedom, autonomy and independence. It assumes that any conflict or anxiety arising within the personal world of the individual can only be dealt with using the resources within that person. An individual may ask for help or advice from another person but, until such assistance is actually accepted, it cannot be used for self-help.*

Counselling skills within the context of nursing

As a common foundation nursing student, you will find yourself drawn into providing psychological support and assistance to people who are trying to come to terms with a life-changing experience and who are experiencing a diversity of personally significant life events (Betts 1995). If you are working in mental health, you will need to develop good listening skills and the ability to help people describe their fears and feelings without being judged. So for your development at this stage in your programme it is wise to be cautious and to develop your skills under the close supervision and support of your mentor.

Qualities of using effective counselling skills

Rogers (1974) suggested that, for counselling skills to be effective, three core conditions of the relationship are necessary:

- Empathetic understanding.
- Congruence or genuineness.
- Unconditional positive regard.

These values are the foundation for a trusting relationship. Without trust in the capacity of clients to help themselves, the nurse is joining forces with those who would keep clients exactly where they are. Respect for the client is linked to trust; it suggests that the individual's rights, beliefs and resources are respected for what they are, without judgement (Ellis et al 2003).

Empathetic understanding

Empathy is often seen as the most critical ingredient of the helping relationship. Carkhuff (1970) argued that, without empathy, there is no basis for helping. Kalisch (1971, p 203) defined empathy as 'the ability to sense the client's world as if it were your own, but without losing the as if quality'. This short definition contains some complex ideas. Empathetic understanding is often described as 'standing in somebody else's shoes', but this is not the full story. Imagine how you might feel at the end of a day if you stand in the shoes of each person you meet in your helping role, experiencing their thoughts and feelings. Empathy involves retaining your own separateness whilst trying to understand the world from the other person's perspective. In order to do this, it is necessary to understand the client's world as if you were inside it, attempting to see it with the client's eyes, but at the same time keeping in touch with your own world. In this way, the helper remains in a position to help, to get close enough to the client's experience to make a difference whilst retaining a sense of objectivity in order to hold on to the process and not become overwhelmed.

Genuineness

This is sometimes referred to as 'congruence' or 'authenticity'. All three of these terms refer to the helper being consistently real in the helping relationship. Corey (2001) suggested that congruent helpers are without a false front and that their inner experience matches their outer expression of that experience and vice versa. In other words, what clients see is who the helper really is. Relating deeply to others is part of the effective helper's lifestyle rather than a role that is switched on and off. Inauthentic helping may appear as unauthentic and lacking in integrity, lacking in the very qualities that make the helper unique as an individual in the relationship. The nurse who adopts a synthetic 'helping mode' when seeing someone in distress may be perceived as patronizing and untrustworthy.

Unconditional positive regard

Unconditional positive regard refers to the idea that there should be no conditions laid down by the practitioner for their acceptance and care for the client. So often we are brought up to believe that we will be accepted if we are good, successful and pleasant, and rejected if we are bad, unsuccessful and unpleasant. The 'unconditional' nature of Rogers' approach means that we are accepted whatever we are, and in our entirety. 'Positive regard' is an attitude of optimistic expectation, stemming from the unconditional acceptance of the person. The three words together, if translated into practice, create a quality and atmosphere in the 'counselling space' that facilitates growth in clients, allowing them to get in touch with the more positive aspects of themselves over time, so that they become more able to help themselves. If we have been lucky, we have experienced the positive effect of someone else who is benign, who believes in us, who accepts us and who is on our side. Such experience releases the potential in us, which otherwise might have remained dormant and unrealized.

From dependence to independence

The paradox that is central to a helping relationship stems from the basic human need to relate, the theme throughout this chapter. It is out of relating to another person that the individual is able to develop a surer sense of 'I, myself' – a common outcome of successful helping. The individual can have no clear sense of identity without relating to others, just as they can have no real independence without having had, at some time, the experience of dependence.

Focusing on the personal world of the patient/client

The focus is on the person and the personal world, especially feelings. Nurses need to listen, think, imagine and feel in the helping relationship, the space between themselves and the patient/client, so that they get as good an idea as possible of what it is like to be that person, as they are, in the present. This empathy has a 'with you' quality

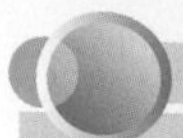

Case history 7.10

Focusing on the personal world of the patient

Patient: Why did this happen to me?

Nurse: (Silence, then:) It's difficult to understand.

Patient: But why me?

Nurse: (Silence, then:) I can see how angry you feel.

Patient: That's not much use, is it?

Nurse: (Quietly accepting the expressed feelings.)

This kind of exchange allows for an acceptance of the patient's feelings (unhappiness and anger in this case) rather than brushing them aside, retaliating or referring to people who are worse off.

about it, which goes beyond intellectual understanding and sympathy, concentrating as it does on 'being there' with and for the patient rather than 'doing something' for him. It enables the nurse to 'hold' a patient's fears and anxieties, without being tempted to try to give answers or solutions (see Case history 7.10).

Commitment in a helping relationship

To be an effective nurse and to develop effective helping relationships requires a commitment to patients/clients, to their well-being and best interests. A word such as 'commitment' can sound heavy and serious, but it describes quality rather than quantity. Such real human contact can happen over a few seconds of time or over a much longer period. In this type of intervention the nurse is available and open, rather than distant or insincere. It immediately becomes clear that such a commitment involves the resources of the inner private world of the nurse as well as skills and knowledge. It necessarily involves a willingness to be affected emotionally by the patient and to be somewhat vulnerable (which is often confused with being weak), but it also involves a certain toughness and resilience. It hardly helps the client if the nurse is overwhelmed by the feelings that are expressed and becomes *too* involved, losing the objectivity that is also needed. There is an optimum 'therapeutic distance' between nurse and patient that allows the best possible helping to take place.

Listening and responding skills

These skills are transferable to all types of helping but are included in this section because of their paramount importance in therapeutic interventions. What are now examined are the skills of communication; that is, what nurses might actually do and how they might behave with other people, in practical rather than theoretical terms. It has been noted that a nurse might be called on to make contact with several categories of people during the course of a day: doctors, patients, fellow nurses, relatives. The focus in what follows is the particular relationship and communication between a nurse and patient. It is assumed that the nurse regards relating to the patient as part of the patient's total care.

The context in which an interaction takes place affects its content and quality. This seems obvious when gross differences are considered, such as the difference between talking to someone in a bar as opposed to in their own home, but more subtle differences might be overlooked, such as the contrast between a ward in a hospital and a day room (a move from one to the other might be beneficial). Community nurses might complain that the television set is left on during home visits, but they also find it difficult to suggest that it be turned off.

Certain features of the setting may militate against effective communication. The principles that are urged here are for nurses to be sensitive to the ways in which the setting affects any interaction, and for them to endeavour to make the most strategic use out of what are often far from ideal settings.

Listening and attending

To listen to someone with attention and commitment is a caring response that is all too rare. It is the basis of all effective communication on a one-to-one basis and requires hard work on the part of the listener. This work involves much more than accurate recording of what is said. It involves making accurate perceptions through several senses, looking for patterns and checking creative ideas against new information. It also requires flexibility and a willingness to give up preconceptions about the person in the face of the evidence.

To some extent, listening and attending are insufficient in themselves. A further component involves the transmission of the message that one is listening and attending to the other person. This is achieved through a combination of verbal and non-verbal channels.

Silence

The possibility of silence is often referred to with anxiety by those wishing to help others. Paradoxically, the capacity to be comfortable with silence is often a good indicator of listening skill. It normally means that listeners are able to contain their own anxiety (if any) and to concentrate on the other person. The rush to 'help' another person with words or gestures is often misplaced and can have its roots in our attempt to deal with our own feelings of awkwardness. An acceptance of silence, on the other hand, can be an eloquent recognition of the patient's need for someone to *be* there rather than for something to be *done*.

Encouraging

Some people who are able to talk freely about their ideas and feelings need only the slightest encouragement to explore these further. This encouragement may be given by minimal prompts such as 'Mm' or 'Aha', a nod or a smile, depending on the listener's own conversational style. Other people will falter without such feedback, needing reassurance before they continue talking. Some seem to need no encouragement at all, but a compulsive way of talking may indicate that real relating is difficult for the patient and may cover painful feelings.

Responding

The two empathetic responding skills of paraphrasing and reflection of feelings are paramount to effective listening.

Paraphrasing consists of a repetition of the core message communicated by the other person translated into the listener's own words. This involves attention to the emphases and meaning of content of what has been said and allows for some personal interpretation and imaginative input on the part of the listener. It can often be helpful to use an image that catches the emotional force of the message: 'It's as though you feel trapped, with no way out'. The patient may accept the image and elaborate further or may wish to modify it in some way to make it more suitable.

To *reflect* back to patients their own expressed emotional reactions is a potent form of empathetic responding. It gives clear feedback that what has been said and felt has been received and understood. It lets the patient know that any implied message that has not been directly expressed has also been understood. The patient's question 'How long will I be in here, nurse?' may have several layers of meaning behind it. The nurse's answer, if the several layers have been successfully decoded, will reflect back something of the underlying feelings as well as giving a direct answer to the question. This response might be: 'It's normally about 3 days . . . You seem a bit concerned about it'.

Summarizing

Summarizing what has been said after a suitable interval serves a similar purpose; that is, consolidating information and verifying whether or not the sense the listener has made of it coincides with the intended message: 'Let me see if I've got this right. What you seem to be saying is . . .'. To some degree a summary is an extended form of paraphrasing but requires a broader perspective. The key to effective summaries is a filtering process that highlights the significant experiences, reactions and themes expressed in the patient's dialogue. For patients to hear what they have just been saying in summary form from somebody else often feels reassuring, but may also offer fresh insights as different experiences are connected in a thematic way, a process that Egan (1998, 2002) terms 'connecting islands'.

Asking open questions

Asking open rather than closed questions – as in 'Can you say a little more about how you felt when . . .', rather than 'Did you feel angry when . . .' – can help patients to explore their experiences. The first form of question makes a demand on patients to examine experience and to express it in their own language. The second invites a yes/no response, which is less exploratory and potentially less useful to the patient. Often students on counselling skills courses will start by assuming that asking a lot of questions of the individual will somehow help understanding. Such questioning may be a way of coping with the uncomfortable feeling of being unskilled by *doing* lots of things verbally. The idea that a timely open question indicates more skill in communication than does asking a large number of closed questions is difficult for the relative novice to accept. Of course, closed questions do have their place, such as requests for factual information during an admission interview.

A dialogue illustrating listening and responding skills

Of course, closed questions do have their place, such as requests for factual information during an admission interview. Case history 7.11 illustrates some of the listening and responding skills in action.

Supporting

Heron (2001) asserts that a supportive intervention is an exchange that affirms the worth and value of other people. He regards it as an attitude of mind that underlies all the different communication strategies previously mentioned. In many ways this relates to the values or qualities previously discussed such as unconditional positive regard, empathetic understanding and warmth or respect. Rogers (1974) saw this type of helping as 'a way of being present with another person' and sometimes this is simply what is needed. Nurses are often required to be pragmatic and this can lead to an over-reliance on being active in doing things for patients. A pure supportive interaction is as much about *not* doing the things that are habitually accessible as merely being present with another in a qualitative way as they experience their particular situation (see Case history 7.12). In some ways this tactic is simple, but the difficulty is learning as a professional helper that sometimes the most helpful intervention is to do nothing more than communicate one's presence to the patient or carer. In this spirit, the supporting tactic

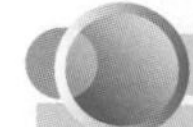

Case history 7.11

Listening and responding skills in action

The general practitioner (GP) has referred Mr White to the practice nurse. Mr White has been under pressure at work over the past 18 months, resulting in a series of minor ailments and conflict within his relationships with his family. The GP thought that the nurse might be able to help with stress-management strategies. The following dialogue is an extract from the interaction:

Practice nurse: How has this increased pressure affected you? (*Open question*)

Mr White: The worst part is that I feel tired all the time. When I get home in the evenings, I don't feel like communicating with my family. All I want to do is go to sleep. I used to be so full of life, but now I'm not much company.

Practice nurse: It's as if your batteries are run down and you have nothing left at the end of the day. (*Paraphrase: repeating back the core message in her own words*)

Mr White: Yes, but I feel so bad about it. I don't like what I'm doing, but I can't seem to stop it. It's not my family's fault, and I feel guilty about the way I treat them.

Practice nurse: So it's like you feel powerless but you still blame yourself for what is happening. (*Reflection of feelings*)

Mr White: I suppose it's like I'm putting my job before them. I'm sure my children see it that way . . . it's like a battle between work, and what's expected of me there, and my family . . .

Practice nurse: Mm, mm. (*Minimal encouragement*)

Mr White: It's such a difficult balance. If I slack off at work, I run the risk of losing my job, and that would be of no use to my family. If I don't, my family and my health suffer . . .

Practice nurse: (*Remains silent for some time – she can sense that the silence is far from empty*)

Mr White: It's like a no-win situation . . . I can't think how things could be improved.

Practice nurse: So far you have talked about the difficulty of balancing work and home life, of how exhausting your lifestyle is at the moment, and of how little control you seem to have over changing things. You seem to feel stuck and pessimistic about finding any solution. Is that how you see things? (*Summarizing the main points that have been brought up and checking her understanding is accurate*)

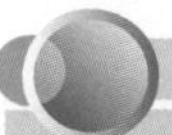

Case history 7.12

Being present as a form of supportive communication

Kelly is a 35-year-old woman with a learning disability. The extent of her learning disability is quite severe, although she can communicate verbally in a limited capacity. Kelly lives in a small community home and has recently been told by a relative that her mother has died following a long illness. Since receiving this news, she has spent most of the time alone and very quiet. Her isolation is plain for all to see. One of the female carers has a particularly close relationship with Kelly. She instinctively knows that Kelly's needs can be best met by just sitting with her, holding her hand and letting her know that she is with her as she goes through the pain of her recent loss.

is placed at the extreme end of the continuum illustrating that the patient is in control.

Transcultural communication

Leininger coined the term 'culturally competent care' in 1960. According to Leininger (Leininger & McFarland 2002), culture has a powerful impact on individuals, groups and entire societies, influencing all aspects of human life. Nurses are living and working in a global world. Global interaction is bringing people into almost instant contact with strangers through rapid transportation, communication and many new technologies within and outside health care systems. The ethnic and racial composition of the population of the UK has been changing dramatically for the past decade. Nurses and other health care providers practise in a multicultural environment. The misunderstandings that develop in health care settings can occur between providers, as well as between patients and providers from different cultural backgrounds. Therefore, there is a growing demand for transcultural communication. Patients from different cultures may communicate their pain, anxiety, fear and other powerful feelings and emotions in different ways. Thus nurses need to assess their patients carefully in order to accurately decode their transcultural communication, both verbal and non-verbal.

All nurse–patient communication is to some extent bicultural, even when the nurse and patient are from the same culture. The patient's terminology, perspective, perceptions, and expectations represent the lay culture, whereas the nurse's terminology, perspective and perceptions represent the subculture of nursing. Consider patients and coworkers from other cultures as individuals first with unique experiences and expectations, and then consider them as members of different cultures.

Communication strategies within different patient/client groups

The importance of communication, as well as general principles and strategies of effective communication, have been discussed above. In this section, specific strategies that can guide you when you look after patients from a specific age group or with a specific communication barrier are discussed.

Communicating with children

We all know that children are not miniature adults. Their normal growth and developmental stage should be considered when communicating with them. For example, newborns are unable to talk, therefore they depend on non-verbal communication. They communicate their needs by crying; they cry when they are hungry, tired or need a nappy change. They are calm and quiet when their needs are met. During your clinical placement you may find that at times you will look after a newborn baby. Have a look at Box 7.6 for some basic elements of caregiving to babies.

Preschool children believe that the world revolves around them. This is why their communication is direct and literal. It is important that you understand that preschool children express their feelings through play. Therefore pictures can be an excellent tool to use when communicating

Box 7.6

Strategies that can be employed when looking after a baby

- Be calm, as newborns respond well to a calm caregiver.
- Remember the infant's crying is a way of saying 'I am not comfortable', or 'I feel sick'.
- Infants respond well to a low comforting voice.
- Infants like to be gently patted on their back or bottom as they interpret repetitive motions as comforting.
- Older infants may respond better when their parents are near.
- It is always helpful to ask parents what the infant's likes and dislikes are.

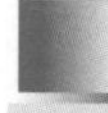

Box 7.7

Strategies that might be helpful when communicating with young people

- Talk to young people like adults even though they are not yet adult.
- Address them formally by calling them by their surnames, and calling them by their first name if they ask you to do so.
- Clarify slang if you do not understand.
- Ensure privacy during any intervention, including history-taking and physical examination (Cox & Lee 2004).

with preschoolers (Cox & Lee 2004). Remember, preschoolers communicate better with non-verbal expression of their feelings, but they are able to talk, so do encourage them to ask questions and keep your answers simple and concrete (Cox & Lee 2004).

School-age children, on the other hand, can talk and are capable of understanding cause and effect. They usually want to know why something is done and how things work (Cox & Lee 2004). It is at this stage that children start to understand the concepts of life and death. When communicating with school-age children it is important to remember to provide information in a manner that they can understand. Simple written material can be very helpful. Remember, it is important that you explain something to the child and then follow up by asking questions and verify how much was understood and clarify incorrect information.

Young people (teenagers) are no longer children but not quite adult (Cox & Lee 2004). This explains why their behaviour is sometimes child-like and at other times very adult-like. Teenagers' friends are very important to them and their opinions are valued. On the other hand, adults, particularly parents, are seen as out of touch and therefore their opinion are not valued. It is common for teenagers to use slang when talking about or to their peer group, which can certainly make communication with them difficult (see Box 7.7).

Communicating with older adults

Similar to other age groups, older people need to be treated as individuals in relation to communication. The factors that need to be considered when communicating with older people include their cognitive ability, level of orientation, sensory deficits such as sight, hearing loss and decreased sense of touch, as well as their medication, which can affect cognitive functioning (e.g. pain medication, sleep medication, sedatives) (Cox 2004). Older people tend to be sensitive to issues relating to personal information such as financial or sexual information, or any information held to be very personal by the individual older adult. It is good practice to address older adults by title and surname and speak slowly and clearly. A helpful strategy when communicating with older adults is to avoid using medical or street jargon (Cox 2004).

Communicating with people with learning disabilities

It is important to be aware that many people with severe learning disabilities have difficulties with communication. In some cases, communication problems are caused by other problems, such as hearing loss. Difficulties might also be related to autistic spectrum disorders. More often, though, the reasons for someone's difficulties have not been properly investigated or diagnosed. Therefore the effectiveness of communication depends on the relationship between the people involved, the nurse's knowledge of the disabled person and the opportunities people have to use their communication skills. Communication is a two-way process, thus it is crucial that nurses and health care professionals strive not to contribute to the individual's difficulties. Some of the things you should keep in mind:

- Do not underestimate hearing difficulties.
- Do not overestimate language skills.
- Do not be too reliant on verbal exchanges.
- Do not ask questions.
- Do not give directions and/or instructions in overly complex ways.

Most people learn to communicate as part of their natural development, but people with learning disabilities often need specialist help and support in order to be able to communicate effectively with others. With training and support, many people with learning disabilities can learn to use alternatives to verbal communication which suit them as individuals (e.g. showing someone a towel and bathing costume to indicate a trip to the swimming baths, or showing someone how to fetch a glass if they want a cold drink).

Record-keeping and using information technology

In nursing, documentation is the only way to show that procedures are carried out, treatment plans are completed and medications are administered. If it isn't written down, it didn't happen. The importance of keeping accurate records cannot be overemphasized.

Accurate record-keeping is essential for ensuring the delivery of appropriate and effective care and protect the welfare of the patients by promoting continuity and consistency of care. Furthermore, accurate and comprehensive record-keeping is also concerned with nurses protecting themselves from litigation. Therefore a high standard of documentation is vital and it must clearly communicate a nurse's judgement and evaluation. Record-keeping should not be regarded as an administrative task; rather, it should be an integral part of the holistic care package.

How to write a clinical incident report

A complete record should provide the reader with all the information required to reach the same conclusions as the health professional who wrote the notes. Charting should provide a thorough picture with the following components:

- Factual information.
- Accurate and reliable.
- Complete details.
- Brief and concise.
- Timely with current data.
- Logical organization of material.

When documenting the care that has been provided you need to record the actions taken to meet the patient's/client's needs. For example, when giving medication, the following details must be included:

- The name of the medication.
- The dose administered.
- The administration route (e.g. oral, IM, IV).
- The site of administration (e.g. right antecubital).
- The date and time administered to the patient/client.
- The name and signature of the clinician.

In general, it is good practice to record facts rather than opinions and to avoid confusing generalizations such as 'patient doing well'. Documentation is an important tool in the delivery of quality care and the prevention of charges of negligence. Therefore following the policies of the institution in which one practises is of utmost importance.

Confidentiality

The concept of confidentiality relates to the expectation of a patient that their health information will be kept in confidence. Health records include information obtained by nurses and other health care professionals through observation, assessment, treatment or conversation that is considered confidential information and is protected by law. Confidentiality of verbal and written communication within health care is essential to achieve an open dialogue between the patient and the providers of care. The sense of trust between patient and health care provider lies at the heart of the confidentiality concern. Furthermore, consent forms for the release of health record information must be signed in the presence of a witness. Disclosing information from the health record without the patient's consent constitutes a breach of confidentiality.

Information technology

In the past 10 years or so the NHS has seen radical changes in the way information is used and shared. The mandate for greater accountability and public involvement is being addressed in the UK through a variety of initiatives underpinned by a developing an electronic infrastructure (www.connectingforhealth.nhs.uk). Using information technology to record patient data provides the opportunity for health care organizations to improve quality of care and patient safety. It also allows the information to be shared amongst all of the health care team. Furthermore, access from remote sites by many people at the same time is possible and retrieval of the information is almost immediate.

Information technology supports accountable autonomy and collects and disseminates information that assists health care professionals in decision-making. Like traditional paper-based systems, electronic health records document admission histories, laboratory test results, X-rays, patient orders, treatments, assessments and beyond, depending on the system your institution uses. Electronic records may be accessed from many places and from any computer on the network, which makes the health care professional's job important in safeguarding confidentiality. The following practical strategies can be used as a guide as your first line of defence for you to protect your patients' privacy (Roberts 2002):

- *Log off.* Remember if you forget to log off a computer on which you were working, anyone can look at anything and enter information under your electronic signature. The computer has no way of knowing that you are not the one at the keyboard; in fact, the computer interprets that it is you who is at the keyboard because you logged in!
- *Remember your password and keep it private.* It is best to pick a password that is easy to remember and keep it in a private and safe place. Never 'loan' your password to another nurse or 'borrow' another person's password. If you loan your password to another nurse, it means you are responsible for what is being documented by that person, including any medication errors!
- *Keep outsiders away from the computers.* It is good practice to tilt the computer screen away from where it could be read by passers-by.
- *Don't go where you shouldn't go.* Don't breach confidentiality by accessing information that you are not supposed to access such as your own laboratory results. This breach could result in administrative penalties, including dismissal.

Conclusion

With the increasing recognition of the patient as a person who happens to be ill, therapeutic interaction is now being viewed as a combination of key communication skills and a human personal relationship between two or more people, the quality of which significantly affects any treatment or caring intervention. These behavioural and relational aspects of communication, when combined, enable a therapeutic relationship to be established.

The communication process has three components – the sender, the receiver and the message –

and, for communication to take place, the message must be not only be received but also understood. The style of the interaction will be influenced by personality and culture. Nurses must be encouraged to be flexible to the needs and communication style of patients, colleagues and family, in order to strengthen their relationships with them.

The key factor in effective communication is making the right choice of intervention based on an empathetic assessment of the individual, the situation and resources. It is possible to classify the available strategies using the acronym TACTICS (taking action, advising, challenging, teaching, informing, counselling and supporting). Having made the correct choice, nurses need to utilize developed micro-skills to ensure the communication is effective. The nurse who is developing the quality of interaction within the work setting is one who has realized both the importance of communication skills and their place in professional effectiveness.

References

Ambady N, Koo J, Rosenthal R, Winograd C 2002 Physical therapists nonverbal communication predicts geriatric patients' health outcome. Psychology & Aging 17(3):443–452

Argyle M 1996 Bodily communication. Routledge, London

Barkauskas V, Baumann L, Darling-Fisher C 2003 Health and physical assessment. Mosby, London

Benner P 2001 From novice to expert: excellence and power in clinical nursing practice. Addison-Wesley, Menlo Park, CA

Betts A 1995 The counselling relationship. In: Ellis R, Gates R, Kenworthy N (eds) Interpersonal communication in nursing: theory and practice. Churchill Livingstone, Edinburgh

Blows WT 2001 The biological basis of nursing: clinical observations. Routledge, Abingdon

Blows WT 2003 The biological basis of nursing: mental health. Routledge, Abingdon

Blows WT 2005 The biological basis of nursing: cancer. Routledge, Abingdon

Boud D, Keough R, Walker D 1985 Reflection: turning experience into learning. Kogan Page, London

Bower SA, Bower GH 1991 Asserting yourself. Addison-Wesley, Reading, MA

Bradley J, Edinberg M 1990 Communication in the nursing context. Appleton-Century Crofts, Connecticut

British Association for Counselling 1992 Code of ethics and practice for counsellors. British Association for Counselling, Rugby

Burnard P 2002 Learning human skills: An experiential and reflective guide for nurses and health care professionals, 4th edn. Heinemann, London

Carkhuff RR 1970 Helping and human relations. Holt, Rinehart and Winston, New York

Carlson NR 2004 Physiology of behavior, 8th edn. Allyn and Bacon, Boston, MA

Corey G 1986 Theory and practice of counselling and psychotherapy. Brooks Cole, Pacific Grove, CA

Cox C 2004 Assessment of disability including care of the older adult. In: Cox C (ed) Physical assessment for nurses. Blackwell, Oxford, p 216–222

Cox C, Lee P 2004 Assessment of the child. In: Cox C (ed) Physical assessment for nurses. Blackwell, Oxford, p 179–215

Davidhizar R, Newman J 1997 When touch is not the best approach. Journal of Clinical Nursing 6(3):203–206

Department of Health 2003 Essence of care. Benchmarks for communication between patients, carers and health care. Department of Health, NHS Modernisation Agency, London

Egan G 1998 The skilled helper, 6th edn. Brooks Cole, Pacific Grove, CA

Egan G 2002 Exercises in helping skills: A manual to accompany the skilled helper, 7th edn. Brookes/Cole Publishing Company, London

Ekman P, Friesen W 1987 Measuring facial movements with the facial action coding system. In: Ekman P (ed) Emotion in the human face. Cambridge University Press, Cambridge

Ellis R, Gates R, Kenworthy N 2003 Interpersonal communication in nursing: theory and practice. Churchill Livingstone, Edinburgh

Gates B 1994 Advocacy: a nurse's guide. Scutari Press, Harrow

Gumperz J 1968 The speech community. International encyclopaedia of the social sciences, 2nd edn. Macmillan, London

Hall E 1966 The silent language. Columbia University Press, New York

Harrigan J, Wilson K, Rosenthal R 2004 Detecting state and trait anxiety from auditory and visual cues: a meta analysis. Personality and Social Psychology Bulletin 30(1):56–66

Hartrick G 1997 Relational capacity: the foundation for interpersonal practice. Journal of Advanced Nursing 26(3):523–528

Henley N 1977 Body, politics, power, sex and nonviable communication. Prentice Hall, Englewood Cliffs, NJ

Heron J 2001 Helping the client. Sage, London

Hewison A 1995 Nurses' power in interactions with patients. Journal of Advanced Nursing 21(1):75–82

Kagan C, Evans J, Kay B 1986 A manual of interpersonal skills for nurses: an experiential approach. Harper and Row, London

Kalisch BJ 1971 An experiment in the development of empathy in nursing students. Nursing Research 20(3):201–211

Kemmis S 1985 Action research and the politics of reflection. In: Boud D, Keough R, Walker D (eds) Reflection: turning experience into learning. Kogan Page, London

Kindlen S 2003 Physiology for Health Care and Nursing, 2nd edn. Churchill Livingstone, Edinburgh

Leininger M, McFarland M 2002 Transcultural nursing: concepts, theories, research, and practice, 3rd edn. McGraw-Hill, London

Lilly C, Sonna LA, Haley KJ et al 2003 Intensive communication: four-year follow-up from a clinical practice study. Critical Care Medicine 31(5):394–399

Murray R, Huelskoetter M 1991 Psychiatric/mental health nursing. Appleton and Lange, Los Altos, CA

National Health Service 2000 Help available to carers from the health service. Online. Available: www.nhs.uk/

Orem DE 2001 Nursing concepts and practice, 6th edn. Elsevier, St Louis

Peplau H 1988 Interpersonal relations in nursing. Macmillan Education, Basingstoke

Phelps S, Austin N 2002 The assertive woman, 4th edn. Impact Publishers, San Luis Obispo, CA

Ricketts T 1996 General satisfaction and satisfaction with nursing communication on an adult psychiatric ward. Journal of Advanced Nursing 24(3):479–487

Riley J 2004 Communication in nursing. Mosby, St Louis

Roberts DW 2002 How to keep electronic health records private. Nursing 31(10):95

Rogers C 1974 On becoming a person, 4th edn. Constable, London

Schön DA 1983 The reflective practitioner: how professionals think in action. Temple Smith, London

Seeley RR, Stephens TD, Tate P 2006 Anatomy and physiology, 7th edn. McGraw-Hill, Boston

Shier D, Butler J, Lewis R 2004 Hole's human anatomy and physiology, 10th edn. McGraw-Hill, Boston

Stein-Parbury J 2000 Developing interpersonal skills in nursing, 2nd edn. Churchill Livingstone, Edinburgh

United Kingdom Central Council for Nursing, Midwifery and Health Visiting 1987 Scope in practice. UKCC, London

Wainwright G 2003 Body language. Hodder and Stoughton, London

Walker D 1985 Writing and reflection. In: Boud D, Keough R, Walker D (eds) Reflection: turning experience into learning. Kogan Page, London

Watson O 1980 Proxemic behaviour: a cross cultural study. Monitor, The Hague

Waugh A, Grant A 2006 Ross & Wilson Anatomy and physiology in health and illness, 10th edn. Churchill Livingstone, Edinburgh

Whitcher S, Fisher J 1979 Multi-dimensional reactions to therapeutic touch in a hospital setting. Journal of Personal and Social Psychology 37(1):87–96

Wilkinson S 1992 Confusions and challenges. Nursing Times 88(35):24–28

Wilkinson S 1999 Schering Plough Clinical Lecture Communication: it makes a difference. Cancer Nursing 22(1):17–20

Chapter Eight

8

Food and nutrition

Hannele Weir, Alison Coutts

Key topics

- The meaning and function of food
- Obtaining food and providing food that meets people's needs
- Food policy
- Food availability
- Eating to promote health
- Introduction to the digestive system
- Nutrients and micronutrients in our diet
- Screening and assessment to identify nutritional needs
- Food and the life-cycle
- Children and food
- The older adult and nutritional needs of older adults
- Planning, implementation and evaluation of care
- Food and malnutrition: obesity
- Diet and cardiovascular disease
- Assistance with eating and drinking

Introduction

In this chapter we introduce you to some of the complexities that are involved in delivering food to our tables and some of the factors that you need to consider when offering meals to your patients/clients. We first discuss some of the current policies that affect how and where food is produced and sold. We also consider the different factors that influence what we eat. By understanding how socioeconomic factors impact on the extent to which people can choose what food they can grow and what food is available to them to eat, you will begin to appreciate the difficulties that many people have when they want to eat a healthy and nutritious diet.

We also introduce you to some of the different nutritional components of a healthy diet and how they promote health and well-being, as well of some of the problems that might occur if there is deficit in the diet or if there is a malfunction of the digestive system. To do this we briefly introduce you to the structure and function of the gastrointestinal system.

In the last section of the chapter, we introduce you to the important dietary needs of different groups of people through their lifespan. Throughout the relevant sections of this chapter we use examples to illustrate potential risk factors. We hope you will use this chapter as a starting point to find out more about how nutrition and disease are related and to use specialist texts to understand how to help people with specific dietary needs. You will find some suggestions in the supplementary reading list at the end of the chapter. You might also find it helpful to read the latest research regarding food and nutrition on the government website (www.food.gov.uk).

Food has a social meaning

Food is made up of substances that we eat or drink and are digested and absorbed to help the body grow and then to function effectively by maintaining its cells, tissues and organs in good repair. We are describing nutrition as all the macro- and micro- (at the level of the cells in the body) processes that help us to ingest and assimilate food into our cells. The Department of Health (2003a) defined a key responsibility of nurses as ensuring that patients/clients are 'enabled to consume food orally which meets their individual need'. This implies that nurses must be knowledgeable about the important components of a healthy diet, as well as be sensitive to specific needs of their patients, and to take responsibility for ensuring their patients are able to eat and drink while under their care.

Food plays an important part in our social lives and in our spiritual lives, with several religions using food as an important symbol in their rituals, which provide guidelines on food that is acceptable or forbidden. This wider meaning of food needs to be acknowledged when caring for people in hospitals or institutions, or even in their own homes. With so many people relying on external agencies to provide their food ready-prepared, the social and religious aspect of food is often overlooked.

In times of civil war, famine and disasters that involve thousands and sometimes millions of people, public attention is focused on the social processes surrounding food production and consumption and the complexities involved in providing and delivering food. Publicity surrounding food production as a commercial and industrial activity has also raised awareness of the conditions under which some food is produced.

Another perspective on food as a commodity is the way it has been used to signify the social standing of both consumers and producers. For example, eating jellied eels or oysters used to be associated with the poor in England; then, when these foods became scarce, they were seen as the food of the wealthy. In some countries, being able to eat meat every day is often seen as a sign of wealth as most of the population do not have the resources to own animals or to buy meat. Thus, if they have the necessary resources, they rely on home-grown vegetables and fruit for their dietary staples. In other countries, many people are not so fortunate. Those who have access to land can enjoy a more secure life, and their ability to consume particular foods demonstrates their social status and thus power to acquire such food.

So you can begin to recognize that the social meaning of food goes beyond the rudimentary production/consumption process for physical survival, and that food is a marker of human social activity and identity, distinguishing people's social status, religious affiliation and cultural practices, and distinguishing those in society who are politically powerful, empowered by their political state or those who are powerless. For the powerless who are struggling to find sufficient food to stave off starvation, irrespective of whether their food is nutritious, there is little choice about what they eat. Their plight contrasts starkly with those populations whose dietary needs can be met relatively easily but because of external influences are struggling to balance the tension between seeking out food that is novel while living in fear of food that might be harmful (Fischler 1980, cited in Beardsworth and Keil 1997). In Western society, where the organization and management of food production and food availability is managed predominantly by large commercial organizations, the challenge is to ensure that food is actually healthy rather than causing disease. Many diseases affecting people in Western societies are attributed to the high content of fat, salt and sugar in many pre-prepared food products.

In post-agricultural societies, many people have the luxury of choosing the origin, quantity, type and content of what they consume. The White Paper on public health ('Choosing health: making healthier choices easier'), published by the Department of Health (2004), states that people want to be healthy. Throughout history, societies have experienced shortage and abundance of food. With greater awareness of the worldwide economy, there is the dichotomy of societies experiencing extreme shortages and famine, whilst others have excess. Although, because of climatic and political reasons, this may always have been the case, the 20th century was probably the first to have the resources to eliminate starvation, but this has not been done (Leather 1996).

Food policy

What is food policy?

Food policy embraces all those policies affecting food, food economy, supply and demand. Food policy is concerned with the global market, international laws and regulations governing the selling of food (Caraher 2000). As Lang & Heasman (2004) note, there is no one food policy or one food policy-maker, but that food policy-making is a social process as well as being highly politicized and contentious.

In the UK in the 1960s and 1970s, food policy was aimed at food security, ensuring that everybody had enough to eat – a legacy from the 1939–1945 world war when governments had struggled to ensure there was sufficient food for everyone to have their essential nutritional needs met. This was achieved by imposing a system of rationing essential foodstuffs, such as meat, eggs, butter, sugar and tea. By contrast, a world food crisis between 1972 and 1974 highlighted the global availability of, and access to, food. Maxwell & Slater (2004, p 3) argued that concern about food security is not sufficient and we need to extend attention to food policy. The lack of a coordinated approach to food reflects the causes of the changes in the food system and food policy. These are driven by urbanization, technical change, income growth, lifestyle changes, mass media and advertising and also fluctuating changes in relative food prices (Maxwell & Slater 2004, p 30). Such shifts are bound to lead to battles of interests, knowledge and beliefs (Caraher 2000, p 429; see also Lang & Heasman 2004). Successive governments in the 1980s and 1990s were in favour of self-regulating markets and food industry. As Caraher (2000) points out, cheap food was produced at the expense of quality and that led to food safety being compromised. Examples of this are the bovine spongiform encephalopathy (BSE) crisis, foot and mouth outbreaks in cattle, swine fever and more recently avian influenza. Despite unsound practices, such as condemned meat being resold, such practices have continued during subsequent governments (Caraher 2000). These examples highlight the difficulties of monitoring food production and the level of scrutiny required to ensure that only food that is fit for human consumption is sold.

Baggott (2000, p 193) noted that pressure for changes in regulations governing food safety and nutrition and calls for better health education resulted in demands for greater regulation of commercial activities, with improvement in standards. Despite this, there are 'powerful counter-pressures' that inhibit more-informative food labelling and allow the continued use of food additives. These commercial interests also favour international free-trade agreements (Baggott 2000, p 194).

Food policy and politics

In recent years, there have been a number of publications focusing on where our food comes from, how is it produced and how it is processed and what the politics of producing and selling food are (see, for instance, Lang & Heasman 2004, Lawrence 2004, Schlosser 2002). Schlosser's (2002) account of the food industry practices in the USA makes worrying reading. We get the impression that customers and consumers have very limited choice or control over the fundamental quality of food. Lang & Heasman (2004) and Lawrence (2004) likewise have taken an in-depth look at the interests involved in food production and processing with a view to future developments. Lang & Heasman (2004, p 277) refer to the Nordic countries where health interests have made an impact on policy and where 'public and environmental health can be fused with food and agricultural policy'. This means that the known health implications of food eaten by people are taken into account when formulating policies as a proactive measure in order to minimize harm to those not yet affected by certain practices. So, for instance, the North Karelia Project in Finland in the early 1970s was initially a response to one of the highest coronary heart disease rates in the world, but which resulted in not only people being asked to change their eating habits, but the food industry response was to offer low-cholesterol options in food available. Thus, for example, fat-free and semi-skimmed milk came about. The implications of the project have been far-reaching in many ways, and not always in ways that could have been anticipated (see, for instance, Lang & Heasman 2004, Puska 2002, p 5–7).

Modern society and food policy

In many Westernized, post-agricultural societies, the way food is produced has changed radically. Many European nations (for example) are no longer able to produce sufficient food for their population and, as a result, other nations supply them with their staple and supplementary foods. This creates a dependence that has led to the Common Agricultural Policy, which seeks to determine which countries will be the main producers of food and which will become the main purchasers of food. One consequence of this has been the huge distances that some foodstuffs have to be transported to the purchasers (see Activity 8.1).

Lifestyle and food policy

Another factor that is impacting on the food we eat is the change in lifestyle that has taken place in many post-agricultural societies and countries. A significantly larger percentage of the population now live and work away from agricultural work, food production and the primary marketing of food. With the change in the structure of these societies, people tend to eat meals that have not been prepared at home but which have been purchased. More people tend to eat processed food from supermarkets rather than buying staple food at local outlets and using it to cook their own meals at home. With so much mass production and consumption of prepared food, the risk of contamination of such products is much greater, leading to increased concerns about food safety.

One consequence is 'cash crop' farming in poorer countries for consumption in richer countries, sometimes for out-of-season vegetables and fruit. A 'cash crop' is food that is grown to sell (probably for a consumer many miles away) to make a profit in cash, rather than growing food for the farmer's own family or community. Prawn farming is an example. Intensive farming of prawns for export has caused untold damage. Not only has this resulted in environmental pollution, food shortage for the local poor populations in South-East Asia and South America as natural fish stocks have been destroyed or depleted, but people in Western countries end up eating prawns grown with the help of antibiotics and growth hormones (Lawrence 2004).

Activity 8.1

When you next go shopping for food, read the information on the packaging, or on the display card, to find out the country of origin of the foodstuffs listed below. Don't worry if there are several brands or types of the foodstuff; it is interesting to see whether they come from the same country.

- Rice.
- Flour.
- Sugar.
- Apples.
- Potatoes.
- Carrots.
- Chicken.
- Beef.

If the food item is available in different forms (e.g. organic or otherwise), see if it is available from more than one country. (NB: If the country of origin is not on the food label, you may find that the supermarket has a website giving this information.)

Consider how many food miles have been used to bring these products to your shop.

Consider whether any of them could have been grown in this country.

As a result of the change to the global production and management of food, food has become a commodity whose value see-saws from day to day depending upon financial market fluctuations. So food policy is no longer the province solely of ministries of agriculture but is discussed in ministries and organizations concerned with trade and industry, consumer affairs, food activist groups and non-governmental organizations (Maxwell & Slater 2004).

Activity 8.2

- Who is the focus of food advertisements?
- Watch some commercial children's television (Saturday morning is a good time).
- What are the implications of the advertisements that are promoted at this time?
- What might be the impact on children's health if they have a diet of these advertised foods?

The food industry

In our commercial, capitalist world, companies compete with each other to establish a market for their goods and to achieve profit margins that enable expansion of the industry. Food manufacturers are equally engaged in these kinds of trade wars, and market products designed to attract the maximum number of purchasers.

Several food manufacturers have been criticized for the nutritional quality of their products, or in the case of alcoholic drinks, their target markets (see, for instance, Lang & Heasman 2004, Schlosser 2002). Some companies have responded by changing their products to reflect current trends in eating healthy foods, such as offering salad alternatives in the range of fast foods available. Selling food products as having a nutritional value is beginning to become more widespread in supermarkets as a marketing strategy; for example, 'free from' ranges for people with special dietary needs, or the increased sales in organic food products indicates that trends can be changed if there is sufficient popular support, often as a result of television programmes. There seems to be some ambiguity in the way the public approaches food. On the one hand, people are aware of risks involved in food consumption and are knowledgeable of the global food scarcity; on the other hand, there is the competition for consumers and shoppers. This may explain the so-called 'price wars' between the major supermarkets (see Lawrence 2004, for example).

The huge financial power of the international food industry can lead to a level of political influence that may not work in the best interests of the population (Schlosser 2002) and even that major democratic governments are unable to control. For instance, Schlosser (2002) argues that the US Congress should ban food advertising directed at children and that tougher food safety laws should be passed (see Activity 8.2). However, moves such as these have been bitterly opposed.

Obtaining food

Choice and consumption of food in the developed countries reflect the powerful economic position of these countries. What people eat depends on availability and acceptability (Fieldhouse 1996) of foodstuffs. Whilst poverty may be associated with people at risk of dying from lack of food, in Western countries people tend to experience *relative* poverty where lack of money and food and other consumables compares unfavourably with other people's purchasing power. People on low incomes spend proportionately more on food than do better off people (Beardsworth & Keil 1997). In the USA, the richest country in the world, it was estimated that 12 million families in 2003 worried they did not have enough money for food and in nearly 3.8 million families someone skipped meals because they could not afford them. These figures represent a 13% increase on year 2000 (Center for Family Policy and Practice 2004).

The economies that people in poverty have to exercise can override concerns about the quality of food. Whether eating healthy food is more expensive than less healthy alternatives is debatable and depends on what ingredients are used. For instance, cheaper food has to be acceptable in terms of cultural and religious customs and beliefs, as well as palatability; people also need appropriate cooking facilities and money for fuel to make use of the cheaper cuts of meat or pulses that need longer cooking times. People used to be able to make use of seasonal fruit and vegetables that were cheaper at times of harvest. The way in which market prices and profits are determined seems to have negated such seasonal advantage in this country.

Food shopping commands a large proportion of weekly income, particularly of those on low incomes. Savings on food release money for other expenditures. Working out the cost of a 'healthy' or 'nutritious' food basket can be complicated. Different countries have a slightly varying number of basic food items. Whether the food is imported or locally grown, and thus the length and type of transport, add to the cost. Different stages of production and processing, whether organic or conventional, and locally or globally sourced, also affect the real cost of the food basket (Center for Family Policy and Practice 2002). Activity 8.3 explores concerns regarding buying food.

Whilst it is possible to improve diet without spending excessive amounts of money, food is a discretionary item of expenditure (Baum 2002) and often it constitutes the first part of the household budget to be reduced in order to save money. People with low incomes eat a 'flexible' diet (Walker 1993). This means variability in quality and quantity. Cheaper meat products and processed food tend to be higher in fat, sugar and salt content, unlike healthier vegetables, fruit and lean cuts of meat, grain and cereal.

Most people in the UK purchase their food from shops with no knowledge of the producer. The consumer is therefore reliant on the information provided by the producer about food. In the UK, £800 billion is spent on fruit juice, very likely because it has a healthy image. But, in 1993, a company in the USA was fined (and the owner imprisoned) for selling adulterated fruit juice as 100% fresh (Patel 1994). 'Flavor Fresh' was concentrated, then diluted, had sugar, cheap citric acid and amino acids added with pulpwash and preservative. The product itself was not illegal; the problem was in the labelling, which should have said 'made from concentrate', as well as declaring the other additives. However, as the producer can charge 20% more for a pure product it may be tempting to withhold full information. This case is not unusual. Between 1986 and1994 the FDA (Food and Drug Administration) successfully prosecuted 10 companies. Prosecution usually occurs as a result of employees whistle-blowing, or occasional random tests.

Activity 8.3

Spend a few moments jotting down the factors that influence your choices when shopping for food.

- Are these factors associated with food cost, distance from the food store, the dietary preferences of you and the people you are shopping for?
- What foods on your list are seasonal?
- When you go to your local food shop and get to the checkout, look at the food baskets of your fellow shoppers. To what extent do they differ from the content of yours?
- What are the chief foodstuffs that they are buying?
- How do these foodstuffs relate to your concept of a healthy diet?

Food Standards Agency of the UK

In the UK, the government's food policy is based on advice from the Food Standards Agency (FSA), which was established in 2000 following the bovine spongiform encephalopathy (BSE) epidemic. The FSA is the only body that deals with the quality of our food, which was previously the responsibility of MAFF (Ministry of Agriculture, Fisheries and Food 2002), which is also concerned with farm incomes. The FSA is answerable to the Department of Health, although its (quite generous) budget comes from MAFF (MAFF 2002).

The functions of the FSA include:

- Commissions research (£25 m).
- Publishes advice to ministers.
- Raises money from the food industry.
- Defines balanced diet; asks health ministers to overrule MAFF.
- Offers guidelines to consumers and companies about labelling.

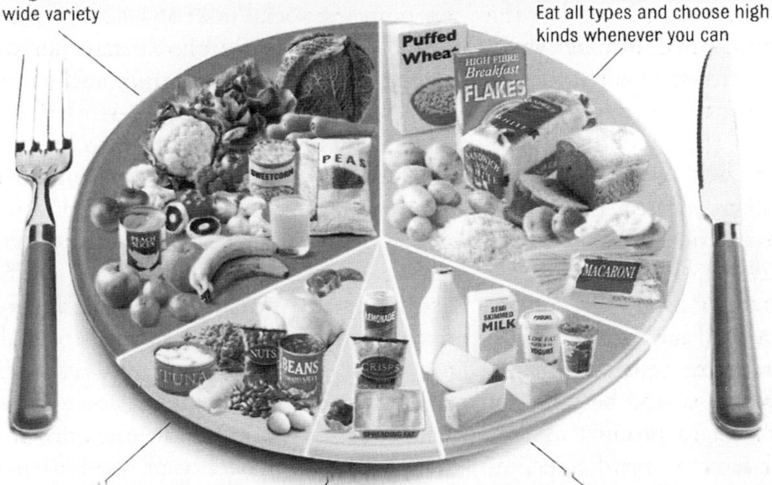

The National Food Guide

The Balance of Good Health

Fruit and vegetables
Choose a wide variety

Bread, other cereals and potatoes
Eat all types and choose high fibre kinds whenever you can

Meat, fish and alternatives
Choose lower fat alternatives whenever you can

Fatty and sugary foods
Try not to eat these too often, and when you do, have small amounts

Milk and dairy foods
Choose lower fat alternatives whenever you can

Figure 8.1 • The balance of good health 'plate'. (Reproduced with kind permission from the Health Education Authority 1994.)

The FSA works at three levels: at a national and international level to influence food regulations; at a community level to influence people's food choices to become more health orientated (see Figure 8.1); through health education campaigns.

Food labelling

Labelling of foodstuffs is not compulsory, unless specific claims are being made (e.g. 'low fat' or 'high fibre'). However, many food firms recognize that labelling their products increases public confidence. Legislation requires that information about nutrients must be provided in one of two ways as outlined in Box 8.1.

Lists of ingredient might not be comprehensive; for example, 'raising agents' or 'flavourings' need not be fully listed. This is a particular concern for vegans/vegetarians and for allergy sufferers as the ingredients they wish to exclude may be omitted

Box 8.1

Labelling of nutrients that must normally be tabulated on food packaging

Group 1: energy in kilojoules (kJ) and kilocalories (kcal), and the amount of protein, carbohydrate and fat in grams (g).

Group 2: as for group 1, but the carbohydrate is divided into sugars and others, fat into saturated and unsaturated, and fibre and sodium.

Vitamin and mineral content: can only be identified if it is in significant amounts, such as a proportion of the recommended daily intake (or Reference Nutrient Intake).

Information must be given per 100 g or 100 ml, and the overall portion size or number of average portions must be stated on the packet.

from the list. (The FSA would like to address this issue.) Many of the terms used in packaging have no meaning (e.g. 'fresh' or 'traditional').

Where foodstuffs are being sold for a particular nutritional use (known as PARNUT foods), the labelling regulations are more strict, although these are sometimes open to controversy as they could mislead people into believing they are eating food that is recommended for their condition. An example could be diabetic jams, when it is probably healthier for the diabetic person not to eat products with a high glycaemic index (see the Food Standards Agency 2004).

The FSA would like to make labels less confusing. For instance, '90% fat-free' can be interpreted in several ways and a more accurate form of labelling, such as 10% fat content, would be safer for consumers. Similarly, labelling a product as 'fat-free' or 'low fat' should have a specific recommended meaning such that low fat would mean 3 grams per 100 grams and fat-free would mean less than 0.15 gram per 100 grams.

The FSA would also like information to be provided regarding the presence of potential allergens and to clarify labelling on genetically modified (GM) foods as well as improved strategies to detect such substances.

Marketing terms such as 'fresh' and 'traditional', which actually mean nothing, are also descriptions on which the FSA would like more clarity and restriction. There is no restriction on how food companies can name their product, or promote its image or promote a food as being 'healthy'.

The meaning and function of food

Food represents more than just bodily fuel and nutrition. Lupton (2000) notes that the aspects of food found most pleasurable and valuable by an Australian study were to do with nostalgia and tradition, and the social enjoyment and happiness of being together with family. The social nature of eating together signifies the importance of such occasions beyond the basic function of food. In health care practice, the positive feelings and sociability that eating together engenders could be enhanced by encouraging mobile patients in hospitals to eat in the day room, depending on the facilities. In nursing homes, meals are often served to residents in a communal setting with the aim of encouraging social interaction.

How importantly people rate health considerations in choosing, preparing and eating meals is reflected in Lupton's (2000) study. Nearly all the participants indicated a strong concern as to the 'healthiness' of meals and seemed to make a connection between 'healthy' and home cooking, which covered basic nutritional needs with 'variety' and 'balance' in food choices. A significant point about healthy meals was that they were seen as a major aspect of family relationships and beginning a cohabitating relationship. These relationships seemed to mark more home-cooked and balanced meals (Lupton 2000). We can draw a conclusion that the social context of food preparation and consumption bear significantly on the type of food (quality) prepared and the pleasure-enhancing way it is eaten. Thus a 'proper meal', consisting of meat and vegetables, brings together the ideal of a 'close family' and health (Lupton 2000). Kemmer (2000) notes that, through food men and women can show their feelings for one another and also that traditional gender roles are expressed in food preparation. However, the increasing number of women in paid employment outside the home seems to have encouraged men to get involved in meal preparation more often (Horrell 1994, cited in Kemmer 2000).

It might be tempting to blame women for the falling standards in our nutrition. However, the picture is more complex than that. Social change affects the way people live their lives. Many women feel that they have little choice in going to work and that in so doing they are, indeed, providing for their families.

Contemporary cookery books and the cooking industry reflect trends in our attitude to food and cooking. There has been a whole industry burgeoning around cooking. Cookery books are amongst the bestsellers in bookshops, and the television channels are competing with each other for viewers for their cookery programmes. However, their impact on promoting home cooking has not been studied.

Food as a social ritual

Most people have at least some opinion as to how food should be prepared, served and eaten. They also have a view about what foods are appropriate on different occasions. Some have a religious significance and some religions have strict dietary rules (see Box 8.2), in some cases originally designed to protect people from food poisoning.

As a nursing student, you will need to ask your patients/clients (or their family) about their beliefs and preferences, and be guided by this. Most people know that eating is essential to life, and for many people eating in the correct way is just as important. It may be useful to consider the point that, although the rules may be important for various reasons, including safe eating, it is not always clear if they are practised for religious reasons or whether they are culturally constructed.

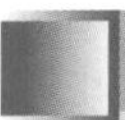

Box 8.2

Religious dietary laws

Many religions and cultures forbid the taking of pork. The reasons for this are complex and varied. Pork is likely to lead to problems with food poisoning, which is a particularly serious matter in hot climates. Furthermore, there is an incident described in the Bible where Jesus sends demons into a herd of pigs (see Matthew chapter 5, verses 8–14). For these and possibly other reasons people may believe that pork is 'dirty'.

Many Muslims teach that some food, like pork, is 'harram' or un-pure. In order to be 'halal' or suitable for eating, food has to be correctly prepared. In the case of meat, the animal has to be slaughtered in a particular way. The Jewish term for food that is satisfactory to eat is 'kosher'.

Christians, particularly Roman Catholics, teach that Friday is a time for special meditation and prayer. Part of this may include eating more simply, often by excluding meat, or substituting meat with fish. This is why many people choose to eat fish on a Friday, even if the original rationale is forgotten.

Many religious people include periods of fasting, believing that this assists in prayer and concentrating on one's soul. Muslims teach that the month of Ramadan is a time when food should not be taken in daylight hours. The time of Ramadan varies, and it can be quite arduous if it falls in the summer. Christians used to use Lent as a time for fasting, or abstaining from animal products, largely because they were scarce.

These periods of fasting are often followed by celebrations, such as Easter, and, in Islam, the Eid. At these times, eating forms an important part of the festivities.

Most religions make exceptions to the fasting requirements for those who are ill, lactating, menstruating or pregnant.

Dietary preferences

Many people choose to reduce or omit animal products from their diet. Such people are often referred to as vegetarians or vegans. The rationale for vegetarianism is varied and will influence the exact type of vegetarian diet chosen. For example, some people are concerned about animal welfare, but may perhaps eat meat if they are satisfied about the standards of animal husbandry (Royal Society for the Prevention of Cruelty to Animals 2004).

The Royal Society for the Prevention of Cruelty to Animals has started the 'freedom foods' scheme, which identifies meat derived from animals in cases where the farmer has met certain criteria. Others feel that the costs of raising an animal to eat makes it morally wrong when so many people cannot get enough to eat; these people may accept meat that has been raised in areas, such as high hill land, that are unsuitable for arable purposes. Still others believe that fruits and vegetables are particularly healthy and choose to eat vegetarian or vegan food, although some may accept meat as an occasional treat or as a courtesy. Many devout religious people believe it is wrong to kill any sentient being and observe a strict vegan or vegetarian diet, whilst others who find it difficult to obtain meat that has been treated according to religious laws, or who are unsure about how the meat has been prepared, choose a vegetarian diet.

The food we need

So far, we have discussed the social and cultural aspects of food and nutrition. In this section we consider what we mean by nutrition. Nutrition is concerned with the quality of our diet and whether it will help us sustain a healthy lifestyle or whether it will lead to physical and emotional problems. The World Health Organization (cited in Lawrence 2004) reported that 60% of deaths around the world are related to increased consumption of fatty, salty and sugary foods arising from changing dietary patterns (Lawrence 2004). This indicates that the changes that have taken place in Western diets are also taking place on an international and worldwide scale, due to the marketing and distribution patterns of international food companies. The same kind of dramatic rise in consumption of fats and sugars has occurred in China and India as these countries have moved away from an agricultural economy and towards greater industrialization and urbanization, and thus increased disposable income of its population (Lawrence 2004). These changes in dietary patterns are resulting in a rise of cardiovascular disease, diabetes and obesity. By contrast, approximately 1.2 billion people in the world have too little to eat (Kew Magazine 2005, Lawrence 2004).

So what are the essential components of a healthy diet and where can they be obtained? Most essential components of a diet can be classified into micronutrients and macronutrients.

The micro-elements are the vitamins and minerals that are essential for a healthy life and which many people believe they can take as supplements to their normal diet as a strategy to increase their health or reduce the incidence of illness. Research so far has discovered that these micro-elements are responsible primarily for the normal development and functioning of cells.

The macro-elements are substances known as proteins, carbohydrates, fats or lipids. These macronutrients form the key building-blocks of cells; they also provide energy for the cells to function and consequently for the body to function, and so for you to live, breathe, digest, think and move (Figure 8.2).

In the following sections, we first explore what is meant by energy then discuss the different nutrients that are needed in your diet.

Energy

Have you ever noticed that you feel warm while eating or that, if you are very hungry, you often feel cold and more sensitive to pain?

Energy is important because we need it for almost all functions of the body. On a macro-level these daily functions require the heart to pump blood around all the tissues in the body, the lungs to absorb oxygen and to excrete carbon dioxide, the kidneys to filtrate blood and form urine, the intestines to absorb and excrete foods, the muscles to contract and expand and the brain to function. Each of these vital organs produces other substances that are also essential to the good functioning of the body.

The basal metabolic rate (BMR) is the amount of energy required by the body when at rest (but not asleep). Additional activities such as moving and even thinking require extra energy. The BMR is not fixed as it will go up in extreme cold temperatures as the body increases its use (burning) of energy to keep the body temperature constant at the optimum temperature for its cells to function (37°C), and also for eating. When someone fasts or is starving, their BMR reduces and the person may feel cold and sleepy as the body tries to save energy to conserve its resources for essential cellular function (you can read more about temperature regulation in Chapter 9). The change in BMR caused by eating or not eating is important as it explains why starvation diets rarely work. The effect of eating can be seen particularly when taking breakfast, as the food intake causes the BMR to rise and thus 'kick starts' the metabolic functions of the body. Pollitt (1995) argues that children of school age who have eaten breakfast are able to outperform those children who have not. Probably the same is also true for adults, which is why almost all effective weight-loss regimens include breakfast.

So what is energy?

Energy is the ability (or potential ability) of the body to function effectively and to enable it to

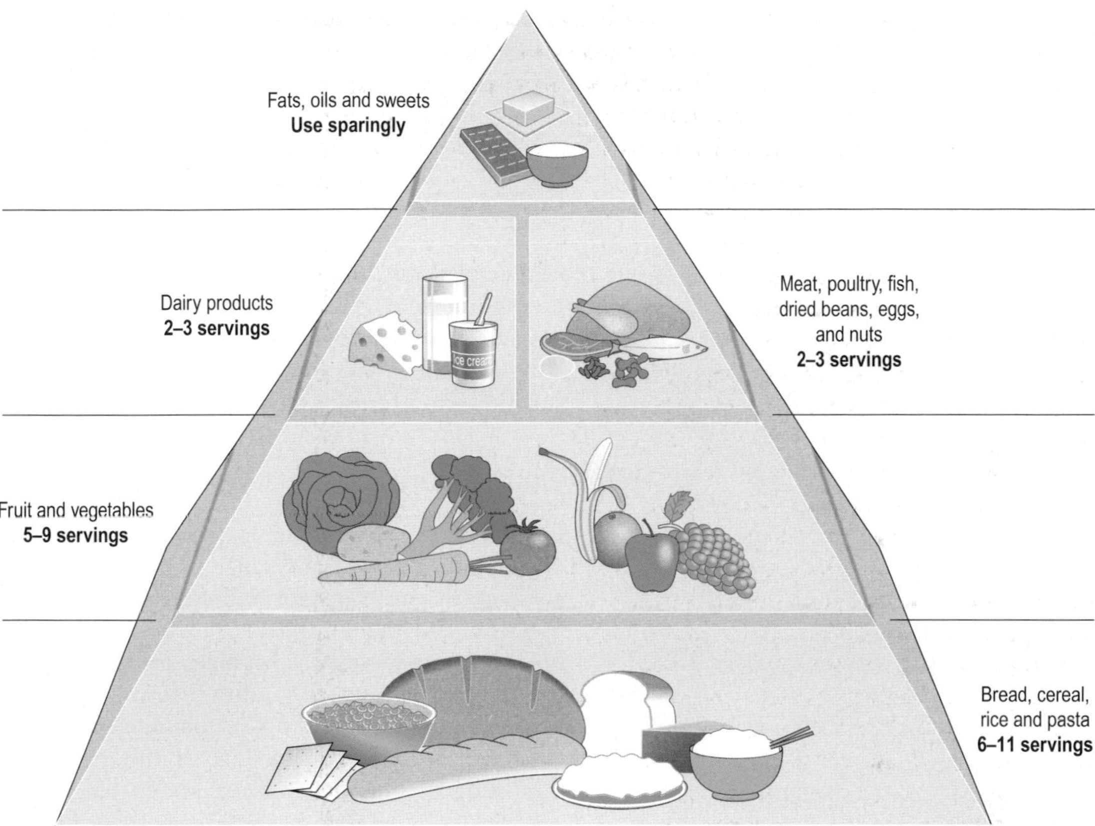

Figure 8.2 • The main food groups and their recommended proportions per day within a balanced diet. (Reproduced with kind permission from Waugh & Grant 2006.)

carry out our daily activities. Most of this body work is conducted within the millions of cells that make up our bodies. Within each cell there are special structures called 'mitochondria' (singular: 'mitochondrion'), often known as the power house of the cell because of their essential role in undertaking the activity of metabolism (Figure 8.3). In order for a cell to carry out its metabolic work, it usually requires energy. The mitochondria use a particular compound that facilitates this energy production; this compound is called adenosine triphosphate (ATP). The mitochondria can manufacture ATP by using oxygen that has been delivered via the red blood cells to the tissue cells, along with another product of nutrition, glucose. (Sometimes the mitochondria produce energy using different products, but this normally only happens as an emergency if there is a shortage of oxygen and glucose.) In the process of manufacturing ATP, the mitochondria also produce several waste products, one of which is energy in the form of heat, another is carbon dioxide and another is water. The water helps transport the carbon dioxide out of the mitochondria and the cell into the capillary blood from where it is transported via the veins, through the right side of the heart and then on to the alveolar capillaries in the lungs to be excreted in the breath.

The process of ATP manufacture is called a metabolic pathway; Figure 8.4 summarizes this process. Energy production is carried out in the mitochondria of all cells, except red blood cells (because red blood cells only have minimal energy requirements).

Humans are described as being in energy balance if the energy they are taking in through their diet

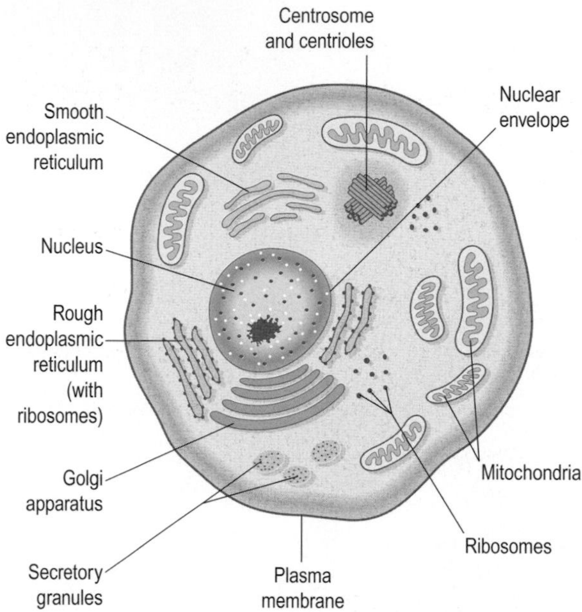

Figure 8.3 • A typical cell showing the mitochondria. (Reproduced with kind permission from Waugh & Grant 2006.)

$C_6H_{12}O_6 + O_2 \rightarrow ATP + CO_2 + heat + H_2O$

Translated as:

glucose + oxygen → ATP + carbon dioxide + heat + water

Figure 8.4 • Production of energy in the mitochondria.

is about the same as the amount of energy being used. So sports people prepare themselves before a sporting event by taking large quantities of high-energy foods. As a result of an evolutionary response to times of hunger, the body has the ability to store energy reserves during times of plenty, usually in the form of adipose tissue (fat) deposited under the skin, or in the buttocks, or over the abdominal organs. If inadequate energy-providing foods are taken, for example during periods of famine or food shortages, or starvation (such as in hospitals), then the body has the ability to maintain its cellular function, and thus life for a period of time, by drawing upon its reserves until they are exhausted, when death will take place.

Carbohydrates and proteins both yield approximately 17 joules (J) of energy for each gram (g) of food consumed. Fats, and also alcohol, yield 30 J/g, and so are a dense source of energy.

Macronutrients

Macronutrients are essential for the effective development of cells and tissues and they all have the ability to be used for energy production, although they also have different and unique functions in a healthy diet.

Carbohydrates

Carbohydrates all contain carbon, hydrogen and oxygen. There is a wide range of foodstuffs that are high in carbohydrate and they are the most plentiful. The main purpose of carbohydrates is to provide the necessary substances for energy production and they are the simplest form of nutrient to transform into energy. Carbohydrates are subclassified, according to the size of the molecules, into monosaccharides, disaccharides and oligosaccharides. These all taste sweet and are present in almost all sweet-tasting foods, including cakes, sweets and fruit (Table 8.1).

Polysaccharides are large complex molecules composed of many monosaccharides. They do not taste sweet. The chief examples are amylose and amylosepectin, which together constitute starch (found in plants) and glycogen (found mainly in animals). In the Western diet the most important sources of polysaccharides are potatoes, rice and wheat products such as bread and pasta.

Most carbohydrates are at least partially broken down in the gastrointestinal tract to mono- and disaccharides. However, the rate at which this takes places varies and this is very important for human health. Some carbohydrates are very quickly and easily broken down to mono- and disaccharides, whereas others take much longer. The speed at which dietary carbohydrate appears as blood glucose is referred to as the glycaemic index. Foods with a high glycaemic index are quickly broken down and lead to a rapid rise in blood sugar, which provides an energy burst,

Table 8.1 Some simple carbohydrates and their dietary source

Type of carbohydrate	Number of carbon atoms or monosaccharides	Examples	Source(s)
Monosaccharide (a one-sugar unit)	Six carbon atoms: known as a hexose Five carbon atoms: known a pentose	Glucose Fructose	
Disaccharide	Two monosaccharides chemically bound together	Sucrose (consists of glucose and fructose) Lactose (consists of galactose and glucose) Maltose (consists of two glucose molecules)	Table sugar Milk Many cereals
Oligosaccharide	Composed of two, three or four monosaccharides		

followed by a rapid drop in blood sugar, leaving the person hungry. Those foodstuffs that take longer to be digested by the gastrointestinal system are identified as having a low glycaemic index. They are absorbed into the bloodstream more slowly and so lead to a slower but more sustained rise in blood sugar. Normally it is better to choose foods with a low glycaemic index, as they provide energy over a longer period of time. Foods with a high glycaemic index can cause wide swings in blood sugar, which might lead to long-term health problems. A simple guide to high or low glycaemic foodstuffs is the size of the molecules. Most foodstuffs with large molecules have a low glycaemic index, but there are important exceptions to this. Note, for instance, that baked and roast (but not boiled) potatoes have a high glycaemic index, and so would lead to a rapid increase in blood sugar, whereas milk and yoghurt have a low glycaemic index, leading to a slower and more sustained rise in blood sugar (see Table 8.2). Try Activity 8.4 and calculate what your typical daily glycaemic index intake might be.

Activity 8.4

Make a list of what you have eaten over the past 24 hours. If you can remember what drinks you have had, include these in your list.

Working through the glycaemic index of foodstuffs listed in Table 8.2, determine how the different food items are categorized.

Now consider whether your dietary intake is mainly from the high, medium or low categories of the Glycaemic Index.

Consider which high-GI foodstuffs you could exchange for medium- or low-GI foods to give you more energy for longer each day.

Fibre

Fibre includes any foods that cannot be absorbed or broken down by enzymes in the human digestive tract and are usually complex carbohydrates (e.g. some forms of starch). Fibre is therefore not a true nutrient. Foods rich in fibre include most fruit and vegetables, and wholemeal foods such as brown rice and wholemeal bread. However, fibre does play an important role in regulating gastrointestinal function, and a lack of fibre can lead to constipation and other difficulties.

Proteins

Proteins are an important component of a healthy diet. They are found in a range of foodstuffs, but particularly in animal products and some pulses and cereals. High-protein foods include meat, fish, dairy products and eggs. Proteins are normally

Table 8.2 Foodstuffs with high, medium and low glycaemic index (GI)

High-GI foods			Moderate-GI foods			Low-GI foods		
	GI > 59	COH (g/portion)		GI = 40–59	COH (g/portion)		GI = 1–39	COH (g/portion)
			Breakfast cereals					
Cornflakes	84	26	All Bran	42	19			
Rice Crispies	82	27	Sultana Bran	52	20			
Cheerios	74	23	Porridge (with water)	42	14			
Shredded Wheat	67	31	Muesli	56	34			
Weetabix	69	30						
			Grains/pasta					
Couscous	65	77	Buckwheat	54	68			
Brown rice	76	58	Bulgar wheat	48	44			
White rice	87	56	Basmati rice	58	48			
			Noodles	46	30			
			Macaroni	45	43			
			Spaghetti	41	49			
			Breads					
Bagel	72	46	Pitta bread	57	43			
Croissant	67	23	Rye bread	41	11			
Baguette	95	22						
White bread	70	18						
Wholemeal bread	69	16						
Pizza	60	38						
			Crackers, biscuits and cakes					
Puffed crispbread	81	7	Digestive	59	10			
Ryvita	69	7	Oatmeal	55	8			
Water biscuit	78	6	Rich Tea	55	8			
Rice cakes	85	6	Muffin	44	34			
Shortbread	64	8	Sponge cake	46	39			
			Vegetables					
Parsnip	97	8	Carrots	49	3			
Baked potato	85	22						
Boiled new potato	62	27						
Mashed potato	70	28	Boiled potato	56	30			
Chips	75	59	Peas	48	7			
Swede	72	1	Sweetcorn	55	17			
Broad beans	79	7	Sweet potato	54	27			
			Yam	51	43			

(Cont'd)

Table 8.2 Foodstuffs with high, medium and low glycaemic index (GI) *Continued*

High-GI foods	GI > 59	COH (g/portion)	Moderate-GI foods	GI = 40–59	COH (g/portion)	Low-GI foods	GI = 1–39	COH (g/portion)
Pulses								
			Baked beans	48	31	Butter beans	31	22
						Chick peas	33	24
						Red kidney beans	27	20
						Green/brown lentils	30	28
						Red lentils	26	28
						Soya beans	18	6
Fruit								
Cantaloupe melon	65	6	Apricots	57	3	Apples	38	12
Pineapple	66	8	Banana	55	23	Dried apricots	31	15
Raisins	64	21	Grapes	46	15	Cherries	22	10
Water melon	72	14	Kiwi	52	6	Grapefruit	25	5
			Mango	55	11	Peaches (tinned)	30	12
			Orange	44	12	Pear	38	16
			Papaya	58	12	Plum	39	5
			Peach	42	8			
			Plum	39	5			
			Sultanas	56	12			
Dairy products								
Ice cream	61	14	Custard	43	20	Full cream milk	27	14
						Skimmed milk	32	15
						Yoghurt (low fat fruit)	33	27
Drinks								
Fanta	68	51	Apple juice	40	16			
Lucozade	95	40	Orange juice	46	14			
Isostar	70	18						
Gatorade	78	15						
Squash (diluted)	66	14						
Snacks and sweets								
Tortilla/Corn chips	72	30	Crisps	54	16	Peanuts	14	4
Mars bar	68	43	Milk chocolate	49	31			
Muesli bar	61	20						
Sugars								
Glucose	100	5	Honey	58	13	Fructose	23	5
Sucrose	65	5						
Maltodextrin	105	5						

Source: BUPA website (www.bupa.co.uk/health).
COH, shorthand for carbohydrate.

used primarily for tissue development; however, in times of shortage of carbohydrate foods, the body can convert proteins into energy. This is one of the principles of some diets.

Proteins are large, complex molecules that are made up of smaller components called amino acids. All amino acids contain nitrogen.

Dispensable and indispensable amino acids

Approximately 20 different amino acids occur in nature and these are often classified as indispensable and dispensable (previously known as essential and non-essential) amino acids. Both indispensable and dispensable amino acids are required for human health, but the dispensable amino acids can be manufactured in the liver from other amino acids. Indispensable amino acids can only be obtained from eating the appropriate foodstuffs. Of these indispensable amino acids, eight are essential for adults, and because the liver of infants is too immature to manufacture histidine, they have to have these provided in their food.

Proteins are essential for the manufacture of cells and tissues, as well as of many chemical messengers such as hormones and neurotransmitters. When people have suffered an injury, such as surgery, a burn or loss of tissue, they need additional intakes of proteins for repairing or growing new tissue.

Sources of protein

You can obtain proteins from both animal and plant sources, although the amino acid profile in animal sources is closer to what is required for humans. In fact, proteins from animal sources used to be referred to as first-class proteins, and those from plant sources as second-class proteins. However, with increased understanding of nutrition, animal proteins are now referred to as proteins of high biological value and plant proteins as proteins of low biological value. Vegetables rich in protein include lentils, potatoes, rice and legumes (peas and beans). Vegetarians and vegans who do not eat meat products can obtain the necessary range of indispensable amino acids by eating a wide variety of plant foods.

Lipids

Fats are more correctly known as lipids because they consist of two main types: fats, which are solid at room temperature, and oils, which are liquid at room temperature. Lipids are essential to bodily function and can be found in a wide range of body tissues:

- In cell membranes.
- As insulation to nerve tissue, thus enabling the electrical impulses to travel faster. The brain is largely composed of fatty tissue.
- As an essential part of the transport system for fat-soluble substances such as vitamins.
- As a vital component of some of the messenger hormones.
- As insulation to the body as a whole, and between some organs and muscles; excess fat intake is stored in these tissues as a resource in times of famine.

Lipids as an energy source

Lipids are also a rich source of energy, yielding almost twice as much energy for their weight as proteins or carbohydrates.

Most lipids in our diet and in our body are composed of triglycerides. A triglyceride molecule consists of a glycerol 'backbone' supporting three fatty acids. Fatty acids are (often long) chains of carbon atoms, with hydrogen atoms (and oxygen in the acid part) attached. Carbon has the capacity of chemically binding up to four other atoms. Each carbon atom will be attached to two other carbon atoms in the chain; if the remaining capacity binds hydrogen atoms, then the fatty acid is said to be 'saturated'. If the carbon atoms have 'spaces' that are not occupied by a hydrogen atom, the fatty acid is said to be 'unsaturated'.

Lipids are not water-soluble, yet the dietary intake of lipid nutrients needs to be transported in the bloodstream. This is achieved by attaching the lipids to plasma proteins, so making a lipoprotein. Adipocytes (in the adipose tissue, about half of which is subcutaneous) remove the fatty acids and glycerol from the bloodstream for up to 4 hours after a fatty meal has been eaten and store approximately 85% of the body's energy in the form of triglycerides. The normal distribution of adipose tissue constitutes 21% of the average female body mass and 15% of the male body mass. It contains approximately 2 months' supply of energy reserves against famine or seasonal changes. With changes in dietary habits and relative affluence in many societies, these percentages have changed considerably.

Between meals, as the blood glucose level begins to fall, the body starts to mobilize its reserves by releasing hormones such as glucocorticoids, human growth hormone and adrenaline (also known as epinephrine), which trigger the adipocytes to release glycerol and fatty acids back into the bloodstream (Martini & Welch 2005). Initially, the glycogen in the liver is converted back to glucose, but this supply is not abundant, and, with prolonged fasting, the individual will utilize adipose tissue and finally protein tissue, particularly skeletal muscle.

Recommendations for dietary lipid intake

Current recommendations state that we should take about 33% of our total energy requirements from lipid (MAFF 2002), yet most people are taking approximately 40% of their energy requirements as lipid. However, most of this (80–90%) should come from unsaturated fatty acids, and only 10% from saturated fatty acids. This is because saturated fatty acids encourage the formation of low-density lipoproteins (sometimes called 'bad cholesterol') in the liver, which are associated with the formation of atheroma (see below). Unsaturated fatty acids, however, are associated with the formation of high-density lipoproteins ('good cholesterol'), which are at the least not harmful to arteries, and may even protect them. Foods that are high in unsaturated fatty acids, particularly polyunsaturated fatty acids, are usually liquids (oils) from plants or fish. 'Fat' from animals tends to be solid and high in saturated fatty acids.

There is some interest in the position of the first carbon to have a double bond within the unsaturated fatty acid molecule (see, for example, Small 2002). Thus, in omega-3 fatty acids the first carbon with a double bond is at the third position, counting from the glycerol backbone. The liver cannot make a fatty acid with a double bond nearer than the eighth position, so the liver cannot make omega-3 or omega-6 fatty acids; these are therefore considered essential fatty acids. Omega-6 fatty acids are reasonably abundant in the diet, and come from seeds and cereals. Omega-3 fatty acids are found predominantly in oily fish such as herring, mackerel, pilchards, salmon and sardines. For many people their dietary intake of omega-3 fatty acids probably needs to be increased, particularly as a diet rich in omega-3 fatty acids may offer protection from a wide range of problems, including allergies, cardiovascular disorders and even mental health problems (Small 2002). Follow Activity 8.5 and try to identify which types of lipids are in your diet.

Lipids and atheroma

One of the much publicized effects of lipids in the diet is the development of atheroma. Atheroma is a condition in which a layer of lipid material develops on the inside walls of the artery. This has the effect of reducing the diameter of the lumen of the artery and so restricting the flow of blood. This causes a reduction in the flow of blood to the tissues the artery serves, and also, if the atheroma is extensive enough, raises the blood pressure throughout the circulation. These changes are clearly dangerous to the health of a child and subsequently the adult. The problem is related to the amount and nature of the lipid and fat intake rather than the inclusion of fats and lipids in the diet.

Activity 8.5

Look in your kitchen store cupboard and in your fridge and make a list of the different types of foodstuffs, fats and lipids that you are using on a daily or weekly basis.

Check the labels to determine whether the foodstuffs contain saturated or unsaturated fats and in what proportions.

Does your diet contain mainly saturated or unsaturated fats?

What might the impact of this intake be on your health, now and in the future?

Micronutrients

In this section we give you a brief introduction to some of the main vitamins and minerals that are essential for health, and their main sources.

Vitamins

Vitamins are organic compounds that are made by plants and some animals, but cannot be made by humans. As they are essential in small quantities for the maintenance of health, we must find them in the food that we eat. Vitamins can be classified as lipid-soluble (vitamins A, D, E and K) and water-soluble (the B group and vitamin C). This means that lipid-soluble vitamins are more commonly found in fats, such as fish oil, dairy fats and some vegetables that have a high lipid content (e.g. avocados). The body is only able to absorb lipid-soluble vitamins if it is able to absorb other fatty substances from the digestive system at the same time. Water-soluble vitamins are more vulnerable to being lost from the diet as they can leach out into the cooking water, which is why it is often better to steam green vegetables, for example, to conserve the vitamins in them.

Some people choose to take vitamin supplements, often in large quantity. If the vitamin concerned is water-soluble, this is probably harmless and may be helpful, as any excess vitamin is lost in the urine. For instance, many people take generous supplements of vitamin C, believing that it will help ward off infections, including the common cold (New Scientist 2005). There is indeed evidence that supplements may assist in reducing the length of the incidence but not reducing its occurrence.

However, taking large quantities of lipid-soluble vitamins is not recommended, as these can accumulate in the liver, and be potentially toxic.

See Table 8.3 for a brief summary of the chief sources and action of some of the vitamins discussed in the sections below.

Vitamin A

Vitamin A is a lipid-soluble vitamin; it is essential for the correct functioning of the eye. If there is an inadequate intake of vitamin A, the person will suffer from a loss of night vision. In many parts of the world, children's sight has been permanently damaged by lack of vitamin A. It is not abundant in the diet, and is often taken in the form of beta-

Table 8.3 Some vitamins, their action and chief sources

Vitamin	Source	Function	Deficiency	Notes
Vitamin A (retinol)	Liver, dairy produce, eggs	Vision, particularly in low light	Poor vision, even blindness	Avoid excess, particularly in pregnancy
Folate	Offal, yeast extract, leafy green vegetables	Essential for rapidly dividing cells		Should be supplemented in very early pregnancy
Vitamin B_{12}	Many animal, dairy and egg products	Manufacture and function of red blood and nerve cells	Pernicious anaemia	Requires intrinsic factor for absorption
Vitamin C	Fruit and coloured vegetables	Maintenance of connective tissue	Scurvy	Is readily destroyed by storage and cooking
Vitamin D	Margarine	Promotes mineralization of bones	Rickets, osteomalacia	Is synthesized from action of sunlight on skin
Vitamin E	Vegetable oil, nuts and seeds	Antioxidant	Rare	

carotene, which is present in milk, cheese, carrots, cabbage, peppers and sweet potatoes. Supplementation, however, should be undertaken with caution. For instance, excessive intake of vitamin A has been associated with damage to unborn children (Kmietowicz 2003). One of the oldest skeletons found, the bones of Lucy, which were discovered in Olduvai gorge in Kenya, were found to contain high quantities of vitamin A and it is believed that she died as a result of vitamin A poisoning, probably from eating animal liver, where it is stored.

B group vitamins

These are water-soluble vitamins and all act as co-factors, which enhance enzyme activity.

Folate (which is a form of folic acid) is one of the B group of vitamins. Folate has been the subject of much interest since it was established as preventing neural tube defects in the growing embryo (Wald 1991). Other research studies have demonstrated that taking folate can reduce the incidence of cardiovascular disease in older adults. In the UK, the best source of folate has traditionally been flour and therefore bread, but more recently the folate content of flour has declined, so some countries now add folate to flour and flour-based products.

Vitamin B_{12} is essential for the formation and functioning of all cells. Its absence in the diet is most noticeable for its effects on red blood cells, and the condition is called pernicious anaemia. It is abundant in all animal-based foods, but people who eat a diet with no eggs or diary products (vegans) may develop signs of deficiency. However, deficiency is more likely to occur through a lack of intrinsic factor.

Vitamin C (ascorbic acid)

This is a water-soluble vitamin and is essential for the maintenance of connective tissue. If it is lacking in the diet, bleeding will occur from the small blood vessels under the skin and mucous membranes, and if left untreated this will develop into scurvy, which can be fatal. Vitamin C is widely available in fruit and vegetables as well as in milk and liver. As a water-soluble vitamin it is easily lost when the vegetable is stored or in the cooking water.

Rich sources of vitamin C are fresh citrus fruits, black fruits such as blackcurrants, and green leaf vegetables.

Vitamin D

Vitamin D is a fat-soluble vitamin that is found in oily fish, fish liver oils, animal liver, fortified margarines, butter milk and breakfast cereals. The form of vitamin D from these sources is known as cholecalciferol. Another source of vitamin D is through the action of ultraviolet B-rays in sunlight on 7-dihydrocholesterol found in the skin. This source of vitamin D may not be available for members of certain cultural groups (who for social, cultural or practical reasons are unable to expose themselves to enough sunlight) and also for individuals in long-term residential care. We need vitamin D to absorb calcium and phosphate from the intestine and this can be inhibited by some foods. Calcium and phosphorus are essential minerals that form healthy bones and teeth. Calcium is also an essential mineral for effective neuromuscular function as well as cell development.

Children who lack any of these nutrients tend to develop deformed long bones (rickets), adults develop osteomalacia, or bones that are principally made up of collagen and have a deficiency of the calcium and phosphorus that gives them their density and hardness. If there is a shortage of vitamin D, the body is unable to absorb calcium from the diet, and under the influence of parathyroid hormone it tries to maintain the level of calcium in the body by leaching existing calcium from the bones, causing osteoporosis. Adding calcium supplements to the diet of people with a predisposition to osteoporosis reduces bone loss and the risk of them developing fractures.

Vitamin E

Vitamin E is a group of fat-soluble substances called tocopherols; they are widespread in the diet and deficiency is rare.

Vitamin K

Vitamin K is a fat-soluble vitamin that is unusual in the diet, but deficiency is rare in otherwise healthy people as most people have bacteria in their large intestines that can manufacture vitamin K as a by-product, which is then absorbed and utilized in the body.

Micronutrients and the diet

One of the best ways to ensure that the required micronutrients are received is to eat plenty of fruit and vegetables. Studies consistently show that people who eat five or more portions of fruit and vegetables are healthier than those who do not (outlined in Vines 1996). The effect is quite strong, and not fully understood. Certainly fruit and vegetables tend to be rich in vitamins and minerals and low in fat, but high in fibre. However, there are probably other compounds that we are only just learning about that are present in fruit and vegetables and that are very beneficial to health.

It has been shown that quite limited intervention encouraging greater consumption of fruit and vegetables can have impressive outcomes in terms of blood cholesterol and other indicators of health (Steptoe et al 2003). The evidence is now so convincing that 'five a day' is government policy, and there are many initiatives designed to increase the intake of fruit and vegetables (Department of Health 1998). For instance, all schoolchildren between the ages of 4 and 6 years should receive one piece of fruit on each school day. Some people regard the 'five a day' target as unreasonably high. These people should have it explained to them about the wide range of foods that 'count' as fruit and vegetables; the food can be in any form, including tinned, frozen then cooked, dried or pureed. However, potatoes, in any form, do not count; they form a very useful part of the diet, but have a different role. People are often surprised to learn that tinned baked beans, dried fruit and fruit juices all contribute to a healthy diet.

Minerals

Minerals are also micronutrients that are required by the body in small quantities. Minerals are of inorganic origin (i.e. they are found in rocks and soil). Of course, unlike animals, humans do not normally lick rocks to obtain these nutrients; instead, they get them from water, or from plants and animals that have ingested them. One of the most important minerals in the body is iron, as it is essential for the formation of haemoglobin and thus the transport of oxygen around the body.

Calcium and magnesium are important for bone development and muscle contraction.

Table 8.4 lists some of the more important minerals, their sources in food and their action.

Table 8.4 Some common minerals, their action and sources in food

Name	Source	Function	Deficiency	Notes
Iron	Red meat, cereals and cereal products	Formation of haemoglobin	Anaemia	Deficiency is common in this country
Calcium	Milk, yoghurt, cheese	Healthy teeth and bones, muscle contraction	Rickets, osteomalacia, osteoporosis	Requires vitamin D for absorption and deposition
Zinc	Cheese, meat eggs	Wound healing, enzyme activity	Poor wound healing, ?depression	
Sodium in the form of sodium chloride ('salt')	Abundant, particularly in cooked/processed foods	Water balance, nerve and muscle function	Heat exhaustion	Most adults take too much, which may damage cardiovascular health

Iron in the diet

About half of the body's stock of iron is found in the haemoglobin, the oxygen-carrying pigment in red blood cells. An inadequate intake of iron is associated with the onset of iron-deficiency anaemia. Women need more iron due to some loss in menstrual flow, yet paradoxically they tend to take less iron in their diet. Thus women of child-bearing years should take about 14.8 mg of iron daily, although they actually get about 12 mg (Caraher 2000, Dallman 1986). This makes iron the nutrient most likely to be lacking from the Western diet.

Sodium

Sodium, in the form of salt in the diet, was once highly prized because it was so difficult to obtain. With changes in Westernized eating patterns, salt is too plentiful and many proprietary foodstuffs contain large amounts of unnecessary added salt, about 75% of which is hidden. Salt is needed as part of the extracellular fluid that bathes the cells throughout the body and is important to normal cellular activity. Excessive sodium is a principal cause of high blood pressure and heart disease (Brewer 2002). This is because the body has a sophisticated mechanism in the kidneys for monitoring and retaining levels of sodium and sometimes the threshold level is re-adjusted incorrectly to retain salt unnecessarily.

How the body digests nutrients

Apart from the cardiovascular system, the digestive tract is the longest organ in the body. It is a system designed to process foodstuffs, by both mechanical and chemical activities, into micro-substances that can be absorbed through the cells in the walls of the stomach and intestine and so into the bloodstream. To assist in this process, the gastrointestinal tract is able to produce a range of chemical substances and is linked to other organs that produce supplementary chemicals. It also has an excellent supply of arterial and venous blood to ensure that there is a transport system for the foodstuffs and liquids that have been processed.

The digestive system is essentially a tube made up of a mucous membrane which has a very rich supply of blood that is sandwiched between this membrane and a double layer of muscle tissue (see Figure 8.5). The advantages of having a good blood

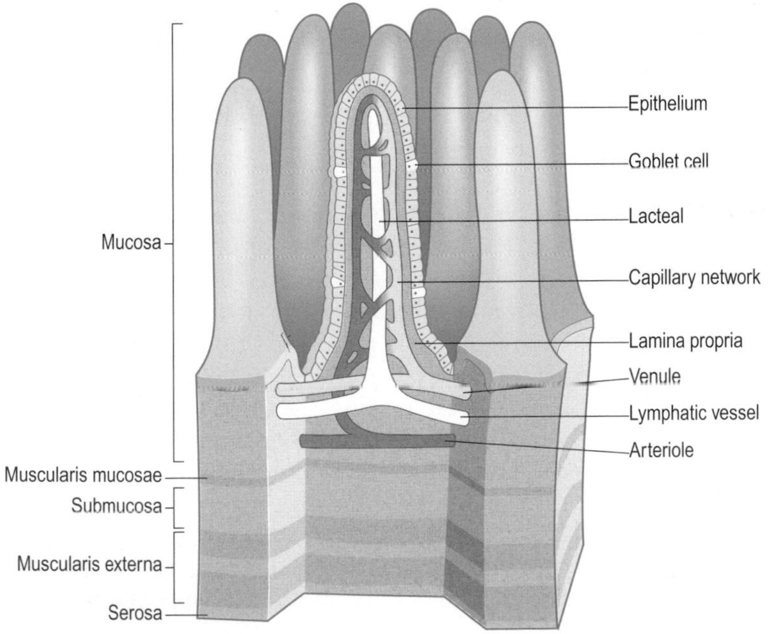

Figure 8.5 • The different tissue layers of the intestinal wall.

supply to the digestive system means that digested foods can be absorbed into the bloodstream very quickly and used to create cells and tissue. For example, it only takes 2 days for the constituents of a meal to be used to form hair.

The closeness of the capillaries to the surface of the mucosa of the digestive system means that they are more sensitive to injury, and consequent bleeding can be seen quickly. However, because of the rich blood supply, once the bleeding has stopped, healing is normally rapid.

Most of the digestive tract has two layers of muscle: an inner layer of smooth muscle that encircles the lumen and an outer layer of longitudinal (striated) muscle that runs down its length. The movements of these muscles are under the control of the autonomic nervous system and so cannot usually be voluntarily controlled; however, these movements can often be felt and may be described as 'hunger pangs' (before food) or 'indigestion' (after food). As well as peristalsis (see below), the muscular wall is responsible for thoroughly mixing the food with the secretions of the digestive tract and the liquids that have been swallowed. In some parts of the intestinal tract the layer of striated muscle creates 'pleats' in the smooth muscular tube, so making the overall length of the tube shorter, at the same time retaining a large surface area for fluids to be absorbed. The terms small and large intestine refer to the diameter of the lumen (tube) not its length; the small intestine is longer than the large intestine and is coiled inside the abdominal cavity. The diameter of the lumen of the intestine influences the rate at which material moves. Food moves more slowly through the wide-lumen large intestine, and this provides time for the water in the digested matter to be reabsorbed.

The main components of the digestive tract (shown in Figure 8.6) are:

- Buccal cavity and pharynx.
- Oesophagus.
- Stomach and duodenum.
- Small intestine and gallbladder.
- Large intestine, rectum and anus.

The mouth or buccal cavity

Food and drink are usually taken into the body via the mouth (Figure 8.7). This is a mucosa-lined cavity whose walls are unusually strong. Most of the space within the mouth is taken up by the tongue, a muscular organ that has the job of moving the food around the mouth and mixing food with liquid to form a bolus (ball), making it easier to swallow.

The tongue houses most of the 10000 taste buds (Marrieb 2005). These are chemical receptors which respond to certain components in the food that have been dissolved through combining with liquid either from saliva or from ingested drink. Some additional chemical receptors can be found in the mucous membranes of the walls of the mouth. There are probably five different types of taste bud, concerned with identifying different flavours: sweet, salty, bitter, sour and the more recently described 'umami' (Coughland 2000), which is a savoury, meaty flavour. Taste buds are genetically controlled, and we appear to have evolved a particular liking for sweet flavours (Wehner 1999), although some people have a stronger genetic predisposition to identify salt in food.

Dental health and disease

Human fondness for sweet things has an impact on dental health. The teeth lie in sockets in the gum-covered margins of the jaw. The first deciduous (or milk) teeth appear at about 6 months of age, and all 20 are present at about 24 months of age. From about 6 years of age these milk teeth are replaced by adult teeth. The third molars (or wisdom teeth) appear by about age 25 years. A complete set of permanent teeth is 32 teeth, but some people never grow their third molars (Marrieb 2005). Oral health (the condition of teeth and gums) is an aspect of health which, despite the addition of fluoride to drinking water, seems to be declining. The very young have poor dental health (Anderson et al 2005), so have children of school age (Peres et al 2005) and older adults (Baily et al 2005). This is important, because poor oral health

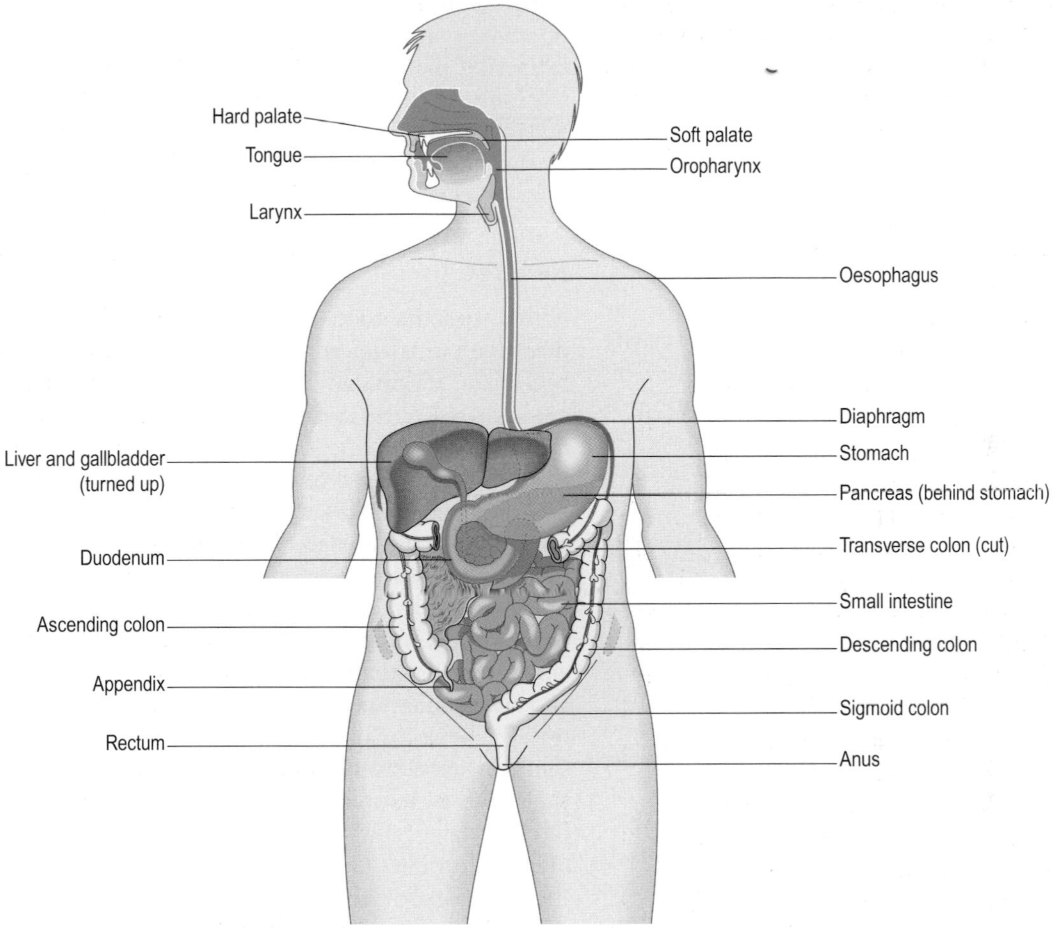

Figure 8.6 • The digestive tract. (Reproduced with kind permission from Waugh & Grant 2006.)

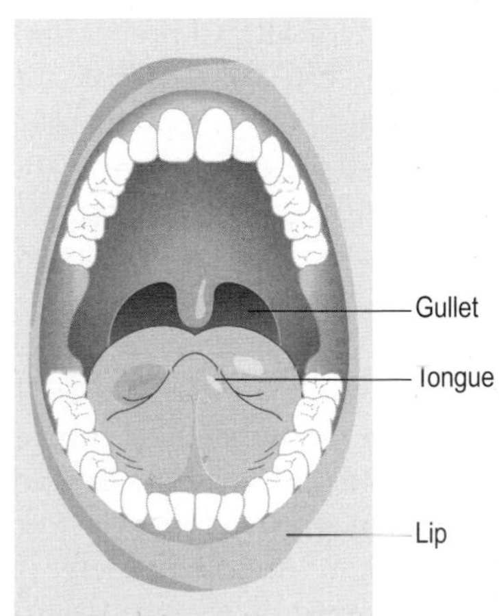

Figure 8.7 • The buccal cavity.

is often linked to serious disorders such as cardiovascular disease (Abnet et al 2005), although the link may not always be causative. Poor dental health can also complicate other disorders, particularly chronic disorders (Foster & Fitzgerald 2005). Oral care is of the utmost importance for all our clients, but has been found to be especially important for older adults (Baily et al 2005) and patients receiving anti-cancer treatments (Karagozoglu & Ulusoy 2005). Cleaning teeth is quite a demanding neuromuscular exercise, requiring both strength and dexterity. It is not surprising that most patients seem to require at least some help in achieving it (Baily et al 2005).

Processing of food in the buccal cavity

The teeth are designed to bite and then grind the food up and mix it with saliva. Saliva has a role in moisturizing foods and keeping the mucous membranes clean. Saliva contains one digestive enzyme, amylase, that starts the digestion of starch.

The tip of the tongue lifts up the bolus of food (see above) and moves it towards the soft palate. These eating activities are voluntarily controlled, but once the food touches the soft palate the autonomic nervous system coordinates activity (Marrieb 2005) and voluntary control is lost. This is probably as well, as swallowing (deglutition) is complex and it is imperative that food does not 'go down the wrong way' and enter the bronchus, causing choking and coughing.

Swallowing involves 22 sets of muscles and is coordinated by the medulla of the brain.

The oesophagus

Once food leaves the mouth, it passes through the pharynx and is moved along the digestive system by an involuntary wave-like action caused by the contraction and relaxation of the longitudinal muscle layer in an action known as peristalsis, passing down the oesophagus to enter the stomach (Figure 8.8 is a cross-section of the oesophagus showing the muscle layers). Perceived problems in the gastrointestinal tract account for a great deal of anxiety and discomfort in our population. It is estimated that dyspepsia (discomfort in the upper gastrointestinal tract, such as 'heart burn') affects 40% of people in a year, and that treating problems in the gastrointestinal tract takes approximately 10% of a general practitioner's time.

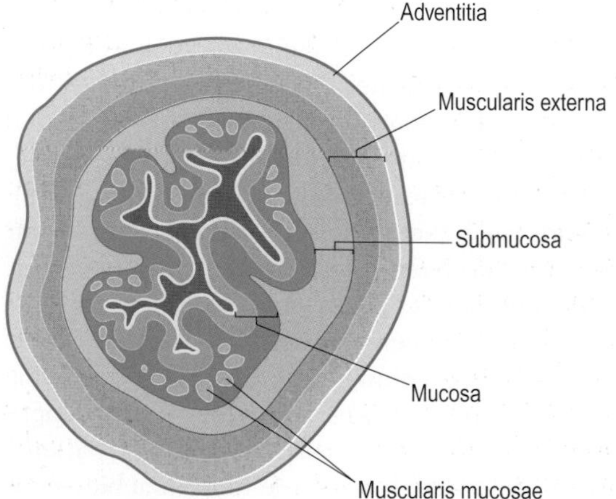

Figure 8.8 • Cross-section of the oesophagus showing muscle layers.

Reverse peristalsis: vomiting

Sometimes the food does not remain within the digestive tract, and is returned forcibly out of the body in an action known as vomiting. Vomiting (or emesis) is a natural response when eating something that the body identifies as being toxic. It is also a side-effect of several medical disorders and can be a side-effect of several drugs. Vomiting occurs when the emesis centre in the brain is stimulated by the presence of toxins or other irritants in the digestive tract, and sometimes by extremes of emotions. The emesis centre stimulates the abdominal and diaphragmatic muscles to contract, and the sphincters in the upper digestive tract to relax. The individual feels nauseated and often salivates excessively. They then typically elevate their chin and straighten their back; all this facilitates a straight and wide passage for the expulsion of the contents of the stomach and, possibly, the contents of the upper small intestine. The process can be remarkably efficient, and is part of our defence against poisoning. However, when it occurs following surgery or as a result of disease, it is important to treat it medically to prevent an excessive loss of fluids and electrolytes that are essential to body function. This is particularly important with babies and young children who are less tolerant of loss of fluids. Helping someone who is feeling nauseated or who is vomiting is an important nursing priority.

Assisting someone who is nauseated or vomiting

The most important role of the nurse is to ensure the person does not inhale their vomit. If the person is conscious and is able to lean forward over a container they can discharge the vomit safely. If the person is unconscious, then it is essential to position them quickly (providing they do not have a spinal injury) into the recovery position so the vomit is able to flow out of the mouth. If there is a danger of spinal injury then an alternative position is to keep the person on their back but to lower the head and turn it to the side, making sure that the vomit drains outwards. If the person is receiving health care attention, it is a good idea to measure the amount of vomit and make a record of the volume and its appearance in the patient's records.

The acidic taste of vomit is extremely unpleasant and may cause further vomiting, so it is important to provide a mouthwash of either fresh cold water, or of water containing a solution of mouthwash, and a clean bowel to spit it into. These should be placed by the patient's bedside, within easy reach so they can use it again if they continue to feel nauseated. Often it helps the patient to feel more comfortable if their face and hands are washed with warm water to refresh them.

The stomach

The stomach (Figure 8.9) is a deeply folded cavity that will hold food for between 4 and 6 hours. The muscular layers of the stomach (known as the muscularis) include an extra, oblique, layer, which through its contraction and relaxation activities causes the food to be churned and mixed thoroughly with the many different gastric secretions

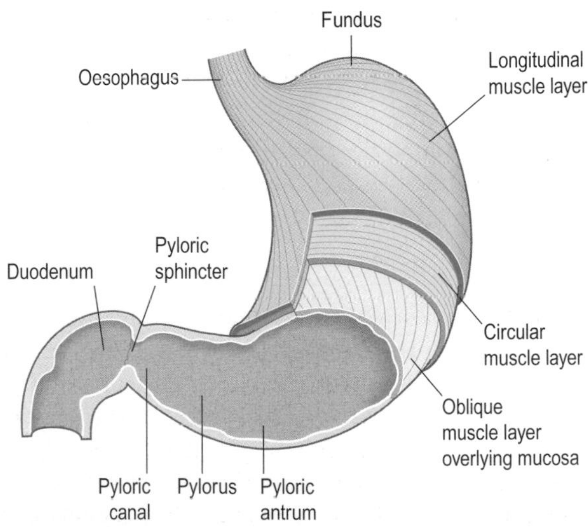

Figure 8.9 • Main structural features of the stomach.

and the mucus. The stomach secretes hydrochloric acid, creating a very acidic environment (it has a pH of about 2); this is an important defence for our bodies against bacteria that might be in the ingested food because they are normally unable to survive in such an acidic environment. The stomach has mucosa that is normally protected against the hydrochloric acid, but if acid is regurgitated outside the stomach it can cause considerable damage to the mucous membrane of the oesophagus, penetrating down to the blood supply beneath the mucosa and causing bleeding. Normally, there is a valve between the oesophagus and the entrance to the stomach which remains closed until peristaltic action pushes food through from the oesophagus, or reverse peristalsis occurs in vomiting.

Another chemical found in the gastric secretions is pepsin, a digestive enzyme that will break down proteins. Pepsin is developed in two stages. It is released from the gastric mucosa as an inactive substance (or precursor) called pepsinogen. When pepsinogen comes into contact with the acidic environment in the stomach it is converted to pepsin. As a result of the action of pepsin on protein-rich food, the protein is broken down into chains of polypeptides. These are then broken down still further into amino acids when they reach the small intestine.

The presence of the enzyme pepsin means that substances that are proteins (e.g. insulin) cannot be given orally.

The mucous membrane of the stomach also produces many hormones that affect different parts of the body; these hormones are associated with general feelings of well-being, or otherwise, after a meal, or to indicate hunger.

After the foodstuff has been subjected to considerable churning and mixing with the pepsin and hydrochloric acid in the stomach, it becomes a watery mixture called chyme. Chyme is squeezed through the pyloric sphincter into the duodenum where it is mixed with a neutralizing agent called bile. Bile is manufactured in the liver and stored in the gallbladder (Figure 8.10). The gallbladder contracts in response to food entering the duodenum and squeezes out bile, which has a high alkaline content to neutralize the acidity and also to begin saponification of lipids and fats that are in

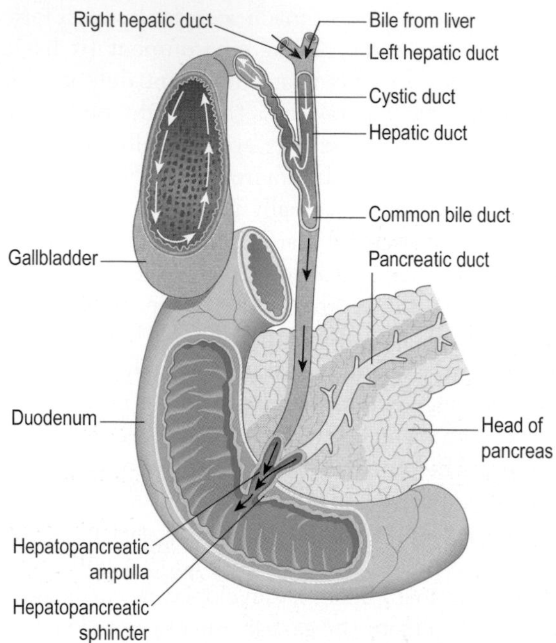

Figure 8.10 • Passage of bile from the liver to the gallbladder and via the bile duct to the intestine. (Reproduced with kind permission from Waugh & Grant 2006.)

the chyme. (Saponification is a chemical reaction between fat and the bile, which begins the breakdown of the fat (likened to the effect of soap or washing-up liquid on fat), thus aiding absorption and metabolism.)

Abnormalities of the stomach and duodenum

Pyloric stenosis

Some infants, often boys, are born with an abnormally tight pyloric sphincter, making it difficult for chyme to pass through into the duodenum; as a result, reverse peristalsis occurs, causing projectile vomiting, which is characteristic of the disorder. Rarely, some adults develop pyloric stenosis as a result of ulceration of the gastric or duodenal mucosa; they develop similar symptoms.

Vitamin B_{12} deficit

Vitamin B_{12} is absorbed as a result of intrinsic factor that is manufactured in the gastric mucosa, but some people lack the necessary hormones to do so, resulting in a form of anaemia. This is when the bone marrow has insufficient vitamin B_{12} to make the red blood cell membrane and so creates fewer, but larger, blood cells, resulting in macrocytic (large cell) anaemia. People who develop this form of anaemia are often unaware that it has happened until the disorder has become quite severe and their haemoglobin level has dropped from a normal level of 12–14 mg/100 ml to 4 or 5 mg/100 ml. By this time the body has been working to compensate for the loss in vitamin B_{12} for the manufacture of other cells and the sufferer is experiencing symptoms of abnormal cell development, such as a sore, red tongue, or loss of sensation in their lower limbs.

Cholecystitis (inflammation of the gallbladder)

Cholecystitis is a common disorder, particularly among women. The gallbladder becomes inflamed, causing a reduction in its capacity to store bile. Sometimes repeated inflammation of the gallbladder (known as cholecystitis) leads to the bile stored in the gallbladder to become more concentrated. This can then cause some substances, most often calcium and cholesterol, to become densely concentrated and form stones. These stones initially cause inflammation of the cystic duct; eventually, gallstones are formed which can completely block the exit from the gallbladder. The gallbladder often reacts to the call to excrete bile by going into spasm as it tries to excrete the stone and excrete bile. Without bile being excreted and mixed with the chyme, its saponifying action means that fats and lipids cannot be reabsorbed through the intestinal villi into the lymph vessels. Also, the chyme does not become deodorized by the bile, so stools are passed that are pale, smelly and fatty.

The small intestine

The small intestine is made up of different parts to distinguish its different activities. These parts are the duodenum, the jejunum and the ileum. Most of the digestion of foodstuffs in the chyme takes place at the beginning of the small intestine, in the duodenum and jejunum. In the ileum and the colon, absorption of substances becomes the key function of the intestinal tract.

Breakdown of nutrients into simpler chemical forms

Digestion is the process by which foods are reduced to simple forms (e.g. amino acids, glucose, fatty acids) so that they can be absorbed into the bloodstream and transported to cells throughout the body. To assist with digestion, there are two vital organs that manufacture specific enzymes: the pancreas and the liver.

The pancreas is located beneath the liver and functions as both an endocrine organ (i.e. is capable of excreting hormones directly into the bloodstream) and an exocrine organ. It is this exocrine function that is important for digestion as the enzymes are fed into the duodenum via the pancreatic duct.

The pancreas manufactures and secretes two distinct types of chemicals:

- *Endocrine chemicals*: these are specifically involved with energy production: insulin, for the regulation of glucose in the blood; glycogen, which is released in emergency situations.
- *Exocrine enzymes*: these are used for the breakdown of polypeptides into amino acids and for breaking down large complex molecules into simple forms, ready for absorption.

Absorption of nutrients into the blood

Once the nutrients have been broken down into their essential components, they are absorbed through the cells in the walls of the intestine, which has an increased surface area due to the presence of intestinal villi. These villi have an excellent blood supply and are made up of cells designed specifically for absorbing small molecules (e.g. amino acids and monosaccharides), which can then directly enter the capillary vessels (see Figure 8.11). The capillaries of the intestinal villi drain into the hepatic portal vein, which takes the nutrients to the liver.

The liver is the most important organ for manufacturing a range of essential substances, including plasma proteins that are essential for maintaining the volume of the blood and for carrying vitamins, minerals and lipids around the body to cells, and for manufacturing blood-clotting agents. So it is essential that the liver is the first destination for all incoming nutrients; as a result, the digestive system is supplied with one-fifth of the volume of blood from each heart beat of blood (known as cardiac output). In times when blood is needed for more urgent requirements, such as 'fright and flight' (in modern terms this would be during exercise), or if there is a severe loss of blood due to haemorrhage, the body cuts down the blood supply to the digestive system and diverts it to where it is needed most.

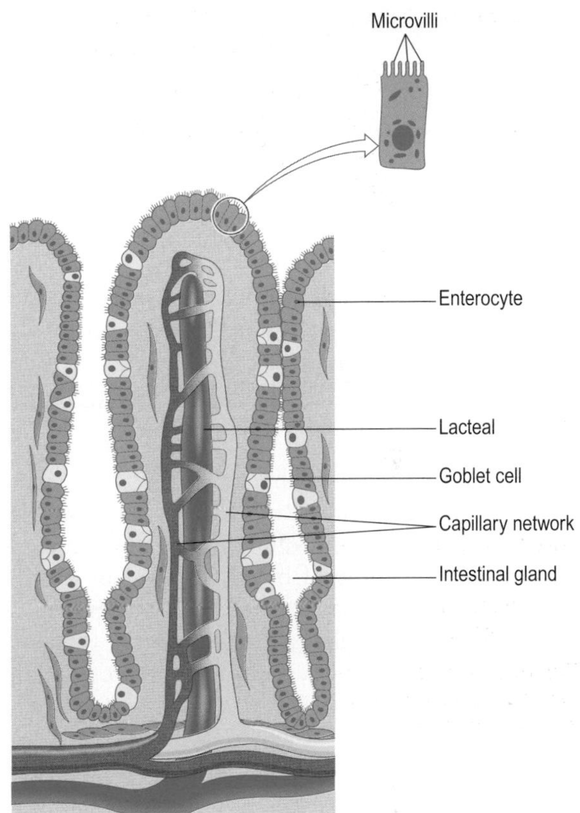

Figure 8.11 • An intestinal villus. (Reproduced with kind permission from Waugh & Grant 2006.)

Absorption of lipids

You will see from Figure 8.11 that the villus is supplied with a capillary and a lymphatic vessel (the lacteal). The lymphatic vessel is designed to absorb fatty acids that have been transported

Activity 8.6

Think about what has happened to food in the stomach and the action of the different enzymes, and remember that tissue is also a combination of protein and fat.

- If a patient has part of their ileum removed and needs to wear an ileostomy bag to drain their faecal material, why is this material watery and greenish in colour?
- Why would the patient need an increased intake of liquids?
- Why would the skin around the ileostomy site be more likely to become red and painful if there is a leakage of faecal materials?

across the cell wall of the intestinal villus. Fat-soluble lipids cannot easily enter the watery environment of the blood until they can be mixed with a larger volume of blood, so they are transported in chylomicrons (small fat globules) from the intestine through to the lacteals of the villi and then transported via the lymphatic system to the cisterna chyli (or fatty lymph cistern), which is located in the thoracic cavity. This excretes chyle (fatty lymph) into the blood at the jugular vein. Immediately after a fatty meal, the blood has a higher density of chylomicrons, giving it a milky appearance. Over the subsequent 4–6 hours these lipids are removed from the blood either to support cellular function or to be stored in the adipose tissue for future use (Martini & Welch 2005).

Activity 8.6 will help you to apply your reading about the physiology of the small intestine to the care of a patient who has had part of their intestine cut out (resected).

Disorders of the small intestine

The most common disorders of the small intestine are due to inflammatory processes. Inflammatory bowel disease is an important group of chronic disorders characterized by inflammation of part of the bowel, rendering it less able to carry out its functions, which often results in dehydration or malnutrition. The cause of these distressing pathologies is not fully known, although the tendency to develop them is partly genetically determined (Newman & Simonovitch 2005).

In people who are on a starvation diet, or who are being fed parenterally (through an intravenous line), the intestinal villi begin to atrophy (see also section on nutrition and recovery from illness, below). This can have consequences if the person then resumes eating a normal diet.

The large intestine

By the time the processed chyme has passed along the small intestine, most of the macronutrients and most of the water have been removed. The faecal material that remains is composed of fibre, fats, bile and water. This material continues to be liquid and brownish-green in colour by the time it enters the large bowel (or colon). One of the key activities of the large bowel is to reabsorb water. If the faecal material lacks fibrous content (roughage), it will take longer to travel along the colon; as a result, more water will be reabsorbed and constipation results. The resulting stool is hard, rendering it difficult and possibly painful to expel. Conversely, if there is an inflammation of the bowel (perhaps due to food poisoning, or an allergic reaction), the material will transit through the large bowel so fast that very little water can be reabsorbed, leading to diarrhoea and the loss of essential water, minerals and some vitamins.

Bacteria and the production of vitamins in the large intestine

The large bowel houses as many as 11 trillion bacteria weighing 1.5 kg. Some 70% of these (probiotic) bacteria are very useful to maintain an ecological balance in the environment (Marrieb 2005). By producing lactic acid they prevent pathogens (other bacteria and yeasts) from colonizing the large intestine. These probiotic bacteria also have an important role in promoting digestion, boosting immunity and making vitamins, as well as extracting some of the nutrients from our food (Brewer 2002). Many of these healthy bacteria are lost when a person suffers from diarrhoea, or as a result of taking an oral course of antibiotics. One strategy to resolve this is to eat yoghurt that contains live

Lactobacillus acidophilus as it replaces the lost bacteria.

Disorders of the large intestine

Constipation

This is probably the most common complaint in Western society, where many people eat a diet low in fibre and low in water. The recommended intake of water is a minimum of 2 litres a day (this does not include coffee or drinks that cause diuresis, or loss of water). Proprietary medicines to counteract constipation are designed either to increase peristaltic action (often causing colic), or to increase the fibre content of the stool. The stool therefore transits through the colon faster and so retains some of its water content, making it easier to defaecate. Many drugs, especially analgesics such as codeine or codeine derivatives, have an effect on the autonomic control of the intestine, causing it to slow peristalsis down, thus allowing increased water reabsorption and consequently constipation. Other causes of constipation can be due to a low intake of water or dehydration; in these situations, the body needs to reabsorb as much fluid as it can in order to maintain the blood and intracellular volumes (see Figure 8.12, which illustrates the secretion and absorption of water in the digestive system).

Faecal material moves along the large bowel slowly: there are only three or four peristaltic waves a day in the most distal (lower) parts of the bowel. As the material is not continually driven along, it tends to stop altogether when it reaches the sigmoid colon, so-called because it is composed of several sharp 'bends'. The faecal material stacks up proximal to (before) the sigmoid colon. Eventually, a more powerful peristaltic wave will occur, and the material moves into the last part of the large bowel, the rectum. The sensation of material in the rectum can be perceived and is understood as the desire to stool; this is usually in response to eating, particularly at breakfast time. This response occurs as a result of food entering the stomach, stimulating peristalsis in the large bowel. It is called the gastrocolic response and is particularly noticeable in babies when they are being fed.

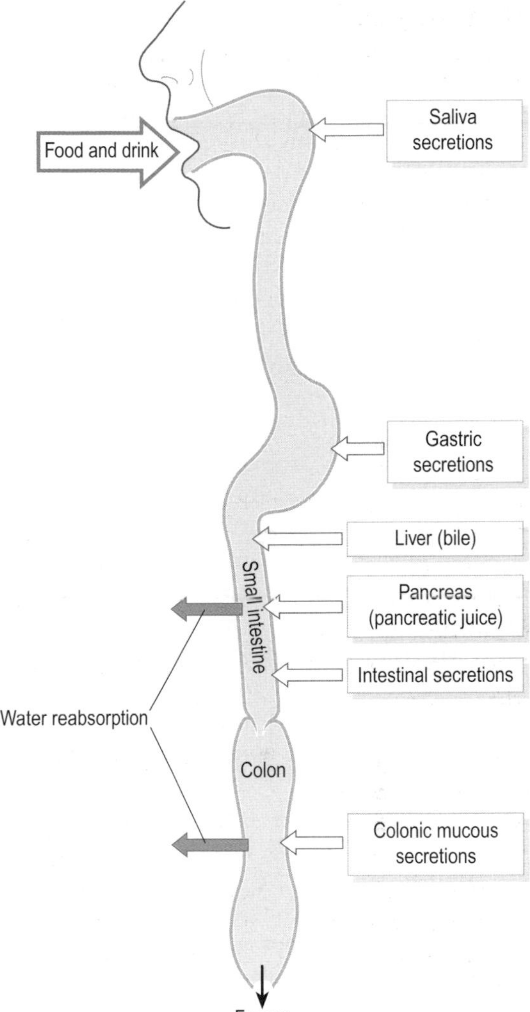

Figure 8.12 • Secretion and reabsorption of water in the digestive system.

Diverticulitis

If someone has suffered from constipation over several years, they are likely to have developed the habit of straining, or raising the intra-abdominal pressure by closing the glottis and pushing downwards. This can lead to ballooning of the smooth muscle of the colon, causing small pouches, known as diverticuli, to develop. Over time, faecal material can become trapped in these pouches and cause localized inflammation as it decomposes, causing pain.

Screening and monitoring to identify nutritional needs

Friedrich Engels, writing during the 19th century on the conditions of the working classes in England when it was in the process of industrialization, noted the significance of poor diet in causing certain diseases such as scrofula (glandular swelling) and rachitis (rickets). His condemnation of the quality of the food available, or lack of it, acknowledged also the lifelong effect of poor food (Engels 1844).

Malnutrition can be either primary or secondary. Engels was recording his observations of primary undernutrition caused by a poor diet, due to insufficient quantities of the macronutrients such as protein, lipid (fat) and carbohydrates. This is sometimes referred to as protein-energy malnutrition, and is now more common in some poorer nations. Micro-undernutrition is a lack of one or more nutrients that are only required in small amounts, mainly vitamins and minerals. This type of malnutrition is common in the UK (MAFF 2002).

Secondary malnutrition occurs when unhealthy intake is caused by disease. Causes can be classified as mechanical, such as the result of dental problems, or an obstruction to the passage of food, such as might occur due to a hiatus hernia of the stomach into the thoracic cavity, or loss of peristaltic action somewhere in the digestive system. Another secondary cause of malnutrition may be due to the inability of the nutrients to be absorbed through the digestive tract, such as in malabsorption syndromes, such as coeliac disease, or where someone has had part of their stomach or colon removed.

There are two levels of assessment health workers need to bear in mind: one is a general assessment of patients'/clients' food habits and diet; the other concerns a more fundamental nutrient deficiency assessment as may be connected with serious health problems and illness. Although the two levels can converge, there is a difference in that people may eat regular meals and obtain their energy intake, but not eat a particularly 'health-enhancing' diet. Those whose diet has changed due to illness may lack both sufficient energy and vital nutrients. In both cases, it is possible to speak of malnutrition meaning 'bad or faulty nutrition' (Stratton et al 2003). This comprehensive definition can be classified into systems of primary and secondary malnutrition: primary malnutrition refers to malnutrition that arises in the absence of disease and can stem from lack of food due to poverty and/or social isolation or, as Stratton et al (2003) point out, in circumstances where demand is not matched by intake, as may be the case in pregnancy, during lactation or physical activity.

With the strong relationship between food and health, it is important for you to be able to assess the nutritional status of your patients. Nutritional screening is a simple process that helps you to identify those patients who need a more rigorous assessment of their nutritional state so that an appropriate dietary plan can be drawn up and implemented. In the UK, nurses and health visitors have traditionally screened people for undernutrition. This was conducted on pre-schoolchildren and children of school age who were screened to check that they were meeting the anticipated milestones of height and weight for their age. Many of these assessments were based on an assumption that undernutrition was primarily associated with poverty. However, the nutritional problems have changed, and screening is now more important to assess whether children are at risk of overnutrition leading to obesity, secondary-onset diabetes and even heart disease. Try for yourself to assess the nutritional status of some children (Activity 8.7).

Activity 8.7

When you are near a group of children, observe their weight for their age.

- Do you see any children who appear to be underweight for their age?
- Do you see any children who appear to be overweight for their age?
- What might be the causes of these children's nutritional status?
- What consequences could arise as a result of their nutritional status, in the short and the long term?

This approach to nutritional assessment is quite difficult to do accurately and the results can be difficult to interpret.

There are three broad approaches that can be taken to nutritional screening: anthropometric, biochemical assessment and dietary assessment.

Anthropometric measurements

These relate to body size and proportion and include body mass index (the most common indicator used) and mid-arm circumference.

Body mass index

Body mass index (BMI) is derived from the person's weight in kilograms divided by the square of their height in metres:

$$\text{Body mass index} = \text{weight (kg)}/[\text{height (m)}]^2$$

A BMI of less than 18.5 is considered underweight, 18.5–25 is normal, 25–29 is pre-obese and over 29 is obese. You may find charts with this calculation already completed in doctors' surgeries. Interpreting the BMI needs to be done with caution as it only works for adults of average stature, and it is less accurate in children. Therefore it is less accurate for young people or people of unusual build, such as athletes.

Activity 8.8 shows you step-by-step how to measure your BMI.

Mid-arm circumference

This is another useful measurement as it does not increase significantly between the ages of 1 and 5 years, and so can be used as a very quick and easy tool in difficult circumstances (e.g. in refugee camps).

Biochemical assessment

Biochemical measurements can be used to determine the levels of certain nutrients such as serum proteins, haemoglobin and glucose. The tests can be complex and require specialist laboratory technicians to carry them out; they are thus usually only used to confirm a diagnosis.

Dietary assessment

People are asked to keep records of their daily intake of food and drink, over a week or a month (see Activity 8.9). The information is then analysed and the volume of nutrients is assessed. This approach tends to be unreliable as it is hard to record every food and drink item accurately, and people may be influenced by an assumption of what they are expected to record. A large-scale study of over half a million Europeans was launched to document their diet and monitor their health and longevity. The study is not yet complete, but will eventually provide information about the relationships between type of diet and health (Coughlan 1991).

The advantage of asking patients/clients to keep a food diary is that they have an opportunity to reflect on the type and quality of food they eat and to begin to identify possible changes with minimal help from health professionals.

Activity 8.8

Follow the steps below to calculate your own BMI:

- Establish what your weight is in kilograms (kg).
- Establish what your height it is metres (m) and square it (m^2).
- Now divide your weight in kilograms by the result of your height squared.

You now have your own BMI. How does it compare with the average range of 18.5–25? If your BMI is outside this normal range, what could it mean?

Activity 8.9

With a group of, say, five colleagues, each keep a record of your intake of food and drink over the same week; try to include information about volume and ingredients. At the end of the week, compare your record with those of your colleagues.

- How easy was it to keep the record, and how much did you guesstimate?
- How did your record of intake compare with your colleagues? What were the similarities and the differences?
- What have you learned from this activity?

In the short term, a recall method may be an alternative means of providing an example of intake of food. It relies, nevertheless, on remembering what has been eaten, for instance, in the previous 24 hours.

Webb & Copeman (1996) provide a useful list of hints that indicate the detail required to ascertain what has been eaten (see Box 8.3). Whilst their focus is on research, the approach could be used as guidance in conducting a short overview during a home visit to an older patient/client. The necessary questions include asking about the time when food was eaten, as well as focusing on specific meals rather than just asking 'What have you eaten today?'. It is important to ask about the quantity and type of food consumed; for instance: how many slices of bread and what kind of bread: what, and how much, was put on the bread; was any fluid taken and, again, how much.

Consider Case history 8.1, which describes a client living in her own home under the care of a community mental health nurse and social services care:

- What nutritional screening could be undertaken to establish Mrs Dewar's state of nutrition and hydration?

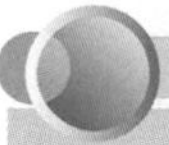

Case history 8.1

Assessing dietary intake

Mrs Dewar is an 80-year-old who is suffering from paranoid dementia. She insists on living in her bungalow, some 20 miles from her daughters. She is under the care of a community mental health nurse, and social services care assistants go into the house to attend to Mrs Dewar four times a day. Mrs Dewar suffers from double incontinence, and has a poor appetite. Today the care assistants reported that Mrs Dewar's incontinence has been resolved. However, Mrs Dewar's skin looks dry and has no elasticity, her tongue is coated, her words are slurring and her breath smells of ketones. The indications are that she is severely dehydrated.

Checking the rubbish bin shows that several of the meals that are delivered each day have been discarded, suggesting that Mrs Dewar has not eaten any food for several days.

Box 8.3

Suggested questions to promote recall of food eaten (adapted from Webb & Copeman 1996)

These hints and suggestions can be useful for any situation, whether determining older adults' intake of food or as an introduction to suggestions for losing weight.

General approach

If you use generic terms like 'dinner', 'tea', 'supper', remember that these have different meanings for people in different social groups, and therefore it may be best to ask about times of day.

Try to ascertain what size portions clients refer to, and what size of plates and cups they use.

If possible, try to get an idea of the ingredients used in the preparation of the meals; this will give some indication of the flavour, vitamin and fibre content. Point to simple improvements that could be made, such as adding shredded vegetables (which otherwise might be rejected), to sauces, even to commercially prepared food.

Remain neutral when receiving the information; the advice comes later when focus is on health education and suggesting changes to the diet.

Specific points

Morning

- When did you first eat today?
- What did you take for food this morning and how much? For example: How many slices of bread? How big a bowl of cereal? Did you have milk with it?
- Did you use margarine, spread, butter, marmalade or anything else on the bread?
- Did you have a drink; what was it and how much (e.g. a cup, a mug, a glass)?

For other intake

Use a similar approach making sure you get an idea of the size of the portions; also, whether other accompanying food was consumed such as salad, bread, dressings.

- Would the questions identified in Box 8.3 be useful to assess Mrs Dewar's intake of food and drink over the past 24 hours?
- What should the community mental health nurse prescribe for Mrs Dewar's care plan?
- What actions could the care assistants take when they visit Mrs Dewar to prevent a recurrence of this state of dehydration and starvation?

Screening should help health care workers to identify patients/clients whose nutritional status is affecting their health and mobility and to then seek help from a dietitian to prescribe a suitable diet. By intervening at an early stage, the patient's quality of life can be improved, and subsequent costs to the health care service can be minimized.

Case history 8.2 illustrates the importance of assessing a patient's needs as soon as possible after admission. After reading this case, consider the following:

- What kind of nutritional screening should have been undertaken during the first 48 hours of Daniel's admission?
- Which health care professional should have been asked to contribute to Daniel's care planning?
- What kind of diet should he have been prescribed to aid his recovery?

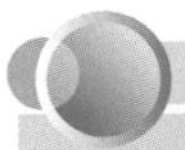

Case history 8.2

Dietary intervention to promote recovery from surgery

Daniel is a 28-year-old of normal height and slight build. He suffered a traumatic injury following a road traffic accident. In the accident his left hand was crushed and he suffered severe lacerations to his left arm. After several operations his hand was restored, although he cannot yet use it and he has been lying in bed for the past 2 weeks while skin grafts are healing. During this period of hospitalization his appetite has been poor and no-one has assessed his body mass index and thus his nutritional status. On his first day out of bed he was weighed, and it was noted that he had lost 20 kg. This weight loss is significant and could explain why his skin grafts have been taking longer than expected to heal.

Nutritional screening can be done opportunistically (Leather 1996, Malin et al 2002) at a point of contact with a relevant professional, but screening does not necessarily identify new needs or problems. This applies especially to those people already known to health workers. Screening procedure may be of little value if it identifies an unmet social, economic or medical need for which there are no resources for intervention. Therefore general screening without any particular indication of an underlying disease process, or other articulated concern, may be of limited value, especially when costs are taken into account.

Malnutrition Universal Screening Tool

It is now accepted practice that all patients should be screened on admission to hospital for a number of risk factors, including nutrition (McWhirter & Pennington 1994). There are several tools being developed, but one of the most widely used is the Malnutrition Universal Screening Tool, or MUST. This has been developed by the Malnutrition Advisory Group, which is a collaboration between a number of interested parties, including the Royal College of Nursing. The tool is available on the Internet (www.bapen.org.uk/the-must.htm) and consists of five steps (Box 8.4).

In summary

Paying attention to needs in both hospital and home is part of overall care. In hospital, nurses can

Box 8.4

The Malnutrition Universal Screening Tool (MUST)

Establish the patient's BMI (MUST provides a means of estimating the BMI if it not possible to measure the patient's height, e.g. if the patient is confined to bed).

Note recent unintended weight loss.

Establish a score for disease states that can affect nutrition.

Use these indications to establish overall risk.

Plan care accordingly.

not only interview patients about their food behaviour and eating habits, but also observe what patients eat. In primary care, assessment is mainly based on verbal interviews and reports, with a possible glance as to what food is on display during a home visit, or, as in case of older people, ask for permission to look into the cupboards, or see if there is evidence of meals-on-wheels having been eaten. Generally speaking, this is what most nurses can do to gain an impression of what their clients are eating.

Thus it is apparent that some sort of screening should be a routine part of assessing patients and planning their care. However, assessing nutritional need is complex and difficult to carry out. As you will have read, there are many tools available to assist with the nutritional or dietary assessment of clients. This in itself suggests that no one tool will be totally effective and, as with all patient assessments, the results have to be interpreted intelligently and clients have to be viewed holistically.

Nutrition in pregnancy

Nutritional needs change throughout the lifespan and as a result of different demands on the body. A mother's state of nutrition during a pregnancy probably has the most significance on the subsequent health and well-being of the child throughout its life.

Beliefs that the mother is able to compensate for any nutritional needs of her fetus by sacrificing her own stores of nutrients have been found to be false. Current research indicates that both the potential father and the mother should pay attention to their diet several months before conception takes place.

A research study compared the nutritional intake of pregnant women from two London boroughs: Hackney and Hampstead (Doyle et al 1989). A detailed record was kept of food intake and the total nutrient load was calculated. The women from Hampstead had greater intake of most of the key nutrients, except energy. The babies born to the Hampstead women averaged 300 g heavier. It is interesting to note that the biggest single difference between the two contrasting diets was that the women from Hampstead were more likely to eat breakfast cereal, many of which were fortified with additional nutrients. This simple addition to the mother's diet can have a profound influence on life prospects of the children. However, as Lang & Heasman (2004) point out, essential nutrients such as calcium, iron, magnesium, folate and vitamin C are more likely to be ingested by the higher socioeconomic groups, thus indicating that factors beyond individual choice significantly impact on food eaten by different people.

Pregnancy and micronutritional requirements

Little is known about the effects of micronutrient deficiency during pregnancy, yet it is an important issue because this form of malnutrition occurs frequently in this country, and what we do know gives grounds for concern. Earlier in this chapter we discussed the importance of folic acid during pregnancy. This is one of the B group of vitamins, and it acts as a co-enzyme in the transfer of carbon atoms during the synthesis of amino acids and nucleic acids. Thus a lack of folate is particularly noticeable in times when new cells are being developed and tissue is being created. Geographical variations in the occurrence of neural tube defects (NTDs) in the embryo reflect differences in the occurrence of folate available in the diet. Such observations led to a research study being conducted to investigate whether increasing folate could reduce the occurrence of NTD in women with a history of previous pregnancies complicated by NTD. Wald (1991) found that by giving these women an increased intake of folic acid (400 mcg/day) reduced the risk of recurrence of NTDs by 70%, a very significant improvement. Further studies (Czeizel & Dudas 1992) showed that NTDs were reduced for all women, not just those with a known risk.

The average diet contains about 200 mcg of folate, which is the Reference Nutrient Intake (RNI) (MAFF 2002). Folate can be increased in the diet through careful selection and cooking of foods rich in the vitamin, such as leafy green vegetables, yeast, nuts, grain (some brands of bread and breakfast cereals are fortified with folate) and bananas. To obtain 400 mcg daily in the diet is quite difficult. Therefore most women are provided with folate supplements as soon as their pregnancy is diagnosed. However, there is a problem: NTDs are one of the most serious and common of all congenital abnormalities and occur when the neural tube fails to fuse correctly, which normally takes place by the end of the third week of gestation. Most women do not realize they are pregnant until after the first missed period, when the pregnancy is already at 2 weeks' gestation and it is too late to start taking extra folic acid.

Folic acid supplements need to be started from the time the baby is planned. Supplementation should continue until at least 3 months' gestation to ensure that all the newly laid down structures in the fetus are achieved with a plentiful supply of folate. However, this may be unrealistic for many women who may not have planned their babies. The answer may be for some staple foods, such as bread, to be fortified with folate, as this is relatively easy to do, and indeed many breakfast cereals are already prepared with artificially increased folate.

Pregnancy and energy requirements

The energy demands of pregnancy are surprisingly modest, just an increase in energy intake of between 0.3 and 0.5 MJ/day (71–120 kcal) is adequate for women who are well nourished. This is approximately equivalent to the energy available in 100 g of banana or 50 g of wholemeal bread. This is quite a small increase in the energy requirements of a non-pregnant, non-lactating woman, which is approximately 8.05 MJ (2480 kcal) energy intake daily. There is some evidence (Doyle et al 1989) that poorer women actually increase their energy intake more during pregnancy than women from more affluent backgrounds, yet their babies are actually, on average, about 300 g smaller at birth.

Relationship of birth weight and health pattern

It is well established that very small babies (under 5½ lb, or 2300 g) are severely disadvantaged at birth. They are prone to cardiac and respiratory problems, and may develop less well intellectually. Babies that are just a little smaller than average (7 lb or 3300 g), however, display 'catch-up' growth; that is to say, they initially grow more than their bigger counterparts, so that by a few months of age they are as big as their peers and seem to do as well. Low birth weight at term and sometimes at 1 year is related to increased risk of some chronic diseases in later life (Livingstone 1997). These include hypertension, coronary artery disease, non-insulin-dependent diabetes and autoimmune thyroid disease. These diseases tend to occur earlier and be more serious in their effect on people who were smaller at birth. These findings were initially greeted with scepticism, but repeated investigations have consistently shown that individuals who were smaller at birth are, indeed, disadvantaged in their long-term health.

Pregnancy and the mother's nutritional health

The benefits of eating well during pregnancy are not reserved just for the infant. The mother can benefit as well. It has been suggested (Newman & Fullerton 1990) that pregnancy-induced hypertension (PIH), previously described as pre-eclampsia, is also linked to nutrition. PIH is characterized by increased peripheral resistance and consequent reduced maternal blood supply to the fetus. This, in turn, can lead to retardation of the growth of the baby, and can even threaten the life of the baby and mother. The cause of PIH is unknown. Women with PIH are often found to have low levels of the plasma protein albumin. Albumin is a most important protein found in the blood as it gives the blood its 'osmotic pull' to facilitate intracellular water to be drawn back into the venous blood. When there are low levels of plasma albumin, water remains in the intracellular spaces of the tissues causing oedema. This means that the overall circulating blood volume becomes lower than normal and the body tries to compensate by retaining as much water as possible by reducing the excretion of urine. A low protein intake in the diet may also contribute to inefficient liver function (where albumin is manufactured), further impeding the manufacture of plasma proteins. However, there are no studies showing a clear link between low protein intake and the development of PIH.

Nutrition in infancy

Is breast best?

All an infant's nutritional needs can be met through breast milk as it has many significant advantages over formula milk (Department of Health 2004). These advantages include:

- The milk is sterile.
- The milk arrives at the perfect temperature and so the risk of scalding the baby does not arise.
- Breast milk contains immunoglobulins that will help protect the infant from the infectious diseases to which the mother already has an immunity.
- Breast-fed infants are five times less likely to be admitted to hospital with common infections in the first year of life; and they are less likely to become obese in later childhood.
- Very early breast milk, colostrum, also includes laxatives, which assist the neonate in expelling muconium.
- Breast milk contains all the nutrients required by the growing infant.
- Emotional bonding between mother and child is stronger.
- Many women find it easier and more convenient to breast-feed as there is no equipment required.
- It costs nothing.

The benefits of breast-feeding also apply to the mother as lactating assists her to return to her pre-pregnant weight, and lactating may give her protection from developing breast cancer later in her life.

For some women, however, breast-feeding is not an option. The World Health Organization estimates that up to 5% of postnatal (puerperial) women cannot breast-feed for physical reasons. Other women, instead of seeing breast-feeding as rewarding, find it messy and painful; some even experience a sense of loss of self (Schmied & Lupton 2001). Anecdotal accounts suggest that male partners sometimes oppose breast-feeding; this may be related to the social construct of breasts as symbols of sexuality.

With the widespread commercialization of formula milk products throughout the world, the consequences have been disastrous in many countries and have been associated with high rates of infant mortality. In many countries where a supply of clean water is not available, mothers have the impossible job of using formula milk without the necessary resources to ensure feeding bottles are clean and the feed is sterile. This results in infants suffering from devastating diarrhoea and vomiting.

In the UK, there is a voluntary code prohibiting advertising of baby milk for infants. However, some manufacturers of formula milk products circumvent this agreement through such practices as sponsorship. Until recently, many health practitioners gave new mothers baby boxes that contained advertising materials and samples from formula milk producers, and health centres were encouraged to make formula milk products available.

'Choosing health: making healthier choices easier' (Department of Health 2004) proposes a new scheme called 'Healthy Start'. This provides eligible women (including all girls under the age of 18 years) who are pregnant or lactating with vouchers that can be ex-changed for fruit, vegetables and fresh or formula milk. The vouchers will also be available to some families of limited financial means.

Weaning

Weaning is an important stage in the infant's development. Physically weaning cannot take place before the baby is 2 or 3 months of age. This is for safety reasons as the baby is unable to push any substance out of its mouth and enables the baby to tolerate being suckled. The extrusion reflex does not develop until after the baby is at least 3 months old. Another developmental consideration is that the immature gut has not developed the ability to digest and absorb solid particles, so any solid foodstuffs have a rapid transit time causing loss of fluids in the form of diarrhoea (Milla 1986). Weaning before 4 months of age can also permanently affect metabolism in such a way as to predispose the individual to developing atheroma (McGill et al 1996) and obesity. Additionally, there is some evidence that weaning after 4 months can protect infants from going on to develop food and other allergies (Arshad et al 1992). As a result, government recommendations are that weaning should not take place until the baby is at least 4 months of age (Department of Health 1994).

Some mothers continue to breast-feed their babies until 2 years of age and even older, supplementing the breast milk with solids and thus providing the necessary iron intake and muscular activity required for normal development of the buccal cavity. During the first few months of life the infant relies on stocks of iron accumulated while in utero. During pregnancy, the fetus has a much higher haematocrit than it needs as an infant. Once the baby is born its excess red blood cells are broken down and the iron is stored for use during the first few months of postnatal life. Eventually these stores will become depleted, and the baby will need to have iron provided in its weaning foods.

Weaning provides the opportunity to introduce the infant to a wide range of foodstuffs and there is some evidence that, between 4 and 6 months, infants will accept almost anything that is given to them (Skuse 1993). Providing the infant with foodstuffs that they can chew and swallow is important to facilitate maturation of the buccal cavity and promote the early skills of speech. However, caution needs to be taken to ensure that the solids do not contain added sugar or salt.

Nutrition and the weaning diet

Infants' nutritional needs are related to the enormous amount of physical and intellectual growth that takes places in their early years. Infants require an energy-dense diet in order to provide high energy, whilst having limited volume in their stomachs (Hardy & Kleinman 1994). Fat has almost twice as many joules of energy for weight than carbohydrate (17 kJ/g instead of 9 kJ/g). Some well-meaning parents are reluctant to provide a diet rich in fat, being mindful of health advice mainly aimed at adults; as a result, some children are suffering from a syndrome that has been termed 'muesli malnutrition' (Livingstone 1997). Indeed, it is possible that the very high content of cholesterol in breast milk actually protects against the development of cholesterol-linked heart disease later in life (McGill et al 1996). As well as the energy component of fat in the diet, the infant requires the essential fatty acids for correct development of the nervous system. It has been suggested (Hardy & Kleinman 1994) that the lack of essential fatty acids explains the consistent finding that malnourished children achieve lower intellectual levels compared with their well-nourished counterparts. Essential fatty acids can only be obtained from lipids (oils and fats) in the diet.

A particular nutrient found to be lacking in the diet of young children is iron (Dallman 1986). As breast milk is deficient in iron, infants need to be eating a significant amount of iron in their diet by 6 months of age, and there is evidence that not all children are getting it (Dallman 1986, Hurtado et al 1999). Initially this can lead to iron-deficiency anaemia, but if the deficiency continues it can be a contributory factor in the development of mild and moderate learning difficulties (Hurtado et al 1999). This is one reason for parents to be very careful if they wish their children to take a vegetarian diet because the iron from animal sources is easier to absorb than that from inorganic sources. It is also worth remembering that vitamin C will maximize absorption of iron from the gut. Proprietary baby foods are often fortified with iron and other minerals, as well vitamins. For this reason, the COMA report (Department of Health 1994) recommended the use of some proprietary foods, whereas before parents were encouraged to use 'family foods' as much as possible. Some foods not specially prepared for infants, such as bread and breakfast cereals, are also fortified with iron and other nutrients.

Weaning foods

Specially prepared baby foods need to be chosen with care. A study (Consumers Association 2000) reported that 40% of baby foods, 60% in the case of breakfasts, contained added sugar, and 40% contained starchy filling. The name of the product was misleading, as the Consumers Association found that one food called 'egg custard with rice' contained more sugar than either egg or rice, and a 'banana and rice pudding' contained no banana, only flavouring.

A varied and nourishing diet during childhood has other long-term implications, apart from the provision of nutrients, and that is programming. Children tend to develop a liking for foods that they are exposed to. In a convincing study, Sullivan & Birch (1994) gave mothers of infants jars of food containing pureed vegetable – either peas or green beans. They asked the mothers to offer this food once a day for 10 days and then, after an interval of 7 days without the food, to offer it again. It was found that, with increased offering of the food, intake increased by about 50% and that this increase was still present after the interval. Adults subjectively assessed from videotapes the extent to which the infant liked the food. They found a strong, positive correlation between the adults rating of liking with intake. The conclusions are clear: even if infants initially reject novel foods, repeated exposure increases acceptance of the food. This occurs because the infants grow to like the food and this liking persists after a brief interval of not being exposed to the food. Parents, however, need to have the confidence and patience to pursue such consistency in offering new tastes to their babies.

As a child reaches 4 or 5 years of age, their rate of growth slows down and remains lower until they reach the adolescent growth spurt. The child's nutritional requirements reflect this change, and are not as great, if expressed by body weight, as in infancy. Thus a 12-month-old boy requires 0.23 MJ/kg/day (56 kcal/kg/day), whereas a 10-year old requires 0.16 MJ/kg/day (38 kcal/kg/day) and a 40-year-old man requires 0.1 MJ/kg/day (22 kcal/kg/day) (MAFF 2002).

Nutrition in childhood

Children's diet is particularly important, and it is now understood that there are at least three aspects in which diet during childhood can contribute to health patterns in the long term: nutritional intake and childhood development and growth; allergies; eating patterns and lifelong eating.

Nutritional intake and disease

Many health problems are related to affluence; particular concern is related to nutrition in relation to energy intake. Indeed, it is possible that childhood nutrition in 1950 was superior to that of today, as rationing caused a reduction in sugary foods and some fatty foods while at the same time the government ensured children received all essential nutrients through provision of fish oil and orange juice to provide vitamin C supplements. 'Choosing health: making healthier choices easier' (Department of Health 2004), in highlighting the problems of obesity in children, quite correctly, goes further than just blaming parents. The question is whether parents should monitor more keenly what their children eat, and to what extent government should regulate the food industry that produces energy-dense food and thus contributes to obesity. The important contributing nutrient to energy is lipids in foods. The lipid part of the diet provides much of the texture and enjoyment of food (Bloom 2003).

Obesity in children

Affluence may be a cause of the increased problem of obesity in childhood. The exact magnitude of the increase has not been reliably calculated for the UK, mainly because there is not yet an agreed definition of obesity in children (Bellizzi & Dietz 1999). However, Chinn & Rona (1994) estimate that children are becoming bigger. The increase is substantial; for instance, English girls seem to weigh an extra 0.5 kg and Scottish girls an extra 1.5 kg over the period 1947–1987 (Chinn & Rona 1994). Some, but not all, of this is related to a small increase in height, but this association has not been replicated (Chinn & Rona 1994). In the USA, it is estimated that 22–30% of children are obese (Troiano et al 1995).

Concerns about childhood obesity and overweight people are not confined to English-speaking countries. Recently, the main daily newspapers in Norway (Aftenposten 2005) and the United Arab Emirates (Gulf News 2005) published basic statistics on the increase in weight and size among their respective populations. A survey carried out by the General Authority for Health Services (GAHS) in the United Arab Emirates found that out of a sample of 24965 people 37.3% were overweight and 36.3% were obese. The concerns expressed by the director of GAHS were related not only to the health implications but also to long-term eating habits and the consequences for the country's economy. The Norwegian newspaper article stated that 15% of boys and 16% of girls between the ages of 4 and 16 years are overweight (using the international definition). Both papers attributed the increase in childhood obesity to lack of physical activity and changes in diet and eating habits: high fat and carbohydrate content in burgers and pizzas (Gulf News 2005) and in cakes, biscuits, chocolate and crisps (Aftenposten 2005).

Obesity in childhood may be linked to genetic factors, but it may also be a behavioural reaction to abundant supplies of nutrients and less-energetic lifestyles (Egger & Swinburn 1997 and Hill & Peters 1998 cited in Baggott 2004).

Body shapes and sizes are also culturally constructed, and may be linked to ideas about wealth and prosperity in societies where famine and disasters can happen, and, conversely, to hoarding of food during the times of plenty (Fieldhouse 1996, p 192). Fieldhouse (1996, p 193) suggests that parental experience of shortage may encourage them to overfeed their children. Also, unhappiness and anxiety are linked to overeating (Fieldhouse 1996). It is reasonable, however, to conclude that the changes in what we eat has led to many children being overfed, and suffering from fast-food malnutrition. Thus, it is ironic that, in the times of relative plenty, the concern is not with over-nourishment but poor-quality nourishment, and this is not necessarily due to ignorance about food. Research conducted by Weir et al (1997) found that the sample of Bangladeshi people interviewed were quite knowledgeable about what food generally speaking is 'good' for you and what is 'bad'. Schoolchildren particularly were aware of what foods are linked to the development of coronary heart disease.

An interesting finding of Chinn & Rona (1994) is that the size of the child is related to the size of the adult, so increases in obesity may be related to family dynamics and lifestyle, such as eating more energy-providing food and leading a more sedentary lifestyle, with no compensating increase in exercise.

Childhood obesity is only weakly linked to health problems in childhood, but it is strongly linked to several health problems in adulthood (Bellizzi & Deitz 1999). Overweight children tend to grow into overweight adults: 'puppy fat' does not exist after the age of 5 or 6 years. Children tend to retain the same percentile ranking for BMI as they grow up (Bellizzi & Deitz 1999). Health problems in adulthood include coronary artery disease (Baggott 2004), hyperlipidaemia, hypertension and reduced glucose tolerance.

Eating disorders

In contrast to the above, there is a small percentage of children and adults who manipulate their diet in an attempt to achieve a particular body shape through unwise dietary practices. These include binge-eating followed by purging, severe energy restriction and fat-free diets. Boys do not seem to be as vulnerable as girls to attempts to lose weight, but can be at risk in the pursuit of athletic excellence. There is a sad irony here in that, just as we are becoming bigger, the ideal body image that is presented through media images is much smaller.

Anorexia is an interesting case of problematic eating, as it appears on the surface. Anorexia nervosa has a long history, although it has been construed and constructed as a late 20th century problem by the popular media. In the medical context, anorexia has been seen as a psychosomatic illness with the problem in the mind–body interaction shifting to a focus more concerned with the 'anorexic body' and biomedical discourse (Mizrachi 2002).

The term 'eating disorders' reflects the medical diagnostic framework within which much of the discussion on problematic diets now takes place. Anorexia nervosa, together with bulimia nervosa, are also seen to accompany the perceived attractions of slimness (Lissau et al 2003) An example is in Denmark, where the prevalence of underweight in young women aged 16–25 years rose by 30% between 1987 and 1994 while, in the same period in the same age-group, the prevalence of obesity doubled (Lissau et al 2003, citing Kjoller et al 1995). Lissau et al (2003) attribute such eating disorders to society's emphasis on looking slim. Writers such as Orbach (1998) and Bordo (2003), however, see in attempts to control body weight something of the complexity of women's need for more control and power, which they associate with thinness (Bordo 2003). By being either obese or anorexic, Bordo (2003) argues, women demonstrate resistance with their bodies to the dominant cultural values and norms: anorectic by outdoing the culture of thinness whilst the obese do not play according to the rules at all.

Medicalized conditions tend to be treated by evidence-based approaches. There is, however, some ambiguity as to how to interpret the evidence and when a condition becomes 'medical'. Frelut & Flodmark (2003), for instance, state that the diagnoses are dependent on symptom lists as in medical syndromes; thus a binge-eating disorder has still to be recognized as a disease. How helpful is it to recognize eating as a medical problem? Can we assume that treatment is always not only successful, which clearly is not the case, but that the problematic issue does not get worse? It may be time to move away from an emphasis on low-fat or other prescribed diets to an emphasis on healthy eating as part of a healthy lifestyle (Lissau et al 2003).

In spite of anorexia being perceived as affecting young women, it seems, on the whole, that women eat more healthily than men. Women of middle age scored highest in relation to 'good diet' as measured by a qualitative description based on a predetermined list of foods (Blaxter 1990). Yet women in nearly all ethnic groups and, in general, the (entire) population in England exceed men in prevalence of obesity as measured by a BMI over 30 (Health Survey for England 1999 cited in Department of Health 2004).

Allergies

There appears to be an epidemic of pathologies related either directly or indirectly to the unhelpful functioning of the immune system. These diseases range from allergic rhinitis (hay fever) to asthma, eczema, insulin-dependent diabetes mellitus and rheumatoid arthritis. As far as food is concerned, there needs to be a distinction made between true allergy, where the food causes an (unhelpful) immune response raising antibodies against the specific allergens in the food, and food intolerance, where the food causes unpleasant symptoms for other reasons (Wood 1986).

Milk allergy

Milk is an important example of the distinction between an allergic reaction and food intolerance. An allergic reaction happens where the milk proteins act as allergens (or antigens) and cause a systemic increased activity in the immune system. It occurs because the infant bowel is 'leaky' and allows large molecules such as proteins to be absorbed (Milla 1986). Very rarely, such cases can lead to anaphylactic shock. Lactose intolerance, on the other hand, is a genetically determined condition in which, sometime after about 12 months of age, the levels of the enzyme lactase available to breakdown lactose, the milk sugar, decreases. This leads to lactose being present in the large bowel, causing osmotic diarrhoea (the result of material, such as glucose, that is highly osmotic, remaining in the large bowel, causing fluid to remain or move into the bowel), flatulence and other unpleasant symptoms.

In the case of milk allergy, there is the possibility of a reaction to any milk products. Since this could be dangerous, milk products should be avoided. However, children often 'grow out' of this condition as the bowel becomes less leaky and whole proteins are not absorbed. Lactose intolerance is lifelong, but only occurs with consumption of milk as such, because in most milk products the lactose has already been broken down.

Alternatives to cows' milk products

In the UK, many infants are now being given soya-based products instead of formula milk and other milk products based on cows' milk, due to concerns about allergy. When soya is offered as an alternative, it is imperative that the infant is given a specifically prepared soya-based product for infant nutrition. There is some evidence (Stehlin 1993) that infants are becoming malnourished as a result of being given soya-based food not intended for infants. It is also possible that these allergic conditions are being overdiagnosed, and infants are being unnecessarily denied milk based on cows' milk. Since soya-based infant milks may not be as nutritionally complete as formulas based on cows milk, more evidence-based information is needed.

Despite this it is important not to expose certain vulnerable infants to allergens. Arshad et al (1992) identified infants whose history suggested they were at considerable risk of developing allergic conditions. They were given a diet free from some well-known allergens, up to the age of 12 months, and were found to be significantly less likely to have developed a range of allergic conditions by that age. However, the long-term benefits of the diet were not explored.

It should also be noted that the diet was quite arduous, particularly for mothers who were breast-feeding (since the mother too had to abstain from certain foods), and a high number of mother–infant pairs did not complete the trial.

It is possible that, by preventing exposure of the infant to allergens for a year or more, their immune system matures and, by the time they are exposed to the allergen, they are able to cope with it, and don't develop the allergy (Arshad et al 1992). On the other hand, if they are exposed to the allergen early on, their immune system may respond, and the child may then go on to develop a lifelong allergy.

Nut and egg allergies

These two foods are particularly prone to causing allergic reactions. Egg protein can cause allergy and, if it occurs, can be extremely troublesome. For this reason, infants should not be given whole egg until 10 or 12 months of age. Cooked egg, such as occurs in many foods, is usually acceptable, since the cooking process will have at least partially broken down the proteins. Nuts also present a choking hazard and, since they are relatively easy to avoid, whole nuts are not usually given to children until 3 or 4 years of age.

Eating patterns and lifelong eating

Studies into the eating habits of school-age children have indicated that those who eat breakfast perform better in certain areas than those children who do not eat breakfast (Pollitt 1995). In a review of several investigations in this area, Pollitt (1995) discovered that children performed better in cognitive tests, particularly those relating to memory and language, if they were provided with breakfast; they were also more stable emotionally. In the USA, approximately 70% of schools offering school lunches also offer breakfast (Food Action and Research Centre 1998). These schools found additional benefits in improved attendance and reduced tardiness. Pollitt's conclusion was that such a programme was definitely justified where there is a large number of poor families. Some attempts have been made to introduce trials of similar programmes in parts of the UK. For example, a primary school in East London offers a self-funding breakfast club. Parents pay a small fee each week for each child, to cover overheads and staffing, and then pay for each food item; for instance, cereal and milk costs 32 p and a carton of orange juice 15 p. Another London primary school (Matuszek 2000) has used lottery funding to start a similar scheme which will ultimately be self-funding.

In the late 19th century, educational authorities were required to provide a midday meal and a third of a pint of milk to all schoolchildren who wanted one. The meal was expected to provide one-third of the child's estimated daily nutritional requirements and was free to families on lower incomes. By 1980 these rules were relaxed and free school milk was abolished. The current situation is that local authorities must provide a midday meal on school days for all schoolchildren who wish it (see Activity 8.10, which concerns school meals and childhood health). Meals are free to those families who receive income support or Job Seekers Allowance; other children are charged a subsidized amount.

Activity 8.10

If you have a child, or know someone with children, try to find out what foods are offered by their school at meal times.

- Try to find out in detail what each child eats for lunch everyday.
- What other food products are available in the school?
- Are there vending machines: If there are, what kinds of foods do they sell?
- What is the overall glycaemic index of the foods available in the child's school?
- What are the nutritional implications of the availability of these foods for the child?
- What might be better nutritional alternatives?

The quality of these school meals has been subject to considerable scrutiny and criticism, with the provision of foodstuffs that are designed to pander to popular fashions rather than to nutritional needs. More recently, the Department of Education has investigated these concerns and are requiring that school meals in England and Wales include fresh food, vegetables and fruit. Scotland has already established its own standards for children's meals in schools: children are to be offered brown bread, two helpings of fruit and two helpings of vegetables (Quarmby 2004).

Some education authorities have re-introduced milk drinks at cost price. The Department of Health has legislated that nursery schools and schools in areas known to support poorer children should adopt the policies outlined in the document 'Choosing health: making healthier choices easier' (Department of Health 2004). This policy document takes a whole-school approach and involves enhancing the quality of school and packed lunches and vending machines, as well as sports and playtime activities.

Lifestyle and lifelong nutritional implications

Food advertising

Children's attitudes to food may be influenced by peer pressure and the effect of advertising. In the USA, children aged between 6 and 11 years watch 23.5 hours of television a week. Kotz & Story 1994 monitored Saturday morning television, and saw 997 product advertisements, of which 564 (56.5%) were for food; this amounts to as many as 3 hours of food advertisements a week, or one advertisement every 5 minutes of television watching. Of the food advertisements, 37.5% were for foods classified as 'fats, oils or sugars' and 23% were for 'high-sugar carbohydrates'; 11% were for fast-food outlets, which tend to serve high-fat meals. The main message of these advertisements was that these foods taste good, and several included a promise of a free toy. Several (7.3%) of the advertisements suggested that the food was in some way fashionable. However, 49.1% of advertisements implied that the food was healthy, often by stating that the food formed part of a healthy meal. By contrast, health education was confined to ten nutrition-related public service announcements. Although controversial, it does appear that advertising has an effect on children's diets (Coon & Tucker 2002). In addition, children who watched a lot of television were more likely to be overweight, to eat foods high in sugar, and to have these foods available in the house.

In the UK, only two of the terrestrial television channels do not carry advertising. The television channels that do survive through advertising can participate in a voluntary code stating that advertisements must not take advantage of children's natural credulity, or raise unreasonable expectations. Other countries, such as Sweden and Norway, have gone further and banned all television advertisements that target children under the age of 12 years (Lang 2001, Lang & Heasman 2004), and there are growing pressures to follow this example in the UK.

Childhood diet and cardiovascular disease in adult life

There is a well-known link between plasma lipid levels and the risk of developing cardiovascular pathologies such as cerebrovascular accident and coronary artery disease. The risk of developing these diseases is greater in an individual with high levels of low-density lipoprotein (LDL) and low levels of high-density lipoprotein (HDL). It appears that atherosclerotic lesions start very early in life. In young children, lesions are seen as fatty streaks in the arteries of persons as young as age 3 years (Berenson et al 1992). It is not certain that these fatty streaks are of clinical significance as they do not occlude the vessel and are reversible; however, it is possible that they could develop into raised, fibrotic lesions. Work from the Bogalusa Heart Study (Berenson et al 1992) indicates that these fatty streaks, particularly when they are located in the coronary arteries, are indeed related to high serum triglyceride levels and very-low-density lipoprotein (VLDL) cholesterol levels, as well as to high blood pressure. Lauer et al (1988) carried out a major longitudinal study of the relationship between cholesterol in childhood (after 5 years of age) and adulthood. They found a high degree of correlation, in that children with a high plasma cholesterol tended to maintain high cholesterol levels into adulthood. The adult levels of cholesterol were unlikely to be above the 90th percentile if childhood levels were below the 50th percentile and, as childhood cholesterol levels rise above the 50th percentile, the adult cholesterol levels also rise. However, this does not in itself indicate that diet in youth and dietary habits are the cause of high or low cholesterol levels, and it is known that there is some genetic predisposition.

Research designed to establish whether dietary intervention was effective in reducing serum cholesterol was carried out in 1995 by the Diet Intervention Study in Children (DISC) Writing Group. Children aged between 8 and 10 years with raised LDL levels were randomized into groups for intervention or normal treatment. Those in the intervention group were given behavioural therapy aimed at achieving a diet in which fat provided only 28% of energy (including up to 8% provided by saturated fat) and cholesterol of less than 75 mg/day. This diet is similar to that recommended for children with a marked family history of coronary artery disease. The intervention consisted of devising a personalized diet based on their current diet, followed by a series of visits to the family. Those in the group receiving normal care were advised that the child's plasma cholesterol was raised, and were provided with written information. No follow-up was organized. After 3 years, the diets of the intervention group were significantly lower in fat and the serum cholesterol levels were also lower. Importantly, the intervention group's diet was equally adequate in other ways with that of the group receiving normal care, in that height growth and iron stores were equal in both groups.

Nutrition and the older adult

There is much interest in the nutritional health of older adults, for two major reasons. The first is to do with the changes that take place as we get older, which influence what we eat and how we utilize food. The second is to do with prevention and cost of health care resulting from impaired health that could be prevented, or slowed down, by appropriate nutrition. For example, Webb & Copeman (1996, p 69) suggest that malnutrition predisposes people to infection, and that infection worsens or precipitates malnutrition, creating a dangerous positive-feedback cycle.

It is estimated that one in four people over the age of 65 years are malnourished, as are 40% of nursing home residents and half of elderly hospital patients (Azad et al 1999, Nourhashemi et al 1999). The nutrients that are most likely to be lacking from the diets of the fit elderly are calcium and vitamins B_6, B_{12} and vitamin D (Scheck & Roubenoff 1999). The reasons for this can be described in terms of physiological changes (e.g. fluid balance and renal function, immune function, ageing of the skeleton and osteoporosis) and changes in their physical, social and psychological environment (e.g. physical fitness and strength) (Webb & Copeman 1996, p 55).

The following discussion generalizes older people and you should not assume that all older people are experiencing the following changes. With the increasing health and fitness of people beyond retirement age and greater longevity, older people are enjoying healthier lives and are more able to maintain a good nutritional intake. However, there are groups of people who are not so able to achieve this nutritional status even at a relatively young old age, and there is also a significant increase in the very old (people of 80 years or more). As a nursing student, you need to be sensitive to the health status of the older people you meet and be observant of their ability to digest their food and thus their nutritional status.

Ageing and physical changes

There are some normal physiological changes that occur with ageing that may lead to a risk of poor nutrition. These include a decreased ability to smell and taste (Rolls 1999), characterized by a decrease in both the number and sensitivity of olfactory and taste receptors and thus a loss of enjoyment in tasting and smelling food. One appropriate response may be to use flavour enhancers, and may explain why some older people add extra salt and sugar to their food, although other flavourings such as herbs and spices would have less problematic consequences.

Dental and oral health

Many older people experience problems with their gums, teeth and jaw, with inevitable consequences. Chewing surfaces can be worn down so that they do not meet effectively. This can hasten the loss of bone from the jaw, which can cause loosening even of healthy teeth. Poor dental health has repeatedly been shown to adversely affect the quality of the diet, particularly for micronutrients (Appollonio et al 1997). However, well-fitting dentures may be as good as natural teeth in enabling a person to enjoy a good diet (Lamy et al 1999). Xerostamia (dry mouth) is common at all ages, but perhaps particularly in the elderly as a result of reduced salivary gland production. Decrease in saliva can be exacerbated by lack of chewing, which normally encourages salivation. It can also be a side-effect of several drugs, or a poor fluid intake. A dry mouth makes food difficult to chew, as well as seeming tasteless as the food particles that give taste need to be dissolved in saliva in order to stimulate taste and smell receptors. All these changes in the mouth can reduce appetite and the older person's ability to eat and enjoy certain foods.

Helping an older person in hospital or at home to have good oral hygiene and effective dental care will enable them to eat and enjoy their food more and thus retain good nutrition. Making food choices that encourage chewing will help keep the mouth clean and the jaw functioning.

Digestive system changes

With age, the entire length of the gastrointestinal tract experiences a reduction of peristaltic strength and an increase in non-peristaltic movements (Christiansen & Grzybowski 1993). This may be due to a diminished blood supply because of poor cardiac output, atheroma causing hypertension, or because of reduced autonomic nervous stimulation, again because of poor blood supply to the nerves. Drinking less than 2 litres of water a day will also have an effect on the bowel. With reduced peristaltic action the transit time of the food chyme is lengthened, which facilitates the absorption of water, with inevitable consequences. Discomfort from constipation can also reduce appetite. These changes will inevitably have an effect on the ability of the digestive system to process and absorb nutrients and to manufacture vitamins, resulting in reduced nutritional status.

Fluid intake

A gradual reduction in body water is a normal aspect of ageing (International Food Information Council 1993) as a result of renal inability to concentrate urine and a subsequent reduction in the sensation of thirst. The person choosing to restrict fluid intake, perhaps as an attempt to minimize frequency of micturition, or incontinence, or symptoms of heart failure and its treatment (which often includes a diuretic), need to be encouraged to monitor their fluid intake and ensure that it is of a minimum of 2 litres a day (Webb & Copeman 1996). Dehydration may be part of the reason why some elderly people suffer from confusion.

Nutritional needs of older adults

There are currently no recommendations for the dietary intake of older adults, who are therefore encouraged to eat the same as adults of any age.

There is, however, one important exception, which is that they require a diet lower in energy. This is because the proportion of an older person's body weight that is made up of lean body mass is reduced, and more is made of adipose tissue and fibrous material. In particular, there is an age-related loss of approximately 15% of skeletal muscle, referred to as sarcopenia. Also, many older people are physically less active than they were when in paid employment or caring for a family.

Older people have a reduced glucose tolerance; that is, a given amount of ingested glucose will cause a greater increase in blood glucose than it would in a younger person. Since appetite is suppressed by blood glucose, it is possible that a small amount of energy results in a feeling of being replete, due to the sharp rise in blood glucose. Indeed, their energy requirements may have been met, for instance, by having eaten biscuits or cakes, without meeting all their other nutritional requirements. Older people need a better quality diet with a greater density of nutrients than younger people, yet the reality for many older people unable to access fresh food is that they survive on a diet of high-carbohydrate snacks.

Vitamins and the older person

A proportion of vitamin D is synthesized by the skin. In order for this to happen, the skin must be exposed to daylight, and this exposure may be reduced in older age due, for example, to restricted mobility. For this reason, older people should increase the amount of vitamin D in their diet to ensure the efficient absorption and use of calcium from the diet. Bone loss is an almost universal aspect of ageing (at a rate of 0.5–1% per annum), and is termed osteopenia or osteoporosis. Osteopenia can be minimized by taking daily exercise, and also by taking additional calcium in the diet. This is because calcium loss increases in women during and after the menopause, and because all older people become less efficient in absorbing calcium. A supplement of 800 mg/day could reduce the incidence of hip fractures (Lau & Wood 1998). Calcium loss can be exacerbated by a diet high in sodium (salt) or high in protein.

Access to fresh food

With increased centralization of shopping facilities that are only accessible by good public transport or by car, many people, especially older people, have their access to food shopping restricted. In addition, they may not be able to carry heavy shopping and so may need to make frequent trips to the shops to meet their needs. Home delivery is a possibility, and doorstep deliveries of milk and, increasingly, other fresh produce, are well established in Britain. However, these services do tend to be expensive. Several major supermarket chains have introduced on-line shopping and home deliveries, but this further reduces the value of social contact and the ability to choose and manage what may be a limited budget.

For people with restricted mobility, meals-on-wheels could provide an effective remedy. However, a study of older people on this sort of programme in the USA (Prothero & Rosenbloom 1999) showed that only 6% were receiving a good diet and 41% were receiving a diet that was inadequate. The study found that diets of the older adults were still dependent on the individual's income and social class, despite the supplied meal being designed to provide up to 50% of nutrients.

Luncheon clubs are invaluable as a means of offering social contact and someone else to cook, and many provide tasty meals at minimal cost (Clarke et al 1999). Other alternatives for the very old are day centres, where the person can be monitored as to their state of health and also be provided with physiotherapy as well as having a social occasion.

Nutrition and recovery from illness

In ideal conditions, patients would be screened for their nutritional status once they had been assessed as in need of surgery and a nutritional plan would be agreed as part of their treatment. Having a good nutritional status prior to surgical trauma promotes recovery and healing. In reality, approximately 40% of patients are malnourished on admission to hospital, and this proportion increases as a result of hospitalization (McWhirter & Pennington 1994). The clinical guidelines produced by the National Institute for Health and Clinical Excellence (NICE) recommend that all patients should be screened for malnutrition or the risk of malnutrition. This is recommended for any patient being admitted to hospital for any kind of procedure, particularly patients who have a body mass index (BMI) of less than 18.5 kg/m^2 or unintentional weight loss of more than 10% within the previous 3–6 months, or who has a BMI of less than 20 kg/m^2 and unintentional weight loss of more than 5% within the previous 3–6 months (NICE 2006).

However, many patients may benefit from extra attention to their diet during their hospital stay and convalescence. Protein, carbohydrate, vitamins and minerals are especially important during any form of physical illness.

Protein

This is required for the formation of all new tissue, including wound healing (Dudek 1997). Additionally, protein is lost during times of immobility due to the body's strategy of degrading tissues that are not being used (e.g. leg muscles). If a patient's intake of carbohydrate is lower than needed, then the body will also start to degrade its protein and fat stores to create energy. This process results in negative nitrogen balance, and can be noticed from increased amounts of creatinine in the urine. As mobility is re-established, protein must be available in the diet to facilitate a positive nitrogen balance. There are a number of studies suggesting that particular amino acids are especially beneficial, but clinical trials have ambiguous outcomes.

Carbohydrate

Energy in the form of carbohydrate is required to maintain and, if necessary, restore normal weight and to provide the fuel for the energy expenditure associated with healing, rehabilitation and so on. Furthermore, a diet rich in energy will be 'protein-sparing'; that is, precious protein will not need to be broken down to provide energy.

Lipids

Little is known about the role of lipids in wound healing other than their importance in the form of fatty acids for cell development and thus tissue regeneration. Fatty acids are also important for the development of prostaglandins (messengers involved in wound healing). Lipids also provide an important source of energy.

Water

Water is required to replace the significant amounts that are likely to have been lost through perspiration, fluid withdrawal and possibly as a result of diarrhoea and vomiting.

Vitamins and minerals

Vitamin C was the first nutrient whose deficiency was noted to have an effect on wound healing, and this was confirmed in a landmark study in 1940 (NICE 2006). It is required to make collagen, a key building-block in tissue repair.

Vitamin A is required for a good immune response and for repair of mucous membranes and wound healing.

B group vitamins are required for cell manufacture, as many of the enzymes involved in this process involve the B group vitamins.

Iron is required for good red cell function. Blood may be needed for replacement of losses during surgery. Furthermore, this is the nutrient most likely to be missing from a Western diet, so it is quite likely that the client was iron-deficient on admission.

Zinc is required for efficient wound healing and for normal immune response.

Supplementary nutrition

Sometimes a patient is unable to ingest their nutritional needs and so these have to be given by a different route. There are two specific routes by which food can be administered: the enteral route, which bypasses the mouth and oesophagus and a suitably processed form of food is delivered directly to the stomach; the parenteral route, in which nutrition is administered directly into the bloodstream intravenously. The latter treatment may be given to patients who are unable to digest

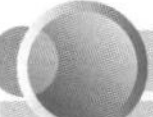

any food at all through their digestive system, usually because of disease. Some patients who are able to eat normally may also need food to be delivered in this way if they are suffering from severe malnutrition and need a high level of nutrients over a short period of time. Others who you may see being provided with either enteral or parenteral feeding are patients who have suffered severe burns, particularly to the face and neck, and need a higher intake of nutrition, or who are unconscious as a result of head injury.

Babies with a congenital abnormality of the mouth, throat or oesophagus may be unable to suck, and food cannot enter the stomach. You will remember from the discussion on the absorption of nutrients through the intestinal villi that the villi start to atrophy if they are not working for any period of time. Increased awareness of the importance of the gut as an organ that influences the maintenance of health and recovery from illness makes it essential that enteral feeding is re-introduced as soon as possible. In these treatments, patients receive a liquid feed directly into the digestive system via a nasogastric feeding tube or a direct link to the stomach through a gastroscopy tube. If it is a baby, it may be possible to give the baby a bottle to suck on and to collect the liquid through a fistula that is above the obstruction. This way the baby receives the nurturing it needs and learns to use its buccal muscles.

Total parenteral nutrition

Total parenteral nutrition (TPN) is a means of getting a rich supply of nutrients to someone who is unable to absorb nutrients from their diet. If food cannot be given directly into the digestive system then TPN is an alternative approach. Artificial food supplements are provided intravenously (parenterally) in a chemical form, which, if the digestive system were working effectively, would normally be absorbed into the blood and delivered to the liver. Indeed, it is possible to provide all of a person's nutritional requirements using TPN.

Nutrition following surgery

Some patients may need to be provided with parenteral nutrition following abdominal surgery, especially if their intestinal tract has been involved. These delicate tissues are likely to become bruised, and peristalsis often stops as a reaction. Normal drinking and eating should not be encouraged until bowel sounds can be heard. These are the 'rumblings' (or borborygmi) of peristaltic action. Another sign of the bowel returning to normal action is when the patient passes flatus. Food and drink should not be given to your patient until these signs are present; otherwise they may well suffer from vomiting as the body regurgitates the food and water.

> **Case history 8.3**
>
> **Supporting dietary intake following surgery**
>
> Mrs Singh has returned from surgery following abdominal hysterectomy (removal of her uterus). She is conscious and has an intravenous infusion of normal saline and dextrose. This is not providing her with any nutrients, but is ensuring she does not become dehydrated. Four hours after her surgery she is complaining of thirst and it is supper time for the patients on the ward.

Now read and consider the case of Mrs Singh (Case history 8.3):

- What factors do you need to consider before letting Mrs Singh have something to eat?
- What kinds of foodstuffs do you think she should have to promote her recovery and healing?

Nutrition in disease: dysphagia and sensory dysfunction

Swallowing difficulties are relatively rare unless associated with neurological damage. It can become a major problem for many patients. Initially, referral to a speech and language therapist, who will assess swallowing function, provide advice about types of food and recommend oral exercises to strengthen muscles, may be sufficient. Patients with neurological damage resulting in their loss of the gag reflex and who are at risk of inhaling food or aspirating fluids need supervision and help when eating to prevent this happening. Eventually, if dysphagia is irremediable, it may be safer to provide enteral tube feeding. It is important to give these patients the sensation of eating to promote the normal digestive processes by giving them very small amounts of food of appropriate consistency for the pleasure of tasting and smelling food; this also stimulates digestive enzymes to be released, increases appetite and helps prevent weight loss.

If you would like to find out more about nutritional support, the National Institute for Health and Clinical Excellence (NICE) has produced guidelines (NICE 2006); you can obtain a copy of these guidelines and others produced by NICE by going to their website (www.nice.org.uk).

Assistance with eating and drinking

Good diet was at the heart of Florence Nightingale's philosophy of care and health promotion, in the hospital and in the home. This was at a time when there was little a nurse could do to alter the outcome of a disease. Nowadays, however, there are many nursing actions that affect a patients' prognosis. There may be a danger of overlooking some of the traditional nursing skills, and assisting patients to eat and drink may be one of these.

Assisting patients at meal-times should be an enjoyable undertaking. It should not be rushed, or the social importance of the occasion overlooked. Assisting patients starts with helping them choose an appropriate diet, one that they will enjoy, that will meet their nutritional requirements and is of a type and consistency that they can manage. Remembering the effect of the gastrocolic reflex is helpful to ensure that patients who are not self-caring have the opportunity to use the toilet and to wash their hands. Patients may also need assistance with mouth care to remove any unappetizing tastes. Dentures need to be made available if necessary, and patients may need assistance in putting on their spectacles, hearing aid and any other appropriate aids so they can enjoy their food to the maximum. Eating in bed and avoiding spills is remarkably difficult, so it is helpful to ensure the patient has a napkin to protect their clothing. If you are feeding a patient, it is important to make this a social occasion that is relaxed and provides an opportunity to share conversation. Sitting alongside the patient at the correct height and so that the patient can see the food is important, as well as keeping the food hot, or cold, as appropriate. If the patient has limited vision, it is helpful to describe the food and to explain where it is located (e.g. by using a clock analogy, peas are at 10 o'clock, potatoes at midday). Some patients may choose to take their meal with a drink and if it is appropriate, perhaps a glass of beer or a glass of wine as this assists in promoting the appetite as well as making it easier to taste and chew the food.

A balance needs to be drawn between encouraging independence and insisting that patients cope on their own so that they don't become frustrated and disinterested in their food. There is a wide range of appliances for people with arthritis or other neuromuscular disorders; these include non-slip mats, plate guards and cutlery with large handles. Drawing on the expertise of members of the multidisciplinary team is helpful as part of planning the patient's care, and occupational therapists and also speech and language therapists have particular expertise.

As feeding patients can be a pleasant activity, and obviously linked with their well-being, the patient's family or friends may like to be involved. This can help carers to learn any necessary techniques that will be needed when the patient is discharged home. The amount of food and fluid that has been taken after eating and drinking may need to be documented, depending on the plan of care.

Eating disorders

Assisting people to eat in situations where their loss of appetite is a result of a voluntary act rather than due to a disease-related loss is complex as they may hold different views as to the meaning of food. They could view it as comfort, enemy, temptation or a means to control.

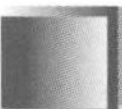

Alcohol disorders

An addiction to alcohol often involving heavy, frequent drinking is a disease that requires medical support if the person is to learn how to control it. Recovery is never complete and can only be managed by complete abstinence of any form of alcoholic drink. Alcoholism has an adverse effect on all organs of the body, particularly the liver and brain. Alcoholic beverages contain variable amounts of energy, and very little else of nutritional value. As a result, addiction is a major cause of malnutrition. There are three reasons for this:

- Alcohol interferes with the brain's regulation of food intake, and limits eating.
- Alcoholic drinks may provide enough energy to satisfy hunger, but fail to provide any other nutrients. Furthermore an addict may concentrate on obtaining relief from the craving for alcohol at the expense of obtaining food. However, the person who abuses alcohol may be overweight.
- Gastrointestinal and liver complications of alcohol intake may interfere with the correct metabolism of food.

Nutritional support for people with alcohol addiction should include vitamin B supplements in particular, as well as a diet rich in protein and carbohydrates.

The role of the health care professional in promoting nutrition

Professionals have the responsibility of being informed about diets and nutrition. Nurses who are in direct contact with families have a particular remit to promote healthy eating (Department of Health 2001). They are in a position to engage on an individual basis and develop programmes focused on a wider community, be it in parent–toddler groups or any other context. The Department of Health also sees nurses as having a public health role to promote healthy choices for the most disadvantaged (see Box 8.5). It is evident that there is a need for improved information and

Box 8.5

Delivering on health priorities

Advice provided by the Department of Health for community specialist health care nurses and health visitors (Department of Health 2001)

What health visitors can do in terms of specific dietary advice

Support people to:

- Eat five portions of fruit and vegetables a day.
- Eat less fat.
- Eat more fibre-rich starchy foods.
- Reduce salt in food by a third.
- Increase the amount of oily fish eaten to at least two portions a week.

Working with individuals

Focus on diet or diet plus physical activity rather than trying to tackle a range of risk factors.

Set clear goals based on theories of behavioural change, rather than providing advice alone.

Sustain personal contact with people or small groups over time.

Give feedback on any changes in behaviour and risk factors.

Working with communities

Map access to healthy foodstuffs as part of the community health assessment.

Work with local people to identify what the issues are and how best to tackle them.

Consider initiatives such as food cooperatives, community gardens, cook-and-eat groups.

Provide nutritional advice that is culturally sensitive and relevant to needs.

Identify training for professionals and local people to acquire skills for different ways of working.

Make use of marketing strategies to increase appeal of health promotion messages to the target audience.

Promote changes in the local environment, such as shops and catering outlets that help people to choose a healthy diet.

Allow realistic time for community food projects to develop.

Evaluate patterns in food purchasing, structural changes and social outcomes in addition to narrow clinical and behavioural measures.

skills for nurses to support people who have nutritional disorders. Prevention of obesity and undernutrition are key priorities to be addressed in Western society (Department of Health 2004).

Recent government policies and initiatives regarding nutrition

Government policies that direct health care professionals to focus on include:

- 'Better hospital food' (2001) and subsequent related campaigns are aimed at improving the quality of hospital nutrition and availability of food (use of locally sourced and, where possible, organic food; food to be available at times suitable for patients; the times when food is served is protected from any clinical activity).
- Breast-feeding and NHS planning and priorities framework aims to increase breast-feeding by 2% each year, for the first 6 months of life. The campaign focuses on encouraging mothers to breast-feed their babies, partly by removing the availability of reduced-priced formula milk in NHS and welfare food clinics and by making fresh milk tokens available to pregnant women.
- 'Healthy start' focuses on children and families in deprived areas and provides vouchers for use in exchange for fruit, vegetables, milk and infant formula.
- Under the '5 A DAY' programme, 4–6-year-olds in local education authority schools will receive a free piece of fruit or vegetable each day.

There are other programmes aimed at improving access to a healthy diet (Parliamentary Office of Science and Technology 2003):

- 'Choosing health: making healthier choices easier' (Department of Health 2004), a Public Health White Paper, has an emphatic focus on nutrition.
- 'Tackling health inequalities: programme for action' (Department of Health 2003b) has identified the role that diet has in reducing the risk of coronary heart disease and cancer.

The main issues that these documents address are concerned with encouraging people to eat more fruit and vegetables. The National School Fruit Scheme and the '5 A DAY' programme are aimed at increasing fruit and vegetable consumption. For instance, there will be 66 local programmes in deprived areas, led by primary care trusts, with the aim of increasing access and awareness of the benefits of fruit and vegetables. Government documents also emphasize the importance of breast-feeding, especially in low-income groups, where mothers are most likely to rely on formula milk; hence the campaign to increase breast-feeding by 2% year on year.

The level of responsibility for risk reduction starts with the Department of Health and then with primary care trusts. Primary care trusts are responsible for commissioning services on behalf of the local population and they no longer have a responsibility to provide the delivery of local services. Agencies employed by the primary care trusts will deliver services through the roles and activities of general practitioners and health professionals, such as health visitors and midwives. Community groups and employers also need to be engaged in this delivery plan. Inevitably, there will be further battles on regulation between consumer groups and health groups with the food and advertising industry.

Conclusion

In this chapter we have demonstrated that there are a number of obstacles to public exhortations to adopt a healthier lifestyle. To achieve any change, the responsibility, impetus and action cannot be left solely to people on their own. Entire organizations, agencies, government and practitioners must join together to bring about change. The emphasis on healthy eating to prevent and reduce obesity is necessary, as indicated by research on the trends of increasing obesity and the health implications amongst populations. However, practitioners need to understand that the cause of obesity is multifaceted and people with weight problems need to be seen in the context of the whole society and its attitude to nutrition and weight, the responsibilities of the food industry in food production and food advertising, and the relevance of psychosocial factors that influence overeating and the sedentary lifestyle that most people have. Counterbalancing these considerations is the right of individual choice and responsibility.

Government policies indicate that it acknowledges its duty to have people and practices in place that support dietary change. However, the complexity of the food industry and factors that influence dietary habits mean that governments must take responsibility for the wider economic context of food production, processing and distribution. Policies are required that involve revision of town planning so that it accounts for lifestyles and access. Improvements in the population's nutrition can only be achieved at three levels of society: the individual, the local community/neighbourhood and the government. All are equally important if improvement in the nutrition of the population is to be expected. The government has demonstrated that it takes nutrition seriously, but a firmer commitment to regulating the food industry is essential to ensure that food production, processing and retailing is oriented towards health rather than commercialism. As we have demonstrated, nutrition and consequently health are too important to be left to decision-making according to free-trade and commercial interests.

References

Abnet C, Qiao YL, Dawsey S et al 2005 Tooth loss is associated with increased risk of health and death from upper GI cancer, heart disease and stroke. International Journal of Epidemiology 34(2):467–474

Aftenposten 2005 Hvalpefett eller overvekt? 7 July, p 12–13. Online. Available: http://www.aftenposten.no/nyheter/iriks/oslo/article1073842.ece

Anderson C, Longbottom C, Pitts N et al 2005 Integrated care approach to targeting caries prevention to pre-school children. Caries Research 39(4):295–296

Appollonio I, Carabellese C, Frattola A et al 1997 Influence of dental status on dietary intake and survival in community living elderly subjects. Age and Ageing 26(6):445–456

Arshad SH, Matthews S, Gant C et al 1992 Effect of allergen avoidance on development of allergic disorders. Lancet 339(8808):1493–1500

Azad N, Murphy J, Amos SS et al J 1999 Nutrition support in an elderly population following admission to a tertiary care hospital. Canadian Medical Association Journal 161(5):511–515

Baggott R 2000 Public health: policy and politics. Palgrave, London

Baggott R 2004 Health and health care in Britain, 3rd edn. Palgrave, London

Baily R, Gueldner S, Ledikwe J et al 2005 The oral health of older adults. Journal of Gerontological Nursing 31(7):11–17

Baum F 2002 The new public health, 2nd edn. University Press, Oxford

Beardsworth A, Keil T 1997 Society on the menu. Routledge, London

Bellizzi MC, Dietz WH 1999 Workshop on childhood obesity. American Journal of Clinical Nutrition 70(1):173s–175s

Berenson GS, Wattigney WA, Tracy RE et al 1992 Atherosclerosis of the aorta and coronary arteries and cardiovascular risk factors in persons aged 6 to 30 years and studied at necroscopy (the Bogolusa Heart Study). American Journal of Cardiology 70(9):851–858

Blaxter M 1990 Health and lifestyles. Routledge, London

Bloom S 2003 The fat controller. New Scientist 179(2407):38–41

Bordo S 2003 Unbearable weight: feminism, western culture and the body, 10th anniversary edn. University of California Press, London

Brewer S 2002 The Daily Telegraph encyclopedia of vitamins, minerals and herbal supplements. Robinson, London

Caraher M 2000 Food policy and public health: a role for community nursing? Community Practitioner 73(1):435–438

Center for Family Policy and Practice 2004. Online. Available: http://www.cffpp.org/archive.html 8 Dec 12 2004

Chinn S, Rona RJ 1994 A commentary: the relation of growth to socioeconomic deprivation. International Journal of Epidemiology 33(1):152–153

Christiansen JL, Grzybowski JM 1993 Biology of ageing. Mosby, St Louis

Clarke DM, Wahlquist ML, Rassias CR et al 1999 Psychological factors in nutritional disorders of the elderly. International Journal of Eating Disorders 25(3):345–348

Consumers Association 2000 Baby food. Which? May:18–19

Coon KA, Tucker KL 2002 Television and children's consumption patterns. Minerva Pediatrica 54(5):423–436

Coughlan A 1991 Europe's search for the winning diet. New Scientist 132(1797):29–37

Coughland S 2000 In good taste. New Scientist 165(2223):11

Czeizel AC, Dudas I 1992 Prevention of the first occurrence of neural-tube defects by periconceptional vitamin supplementation. New England Journal of Medicine 327(26):1832–1835

Dallman PR 1986 Iron deficiency in the weanling: a nutritional problem on the way to resolution. Acta Paediatrica Scandinavica Supplement 323:59–67

Department of Health 1994 Weaning and the weaning diet 'COMA' report. HMSO, London

Department of Health 1998 Five a day. Department of Health, London. Online. Available: www.doh.gov.uk/fiveaday

Department of Health 2001 Health visitor practice development resource pack. Department of Health, London

Department of Health 2003a Essence of care. Department of Health, NHS Modernisation Agency, London

Department of Health 2003b Tackling health inequalities: programme for action. Department of Health, NHS Modernisation Agency, London

Department of Health 2004 Choosing health: making healthier choices easier. White Paper for Public Health. Department of Health, London

Diet Intervention Study in Children (DISC) Writing Group 1995 Efficacy and safety of lowering dietary intake of fat and cholesterol in children with elevated low-density lipoprotein cholesterol. JAMA 273(18):1429–1435

Doyle W, Crawford MA, Wynn AHA 1989 Maternal nutrient intake and birthweight. Journal of Human Nutrition and Dietetics 2(1):415–422

Dudek SG 1997 Nutrition handbook for nurses, 3rd edn. Lippincott, Philadelphia

Engels F 1844 Health. In: Davey B, Gray A, Seale C (eds) Health and disease: a reader, 3rd edn. Open University Press, Buckingham

Fieldhouse P 1996 Food and nutrition: customs and culture, 2nd edn. Stanley Thornes, Cheltenham

Fitzpatrick R 2003 Society and changing patterns of disease. In: Scambler G (ed) Sociology as applied to medicine, 5th edn. Saunders, London

Food Action and Research Centre 1998 School breakfast score card. Food Research and Action Centre, London

Food Standards Agency 2004 Do food deserts really exist? A multi-level, geographical analysis of the relationship between retail food access, socioeconomic position and dietary intake. N09010. Online: Available: http//:www.food.gov.uk/science/research/researchinfo/nutritionresearch 23 Dec 2004

Foster H, Fitzgerald J 2005 Dental disease in children with chronic illnesses. Archives of Disease in Childhood 90(7):703–708

Frelut L, Flodmark CE 2003 Binge eating disorders. In: Burniat W, Cole T, Lissau I et al (eds) Child and adolescent obesity. Cambridge University Press, Cambridge

Gulf News 2005 Two-pronged health and fitness programme to combat obesity. Section Nation 3, 26 July

Hardy SC, Kleinman RE 1994 Fat and cholesterol in the diet of infants and young children: implications for growth, development and long-term health. Journal of Pediatrics 125(5):S69–77

Hurtado EK, Classen AH, Scott KG 1999 Early childhood anaemia and mild or moderate mental retardation. American Journal of Clinical Nutrition 69(1):4–5

International Food Information Council 1993 Tasteful solutions to elderly malnutrition. Food Insights May/June. Online. Available: http://ificinfo.health.org/insight/elderlym.htm 19 June 2000

Karagozoglu S, Ulsoy M 2005 Chemotherapy: the effects of oral cryotherapy on the development of mucositis. Journal of Clinical Nursing 14(6):754–756

Kemmer D 2000 Tradition and change in domestic roles and food preparation. Sociology 34(2):323–333

Kew Magazine 2005 Keeping traditions alive. London: Royal Botanical Gardens

Kmietowicz Z 2003 Food watchdog warns against high doses of vitamins and minerals. BMJ 326(7397):1001

Kotz K, Story M 1994 Food advertisements during children's Saturday morning television programming. Journal of the American Dietetic Association 94(11):1296–1300

Lamy M, Mojon P, Kalykakis G et al 1999 Oral status and nutrition in the elderly population. Journal of Dentistry 27(6):443–448

Lang T 2001 The new globalisation, food and health. In: Davey B, Gray A, Seale C (eds) Health and disease: a reader, 3rd edn. Open University Press, Buckingham

Lang T, Heasman M 2004 Diet and nutrition policy: a clash of ideas or investment. Development 47(2):64–74

Lau EM, Wood J 1998 Nutrition and osteoporosis. Current Opinion in Rheumatology 10(4):368–372

Lauer RM, Lee J, Clarke WR 1988 Factors affecting the relationship between childhood and adult cholesterol levels: the Muscatine Study. Pediatrics 82(3):309–318

Lawrence F 2004 Not on the label. Penguin Books, London

Leather S 1996 The making of modern malnutrition. Caroline Walker Trust, London

Lissau I, Burniat W, Poskitt EME et al 2003 Prevention. In: Burniat W, Lissau I, Cole T et al (eds) Child and adolescent obesity. Cambridge University Press, Cambridge

Livingstone B 1997 Healthy eating in infancy. Professional Care of Mother and Child 7(1):9–11

Lupton D 2000 The heart of the meal: food preferences and habits among rural Australian couples. Sociology of Health and Illness 22(1): 94–109

Malin N, Wilmot S, Manthorpe J 2002 Key concepts and debates in health and social policy. Open University Press, Buckingham

Marrieb EN 2005 Human anatomy and physiology, 8th edn. Benjamin Cummings, San Francisco

Martini FH, Welch K 2005 A&P applications manual. London, Pearson

Matuszek C 2000 Lottery win cooks up a healthy diet. Wimbledon News 21 January:16

Maxwell S, Slater R 2004 Food policy old and new. In: Maxwell S, Slater R (eds) Food policy old and new. Blackwell Publishing, Oxford

McGill HC, Mott GE, Lewis DS et al 1996 Early determinants of adult metabolic regulation: effects of adult nutrition on adult lipid and lipoprotein metabolism. Nutrition Reviews 54(2):S31–S40

McWhirter JP, Pennington CR 1994 Incidence and recognition of malnutrition in hospital. BMJ 308(6934):945–948

Milla PJ 1986 The weanlings gut. Acta Paediatrica Scandinavica Supplement 323:5–13

Ministry of Agriculture, Fisheries and Food (MAFF) 2002 Manual of nutrition, 10th edn. HMSO, London

Mizrachi N 2002 Epistemology and legitimacy in the production of anorexia nervosa in the Journal of Psychosomatic Medicine 1939–1979. Sociology of Health and Illness 24(4):462–490

National Institute for Health and Clinical Excellence (NICE) 2006 Nutrition support in adults: oral nutrition support, enteral tube feeding and parenteral nutrition (Clinical guideline 32). NICE, London. Online. Available: http://www.nice.org.uk Feb 2006

Newman V, Fullerton JT 1990 Role of nutrition in the prevention of pre-eclampsia. Journal of Midwifery 35(3):282–291

Newman B, Siminovitch KA 2005 Recent advances in the genetics of inflammatory bowel disease. Current Opinion in Gastroenterology 21(4):402–407

New Scientist 2005 Vitamin C left out in the cold. New Scientist 187(2506):18

Nourhashemi F, Andrieu S, Rauzy O et al 1999 Nutritional support and aging in preoperative nutrition. Current Opinion in Clinical Nutrition and Metabolic Care 2(1):87–92

Orbach S 1998 Fat is a feminist issue, 3rd edn. Arrow, London

Parliamentary Office of Science and Technology 2003 Improving children's diet. Number 199 Report Summary. July

Patel T (1994) Pure juice, real fraud. New Scientist 1926: 26

Peres K, Armenio M, Peres M et al 2005 Dental erosion in 12-year-old school children. International Journal of Paediatric Dentistry 15(4):249–255

Pollitt E 1995 Does breakfast make a difference in school? Journal of the American Dietetic Association 95(10):1134–1139

Prothero JW, Rosenbloom CA 1999 Description of mixed ethnic, elderly population: demography, nutrient/energy intakes and income status. Journal of Gerontology 54(6):315–324

Puska P 2002 Successful prevention of non-communicable diseases: 25 years' experiences with North Karelia Project in Finland. Public Health Medicine 4(1):5–7

Quarmby K 2004 Food fight. The Guardian Education 14 Dec:2

Rolls BJ 1999 Do chemosensory changes influence food intake in the elderly? Physiology of Behavior 66(2):193–197

Royal Society for the Prevention of Cruelty to Animals 2004 Online. Available: www.rspca.org Dec

Scheck JM, Roubenhoff R 1999 Nutrition in the exercising elderly. Clinics of Sports Medicine 18(3):565–584

Schlosser E 2002 Fast food nation. Penguin Books, London

Schmied V, Lupton D 2001 Blurring the boundaries: breastfeeding and maternal subjectivity. Sociology of Health and Illness 123(2):234–250

Skuse D 1993 Identification and management of problem eaters. Archives of Disease in Childhood 69(5):604–608

Small MF 2002 The happy fat. New Scientist 175(2357):34–37

Stehlin D 1993 Feeding baby: nature and nurture. Food and Drug Administration, USA

Steptoe A, Perkins-Porras L, McKay C et al 2003 Behavioural counselling to increase consumption of fruit and vegetables in low income adults. BMJ 326(7394):855–858

Stratton RJ, Green CJ, Elia M 2003 Disease-related malnutrition: an evidence-based approach to treatment. CABI Publishing, Wallingford

Sullivan SA, Birch LL 1994 Infant dietary experience and acceptance of solid food. Pediatrics 93(2):271–277

Troiano R, Flegal K, Kuczmarski J et al 1995 Overweight prevalence and trends for children and adolescents. Archives of Paediatric and Adolescent Medicine 149(1):1085–1091

Vines G 1996 Five apples a day. New Scientist 1(2054):50

Wald N 1991 Prevention of neural tube defects: results of the Medical Research Council Vitamin Study. Lancet 338(8760):131–137

Walker C 1993 Managing poverty: the limits of social assistance. Routledge, London

Waugh A, Grant A 2006 Ross & Wilson Anatomy and physiology in health and illness, 10th edn. Churchill Livingstone, Edinburgh

Webb GP, Copeman J 1996 Nutrition of older adults. Arnold, London

Wehner P 1999 Sweet sensation. New Scientist 164(2176):14

Weir H, Richardson J, Buxton V 1997 Using health beliefs for community based intervention in heart disease prevention. Research report to the UK Health Education Authority, London

Wood CBS 1986 How common is food allergy? Acta Paediatrica Scandinavica Supplement 323:76–83

Further reading

Garrow JS 2000 Human nutrition and dietetics, 10th edn. Churchill Livingstone, Edinburgh

Useful websites

Age Concern England: www.ageconcern.org.uk

Blood Pressure Association: www.bpassoc.org.uk

British Dietetic Association: www.bda.uk.com

British Heart Foundation: www.bhf.org.uk

British Nutrition Foundation: www.nutrition.org.uk

Child Poverty Action Group: www.cpag.org.uk

Department of Health: www.dh.gov.uk

Diabetes UK: www.diabetes.org.uk

Faculty of Public Health: www.fph.org.uk

Food Standards Agency: www.food.gov.uk

Health Education Trust: www.healthedtrust.com

International Obesity Task Force: www.iotf.org

National Osteoporosis Society: www.nos.org.uk

NHS 5 A DAY Campaign: www.5aday.nhs.uk

Sustain: www.sustainweb.org

Chapter Nine

9

Hygiene

Maria Dingle, Carol Cox, Alex Grayson

Key topics

- **Benchmarks for personal and oral hygiene**
- **The significance of personal hygiene in religious and cultural rituals**
- **Anatomy and physiology of the integumentary system and the mouth**
- **The nurse's role in promoting safety, comfort, privacy and dignity whilst attending to patients' personal and oral hygiene**
- **Thermoregulation**
- **Assisting with elimination of urine and faeces**
- **The system as a first line of defence for the body and some of the potential infective agents such as bacteria (e.g. MRSA), fungi, viruses and parasites**
- **Prevention of cross-infection**

Introduction

In this chapter we discuss the importance of personal and oral hygiene. Keeping oneself clean and well groomed is a normal human activity that is taken for granted in the fit and healthy. As a nursing student, you are likely to meet people who are having difficulty achieving their preferred state of hygiene, especially if they have some degree of dependency, either in a hospital, in their own home or in a nursing home. Maintaining personal hygiene is such an important daily function that the Department of Health (2003) provided a definition of personal hygiene as being the:

> *Physical act of cleansing the body to ensure that the skin, hair and nails are maintained in an optimum condition.*

and of oral hygiene as being the:

> *Effective removal of plaque and debris to ensure the structures and tissues of the mouth are kept in a healthy condition.*

and a healthy mouth as a:

> *Clean, functional, and comfortable oral cavity and free from infection.*

Giving a patient assistance in their personal hygiene can be an enjoyable social occasion for the patient and for the nurse. Assisting someone with their personal grooming can also provide the nurse with an opportunity to assess the patient's physical and emotional well-being and so identify any nursing or health care needs that require attention. Helping someone in this way may appear daunting if you have never had physical contact with a stranger before. If you can develop an attitude that, through the act of washing and making a fellow human being as comfortable and refreshed as possible, you are in a position of privilege and engaged in an act of moderated love (Campbell 1984), then you can transform the experience for your patient as well as for yourself. In the process you are developing the artistic skill that is an essential part of nursing.

Maintaining personal hygiene is such an important activity in society that many religions and cultures have embodied the process in their rituals. So in this chapter we shall be considering some of these different aspects of promoting hygiene and comfort. To help you understand the importance of this process and the kinds of professional observations you should be making, we shall introduce you to the anatomy and physiology of the skin (otherwise known as the integumentary system), the appendages such as hair and nails and the different glands of the skin. Temperature regulation (or thermoregulation) of the body is an important activity of the integumentary system, along with providing the first line of defence against bacterial and parasitic infections. In Chapter 8 you were introduced to the structure and functions of the buccal cavity as part of the digestive process. In this chapter, we discuss the importance of maintaining the health of the mouth and how this can be achieved. When bathing someone or giving any form of assistance, touch is an important technique to develop and we shall explore its significance when delivering care. Throughout this chapter we will be stressing the importance of your role in ensuring that your patient is always protected from emotional, physical, social and spiritual harm, and that their comfort, privacy and dignity are promoted.

Benchmarks for personal and oral hygiene

The 'Personal and oral hygiene' benchmarks developed by the UK Department of Health to support their 'Essence of care' programme (Department of Health 2003) emphasize the importance of assessment when caring for patients so that the nurse can identify the appropriate advice and care that is needed to maintain and promote personal and oral hygiene. As you will have read in Chapter 5, it is important to maintain your patient's dignity and self-respect by ensuring that any care is negotiated with the patient and, if relevant, their carers. Such care plans must be based on your patient's specific and unique needs.

To help you develop a care plan for a patient that is concerned with personal and oral hygiene, you should consider the benchmarks describing best practice listed in Box 9.1.

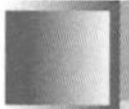

Box 9.1

Essence of care benchmarks

(Department of Health 2003)

Planned care is negotiated with patients and carers and is based on assessment of the patient's individual needs.

Patients have access to an environment that is safe and acceptable to them.

Patients are expected to supply their own toiletries, but single-use toiletries are provided until they can supply their own.

Patients have access to the level of assistance that they require to meet individual personal and oral hygiene needs.

Patients and carers are provided with information and education to meet their individual personal and oral hygiene needs.

Patients' care is continuously evaluated, reassessed and the care plan re-negotiated.

Assessing oral and personal hygiene needs

Anyone working in the health or social care environment, who has received the appropriate training and is considered to be safe to undertake the delegated activity, can assess patients for their oral and personal hygiene needs, but the ultimate responsibility remains with the registered practitioner responsible for that patient's care.

When assessing your patient's needs you should focus on their specific and individual needs, and the assessment should be conducted at the earliest opportunity, carefully recorded in their care notes and signed by the person making the assessment. It may be necessary to discuss your patient's needs with other members of the health care team if there is a specific issue that requires particular attention. An example might be a patient who is noted to have an infestation, or a wound that appears to be infected; in such situations, the infection control nurse needs to be notified. A patient admitted with a decubitus ulcer (pressure sore) may need to be seen by the tissue viability nurse. When planning the care it is important to make use of any relevant research or other source of evidence to support the nursing practice. The care plan should be reviewed regularly to monitor its effectiveness and, if necessary, revised. It is important that an evaluation of the patient's condition is made daily and signed by the key worker for the patient. Care plans may need to be adjusted to reflect the individual needs of patients if there are, for example, religious reasons that prescribe a particular approach.

Indicators of best practice

Infection control arrangements must ensure that the safety of both health care personnel and patients is preserved. If care is being delivered under the supervision of a registered practitioner, it is important that the student nurse is aware of any changes in the person's condition or needs. To ensure this happens, the registered practitioner must make sure there are clear guidelines about what to observe and how to respond if necessary. The care plan should also specify the nature of care and assistance to be provided; this should be based on negotiated agreement with your patient. The aspects of essential care that should be included in the care plan are opportunities for the patient to carry out their personal hygiene particularly before and after meals, before and after using the lavatory (bedpan, commode or urinal), the nature of care they prefer and so on.

Providing health care education is an important aspect of your role as a nursing student. This may require you to check your patient's understanding, to reinforce any health and hygiene principles using information that is based on best practice and to use language that is understandable and culturally appropriate to your patient. You may need to ensure your supervisor is aware of any situations that could cause a breach in best practice and to discuss any issues with your patient and their carers. This is particularly important if there is a risk of cross-infection (Nicol 2004). To ensure that you can recognize situations that may breach best practice guidelines you need to be knowledgeable about the biological, psychological and sociological sciences related to caring for patients' personal hygiene needs and disposal of excreta.

Providing effective psychosocial support that is culturally sensitive is crucial when planning hygiene or elimination needs. Elimination mainly involves the urinary system and the gastrointestinal tract, but it also includes the skin and the respiratory system in the form of sweat loss and exhaled water vapour.

The significance of providing personal hygiene

The social perspective of intimacy

Healthcare providers need to go beyond sensitivity to diversity if they are effectively to assess the health of culturally diverse groups and the individuals that comprise them.

(D'Avanzo & Geissler 2003)

With increasing mobility of the world population you are likely to encounter a diverse range of beliefs and values depending upon your patients' religious and cultural backgrounds. These factors and others, including literacy, social and economic status, have an impact on personal health. Having an understanding of these different factors will help you to deliver care that is sensitive and appropriate to your specific patient. Some of the other factors that you need to consider are the significance of nakedness, different perceptions of the experience of touch and embarrassment in relation to how you bathe and attend to your patients' hygiene needs.

In Western society, the social meaning of nakedness is connected to intimacy, and sexual intimacy in particular. For many people, being naked is to feel deprived of protection. Clothes are used to protect the body and assist the wearer to feel that they are in keeping with what is correct socially. By removing your patient's clothes or denying them the opportunity to wear their own clothes, the relationship between nurse and patient changes and is related to a change in the power–relationship balance. The patient is naked and the nurse is not. Avoiding the embarrassment that this imbalance may cause requires sophisticated communication skills by the nurse.

Touch in delivering care

> *Touch has profound emotional significance. Preceding speech as a form of communication, it takes us back to our earliest experiences . . . Skin is the largest sense organ of the body . . .*
>
> *(Twigg 2000)*

Twigg goes on to note that touch in contemporary Western life is increasingly associated with erotic relationships and, as such, adults and men in particular, live a life of limited touch except for sex. It is this that can lead to embarrassment for the nurse and the patient due to the inappropriate connection between nudity, touch and sex. Twigg also notes that men in particular regard touch in a sexualized manner and that male touch may be interpreted as homosexual. In order to deal with these often unspoken issues, the nurse must give the patient very strong, business-like cues without giving the impression that their feelings of unease are of no importance (see Case history 3.6). For example, there must be no sense, for the patient, that the nurse is in any way affected by the nature of the work or the patient's condition. Being able to deliver care in a professional and aloof manner whilst maintaining a caring attitude takes great skill. Being able to mask any feelings towards the patient is important and finding strategies to cope with such feelings is an essential part of learning to nurse. It is not uncommon to have feelings of personal embarrassment, revulsion, curiosity or attraction, but it is essential to handle such feelings discretely and professionally. By contrast, with frequent involvement in caring for people to meet their hygiene needs, it is possible to forget any personal feelings of inhibition and at the same time to lose the insights into how your patient may be feeling with the result that they may become a work object rather than another human being and consequently dehumanized, to the detriment of good nursing practice. The key concepts for the nurse to keep in mind are communication, dignity and privacy (Twigg 2000).

The symbolic nature of hygiene

This introduction to the principles of providing intimate care when meeting your patient's hygiene needs has explored some of the psychosocial aspects. Washing and personal hygiene have significance other than their main purpose relating to maintenance of health. Water is a very ancient, natural symbol of purification and cleansing in religious and ritual practices.

> *Baths have often been rites of passage into institutions and something of this sense remains in relation to their use by individuals . . . to mark the passage of the day or week.*
>
> *(Twigg 2000)*

There are many different religious and cultural attitudes to personal hygiene. By working closely with your patients and by reading widely about health, religion and ethnicity, you will be able to appreciate the important health issues and how to address them without causing affront to your patients in terms of their belief structure and faith. Many faiths have strict hygiene laws concerning preparation for prayer, meal times and following excretion of waste products. The following sections identify some of the different bathing preferences that you might encounter, but it is important that you find out about your patient's preferences before making assumptions.

Muslim patients

Patients who adhere to the Muslim faith may require running water in which to wash, and so may prefer to be offered a shower. It is considered imperative for people who are Muslim to clean the genital area after going to the toilet and this requires the provision of a jug and washbasin or a bidet. The left and right hands in the Muslim faith have very specific purposes, and for some patients it is considered an insult if these purposes are ignored. A person's left hand is used to provide hygiene, the right hand for nourishment. This can have important implications for a nurse who is left-handed and feeds a patient with their left hand, or the siting of intravenous fluids if it means the patient can not use their hand for the appropriate purpose.

The mouth, hands and feet are cleansed five times a day prior to praying. The sanctity and privacy of the female Muslim patient is considered paramount, and she may require that she is completely covered from head to toe to shield her from the gaze of male visitors, patients or male health care workers who may come into the clinical setting. You need to bear in mind that your patient may object to wearing hospital clothes and you will need to negotiate suitable alternatives.

Hindu patients

Hindu patients may require running water in which to bathe. Hindu religious laws require that the genital region must be washed after using the toilet, so patients will need to know that there is a jug and washbasin within the toilet area or will be made available if they are confined to their bed space. If you are caring for a Hindu patient, you need to make sure that this care is documented in their care plan and that it is carried out. Female Hindu patients may wish to ensure that they can keep their legs, breasts and upper arms covered at all times. They may prefer to wear their own clothing during medical procedures and may object to wearing hospital clothing. Some Hindu patients may wish to wash prior to praying.

Sikh patients

Sikh patients may prefer to shower. The adult, male Sikh patient will have long hair, a beard and be required to wear a turban on his head. The hair of the female Sikh patient is held in a 'bun'. The hair of the Sikh patient must never be cut, as the head is the most sacred part of the body. Devout Sikhs may never completely remove their underclothes. They are required to push their underclothes down leaving them over one ankle, only removing them completely when clean underclothes are in position over the other leg. The Sikh patient may need to wash once or twice daily before praying.

Summary

The above discussion is a huge oversimplification of the religious issues involved with hygiene and religion, and we are indicating only the most frequent nursing interventions that you may need to provide. Reading widely about differing cultures and being open to learning from your patients are important if you are to provide effective nursing care.

> *Help with bathing involves nakedness, touch and the transgression of the normal boundaries of adult life. To receive such help thus represents one of the greatest watersheds of aging or disability . . . Only the very young, or people who cannot manage, are helped in these ways, and this is a powerful source of the infantilizing tendency in care work.*
>
> (Twigg 2000)

Twigg's statement is of great importance, and warns nurses of the dangers of infantilizing patients by robbing them of independence and thus providing poor nursing care. During any episode of delivering hygiene care, it is important to promote and preserve your patient's independent activity as far as possible. Your goal when providing personal hygiene care is to promote your patients' ability to care for themselves, and to assist them only until they have the necessary knowledge or strength to be independent. There is usually some small part of the care delivery process that your patient can undertake independently, unless they are too young or suffering from a chronic condition such as dementia, or if they are unconscious.

Having an understanding of the skin or the integumentary system will help you to appreciate the differences you might notice when delivering personal hygiene, and can alert you to signs and symptoms that may need attention.

Anatomy and physiology of the integumentary system

The integumentary system is considered to be the largest system of the human body. In an adult it is estimated to weigh about 4 kg (9 lb) and has a surface area of approximately 1.5–2 square metres (m^2). Its thickness varies depending upon where it is located and its function, so in some areas it is only 1.5 mm thick and in others it is as much as 4 mm (Marieb 2005). The integumentary system has two well-defined regions: the epidermis and the dermis. Enclosed within these two layers are the organs of the epidermis and dermis and the skin appendages: sweat glands, sebaceous glands, hair and nails. All of these structures provide a warning system, through receptors responsible for pain, pressure and touch, and a defence system of protection so that everyday encounters do not damage the internal structures of the human body. The skin is the body's first line of defence and is also important in the regulation of body temperature and fluid balance.

The structure of the skin

The epidermis is the outermost region of the skin and is composed of layers of epithelial cells that naturally regenerate. Beneath the epidermis is the dermis. This is made up of connective tissue and constitutes the bulk of the skin (Figure 9.1). The dermis and epidermis are firmly attached to each other through a basement membrane. To keep the dermis healthy, it has a blood supply that in some areas of the body is very rich and involves a process

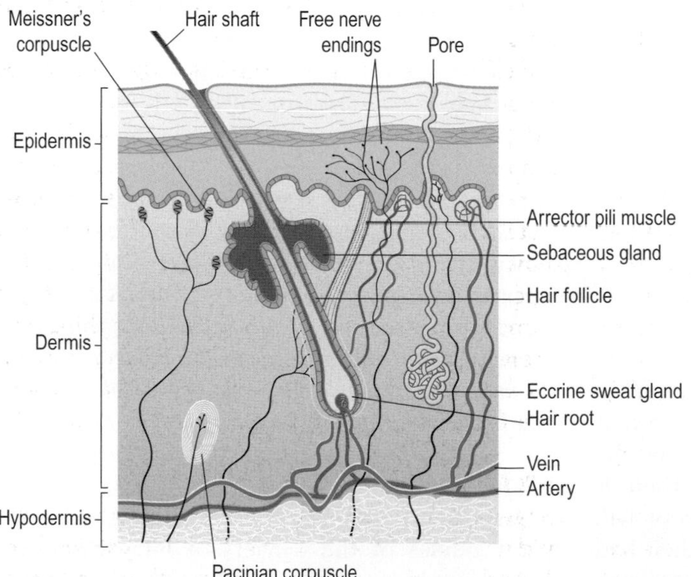

Figure 9.1 • A cross-section through the skin.

called diffusion from dermal blood vessels. Beneath the dermis lies the subcutaneous tissue. This is not strictly considered to be part of the skin, but it does contribute to its protective nature. It is made up of mainly adipose tissue and it anchors the skin to underlying organs. It acts as a shock absorber and provides a storage place for excess lipids and so insulates deeper body tissues.

The epidermis

The epidermis is avascular (without blood vessels), stratified (in layers), squamous (sheds and replaces its cells) epithelium, containing keratin (a protein) and cells that have important functions. These cells are:

- Keratinocytes.
- Melanocytes.
- Langerhans cells.
- Merkel cells.

Keratinocytes

Most of the epithelial cells of the epidermis are keratinocytes. Their main role is to produce keratin, a tough protein that contributes to the protective qualities of the epidermis. As keratin is made within a cell, the cell becomes harder and flatter (Herlihy & Maebius 2003). Without keratin the skin would not be able to provide protection against water loss and provide resistance to biological, chemical and physical damage. Keratin also makes the skin waterproof. Some substances, however, can gain entry to the body via the skin, including steroids, fat-soluble vitamins (A, D, E and K), acetone, lead and mercury (Marieb 2005). This also means that some types of medication can be administered via the skin (e.g. nicotine and glyceryl trinitrate). If the skin becomes excessively dry, then it may crack and provide a route of entry for invading micro-organisms such as methicillin-resistant *Staphylococcus aureus* (MRSA). This would also occur if the skin were subjected to trauma (cuts and abrasions). When trauma occurs, a localized inflammatory response takes place, leading to redness, pain, swelling, increased heat and possible loss of function of the affected area. These features of inflammation arise as a result of increased blood flow (hyperaemia) to the area with an associated dilation of the underlying dermal blood vessels. There is also migration of white blood cells and macrophages to the area in order to destroy any bacteria or other foreign substances present at the site and to initiate the healing process (Marieb 2005).

Melanocytes

Skin colour is made up of a pigment known as melanin; this is produced by melanocytes, which are found distributed amongst the keratinocytes of the deeper layers of the epidermis. Once melanin has been made by the melanocytes, it is transported along slender 'highways' (processes) that protrude from the main body of the melanocyte. It is then exported out of these processes where it is taken up by the surrounding keratinocytes, which become stained by the melanin. Differences in skin colour appear to be attributed to the amount of melanin made by the melanocytes rather than the number of melanocytes, as all humans have approximately the same number of melanocytes (Marieb 2005). The skin is protected from the harmful effects of ultraviolet light (UV) radiation by the action of melanin. Once melanin is taken up by the keratinocytes it accumulates and forms a shield to protect the nucleus of the cell (and the deoxyribonucleic acid inside the nucleus) from the damaging effects of UV radiation from the sun.

Exposure to ultraviolet light (sunlight) increases the amount of melanin made by the melanocytes and contributes to changes in skin colour. In fair-skinned people who have had exposure to sun burn, particularly in their childhood, these melanocytes are known to change and develop tumours known as melanoma (see Case history 9.1). During exposure to strong sunlight and ultraviolet light, it is important to protect the skin by clothing and where this is not possible to wear a high-protection sun screen (see Case history 9.2); this is particularly important for babies and young children.

Langerhans cells

Langerhans cells are star-shaped and migrate to the epidermis from the bone marrow. They are a form of macrophage (a white blood cell that can ingest

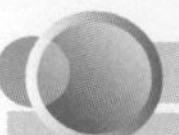

Case history 9.1

Caring for a patient with a mole on her back

Andrea is on placement in a gynaecology ward and is caring for a glamorous 30-year-old fashion model, Jerry, who has been admitted for minor surgery the next day. While Andrea is chatting to Jerry, she notices that she has unseasonably brown skin and discovered that Jerry uses a sunbed every week to top up her tan, because of her naturally pale complexion. Andrea is a bit concerned to hear about this as she knows that the incidence of malignant melanoma is rising in the UK, particularly in younger people. She asks Jerry if she has any itchy moles that she has noticed. Jerry shares that she does have one on her back that seems to be getting larger, and tends to bleed if she scratches it. Andrea realizes that these are the signs of skin cancer and that Jerry ought to be seen by a dermatologist or melanoma specialist as quickly as possible.

The house officer comes to see Jerry's mole and decides that it does need to be investigated further as a matter of urgency, and makes the necessary arrangements.

Andrea is curious to know more about these kinds of skin lesions as she thought it was only older people who are at risk, so she arranges to spend an afternoon in the melanoma clinic and observe patients being seen. She also visits the website of the National Institute for Health and Clinical Excellence (www.nice.org.uk) to see if there are any guidelines on treating people with skin tumours. On the website under 'cancer service guidance' she finds 'Skin tumours including melanoma. Improving outcomes for people with skin tumours including melanoma' (NICE 2006). This document provides an overview of the incidence of skin tumours as well as guidance on best practice in their management.

foreign protein such as bacteria) and are important for activation of the immune system. They too have slender processes protruding from a main body and these processes extend between the keratinocytes. Langerhans cells are responsible for the normal response of the skin to chemical or physical damage to the skin, and alert the lymphocytes of the immune system to their presence.

Merkel cells

Merkel cells are found where the epidermis and dermis meet. There are not so many of these and they are semicircular in shape. Adjoining each one is usually a sensory nerve ending. This arrangement is known as a Merkel disc and operates as a sensory receptor (touch).

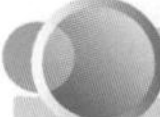

Case history 9.2

Caring for a patient with a mole on his face

First-year nursing student Michael was assisting Mr Marsh (a 65-year-old retired teacher) with his daily shower following knee surgery. Mr Marsh had had a kidney transplant 10 years previously and was taking immunosuppressant therapy to prevent his kidney being rejected. Michael noticed that Mr Marsh had a pale raised skin lesion on his forehead and asked him if he had noticed it. Mr Marsh thought it was probably a basal cell carcinoma as they are common in people who are taking immunosuppressants. Mr Marsh said he normally tried to protect his skin from the sun as these carcinomas tend to pop up quite often. In fact, he had already had three removed from his face and hands. Michael had read about skin cancers and was interested to speak to Mr Marsh about his experience of them. Mr Marsh was hoping that the house officer would arrange for him to be seen by the dermatologist or the melanoma specialist so that he could have it removed with a dose of radiotherapy. Michael agreed to talk to his mentor about it and perhaps get the house officer to come and see Mr Marsh. He documented his findings and his actions in Mr Marsh's care notes.

The layers of the epidermis

The layers of epithelial cells found in the epidermis are divided into four or five sublayers. Most areas of the skin have four layers, but in areas where there is a great deal of friction and wear, such as the heels or soles of the feet, there are five layers (Richardson 2003). The cells that compose the epidermis are capable of regenerating, and their progeny migrate from the basal layer to the surface, or stratum corneum, as they age.

From the base of the epidermis to the topmost visible layer, the layers of the epidermis are:

- Stratum basale (germinativum).
- Stratum spinosum.
- Stratum granulosum.

- Stratum lucidum.
- Stratum corneum.

Of these, the two most important are the stratum basale and the stratum corneum.

Stratum basale

This is the deepest layer of the epidermis and is the region in which new epithelial cells (keratinocytes) are constantly being made. A small percentage of the cells in this layer are stem cells that continually produce new keratinocytes via mitosis (cell division). Each stem cell divides approximately every 19 days and produces one daughter cell and one stem cell. The stem cells remain in the stratum basale and the daughter cells migrate towards the stratum corneum. It can take about 14 days for the daughter cells to reach the stratum corneum, and another 14 days to move through it (Haake et al 2001). Melanocytes are found here as well as some Merkel cells. As the epidermis does not have blood vessels, the cells in this layer receive their oxygen and nutrient supply via diffusion from the blood vessels in the dermis below. The further these daughter cells move from the basal layer towards the stratum corneum the fewer nutrients they receive and so they age and eventually die and are shed from the body (on a daily basis, millions of cells are lost through wear and tear).

Stratum spinosum

As the daughter cells move into this layer, they become less able to divide and are connected to each other via specialized intracellular connections called desmosomes. This layer is between five and twelve cells thick and it is here the cells become filled with keratin-rich filaments that become arranged around the nucleus.

Stratum granulosum

In this layer, which is between three and five cells thick, the keratinocytes are flattened. As well as containing the keratin-rich filaments, they also contain keratohyaline granules. These contribute to the formation of keratin in the upper layers of the epidermis. Lamellated granules are also evident within the keratinocytes here and they contain a glycolipid that has waterproofing qualities. The glycolipid is secreted into the extracellular spaces and helps to slow down water loss via the epidermis (Marieb 2005). Other changes that take place include loss of the intracellular organelles and the nucleus (Penzer 2002). By this stage in their progress to the upper layer of the dermis the keratinocytes are dead and they form an important part of the stratum lucidum.

Stratum lucidum

This layer provides protection to the more delicate tissues beneath the dermis. It is much thicker and is found in areas that are subjected to pressure or frequent wear and tear such as the soles of the feet and the palms of the hand or calluses.

Stratum corneum

This is the thickest layer of the epidermis ranging from either 15 cells thick on the upper arm, to hundreds of cells thick on the palms of the hands and soles of the feet. The cells in this layer are fully keratinized, dead cells and are continually being sloughed off as a result of friction (via washing, putting on clothes and taking them off, scratching, etc). However, as these cells are lost, they are constantly replaced by cells that have been moving up through the lower layers of the epidermis from the stratum basale. On average, an adult can shed 18 kg (40 lb) of skin cells in a lifetime (Marieb 2005).

The dermis

The dermis is connected to the epidermis through a basement membrane, covered with the basal layer. This basement membrane provides the skin with some protection from stretching and shearing forces. The dermis is made up of connective tissue, making it flexible and strong and has two distinct regions: the uppermost papillary layer and a lower reticular layer. It is richly supplied with nerve fibres, lymphatic vessels and blood vessels, and also contains oil and sweat glands, hair follicles and sensory receptors. These structures are embedded in a gel-like matrix called the 'ground substance'.

The ground substance

The ground substance is a formless gel-like substance made up of proteins, interstitial fluid and proteoglycans (Marieb 2005). It fills the spaces between the fibres and cells of the dermis. The proteins act like glue, allowing the cells to adhere to other structures of the matrix, and the proteoglycans help to trap water. Nutrients and other substances are able to diffuse through this watery ground substance. Embedded within the ground substance are three different types of fibres (see Table 9.1).

The layers of the dermis

The papillary layer

This is a thin layer of connective tissue that is highly vascular with a loose arrangement of fibres. Some sensory receptors are found in this layer; for example, Meissner's corpuscles, which are stimulated by light pressure (e.g. stroking) applied to the epidermal surface. There are also pain receptors in this region.

The reticular layer

This constitutes 80% of the dermis (Marieb 2005). The fibres in this layer are more densely packed. In the lower part of the reticular layer may be found other sensory receptors; for example, Pacinian corpuscles, which are stimulated by heavy pressure applied to the epidermal surface. It is within this layer that many of the other structures of the skin are embedded (e.g. hair roots and sweat glands).

Cells of the dermis

These include fibroblasts, macrophages and mast cells.

Fibroblasts

These are mitotic cells that are responsible for making the fibres of the dermis.

Macrophages

These are cells that actively phagocytose (engulf) foreign substances such as bacteria, dust etc. They are especially important in the process of wound healing in the skin.

Mast cells

These contain large numbers of granules of histamine. The role of mast cells is to initiate an inflammatory reaction as part of the first-line defence mechanism when foreign substances (e.g. an insect sting, chemicals from a plant or animal bite, or bacteria) have invaded the dermis. Once activated, mast cells release histamine. Histamine then initiates the local inflammatory response. Blood vessels in the immediate area around the invasion, or tissue damage, dilate and become more permeable. Fluid then leaks out of the blood vessels into the surrounding tissue causing a localized oedema. Histamine is also involved in the local anaphylactic reaction which may be seen in the skin when it comes into contact with an allergen, as indicated by dermatitis, which some people contract from contact with hand soaps or detergents.

Table 9.1 Fibres within the ground substance

Fibre	Composition	Action
Collagen fibres	Protein	Provide the dermis with its tensile strength Able to bind with water providing hydration to the skin
Elastic fibres	Protein called elastin	Provide the dermis with its ability to stretch and recoil Are visible when the person has lost weight (such as after pregnancy) and leave marks known as stretch marks
Reticular fibres	Finer than collagen and elastic fibres	Provide support for the structures found within the dermis (e.g. blood vessels)

The skin appendages

Hair

In humans, hair does not appear to have any physiological function. Eyebrows and eyelashes do protect the eyes by preventing dust and sweat from entering them. Adults have two type of hair: vellus, which is usually fine and pale and covers the body; and terminal hair, which covers the scalp and is found in the eyebrows (Marieb 2005). At puberty, terminal hair begins to grow in the pubic and axillary regions of both males and females. Areas of the body that do not have hair include the palms of the hands, the soles of the feet, the lips and around the nipples.

You will see from the diagram of the skin in Figure 9.1 that each hair has a root surrounded by a bag-like structure called the follicle embedded in the dermis. The hair follicle is derived from the epidermis and is composed of epithelial cells that are surrounded by a dermal connective tissue layer. Extending down from the root is the hair bulb where new hair cells are made through a process known as mitosis. These newly made cells produce keratin, which is the hard kind to give the hair durability, take up melanin from the melanocytes found in this region, to gain their hair colour, and then become part of the hair shaft. Our unique hair colour is through the action of these melanocytes found in the base of the hair follicle. Our genetic profile will determine how these different coloured melanins combine to create the hair colour. With age, melanin production decreases and the hair follicles can only generate grey and white hair. In times of famine or starvation many people develop a condition caused by a protein deficiency, known as kwashiorkor. It is characterized by the hair becoming coarse and losing its pigmentation. Some endocrine disorders cause similar changes to the hair.

On average we lose about 50 hairs every day. This process takes place in much the same way as we lose epidermal cells from the skin. Sometimes people lose more hair and this can indicate ill health or vitamin deficiency such as vitamin A deficiency, stress, fever, surgery, emotional trauma (Marieb 2005, Penzer 2002). By contrast, during pregnancy, there is an increase in hair growth, followed by hair loss in the 3 months after giving birth. Some medications such as minoxidil and phenytoin, may also increase hair growth (Quinn 2000). It seems that as humans grow older their hair growth starts to slow down, often in the fourth decade of life. This phenomenon appears to be related to atrophy of the hair follicle so that, as hair is lost, it is not replaced as quickly as it is when younger, leading to thinning of the hair or, more frequently in men, baldness (alopecia), and may be genetically determined (Marieb 2005).

Hair and heat retention

Heat retention can be assisted through the smooth muscle cells collected around the base of the hair follicle. These smooth muscle cells (called the arrector pili) contract and pull the hair follicle into an upright position. If you are exposed to cold temperatures, you can see this response with the effect of 'goose bumps' or 'goose flesh', caused by the surrounding skin of each hair being raised into a dimple. This action then traps a layer of warm air against the skin surface. Its effect is thought to help to maintain body temperature. However, its value for humans is questionable, as they have very little body hair compared to fur-coated animals for which this effect is undeniably important.

Sebaceous glands

Sebaceous glands are found all over the body except in areas such as the palms of the hands and the soles of the feet (Marieb 2005). They produce an oily substance called sebum, which is secreted either into a hair follicle or directly onto the skin surface. The sebum provides lubrication for the skin and hair, keeping them soft and moist. Without sebum the skin may become dry or the hair brittle. Many adolescents are only too well aware of the action of these sebaceous glands on their face, neck and back of the body when hormonal changes take place. Acne appears to be caused by an overproduction of sebum with an associated infection of the gland (caused by the bacteria *Propionibacterium acnes*), leading to a localized inflammatory response (Botek & Lookingbill 2001). Whiteheads are closed, blocked sebaceous glands and babies often have a lot of them over their face. Blackheads are simply the accumulation of oil and dust in the sebaceous gland, giving it a black appearance (Martini & Welch 2005).

Other factors that appear to affect sebaceous gland activity include fasting and age, which cause sebum secretion to decrease. Sebaceous glandular activity is high at birth, slowing down in early childhood and rising again at about 6–8 years of age. Maximum secretion occurs in the late teens and early twenties with a slow decline into old age (Botek & Lookingbill 2001) (see Case history 9.3). With sebum production low in young children and in the older adult, appropriate skin and hair care for patients in these age groups becomes extremely important.

Case history 9.3

Marianne advises a teenager about skin care

Nursing student Marianne has been on placement in the outpatients clinic; some of the placement has been in a dermatology clinic. During her last shift, Marianne had an opportunity to speak with Rehana aged 13 years, who is concerned about the recent development of blackheads (comedones) on her nose and chin. Rehana has also noticed that spots are appearing (papules and pustules) on her face and neck. Marianne explains that the changes are due to normal hormonal influences causing an increase in the production of sebum through enlargement and overproduction of the oil glands. Marianne also knows that when the oil glands are overactive and the canals become blocked, bacteria that normally live on the skin and in the oil multiply, leading to inflammation and infection.

Marianne suggests that Rehana should wash her face with a mild antibacterial soap twice a day and if her skin becomes more oily over the next few months she should wash her face more often. Marianne stresses that over-washing and the use of exfoliates tends to irritate the skin and will make acne worse; therefore, Rehana should not use any abrasive cleaners/pads.

Rehana then asks Marianne how often she should wash her hair. Marianne knows that the oilier a person's hair is the more often they should shampoo it; also that it is best to keep the hair off the face so that the oils from the hair are not transferred to the face. Rehana is concerned about her appearance and has taken to wearing an oil-based foundation cream as it provides a more effective cover for her acne. Marianne encourages Rehana to use a light cosmetic that is water-based and suggests she checks the ingredients to ensure that the first ingredient on the label is listed as water. Greasy applications such as cold creams, Vaseline and vitamin E products should be avoided.

Sweat glands

There are approximately 2.5 million sweat glands in the human body; there are two main types: the eccrine glands and the apocrine glands (Marieb 2005).

Eccrine glands

Living in a temperate climate, our bodies each produce daily an average of 900 ml of a watery substance with a low (acidic) pH of 4–6. This acidity maintains the ecology of the surface of the skin by creating a hostile environment for the bacteria that normally occur there (Marieb 2005). This acidic sweat is produced by the eccrine glands, of which there are between 144 and 339 per cm^2 of skin (Kuno 1956, cited by Hurley 2001), located all over the body. You may have noticed that your own sweat has a salty taste due to its composition of various salts (0.1–0.4% of sodium, potassium), small amounts of normal waste products from protein metabolism (urea, ammonia, uric acid), vitamin C and lactic acid. Sweat is colourless and odourless.

You will see from the diagram of the skin (Figure 9.1) that each sweat gland is a coiled tube embedded in the dermis, where the sweat is manufactured, and has a duct that extends to the skin surface where sweat is released. On contact with the skin sweat normally evaporates through a process of convection from the skin surface. This process takes with it heat from the body, making it an important component in the process of temperature regulation (we shall talk about this further on in this chapter). Deodorants containing aluminium compounds inhibit the production of sweat and act as a bacteriostatic, thereby reducing the odour that arises from the increase in bacteria that would otherwise occur.

Sweating and fluid conservation

Consider Case histories 9.4 and 9.5 concerning sweating and fluid conservation.

- What advice do you think Mrs Bailey should be given about drinking fluids?
- In the case of baby Abrahams, what should be your first action?

Sweat loss can also have important implications for fluid balance of the body. On a hot day, an excess of sweat can be lost, taking with it important salts such as sodium and potassium salts. Normally, as sweat travels up the duct to the skin surface, electrolytes such as sodium are reabsorbed back into the body. However, with excessive sweat loss, the sweat travels so quickly along the duct that much less of the sodium is reabsorbed. Fluid and, in some instances, salt replacement are therefore vital, especially in older patients or babies, and those who are unable to obtain their own drinks. Because a fever may also cause excessive sweating, fluid replacement therapy is fundamental to the care of these affected individuals. In some circumstances, fluid and salts may need to be given intravenously. Babies and young children are particularly vulnerable in hot weather due to dehydration and loss of vital electrolytes, leading to loss of consciousness and death if their condition is not resolved quickly.

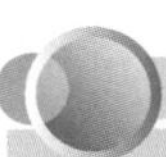

Case history 9.4

Mrs Bailey

Mrs Bailey is an 80-year-old lady who takes tablets for her heart condition. These medications include a diuretic that is intended to ensure that any fluid that she retains due to her heart condition is excreted. However, on this day, the weather is extremely hot and Mrs Bailey is sweating profusely to keep cool. Her urine output is very low, but she has no swelling of her ankles. She is reluctant to drink very much as she believes it could make her heart condition worse.

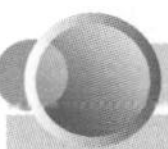

Case history 9.5

Baby Abrahams

You are giving Baby Abrahams a bath. You notice that his skin is very sweaty and that his fontanelles are quite depressed. He is listless and, although he is making repeated sucking noises, his tongue is dry. All these are signs of a baby who is severely dehydrated.

Apocrine glands

The second type of glands that are in the skin are the apocrine glands. These are not so widely distributed over the body and are found predominantly in areas where there are hairs and lymphatic glands, such as the axillary and genital areas. Apocrine glands are larger than eccrine glands and empty their secretions via ducts directly into the hair follicles. The sweat produced by these glands is similar in composition to that produced by the eccrine glands; however, it also contains lipids and proteins, giving it a milky, odourless appearance. If a person is unable to maintain good hygiene of these areas, the bacteria normally living on the skin surface are able to multiply by feeding off the lipids and proteins from the secretions from the apocrine glands. Their subsequent decomposition results in the characteristically musky odour, also known as body odour (BO). The volume of apocrine sweat is quite small, although it increases during pain, or when an individual is frightened or upset and during sexual stimulation (Herlihy & Maebius 2003). It has no role in thermoregulation.

Nails

Nails are a modification of the epidermis and evolve from the stratum basale, which also forms the nail bed. The structure of each nail comprises a body (the transparent visible region), a free edge and a root that is embedded in the skin. Beneath the body of the nail is the nail bed which has a good blood supply, giving nails their pink hue and

Table 9.2 Functions of the skin

Protective function	Active agents	Process
Chemical	Melanocytes pH of the skin	Melanin protects the skin against ultraviolet radiation light from the sun Acidity of the secretions kill off any bacteria
Physical	Intact skin Keratin Glycolipids	Whilst the skin is intact no micro-organisms can penetrate the epidermis Keratin provides durability and toughness Glycolipids provide lubrication and this in turn waterproofs the skin
Biological	Epidermal Langerhans cells Dermal macrophages	Present foreign substances (bacteria/viruses) to cells of the immune system (lymphocytes) Macrophages in the dermis can actively ingest (phagocytose) foreign substances and present them to lymphocytes to be destroyed

the necessary nutrients for regeneration. Like the dermis, the nail is constantly changing its cell structure. This may be noticed if your patient is a child or young adult with a congenital abnormality of the heart or in an adult with a chronic cardiac or respiratory disorder causing severe dyspnoea (breathlessness) such as congestive cardiac failure or emphysema. In patients with these kinds of disorders their nail shape changes, with the finger tips becoming broader and the nail curved, giving a distinctive club shape (Martini & Welch 2005).

Nail growth starts from the nail matrix in the nail bed, with nail cells filling with keratin to provide strength; then as the nail cells move away from the blood supply they die and are pushed outwards across the nail bed, extending the length of the nail body. The hard keratin that makes nails tough gives them the ability to protect the soft distal aspects of the fingers and toes. Without fingernails it is often difficult to pick up or to open objects.

Functions of the skin

You will have gathered by now that the skin has a range of functions:

- Protection.
- Thermoregulation.
- Sensory reception.
- Store and synthesizer of essential substances.
- Excretion.

Protection

By providing a continuous barrier that envelopes all the body structures, the skin provides an effective first line of defence against damage from a range of pathogenic substances. This protective function of the skin takes place in three ways: chemical, physical and biological (see Table 9.2).

Thermoregulation

An equally important feature of the skin is its role in the maintenance of body temperature. Normal core body temperature is 37°C, but it is often within a range of 35.6–37.8°C (Marieb 2005). The maintenance of core temperature is essential for the normal functioning of cellular enzymes within the body. The temperature-control centre in the body is the hypothalamus. It is situated within the brain, just under the thalamus at the top of the brainstem (Marieb 2005).

Decreasing body temperature

The body has two kinds of thermoreceptors, which are able to monitor the core temperature of the body. These thermoreceptors are responsive to information from both peripheral thermoreceptors (in the skin) and central thermoreceptors that monitor the temperature of the blood and these provide the hypothalamus with important information about temperature changes. Once the hypothalamus receives information about an increase in body temperature, various mechanisms are activated in order to promote the loss of heat from the body. These mechanisms use the structures in the skin to activate three specific processes to maximize heat loss: radiation, convection and conduction. Enabling this to happen is the good blood supply to the dermis. The hypothalamus sends chemical messengers to the peripheral blood vessels to dilate, increasing their diameter and thus increasing the flow of blood through the capillaries. This allows more blood to enter those vessels just below the skin surface, causing heat to be lost via radiation, conduction and convection. A good example of this happening is if you take a very hot bath, or shower. You will notice that if you are fair-skinned it becomes very pink, and warm, due to the vasodilation and consequent increased blood supply. You may well feel sleepy as the brain attempts to reduce energy (and thus heat) production in order to reduce the body temperature.

If the vasodilation does not resolve the high temperature, then sweating will occur. Sympathetic nerve fibres activate the sweat glands to increase sweat production. The sweat rises to the skin surface where it then evaporates, absorbing and dissipating body heat in the process.

Providing the surrounding environment is dry, heat loss via evaporation is very effective. However, if there is high air humidity, evaporation is less effective and heat loss is impaired. Generally though, as a result of the above mechanisms, body temperature will return to its normal range.

Increasing body temperature

By contrast, if the core body temperature starts to fall, the hypothalamus responds with contrasting mechanisms to ensure that heat is generated and the core temperature is maintained as far as possible.

With constriction of the blood vessels within the dermis, the blood flowing to the skin is reduced and heat loss is restricted. Because blood flow to the skin has reduced, the skin temperature drops to that of the external environment and will feel cold to touch. If this process is insufficient to maintain the core temperature then shivering occurs. Shivering is involuntary, intermittent contraction and relaxation of skeletal muscle and creates heat within the body. If the person is conscious and mobile, they will also want to move around to generate more energy and heat.

A further strategy of the body is to increase the metabolic rate by secreting a substance called norepinephrine (also known as noradrenaline). Norepinephrine is released from sympathetic nerve fibres, increasing the metabolic rate and thus causing heat production to go up. It also causes the person to feel very energetic (or jumpy) and to move around, thus generating heat. These mechanisms are designed to ensure that body temperature is able to return to within its normal range. However, if this does not happen (e.g. when the person is paralysed, or unconscious or immobile for other reasons) and the body temperature continues to fall lower, then the person will suffer from hypothermia and, unless artificial means of slowly warming them are used, they will gradually lose consciousness and die.

The skin as a sensory organ

The skin has a very good supply of various sensory receptors that are located in the dermis to help the body to monitor external stimuli such as pressure or pain, hot or cold. To protect the body from extremes of heat and cold it has a plentiful supply of nerve cells specially designed to interpret the sensation throughout the dermis – the peripheral thermosensors.

Meissner's corpuscles respond to light touch or caresses of the skin and are located close to the surface of the dermis (papillary layer). The Pacinian corpuscles, on the other hand, sit deep in the dermis and respond to deep pressure and impact to the skin. All these receptors are wired up to the central nervous system and so the brain receives stimuli from these cells rapidly, when the system is functioning effectively. Certain parts of the body that are more likely to be exposed to these kinds of extremes (e.g. the lips and face, fingertips and genital areas) have a higher ratio of nerve sensors and so are more sensitive than other parts (Scanlon & Sanders 1995). People who have damage to the sensory nerve pathways (e.g. those with some vitamin B deficiencies, or neurological disorders) will not feel pain and so are at risk of tissue damage. People who are confused or who have brain damage or cognitive disorders may not recognize the significance of pain and so are also at risk of tissue damage.

The skin as a store and synthesizer of essential products

The skin has the capacity to store excess substances such as calcium and iron and some forms of fatty substances. Sometimes these fatty substances are stored as part of a system of synthesizing other agents such as vitamin D. We need vitamin D to absorb some essential minerals such as calcium and phosphorus, which are derived from our food through the digestive system (small intestine). However, we can not normally take vitamin D in our diet and it has to be derived from a chemical reaction with ultraviolet light sunlight in our skin. The epidermis contains a modified form of cholesterol which when exposed to ultraviolet sunlight is converted to vitamin D. This synthesized vitamin D becomes absorbed via the capillaries in the dermis into the venous blood and is transported around the body to those cells needing vitamin D for their normal functions (see also Chapter 8).

Beneath the dermis is the adipose tissue. This is an essential store for fatty acids and glycerol that has been removed from the lacteals and the bloodstream following a fatty meal and are surplus to the immediate needs of the body (see also Chapter 8). During the subsequent period, or postabsorptive state, the body draws on this store to replenish the level of energy available for normal cellular function. If you take more than is necessary, then the store of fat deposited in the adipose tissue will get bigger (Martini & Welch 2005).

Excretion

The most important organs responsible for excretion of water and water-soluble waste products are the kidneys. However, a small amount of excretion does take place via the skin. You will remember from our description of the eccrine and apocrine sweat glands that they secrete small amounts of urea (produced as a result of protein metabolism), ammonia and uric acid, along with minerals such as sodium and water. You will remember that sweating is greatest on hot days, during intensive exercise or during a fever. In normal circumstances when sweat is excreted and travels up the sweat gland duct to the skin surface, most sodium chloride in the sweat is reabsorbed. However, on a hot day, or if an individual has a fever, there may be a dramatic increase in the amount of sweat produced. In such events, sweat often travels up the duct so quickly that there is less time for the sodium chloride to be reabsorbed and consequently more of it is lost.

Skin in the older adult

Skin changes

If you compare your own skin with that of a child and with that of an older adult, you may notice that there a number of differences. These differences are part of the natural responses to health and illness and ageing. As people age, they notice changes to the structures within the integumentary system. Skin care products are often sold with the promise that they will combat the symptoms and signs of ageing, and some even promise to hold back the natural changes. These changes are associated with loss of collagen and the subsequent loss of elasticity, leading to a greater fragility of the structures and less resistance to wear and thus they are less able to heal and repair injuries. These changes take place at a different rate depending upon the health of the individual. Some of the symptoms that older adults complain of are: skin that is dry and itchy, wrinkling, age spots, loss of sensitivity to temperature changes, increased sensitivity to pain or pressure. Older people living in dry climates tend to develop a condition known as xerosis. This is where the changes in the stratum corneum cause the skin to become dry and scaly; it is therefore more permeable and thus allows more perspiration to be lost (Martini & Welch 2005).

Wrinkling of the skin

With increased ageing, the collagen fibres in the dermis begin to disappear; thus, because these fibres provide structure (or scaffolding) to the dermis, it begins to sag or wrinkle. The loss of collagen also reduces the elasticity of the skin and thus its ability to stretch and recoil. You may notice this in an older patient who has ankle oedema – their overlying skin looks tight and glossy.

Age spots

The production of melanin gives skin its colour. With ageing, less melanin is produced, causing the skin to become paler in some individuals. However, this change is not uniform and some melanocytes produce more melanin, creating localized spots of increased skin colour in areas that are exposed to the sun (Benbow 2002).

Dry, scaly and itchy skin

Many of the conditions that we are discussing in relation to ageing can happen at any age, but as people become older they are at greater risk of such changes developing. With ageing, the skin becomes thinner and translucent, making it easier to see the underlying veins and arteries. This is caused by a slowing in the regeneration of epidermal cells, which also become larger and more irregular in shape (Herlihy & Maebius 2003). The normal daily production of sebum that lubricates the skin and makes it weatherproof diminishes, thus making the skin dryer and reducing its resistance. This can lead to skin problems such as pruritus (itchiness) and dermatitis (inflammation of the dermis), which may become more evident. If the general condition of the person's vascular system is poor, then there may also be a reduction in dermal blood supply, giving the person cold peripheries (e.g. fingers and lips), and the healing of minor wounds such as scratches and cuts may take longer. There are also consequences if the person has surgery, as their ability to heal the incision may be reduced. With these changes, older people are more sensitive to pressure on the skin caused by sitting in one position for any time, or wearing ill-fitting footwear, resulting in sores and ulcers that are very difficult to heal.

Increased risk of damage

Ageing has an effect on the blood supply to all the organs and nerves in the body and this can reduce the effectiveness of the sensory receptors. With loss of the supportive, protective layer of tissues, the skin is at greater risk from damage. Sometimes the individual may be unaware that is has happened if their sensory receptors are not responding effectively. Similarly, with increased fragility of the capillaries and other blood vessels lying unprotected immediately below the dermis, simple knocks or handholds can result in damage to the vessels and result in bruising. Also, some medications (e.g. corticosteroids) can increase the risk of bruising.

Increased risk of infections

There is a reduction in the number of Langerhans cells in the skin with ageing, making it less effective as the body's first line of defence (Benbow 2002). By now you will have realized that any kind of breech in the skin can predispose the person to infections; this risk is greater if the person's natural defences are reduced as a result of ageing.

Hygiene, safety, comfort, privacy and dignity

In her 1992 text, 'The emotional labour of nursing', Smith (1992, p 1) wrote:

> *It was the 'little things' that made the qualitative difference to patients' lives; little things such as dressing in their own clothes, manicuring their nails, making sure their hearing aid worked and their glasses were clean. As one student put it, in the elderly ward, the functioning hearing aid was just as much a lifeline to survival as the intravenous infusion was to the postoperative patient on the acute surgical ward.*

From the above quote it is evident that it is the seemingly insignificant things that make a significant difference to patients (Figure 9.2), and especially when assisting them with their personal hygiene. As Nicol (2004, p 79) indicated:

> *The skin needs to be kept clean in order to prevent infection, but the physical aspects of washing and bathing are only a small part of nursing aims to provide holistic care, which means care that involves much more than just meeting physical needs; it means taking into account the physical, psychological, emotional, social and spiritual aspects.*

Whenever you give care, you need to first explore factors that may affect your patient's ability to carry out their own personal cleansing and dressing and what help they need to undertake these activities. In the process of providing assistance it is important that you draw on your scientific and artistic nursing knowledge (e.g. interpersonal skills, knowledge of anatomy and physiology, knowledge of safe handling and moving) when you help your patient with their personal cleansing and dressing, while at the same time utilizing the principles of prevention of cross-infection.

Skin hygiene is important to prevent infections, but it is also important to remember that you have to be careful that you are not overzealous and wash people (particularly older people) too frequently or use soaps and towels that are abrasive and drying to the skin, otherwise natural oils will be removed from the skin, causing it to become dry and thus at risk of cracking and susceptible to infection (see Case history 9.6). Washing and bathing can provide an opportunity for a social experience between the nurse and the patient, an opportunity to listen to patients' experiences of health and ill-health and so to learn from them whilst also giving comfort and reducing anxiety (Nicol 2004). When preparing to deliver the care, it is a good idea to ask your patient what their normal routine is and to try and follow it as closely as possible. For example, some people prepare to have their main wash at the end of the day, whereas others prefer a morning bath or shower. Most people use the toilet before washing, so it is a good idea to provide your patient with an opportunity to use the toilet or bedpan before you start any procedure.

Patients who are confined to bed usually have a thorough wash each day. This can be refreshing

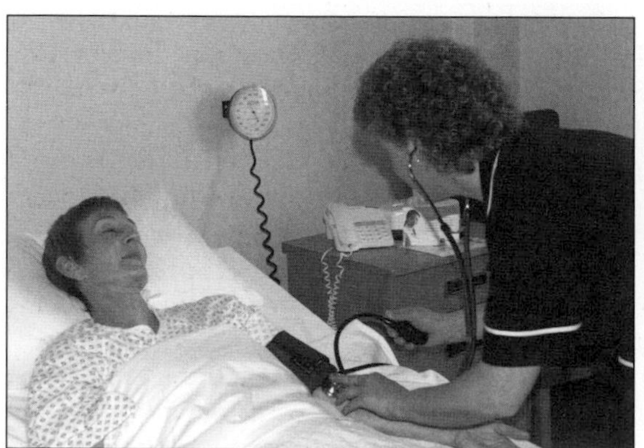

Figure 9.2 • Providing privacy when taking a blood pressure.

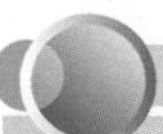

Case history 9.6

Caring for an older adult

Mrs Walton is a 72-year-old widow complaining of dry skin. Sophie is in her first year of nursing and is caring for Mrs Walton over this shift. Sophie has just completed learning about the skin in a recent seminar discussing the care of older people and can recognize the links with her current placement experiences. She discusses with Mrs Walton the water temperature that she prefers and tries to ensure that it is not too hot or too cool by testing it with her elbow and asking Mrs Walton to check if it is alright for her. (Sophie remembers to check that Mrs Walton's sensory receptors for heat and cold are healthy.) They discuss the benefits of using a cream-based bath lotion or a mild cleansing cream when bathing; applying handcream or a massage oil is beneficial to relieve dryness. Using a humidifier in her home might be useful to relieve any atmospheric dryness and Mrs Walton might find it helpful to increase her fluid intake to at least 2 litres of water a day and to avoid drinks that have a diuretic effect such as coffee and tea. Mrs Walton enjoys her evening bath as she finds it helps her to sleep. Sophie also explains that, after her bath, Mrs Walton should apply body lotion to counteract the drying effect of the water, or she may find it better to take a shower.

rather than cleansing. Your patient may be able to do much of this themselves with just a little help from the nurse or their carer, or they may require your full assistance in a procedure known as a blanket or bed bath. It is called this because the bed clothes are removed from the top of the bed, but to keep your patient both warm and protected from exposure they are covered with a blanket. Throughout the procedure it is important to try to expose only the minimum amount of flesh and to keep the rest covered.

Patients who are suffering from the misfortune of incontinence of urine or faeces will need to have their skin cleansed and protected from the damaging effects and their bed linen changed.

Assisting your patient with their personal hygiene

Hygiene is the science of health.

(Perry & Potter 2002)

Personal hygiene is also very closely linked with a person's sense of well-being.

Our lives are, in fact, profoundly bodily based and the rhythms of the body and its care provide an existential foundation for day to day existence.

(Twigg 2000)

Hygiene has, more importantly, been described as a basic human right within a developed country.

(Young 1991)

Assisting with personal hygiene provides an excellent opportunity to assess the patient's physical and emotional state. When patients are critically ill, it is the nurses who provide this care, not care assistants.

(Nicol 2004, p 84)

Planning hygiene care

Before giving assistance with personal hygiene you must make a number of assessments regarding your patient:

- To what extent is your patient able to attend to their own needs?
- What factors might inhibit their ability to be independent?
- Do they have a wound that could inhibit movement?
- Do they have an intravenous infusion or any other invasive cannulation, or catheters?
- Can they initiate actions without prompting or help?
- Do they have any cognitive disability and any peripheral neurological or musculoskeletal damage that might affect independent movement?
- Is it likely to be painful for your patient to move and do they need analgesia?

Assessment of these factors helps you to decide how much your patient is able to do independently and how much help they may need, the type of bath that is required and how much nursing intervention is necessary. If your patient is a child, it may be appropriate to ask the parent to help assist or bathe their child with your support.

If your patient has a mental health problem and is depressed or neglectful of their appearance, then you are likely to need more time and patience to encourage them to attend to their hygiene needs and this may be part of their therapeutic care plan. If you are working in a care home for older people, it is possible that bath time is one of the few times in the day when your patient has any privacy and attention, so this luxury needs to be savoured and made special for them. If your patient is terminally ill then the act of providing hygiene care is a means of providing physical comfort and reassurance to both the patient and to their relatives. Seeing their loved one looking fresh, smart and clean can be very comforting and reassures them that they are being properly cared for.

Assessing your patient's capability and preferences is an important element of the bathing process and helps promote a sense of dignity and respect. Your nursing interventions should be designed to preserve or promote your patient's independence as far as possible and so your ultimate goal of care may be to facilitate your patient's ability to carry out a healthy level of personal hygiene without the need for assistance.

Assessing the state of the skin

One of your main objectives is to maintain the integrity of your patient's skin, so you need to observe for potential and actual risks of skin damage. Discussing these risks will help you to find out if there are any areas of soreness. The risk factors are related to internal (see Box 9.2) and external factors. All of the factors identified in Box 9.2 have a bearing on the likelihood of skin injury and the ability of the skin to regenerate itself in that event (Quinless & Blauer 1992), so you need to be mindful of these potential problems when helping your patient to bathe. External factors affecting risk of skin damage might be associated with the comfort of the bed or chair that the patient is using, especially if it is a hard surface and the patient has limited mobility.

Box 9.2

Internal risk factors to the skin

Nerve damage: leads to loss of sensation such as pressure, heat and cold, or pain, thus leading to risk of damage to the epidermis and dermis and, if allowed to continue, to the underlying muscle.

Dehydration or poor blood supply to the dermis: leads to poor healing or regeneration of the cells and loss of integrity.

Malnutrition: leads to poor integrity and healing of the tissues, and possible loss of the insulating and protecting subcutaneous layer of fat.

Immobility or paralysis: leads to continuous pressure on specific (bony) areas of the tissue and thus damage and death of the tissue if unresolved; immobility might be due to unresolved pain.

Excessive sweating (diaphoresis): leads to rubbing and soreness, especially in deep skin folds such as around the breasts and between the buttocks.

Incontinence of urine and/or faeces: leads to chemical damage to the skin (such as nappy rash found in babies).

Cognitive function: can the patient seek help if they are uncomfortable or wish to use the toilet?

Delivering hygiene care

Planning your work load

It is good practice to make a nursing round of all your patients at the beginning of your shift to find out how they are feeling and how and when they would like you to assist them with their care. You also need to assess whether they need pain relief and to allow sufficient time in your care planning for any analgesia to be effective. Developing a plan of action for your shift, based on your patients' wishes and your priorities, can reduce interruptions and help your work to go smoothly. More importantly, it means that your patients are fully engaged in their care planning. You may find it helpful to check if your patients need to use the toilet or need any medications, such as analgesia; this will mean that they are comfortable and rested while they are waiting for you. If you are caring for children then you may wish to plan your care delivery with the child's parents and when they are going to be available if they wish to be involved. If you are using bathing as a therapeutic activity in a mental health setting, then you will need to plan your time differently than if you are working in an acute care setting.

When you come to give care to your patient, it is important that you explain what you plan to do and obtain their consent. Once you have both agreed a plan of action, you need to check whether they need any medications such as analgesia, and whether they need to use the lavatory. Next you need to assemble all the required equipment, and arrange the environment to ensure that it can be as private and conducive to effective personal hygiene care as possible, including monitoring the room temperature and protecting your patient from draughts (Quinless & Blauer 1992).

The bed bath (Figures 9.3a & b)

The complete bed bath contains all the elements of the partial bed bath, so we will discuss them as if they are the same. The main difference is the extent to which the body is washed. Normally in a partial bed bath it is just the hands, face, axillae,

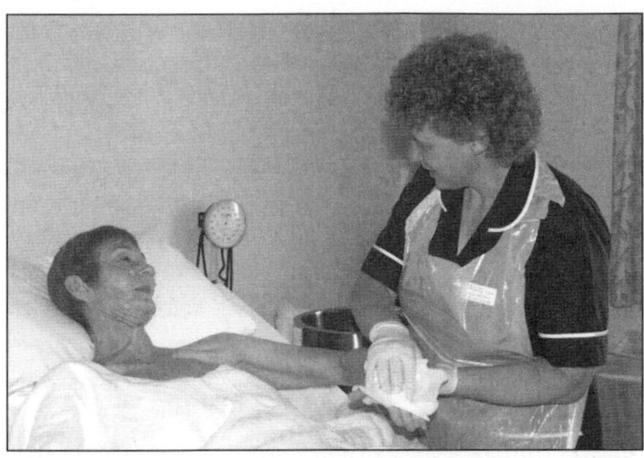

(a)

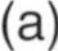

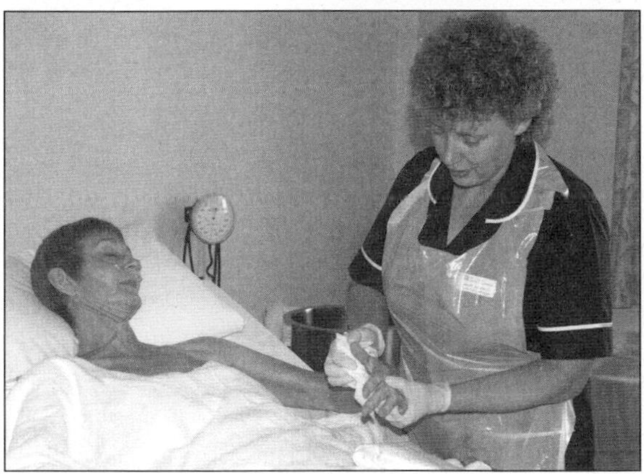

(b)

Figures 9.3a & b • Giving a patient a bed bath.

Box 9.3

Relevant equipment for a bed bath

Generally you will require:

- Sufficient blankets to cover your patient and keep them warm during the procedure.
- Sufficient flannels to wash the clean areas and the 'dirty' areas of the body, so two flannels (washcloths).
- Two bath towels.
- Soap and a soap dish, toothbrush, toothpaste and water and spittoon.
- The patient's toiletry items, including comb and brush, any skin lotion or cosmetics that your patient wishes to wear, nail brush and handcream.
- A cleaned washbowl and water that is hot enough to be the right temperature when washing the patient.
- Clean garments to replace the ones your patient is going to remove.
- A laundry bag and disposable gloves if your care means that you are going to make contact with the patient's body fluids.

and genital and anal regions that are washed. The partial bed bath is used if the patient is too weak to undergo a full bed bath, or as part of other forms of hygiene care such as when your patient has suffered from incontinence or diaphoresis (sweating), or before they rest for the night.

Reflecting on your normal routines when meeting your own hygiene needs will help you to remember what equipment you need to prepare (see Box 9.3). Also, to protect your clothing and prevent the spread of any micro-organisms from the bed linen and the patient you will need to wear a plastic disposable apron (Dougherty & Lister 2004).

Positioning the bed at a suitable height and being able to reach your patient comfortably without causing back strain is important. So you may want to move your patient's bed so you can access it from all directions. Raise the height of the bed to a comfortable working level so that you do not have to bend your spine and place yourself at risk of back strain. Depending upon your patient, your care plan may require the use of cot sides (protective side-rails) on the bed if there is any chance of their falling out of bed while you are not at the immediate bedside. That is not to suggest that patients should be left unattended at any point during washing unless it has been agreed with the patient and you have ascertained that the patient is capable of maintaining their own safety in your absence.

Preparation for the bed bath

Make sure the washbowl has been cleaned with a bactericidal solution to kill all micro-organisms and ensure that it has been rinsed sufficiently to prevent your patient being contaminated with the cleaning agent. Fill the washbowl two-thirds full with warm water (46°C approximately). Taking great care not to spill the water, bring the warm water to the patient's bedside. The water should be comfortably hot for you and your patient.

Keeping your patient covered with a blanket, strip the top bed clothing, either by folding it and placing it at the bottom of the bed or removing it directly into the laundry bag. Using protective gloves routinely is a contentious issue. They are symbolically clinical and may serve to act as a barrier between the patient and the nurse and increase your patient's sense of objectification and vulnerability. They are a potent symbol of the clinical environment, which is often full of equipment and personnel that appear threatening and leave the patient feeling powerless.

> *Power is exercised over . . . bodies which are required to be exposed and immersed in circumstances when they are naked and the administrator is not . . . Equipment reinforces the objectification which is always at play when someone is bathed . . . Equipment both distances the person from the direct human contact, putting a barrier between them and the operator and acting to objectify them . . .*
>
> *(Twigg 2000)*

However, the risk of cross-contamination of potentially harmful micro-organisms, from the nurse to the patient and vice versa, during hygiene care is very great and so the appropriate use of gloves must be discussed with the patient, taking great pains to ensure that your patient does not perceive an affront to their dignity, but understands the necessity for the prevention of cross-infection. Research has shown that, when patients understand why the nurse is wearing gloves, they do not find it demeaning or objectionable and may actually find it preferable (Woloski-Wruble et al 2000). Put on protective gloves if there is going to be any contact with the patient's body fluids.

Delivery of the bed bath

The detailed procedure for delivering a bed bath is described in Box 9.4.

Perineal care for patients

Patients may be embarrassed when a nursing student must wash their perineal area. Their embarrassment may be greater or lesser if the nurse is of the same gender, depending upon their beliefs and attitudes and the professionalism of the nurse. It may be necessary for you to provide someone of the same gender as the patient to chaperone you or to arrange for a different nurse to provide this care. Throughout the process it is important that you are careful to respect and protect the patient's privacy and dignity. You also need to develop a strategy to mask any embarrassment that you might feel and to alleviate your patient's. Part of this strategy is to make sure your patient understands what you are planning to do and ensuring that you have their consent. Ensure you have all the necessary equipment and that you have a bowl of water at a suitable temperature. Put on protective gloves, but explain the necessity for them to your patient.

Delivering perineal care to a female patient

You may be required to provide this care if your patient has just had a baby and had perineal sutures, or has had surgery to the perineal region such as a vaginal hysterectomy, or surgery to the anus and rectum. You may also need to provide it to patients who have an indwelling urethral catheter. Throughout the procedure you need to observe for any signs or symptoms of inflammation (redness, swelling), pain or discharge. If you are able to deliver this care effectively, your patient will feel more comfortable both physically and emotionally and any risk of infection will have been reduced. Keep as much of your patient covered as possible throughout the procedure and wear protective gloves.

If your patient is conscious and able to cooperate, ask the patient to bend her knees slightly and to spread her legs. Separate her labia with one hand and use the other to wash. Use a separate, disposable cloth using gentle downward strokes. Clean from the symphysis pubis at the front of the perineum towards the rear to prevent intestinal organisms from entering the urethra or vagina.

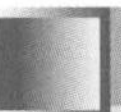

Box 9.4

Delivering a bed bath

Assist your patient to adopt a position that is comfortable and allows them to contribute to the procedure, if they are able to do so (this is likely to be semi-recumbent, supine position). If your patient is able to assist themselves then they need to be positioned so they can either reach the washbowl and equipment or for you to hand them the soapy flannel. Areas of the body that are more pleasant for the patient to self-care are the face and hands, and perineal region. Your discretion and tact in assisting your patient in cleansing the latter is vital.

Help your patient to remove their clothing and any other items, such as support stockings, that will impede your ability to observe and wash the legs and feet. Throughout the procedure it is essential that you take care to keep your patient warm and covered with blankets.

The rest of this procedure is described on the assumption that your patient is unable to assist in the procedure.

Start by washing the face and neck. If your patient has an eye infection, it is better to cleanse each eye separately using the prescribed lotion and cottonwool balls. Use separate eye pads to cleanse and dry each eye to prevent cross-infection and clean from the inner to the outer canthus. The same principle applies to washing the upper body and the perineal area, using separate cloths that are clearly identifiable. The same applies to the towels that you use to dry the perineal area, it should be different to the one used for any other part of the body. Using this principle will reduce the risk of contamination from the anal area.

While you are washing your patient, it is a good idea to talk to them, even if they are unconscious or confused, about topics of mutual interest. Talking to your patients while undertaking care delivery is a good way to reduce both your own, and your patient's, self-consciousness. In the process, it is good practice to observe your patient's condition such as observing for any skin abnormalities, whether their breathing is laboured from the effort of talking or undertaking any self-care; what their level of consciousness or coherence is like and any other factors that might be relevant to their medical condition.

Check whether your patient normally uses soap and water on their face or whether they prefer a cleansing lotion. If you are going to wash their face, place a towel under your patient's chin. Do not use soap to clean the eyes. If your patient tolerates soap on their face it may be applied to a separate face cloth prior to washing their face, ears and neck. Rinse thoroughly because residual soap can cause dry skin and discomfort. Dry the face, neck and ears.

Now wash your patient's chest. Turn down the blanket and cover the patient's chest with a towel. During the washing, rinsing and drying of the patient's chest and axillae you can notice whether there are any skin changes and the quality of respirations without your patient being aware and self-conscious, thereby making the result of the observation more accurate. If your patient is female, make sure you wash and dry carefully under each breast, taking care not to stimulate the nipples, and checking for any redness or soreness. Your patient may want to powder this area and use an underarm deodorant; make sure the skin is absolutely dry otherwise the powder will cake and cause irritation.

Before washing the upper limbs, cover your patient's chest, place a towel under the arm furthest away while keeping the other covered. Bathe and dry the arm using long firm strokes moving from wrist to shoulder. This motion helps stimulate venous circulation. It is nice if your patient can enjoy the sensation of being able to dabble their hands in the water and wash their hands. Observe the colour and temperature of the hand and nails, as a guide to the patient's peripheral circulation. Cover the distant arm and repeat these actions for the other arm. This may be a good opportunity to exercise your patient's joints and muscles to prevent contractures from lack of use. If you are unsure how to do this discuss, your patient's care with the physiotherapist and the registered nurse.

Cover the top half of your patient's body and expose your patient's abdomen. Bathe, rinse and dry these areas using the opportunity to observe the abdomen for signs of distension and tenderness. Make sure the umbilical area is clean and free from dead cells and talcum powder. Cover the patient as soon as washing is complete to maintain body temperature and preserve the patient's dignity. If your patient is able to self-care, this might be the moment to encourage them to wash their perineal area using a separate washcloth and towel and with your discrete assistance (see below).

If the patient is not able to wash their lower limbs themselves, then it is a good time to change the water. Cover your patient completely with the blankets

(Cont'd)

Box 9.4

Delivering a bed bath *Continued*

and ensure they are warm enough. On your return, position yourself and the washing equipment on the side of the bed to prevent back strain. Expose the most distant leg, place the towel underneath it and wash the leg. Flex the leg, wash and dry it, moving from ankle to hip to stimulate venous circulation. Observe the limb for any signs of abnormality in terms of its colour, skin integrity and temperature. Any pain, swelling and redness and heat, particularly in the calf region, may be indicative of deep venous thrombosis, a fairly common complication of reduced mobility, which should be reported immediately to the nurse in charge (Quinless & Blauer 1992). In the event of any of the signs of venous thrombosis, do not massage the limb during bathing, as there is a risk of dislodging the clot, enabling it to migrate in the circulatory system and become lodged in a more life-threatening location (Quinless & Blauer 1992). If your patient's condition merits, put the leg through a range of movements to exercise the joints and improve venous circulation and return and thus reduce the risk of your patient developing joint contractures. Repeat these actions for the other leg. If there are no problems with the flexion and extension of their leg, place the washbowl on the bed and, flexing their leg, assist your patient to place their foot in the water. Soak, wash and dry the foot observing skin condition, colour and temperature as a guide to peripheral circulation. If your patient has diabetes or any form of peripheral vascular disease it is a good idea to check for any skin lesions on the foot or signs of reduced circulation, such as reddening or blanching of the toes.

If the water remains sufficiently hot, assist your patient to lie on their side so you can wash their back. Make sure that they feel secure, or, if they are not conscious, seek the assistance of a colleague to support your patient while they lie in this position, or erect the cots sides. Make sure their head and neck are carefully positioned.

Place a towel alongside your patient's back and wash the back and buttocks with firm gentle strokes. Dry the back. Observe for any signs of redness where there are bony protuberances, such as the coccyx, top of the spine and shoulder blades. Tell the nurse in charge and make a written report in your patient's notes if you observe any signs of skin damage or pressure.

Cover your patient with the blanket. Providing the water continues to be at a satisfactory temperature, it is at this stage that you are going to wash the patient's perineal and anal regions.

Washing the perineal area

This area of care should be seen in some ways as separate from the rest of the wash because it carries with it special risks and significance to the patient. In terms of its significance to the patient, this is possibly the most private part of their body and, as such, the possibility of causing embarrassment and loss of dignity is great. In terms of risk to the patient, there is a great risk of cross-contamination of micro-organisms from the anal region to the genitourinary region. This section of the wash should be carried out using separate water and washcloths. At all times you need to remember the principle of moving from the 'clean' area to the 'dirty' area, so wash from the symphysis pubis to the coccyx.

If your patient is menstruating or losing blood vaginally, then, once you have finished washing and drying her, provide her with a clean sanitary towel and possibly her underpants, making sure to record any vaginal loss on her observation chart and notes.

When you have finished this procedure, help your patient to dress either in their daily clothes or in a fresh set of night clothes, and remake the bed with fresh bedding.

Store away the equipment, remove the bowl and water and clean the bowl thoroughly.

Avoid the anal area. Use a clean section of the washcloth for each wash stroke to prevent the spread of contaminated secretions. Discard the used washcloth in the infected waste. Then using a clean cloth, repeat the above actions to rinse the area. Follow this by using a separate towel to pat the area dry to prevent irritation from rubbing. If your patient has an indwelling catheter, then the area around the catheter needs to be washed carefully ensuring that any crusty exudations are removed, and taking care not to pull on the catheter and cause trauma and pain to the urethra. Dispose of the protective gloves in the infected waste (Dougherty & Lister 2004).

Delivering perineal care for the male patient

You may be asked to deliver this care to patients who have an indwelling catheter, or who have had surgery that might affect the nerve supply to the bladder or perineum, such as major rectal surgery.

Before starting the procedure, make sure your patient understands what you are planning to do and has given his consent. Wear protective gloves and an apron for the procedure and explain to your patient the reasons for doing so. If your patient is not conscious, it is still important to treat him as if he were and that you talk to him throughout the procedure, explaining each step. Ensure you have all your equipment and that you have protected your patient's privacy and dignity. Keep as much of your patient covered as possible throughout the procedure.

Start by holding the shaft of the penis with one hand and wash with the other. Using a separate, disposable washcloth, clean the penis starting at the tip, working in a circular motion from the centre to periphery to prevent organisms being introduced into the urethra. If the patient is not circumcised it is essential to retract the foreskin and clean beneath it. Remember to replace the foreskin in its natural position to prevent damage to the head of the penis as a result of constriction. Wash and dry the rest of the penis using downward strokes towards the scrotum. Wash and dry the scrotal region very gently to avoid causing the patient discomfort. Dispose of the contaminated gloves and washcloths in the infected waste (Dougherty & Lister 2004).

Following perineal care, cover your patient. Dispose of your soiled protective gloves appropriately. Empty the washbowl and clean the bowl.

Showers and baths

Wherever possible it is much better, both psychologically and from the perspective of reducing the risk of contamination, to offer your patient a shower (Greaves 1985). For some people, washing in running water is an essential part of their religious observances, so a shower is preferable to any other form of bathing. Taking a shower is also a more economical strategy as it significantly reduces the amount of water used compared with taking a bath.

However, both strategies can be hazardous unless care is taken to ensure that the patient's safety is ensured. Both the shower cubicle and the bath need to be cleaned before use by a patient and again immediately afterwards, thus preventing any waterborne bacteria to remain. Hot soapy water is normally sufficient. The area surrounding the shower and the bath must be kept dry and free from any risk of slips; it should also be appropriately heated and ventilated.

Showers

People who have difficulty standing unaided will prefer to have a seat to sit on under the shower so that they can bathe independently, and a non-slip mat also increases safety. It is important that your patient has a call-bell close to hand if they get into any difficulty and that you check that they are managing safely at regular intervals (say every 5–10 minutes). Temperature regulation is an essential aspect of showers and it is safer that each shower is fitted to function at a preset temperature to prevent fluctuations and scalding from water that is too hot.

It is often possible for patients recovering from surgery, with dressings, infusions and plaster casts to take a shower providing the affected area is well protected from the water and can be kept dry. If you have any doubt, consult with the nurse in charge of your patient's care. Some people may need constant supervision while taking a shower, in case they become confused or dazed and fall.

Preparing your patient with all the necessary equipment and clothing is an important aspect of the procedure, and it is a good idea to offer to take them to the toilet before they start their shower. Following the shower, make sure they have been able to dry themselves completely; back, legs and feet are often difficult to reach, so your patient may need help. When everything is in order and your patient has completed their toilet, help them return to their bed space or to go to a day room as appropriate, making sure that the shower cubicle is clean, safe and tidy for the next patient to use.

Baths

If your patient is unable to tolerate a shower, then it may be more suitable to offer them a bath. They may need assistance to prepare for this, and may need to use a hoist lift to get in and out of the bath. All such equipment needs to be checked before use to ensure that it is in safe working condition and is clean. Preparing your patient will include taking them to the toilet, and ensuring they have all their necessary washcloths, bath soaps, nail brush, towels, a change of clothing and any hair care materials (combs, slides, etc.), cosmetics, face lotions and/or shaving equipment they wish to use. It is wise to have a non-skid bath mat, floor towel, bath thermometer and cleaning agents to prepare the bath and after use.

Prepare the environment by making sure it is warm and free from drafts, and clean of any debris left by the previous user. A chair by the side of the bath will allow your patient to sit down whilst removing their clothes and afterwards whilst getting dried and dressed.

Clean the bathtub with a suitable bactericidal solution, preferably one containing hypochlorite, as viable organisms can survive in bath scum (Aycliffe et al 2000). Rinse the bath thoroughly to make sure that none of the solution remains to contaminate the patient.

Half-fill the bath tub with warm water at about 40°C. Use a thermometer to verify this temperature. If you do not have a thermometer then dip your elbow into the water to ensure that there is no risk of scalding your patient. But also ask your patient to check the temperature to reassure them that it is safe for them. You will remember that just below the surface of the dermis is a rich supply of blood vessels and that immersion in hot water will cause them to vasodilate, diverting the blood supply from other parts of the body, including the brain, and so could cause your patient to feel faint, dizzy and even have an irregular heart beat (syncope). A non-skid mat could be put into the bath to prevent your patient from slipping when getting in and out of the bath.

You need to escort your patient to the bathroom and provide assistance with undressing if necessary. Supporting your patient in a discrete and tactful manner is important and bath-time can be made into a pleasant social occasion between the nurse and patient if they need to be supervised during the whole procedure. Once your patient is safely in the bath and is able to attend to most of their needs, you need to arrange how long you will leave them alone, but making sure that a call-bell is at hand should they need help. This may require the door to the bathroom to be left unlocked, but with a clear sign indicating that it is in use. If you have any concerns, either do not leave your patient or stay discreetly close by so you can listen for any signs of help required (Dougherty & Lister 2004).

Bathing and hydraulic lifting equipment

If your patient is unable to get in or out of the bath and is unable to use a shower, then an alternative solution is to provide an hydraulic lift to lower and raise your patient in and out of the bath. Using the hydraulic lift requires both technical and interpersonal skills and sensitivity as such lifts are not necessarily the most comfortable system and patients can feel quite vulnerable using them (Twigg 2000). Before using an hydraulic lift, it is important that you learn how to use it safely and confidently at the same time maintaining your patient's dignity and privacy. Figure 9.4a–j illustrates the use of a hydraulic lift to transfer a patient to a chair. The importance of this was highlighted by a recent legal case. In the Queen versus East Sussex County Council and the Disability Rights Commission [2003], the precedent was set whereby, in certain circumstances, if a patient perceives an affront to their dignity as a result of the use of lifting apparatus, then nurses caring for that patient may be bound by law to use manual lifting techniques. This judgement was passed in spite of the fact that manual handling techniques may endanger the health of the person being lifted and of the nurse who is lifting (Fullbrook 2004). This point is made to stress the importance of giving clear explanations to your patient and the importance of using equipment in a manner that clearly demonstrates your commitment to maintaining

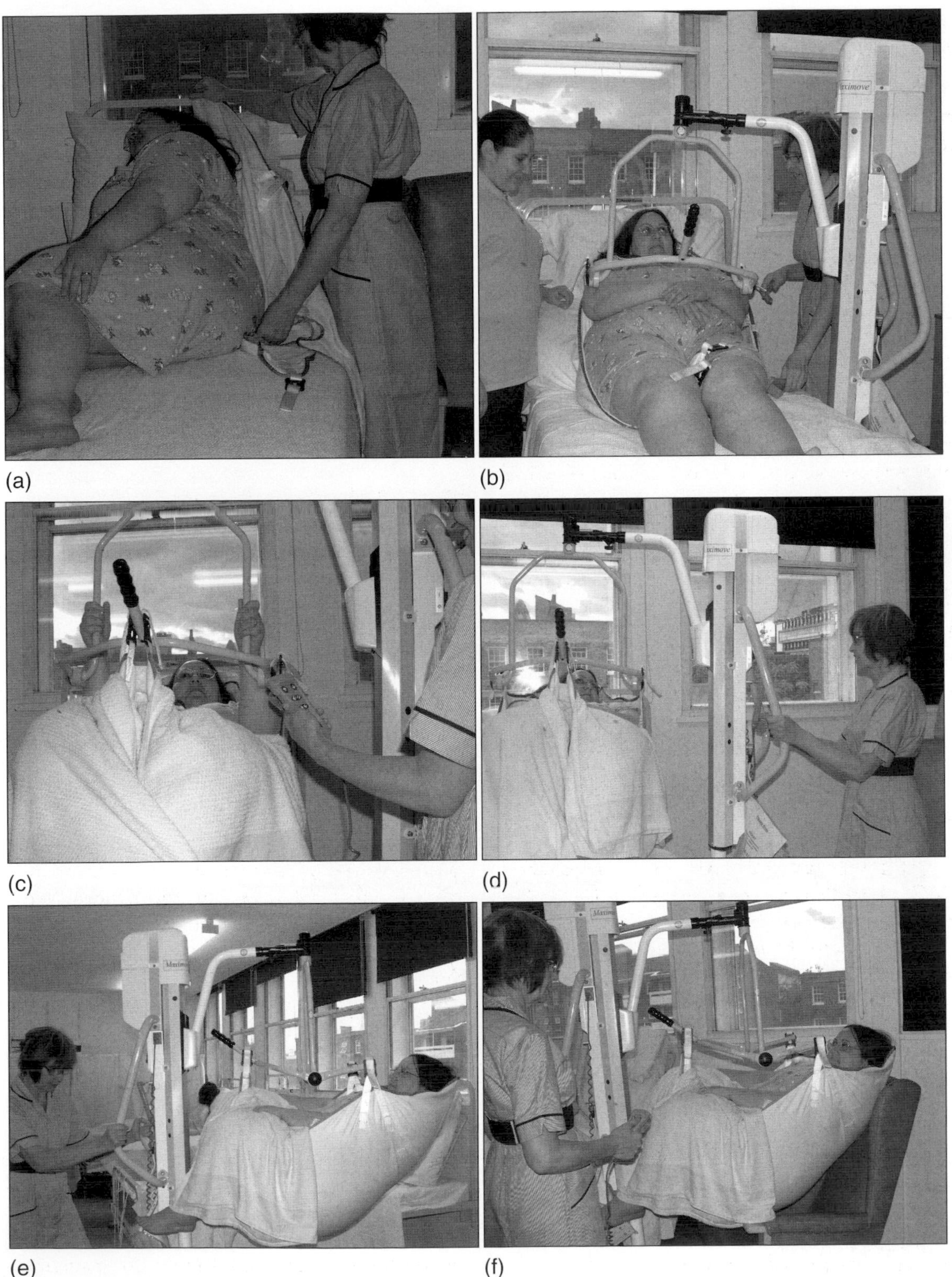

Figure 9.4a–j • Transferring a patient from their bed to a chair using a hydraulic lift.

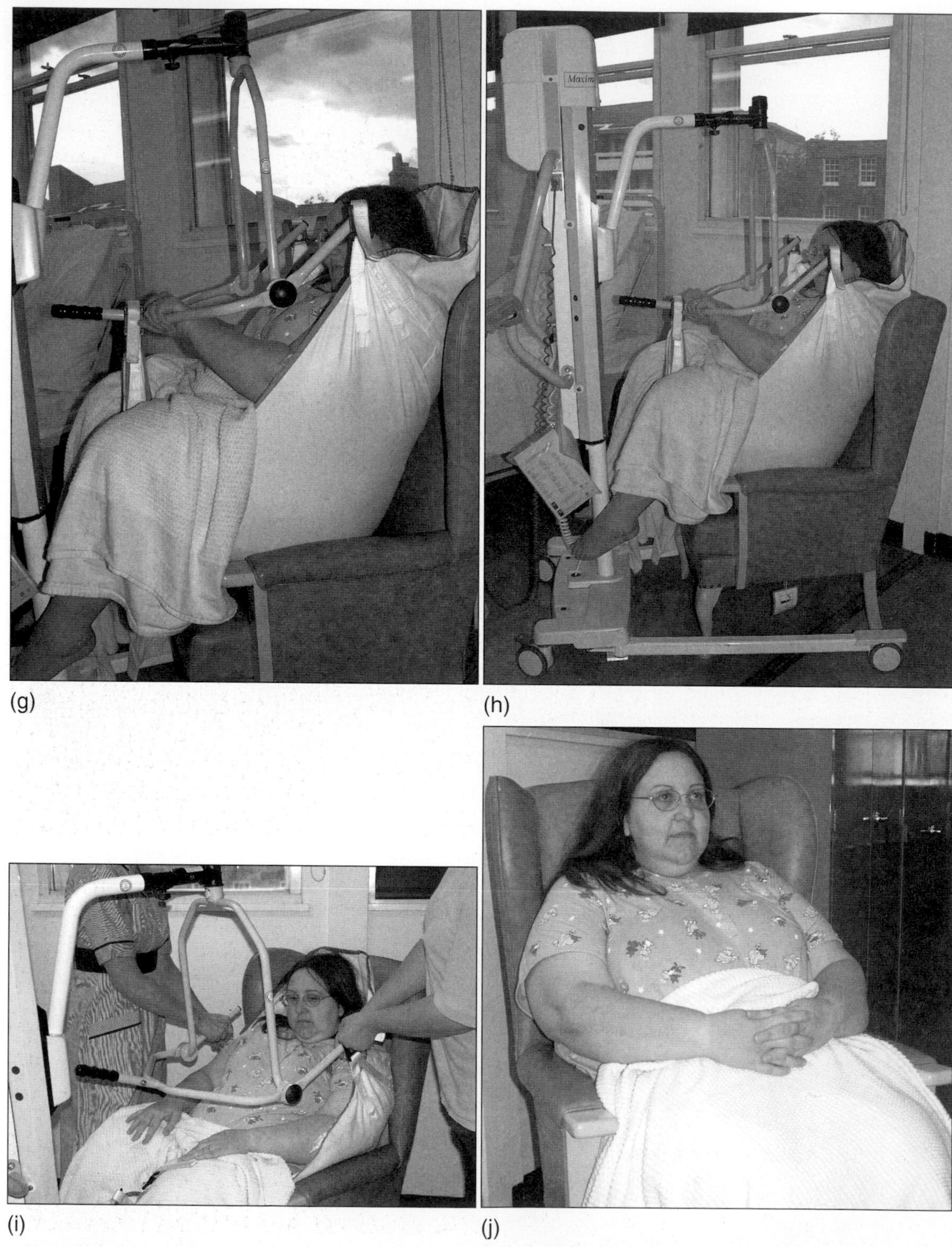

(g) (h) (i) (j)

Figure 9.4a–j • *Continued*

your patient's dignity and safety, whilst protecting your own well-being. When using the hydraulic lift it is important to make sure your patient is comfortable on the seat and does not slide off it, as it would then be very difficult to elevate them out of the bath safely. After use, it is vital that you wash the hydraulic chair down with either hot soapy water or with a hypochlorite solution.

Hair care

Having clean and comfortable hair has a profound impact and importance from a physical and psychological standpoint, and for many people the condition of their hair is a barometer of their sense of well-being (Perry & Potter 2002). Hair care includes combing, brushing, shampooing, rinsing and drying. The combing and brushing of the patient's hair stimulates scalp circulation, removes dead skin cells and debris and distributes natural hair oils throughout the hair. By washing and drying their hair, dirt and old oil is removed, hair condition is maintained and scalp irritation prevented.

The frequency with which hair care is given depends on your patient's personal preference, which may be influenced by the length and texture of the hair, your patient's condition, the duration of their hospital stay and any cultural, personal or religious preferences they hold. You need to be aware that some religions do not allow hair washing or brushing and that in some cultures the head and the hair must be always covered. Facial hair may be of religious significance to some patients. You need to be aware of any cultural and religious preferences of your patient and these should be logged in their nursing care plan and respected. It is good practice to either encourage your patient to groom their hair whenever they wash or for you to do this as part of your normal routine of supporting their personal hygiene.

Washing the bed-bound patient's hair

(Figures 9.5a–c)

If you have a patient who is unable to take a shower (and thus wash their hair), it may be necessary to wash their hair while they are in bed.

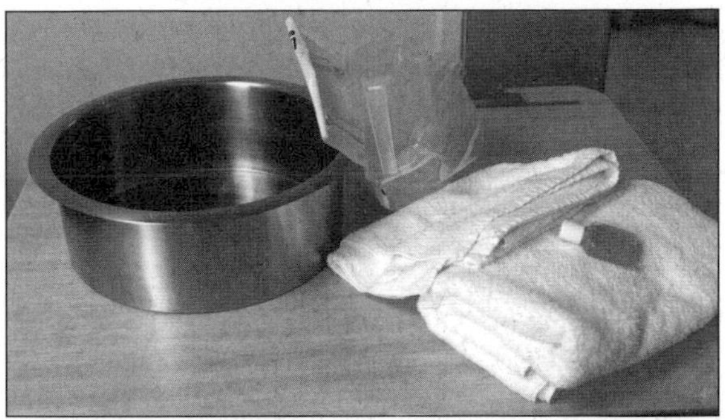

(a)

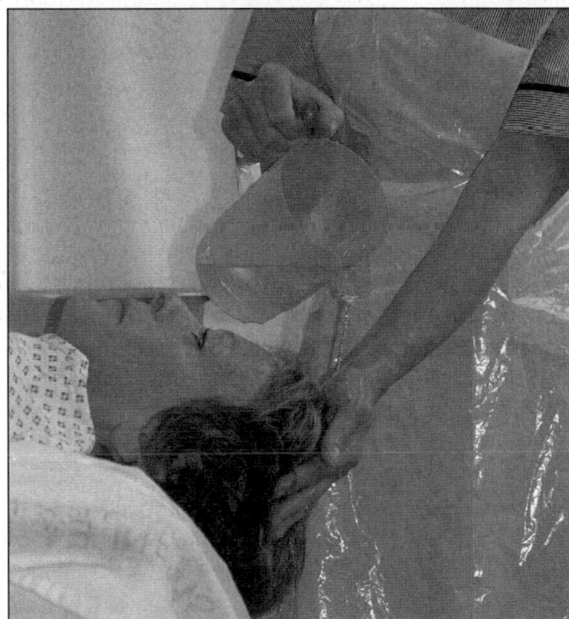

(b)

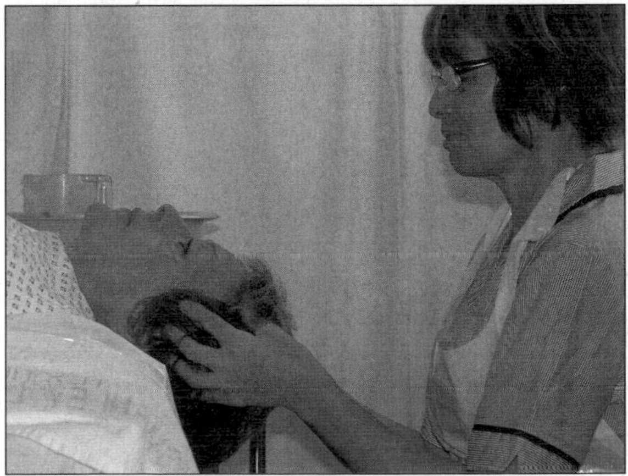

(c)

Figure 9.5a–c • Washing a patient's hair in bed.

Conducting this procedure is often an interesting challenge and can give your patient a great deal of relief and personal satisfaction. It may be possible to wash your patient's hair with them sitting forward and leaning forward over a washbowl. However, this is not always possible.

A second approach is to tackle the problem from the head of the bed. This method should not be used if the patient has any history of neck or back injury because of the risk of aggravating that injury.

First you need to discuss your proposed plan of action with your patient and then assemble all your equipment. You will need plastic sheeting to go across the mattress at the head of the bed and a plastic sheet to provide a conduit for the water to drain into a bucket on the floor.

Remove the head of your patient's bed, then position your patient lying on their back with their shoulders supported by a plastic-covered pillow so that their head is in contact with the plastic drawsheet. A shallow bowl containing warm water can be placed immediately under your patient's head. Water can then be poured over your patient's forehead and the hair bathed in the shallow bowl, any surplus water running down the plastic drawsheet into the bucket. Providing a scalp massage is good for the hair follicles and encourages the sebaceous glands to work, as well as being refreshing for your patient. Don't forget to make sure that all the shampoo is thoroughly rinsed off and the hair is squeaky clean. Your patient may wish to have a conditioner applied to reduce the tangles and to improve its condition, especially if they have dry hair or flaky skin on their scalp.

You can then wrap a towel around your patient's head to reduce the drips and help them sit back into a normal position. Remove all the equipment and if appropriate use a hair drier to dry the hair. Using an electric hair dryer takes some skill to prevent burning the scalp, and it is often better to move the drier over the scalp with your hand immediately beneath the blast of air so you can check if you are leaving it focused on one place for too long.

Any electrical equipment must first have been checked by a qualified electrician, for safety and compatibility with the hospital's electrical supply.

Observations of your patient's hair condition

While attending to your patient's hair care, observe for conditions such as dandruff, psoriasis and head lice. Psoriasis is a skin disease of the stem cells of the stratum germinatum and affects about 5% of the population. Instead of dividing every 20 days, these cells divide in a day and a half, causing areas of red skin covered with silvery, flaky scales. It seems to be an inherited condition aggravated by stress or diet (Martini & Welch 2005). The rash may not itch and is not infectious. It may affect the elbows, knees and back as well as the scalp and fingernails (Walton et al 1994).

Head lice (*Pediculus capitis*) are highly infectious parasitic organisms that are common in institutional settings. They are easily recognized with the naked eye, as are their eggs, which adhere firmly to hair shafts (Walton et al 1994). If you notice anything unusual it is important that you report it to the nurse in charge and document your findings and action in your patient's nursing notes (see Case history 9.7)

If the patient has a beard or moustache, it is very important to assist with its cleaning, grooming and trimming. It is very easy for food particles to become lodged in the beard area, which is both uncomfortable and unhygienic (Dougherty & Lister 2004, Perry & Potter 2002, Quinless & Blauer 1992, Twigg 2000, Watson & Walsh 2002).

Removing facial and unwanted hair

(Figures 9.6a & b)

For some male patients, facial hair may be of religious significance and so it would be a serious matter if they are asked to have it removed; this should only be done if it is deemed to be essential to his medical treatment and only with the patient's consent or that of his immediate family. Many other male patients prefer to have a daily shave and for them it is an important part of preserving their dignity and self-respect. Their type of skin and their normal practice will influence their preference for an electric razor or a wet shave. Your patient may wish to shave after they have completed other aspects of their daily hygiene. Using

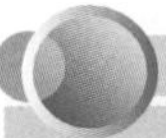

Case history 9.7

Meena's son has head lice

Meena has a 7-year-old son who brings home a note from school that indicates there is an outbreak of head lice (*Pediculus capitis*) in the school. Meena checks her son's hair and scalp and finds white concretions (nits) on the hair shafts. Her son is also complaining of pruritus (itching). Meena is not sure what to do, so when the health visitor and the nursing student visit she asks their advice.

The health visitor tells Meena that head lice are hard to spot but once identified can be removed by combing them out. The hair should be combed in sections using a 'nit comb', if one is available, or a very fine-toothed comb. A 'nit comb' can be purchased at the local pharmacy/chemist.

Mary, the student, has four children of her own and regularly has to deal with this problem. She suggests that the hair may be easier to comb if it is wet. A few teaspoons of olive oil or hair conditioner applied to the hair works well in keeping the hair moist during combing. The oil or hair conditioner should be rinsed off afterwards. It is important to comb the entire length of the hair, beginning at the root combing through to the tip. After each stroke, the comb should be checked for nits/lice. It may be useful to comb the hair over a piece of dark paper, or a bowl of water, which can then be checked for lice.

There are a number of treatments available; these include insecticides and thorough and frequent combing. The insecticides, as well as alternative treatments, can be strong chemicals with the potential to cause side-effects such as scalp irritation. Therefore Meena should only use them for a confirmed head lice infection. The health visitor will check Meena's son today. After it has been confirmed that Meena's child has head lice, Meena should check every member of the household and treat them if necessary. Mary suggests that, due to the risk of side-effects, the whole family should not be treated as a preventive measure. Only members of the family that have a live louse should be treated.

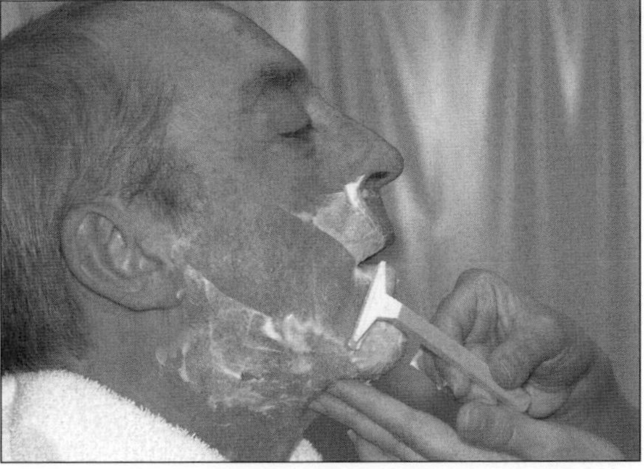

(a)

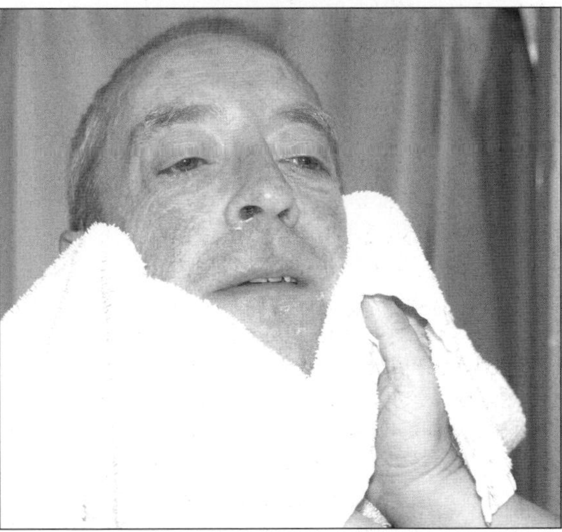

(b)

Figure 9.6a & b • Giving a patient a shave.

warm water serves to soften the facial stubble which, in some patients, can be very coarse and difficult to remove. A well-conducted shave requires some skill and results in the patient feeling refreshed and comfortable (see Box 9.5). The reverse is also true. Many female nursing students may initially feel embarrassed and uncomfortable about performing such an intimate aspect of care, as well as cautious about causing discomfort. If the shave is carried out ineffectively, the patient may be left feeling very sore and uncomfortable. During the procedure it is often hard not to work silently because of the concentration needed. However, if you can make the occasion into a social experience for your patient it reduces the tension and makes it more enjoyable (even if your patient is unconscious).

Using an electric razor is simpler than wet shaving and is generally less likely to cause cuts, so

Box 9.5

Procedure for giving your patient a wet shave

Equipment

- Either a new, disposable razor, or a new blade for your patient's razor.
- Shaving foam.
- Aftershave lotion (if preferred).
- Warm water in a bowl.
- Clean towels.

Procedure

- Explain to your patient what you are planning to do and ensure he has given his consent (if your patient is unconscious, it is still important to tell him what you are planning to do).
- If possible help your patient to sit up (otherwise lying flat is possible).
- Place a towel under his chin and around his shoulders to protect the chest area from water.
- Immerse the clean washcloth in the (hand) hot water and after checking that the temperature is alright for your patient, apply the cloth to his face. This process will help to soften the bristles and make it easier to shave them off. It can also prevent soreness of the skin caused by the abrasion of the razor.
- If your patient tolerates shaving foam then apply some to the bristly areas of the face to be shaved. Some patients have sensitive skin and prefer to use a shaving gel or oil designed specifically for this purpose. You can apply the shaving gel or oil in the same manner as a shaving foam. The advantage of using a gel or oil is that they are usually clear liquids that do not obscure the view of the skin.
- If your patient has a tendency to bleed (this is possible if your patient is suffering from any form of heart failure, liver disease, blood disorder or malnutrition), it may be necessary for you to wear protective gloves. It is not uncommon for men to cut their face while shaving so it could be a normal occurrence.
- Wet the razor and apply it to your patient's face with the handle at an angle of about 45° to the face, using the hand that feels most comfortable. Use the other hand to pull the skin of the patient's face taut.
- Shave in the direction of the hair growth. If your patient indicates that it is acceptable, it may be necessary to shave against the direction of hair growth, but this method should be used with care as it may cause skin irritation.
- Use short strokes of the razor to maintain control and reduce the risk of cutting the patient.
- Pay particular attention to the skin under the nose, as it is extremely easy to cut your patient in this area. Also, bear in mind that the skin under the chin and neck is very delicate and easily damaged by shaving. During the shave, rinse the razor after every four or five shaving strokes to ensure that the blade does not become clogged with soap and hair and become ineffective.
- Once all the facial hair has been removed, use the face cloth to rinse excess soap from your patient's face. Use a towel to pat the skin dry.
- Apply moisturising lotion or aftershave lotion according to your patient's preference
- Dispose of the used razor in the contaminated sharps bin (Dougherty & Lister 2004).

it is safer to use if your patient is taking anticoagulants or has a bleeding disorder. Your preparations for giving a dry shave are the same as those for wet shaving. Your patient may like you to apply a hot washcloth to soften the stubble, but you must make sure his face is completely dry afterwards so that the electric razor does not become clogged. See Box 9.6 for the procedure for giving a dry shave.

With both methods of shaving it is important to press the razor firmly against the skin to ensure a close shave, but not to press too hard as this causes skin irritation. Check with your patient to assess whether your are applying the right amount of pressure (Dougherty & Lister 2004).

Some female patients may wish to shave their underarm and leg hair. The technique for this hair removal is the same as for male facial hair.

Box 9.6

Procedure for giving a dry shave

- Ensure you have your patient's consent and cooperation.
- Check that the razor head is clear of any debris from a previous shave.
- Switch on the razor and hold it in the hand that feels most comfortable. Use the other hand to pull the patient's skin taut.
- Start shaving by placing the razor head on the patient's skin and rotating it in small circles.
- You may need to empty the cut hair from the razor to maintain its effectiveness throughout the shave.
- At the end of the shave ask your patient if he would like you to apply aftershave.
- You do this by shaking a small quantity onto the palms of your hands, rubbing them together to spread it evenly and then applying your hands to your patient's face. It can sting, so beware!

Another dilemma facing nurses is when a female patient has facial hair that is normally removed by using depilatory creams, waxing or plucking, or some other means. A prolonged stay in hospital can result in this aspect of their toilet being neglected. If you have a patient who may wish to have this matter resolved, it is a good idea to discuss the matter with them, and choose an appropriate method of safe removal. When using a proprietary agent, it is important to read the instructions carefully, taking care to test that your patient is not sensitive to any chemical products, and to document your actions and the product used in your patient's nursing notes.

Foot care

Having comfortable, clean feet is an important aspect of personal hygiene. Taking care of your patient's toenails can be a potential risk if your patient suffers from a foot or toe infection, diabetes mellitus, peripheral neuropathy or peripheral vascular disease. In such situations it is essential that your patient receives care from a registered podiatrist, chiropodist or doctor (Watson & Walsh 2002).

If your patient is free from any of these disorders and it is part of their nursing care plan, then foot care can be carried out either separately from the general hygiene regime or as part of it. If your patient needs to have their toenails clipped it is a good idea to soak the feet for 10 minutes in a bowl of warm water; this softens the nails and makes it easier to clip them. After drying the feet, clip small sections of the nail at a time and cut straight across the nail to prevent ingrown toenails. Once the nails are trimmed, they should be filed using an emery board to remove any jagged edges. Keeping the toenails trimmed may prevent accidental scratching injuries being self-inflicted on the patient's legs. If your patient has dry skin, it is a good idea to massage the feet with a foot lotion, a handcream or arachis oil, as this helps the skin to regain its suppleness and increases comfort.

If your patient is suffering from corns and calluses, warts or verrucas, fungal infections, ingrown toenails, foot odour, unusually elongated toenails and paronychia or inflamed tissue around the nail bed, you need to discuss the problem with your patient's key nurse and she will arrange for a podiatrist to visit them (Quinless & Blauer 1992).

Hand care

As a routine part of giving care you need to take care of your patient's hands. People who have been in hospital for some time rarely have the opportunity to scrub their nails or to manicure them. As a result, their nails are often filled with skin cells and other debris. You can use the same principles that are used for foot care when giving the appropriate hand and nail care. You may find it necessary to use a soft wooden stick to gently clean any debris from under the nail (Dougherty & Lister 2004). Giving a hand massage using handcream or arachis oil is relaxing and refreshing for your patient even if they are unconscious and a reassurance to their relatives that they are being properly cared for.

Mouth care

Having a fresh and clean-tasting mouth makes so much difference to your patient's sense of well-being. Patients who are dehydrated or taking medications that reduce the normal production of saliva often experience an unpleasant taste that is hard to remove. Good oral hygiene can help; this also includes dental and gum hygiene. For maximum effectiveness mouth care should be provided after meals to remove food particles and any dental plaque. It can also help to clean and massage the gums and to reduce mouth odour. If a patient is banned from taking oral fluids or has been nauseated or vomiting, providing mouth care, either as refreshing mouthwashes or cleaning their teeth, can help reduce the unpleasant experience and promote a sense of well-being.

The results of poor oral hygiene are significant as it can lead to tooth decay, gingivitis or inflammation of the gums, periodontitis or receding inflamed gums, halitosis or malodorous breath, cheilosis or cracked lips and stomatitis or inflammation of the whole mouth care. Whilst cleaning your patient's mouth it is a good idea to observe for any signs of dehydration or disease. This may be indicated by a dry tongue, whether it is a healthy pink colour or coated with white, black or yellow film, and whether there is any evidence of an infection such as thrush (*Candida albicans*). You can also notice whether your patient's gums bleed when you brush their teeth as this could indicate a gum disease or a bleeding disorder. If you notice any of these signs then you need to notify the nurse in charge and document the findings in your patient's notes.

The structure of the mouth

The mouth is also known as the oral cavity or the buccal cavity (see Figure 9.7). In normal health, the mouth is the first stage in the digestive process and contains structures designed to commence the chemical and mechanical processes of digestion.

The lining of the mouth is stratified squamous epithelium, somewhat like the skin. However, unlike the skin, there is no keratin except in the epithelium of the gums, hard palate and dorsum of the tongue, thus providing extra protection against abrasion during eating (Marieb 2005).

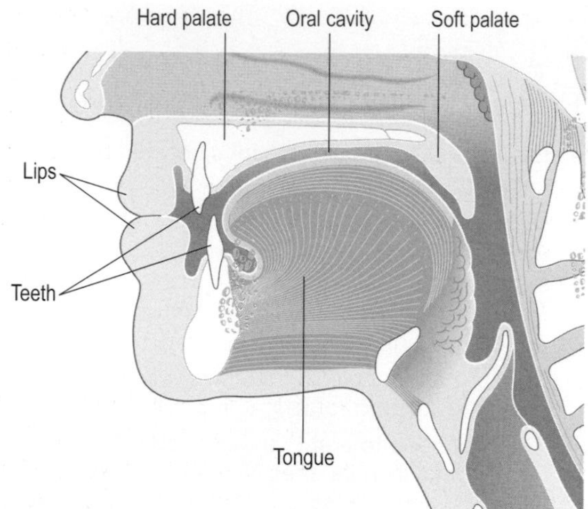

Figure 9.7 • Structures of the mouth.

The lips and cheeks

To provide the strength and movement needed for speech and mastication, the lips and cheeks are composed of skeletal muscle covered by skin and help to keep food between the teeth when eating. The external part of the lips (where lipsalve is applied) has no sweat or sebaceous glands and therefore must be moistened by saliva to prevent them drying out (Marieb 2005).

The palate

The palate forms the roof of the mouth and consists of two parts: the hard palate, which sits towards the front of the mouth; and the soft palate, which sits posterior. The hard palate is rigid with bone so that, during chewing, the tongue can push food against the hard palate to help break food up.

The tongue

The tongue is composed of skeletal muscle and contains taste buds and mucous and serous glands. The taste buds are contained within papillae (small projections) that are located all over the surface of the tongue. Taste buds are important for the recognition of the food that is eaten and they enable us to distinguish between sour, salty, bitter and sweet tastes (McKance & Huether 2002). In the process of chewing and masticating food, the tongue helps to form food into a bolus that can be pushed towards the back of the mouth and swallowed.

Salivary glands

You may have noticed that, when you have a dry mouth, how tasteless food seems and how hard it is to speak. The salivary glands are important for diluting the taste elements in food and thus facilitating the chemical activities that enable taste. We need saliva to masticate food, and people taking medications that reduce the flow of saliva often find it difficult to swallow unless they use drinks to dilute their food. Located around the face and excreting into the mouth are three large pairs of extrinsic salivary glands (see Figure 9.8):

- The parotid glands, located anterior to the ears.
- The submandibular glands, located at the posterior corners of the mandible.
- The sublingual glands, located under the tongue.

There are also small intrinsic salivary glands known as buccal glands. These glands are scattered throughout the mouth (Marieb 2005); they produce saliva constantly to keep the mouth moist.

The association between the sight and smell of food and the production of saliva from the extrinsic glands is strong. Saliva is 97–99.5% water and slightly acidic (pH 6.75–7) (Marieb 2005); it also contains electrolytes (sodium, potassium, chloride and bicarbonate ions), salivary amylase, lysozyme and mucin, which are important for the first stages of digestion of some foods. Box 9.7 provides a summary of the functions of saliva.

If food debris is not removed, then bad breath (halitosis) may develop. Your patient may find it difficult to eat, speak or swallow if saliva production is inhibited, which is likely to occur if they are dehydrated or if they are taking some drugs, especially those for cardiovascular disease such as hypertension. When people are under stress the activity of the sympathetic nervous system normally increases; this can cause a dry mouth because the blood vessels supplying the salivary glands vasoconstrict, thus stopping the supply of fluid to the salivary glands and this in turn inhibits saliva production and release. Some infections of the salivary glands (e.g. mumps and parotitis) will cause swelling of the ducts of the gland and cause pain and loss of salivation.

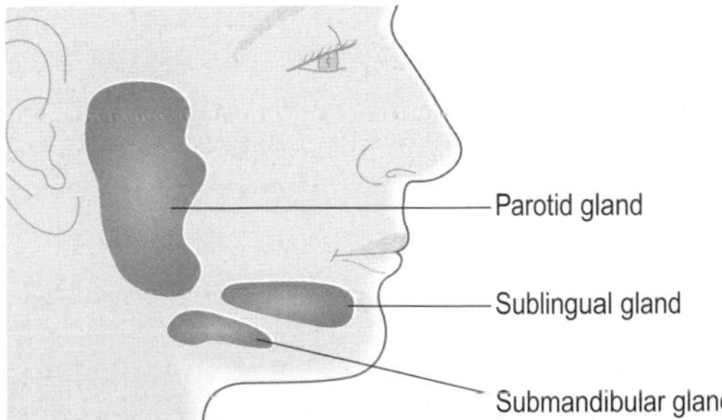

Figure 9.8 • Location of the salivary glands.

The teeth

We need good teeth to tear and break down food mechanically through chewing. This chewing process mixes the food bolus with saliva and so starts the tasting and digestive processes. In the adult there are 32 permanent teeth (20 deciduous teeth develop in childhood; these start to be

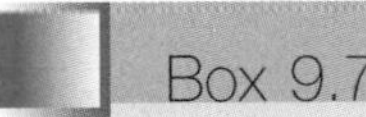

Box 9.7

Functions of saliva

- Cleansing of the mouth by removal of food debris.
- Dissolving of chemicals in ingested food to facilitate taste.
- Moistening of food to help form it into a bolus.
- Beginning the chemical process of carbohydrate digestion via salivary amylase.
- Aiding speech.
- Acting as an antimicrobial via lysozymes.
- Lubricating the mouth via mucin.

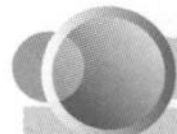

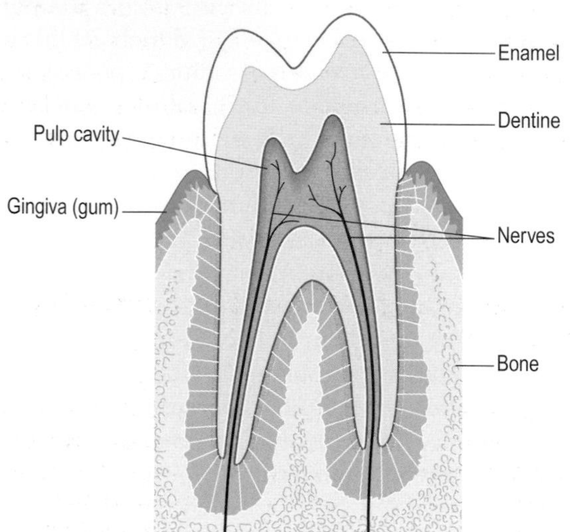

Figure 9.9 • Longitudinal section of a tooth.

replaced with the permanent teeth from the age of about 6 years) (Scanlon & Sanders 1995). If the person does not have teeth or their dentures do not fit comfortably they will have difficulty eating their food unless it has been pureed. It is often possible to use denture adhesives to help with this, although with ageing the mouth shape changes and dentures need to be replaced. It is probable that your patient will know how to remedy any difficulties they might be experiencing if you talk to them about it.

Each tooth is situated in its own socket within the gums of the upper (mandible) and lower (maxilla) jaws (Figure 9.9). A tooth consists of a central pulp cavity that contains blood vessels and nerve endings surrounded by dentine. Dentine makes up the bulk of the tooth and is bone-like in its composition. Surrounding the dentine is a layer of enamel that contains a large amount of calcium salts and is the hardest substance in the body. Enamel helps to protect the rest of the tooth structure providing the teeth are kept clean by regular brushing and flossing.

Dental cavities are caused by the breakdown of the enamel and the underlying dentine by the presence of dental plaque (a sugar, bacteria and mouth debris layer) that coats the teeth if the teeth are not kept clean (see Case history 9.8). Pain occurs when the pulp cavity is breached.

Case history 9.8

Martin is preparing to be a children's nurse

Martin is studying to be a children's nurse and is in his first-year taster placement. He has been undertaking a clinical placement in a general practice surgery. Today, during 'well child' visits, a mother pointed out to the nurse practitioner that her toddler seemed to have cavities (dental caries) in two of the upper teeth. The mother wanted to know what had caused the cavities and what should be done to resolve the problem. The nurse practitioner indicated that generally dental caries occur because of children eating or drinking sugary foods. A simple example is when children are still drinking from the bottle, especially to settle them at night. Milk and fruit drinks contain sugar which remain on the toddler's teeth overnight, resulting in the development of what is commonly known as 'nursing bottle caries'. These generally occur on the upper teeth. The nurse practitioner tells the mother that, in addition to taking the toddler off the bottle, and brushing his teeth twice a day with a soft toothbrush, fluoride is the most effective measure for preventing dental caries. If their drinking water does not have sufficient levels of fluoride than her toddler may need additional supplementation. Toothpaste that contains fluoride should also be used, keeping in mind that only a small amount of toothpaste (about the size of a pea) should be put onto the toothbrush. Modifying the toddler's diet will also reduce the risk of further caries. His intake of sugary foods and drinks should be decreased. If the toddler insists on having something to drink at naptime or bedtime, it is best to give plain water.

Martin has a toddler at home and another baby on the way. He was unaware that giving his toddler a bottle at bedtime could lead to dental caries. Martin intends to discuss this with his wife with the view to changing his toddler's oral hygiene routine.

Gingivitis (gum inflammation) may occur if the dental plaque is allowed to accumulate and then calcify (calculus). This can then cause a breach in the seal between the gums and the teeth increasing the risk of infection. Early gingivitis may manifest as red, swollen and painful gums that bleed easily. If left untreated the bone around the teeth is eroded by the bacteria and may lead to tooth loss. This is known as peridontitis and is detrimental to the overall health and well-being of the patient as it can make eating painful as well as causing a generalized malaise. As indicated in the Department of Health (2003) 'Essence of care' benchmarking toolkit, personal and oral hygiene involves the 'effective removal of plaque and debris to ensure the structures and tissues of the mouth are kept in a healthy condition'. In the section that follows, personal and oral hygiene will be discussed in relation to the skin and mouth.

Delivering mouth care

As with most personal care, you should encourage your patient to carry out as much of their mouth care as possible. However, if your patient is severely debilitated you may need to provide some or all of their mouth care. Before you start the procedure you need to explain your plan of action to your patient and obtain their consent. Ensure your patient is comfortable and does not wish to use the toilet and it is convenient for you to provide this care. Then you need to prepare your equipment (see Box 9.8) and take it to your patient's bedside. Make sure that your patient's privacy is protected. If possible raise the height of your patient's bed to a comfortable working height in order to prevent back strain, and position your patient so they can do as much of the care as they can manage. Wash your hands and put on protective gloves to minimize cross-infection.

The procedure for flossing and brushing the teeth is described in Box 9.9.

Box 9.8

Mouth care equipment

- Soft-bristled brush (this is safer to use).
- Non-abrasive toothpaste (it does not cause damage to the tooth enamel).
- Dental floss and dental floss holder or interdental brush.
- Water.
- A bowl for the patient to spit out any mouthwash or water.
- Protective gloves.

During the procedure it is good practice to observe for any signs of bleeding from the gums, oedema of the gums or tongue, halitosis, secretions and any deposits such as *Candida albicans*, which forms painful white plaques in the mouth, particu-

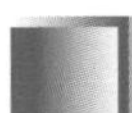

Box 9.9

Procedure for flossing and brushing the teeth

- First check whether your patient has any dentures or an orthodontic plate and ask them to remove them so they can be cleaned separately. Floss your patient's teeth of any food debris by using dental floss in a holder, cleaning between their teeth, taking care not to damage the gum tissue by being too vigorous. After flossing the teeth encourage your patient to rinse their mouth to remove dislodged material.
- Wet the toothbrush and apply toothpaste to it. Place the brush head against the patient's teeth at an angle of 45° degrees. Brush the teeth of the lower jaw from the gum line upwards and those of the upper jaw from the gum line down. Use short and gentle brush strokes to prevent damaging the gums. Take care to brush both facial and lingual tooth surfaces using the tip of the brush to clean the lingual surfaces of the incisors and canines, then brush the chewing surfaces of the upper and lower premolars and molars.
- Encourage your patient to rinse their mouth regularly during the cleaning so as to remove any dislodged matter. If your patient has dry, chapped or uncomfortable lips they may want to have either lip salve or petroleum jelly applied during the brushing phase in order to protect the lips. When you have completed the brushing and rinsing phase, use a mouthwash swab soaked in mouthwash solution gently to massage the gums, buccal surfaces, palate and tongue to clean the mucosa and stimulate circulation.
- During this procedure you should take every effort to protect your patient from gagging. You can achieve this by not being too vigorous with the brush strokes or pushing the brush or swab too deeply into the mouth.
- Dispose of soiled swabs and gloves in the infected waste.
- In some situations, such as when your patient is unable to assist, you may need to use suction equipment to aspirate liquid from the mouth.

larly in patients who are on antibiotic therapy. If you notice anything unusual you must report it to your supervisor and record your observations in your patient's nursing notes (Dougherty & Lister 2004).

Denture care

Good dental care involves removing and rinsing dentures after meals, and daily brushing and soaking of the dentures to remove more tenacious deposits. There are specific products on the market designed for soaking and cleaning dentures that may be used, and your patient may have brought their preferred product for this. During mouth care these prostheses will need to be removed and cleaned in a similar manner as natural teeth. You need to make sure that you have labelled the container with the patient's name and bed number so there is no confusion.

Removing dentures can be quite difficult unless the patient is able to assist you. Care of the mouth of the denture wearer is the same as the suggested care above (Dougherty & Lister 2004).

Assisting with elimination of urine and faeces

Going to the toilet is normally a very private activity. Therefore, your patient may feel embarrassed about needing assistance. If you are embarrassed or lack confidence, your patient may feel embarrassed as well. Whenever you are assisting your patient with their elimination needs you must always maintain their safety, comfort, privacy and dignity to avoid potential embarrassment. You may remember from Chapter 8 that we described the normal response to eating and drinking is the gastrocolic reflex. This is when the stimulus provided by food entering the stomach causes a ripple of peristalsis all along the intestinal tract and thus creates the urge to defaecate. It is a good strategy to make use of this knowledge by offering your patient the opportunity to open their bowels after meals, preferably by helping them to the lavatory or to use a commode if they are not well enough to move.

Patients who have a high intake of fluids as part of their nursing care plan, either orally or intravenously, will need regular opportunities to pass urine. Similarly, people who are taking medications such as diuretics that cause them to pass urine will need to have more frequent opportunities to use the toilet if they are not able to do this unassisted. Many patients know the routine of their body, especially if they have been taking diuretics for some years, and they can tell you when they are most likely to need this assistance; this should be recorded in their nursing notes and acted upon as part of their routine care. You may find it helpful to keep a chart as a reminder if your patient needs help to go to the toilet.

Some patients may need assistance with cleaning their perineal and rectal area following elimination. As you read earlier in this chapter, in some religious practices this must be done with running water. Whatever system is observed it is important that effective and gentle hygiene is practised. Research has demonstrated that vigorous cleansing beyond normal hygiene practice is not necessary and may increase the risk of infection (Pellowe et al 2001).

Personal hygiene and parasites

Humans are host to organisms and micro-organisms, some of which are beneficial and some that are dangerous if they move out of their normal environment. Organisms that are capable of causing disease are called pathogens or infectious agents, and include bacteria, viruses, fungi, protozoa and parasites. However scrupulous we are in maintaining our personal hygiene, it is inevitable that every human being will host many parasites. A parasite is any organism that, for all or part of its life, derives an advantage by living on or in another organism. The human body can provide a home and nourishment for bacteria, viruses, fungi, protozoa, lice, worms and fleas. Some of these may be pathogenic if displaced, such as when as a result of a cut or an abrasion they can move through the surface of the skin. The advantage for these parasitic organisms is usually nutritional. It is a very successful mode of living and the number of parasitic organisms outnumbers those being parasitized. It is interesting that the population of worms living in human intestines is greater than the total number of humans (Youngson 1994). As far as we know, parasites do not usually offer any advantage to the host, but those that do are referred to as saprophytes. In many cases the parasite can be pathogenic to the host. Some organisms regularly inhabit areas of the body without causing disease and constitute the normal body flora. These are called commensal organisms. Commensal organisms may play an essential role in the functioning of the body. For example, as a result of bacterial action in the intestine, vitamin K is produced and this vitamin is essential to facilitate blood clotting (Watson & Walsh 2002). If commensal organisms become relocated to different areas of the body they may cease to be commensal and become pathogenic.

Infection is the term used to describe the multiplication of a pathogenic organism within the host's body tissues. The outcome of infection is the balance between the ability of the pathogen to adhere to, invade and damage the host's body tissue, versus the host's defence mechanisms. In the following sections we provide a brief outline of some of the organisms that parasitize the human body. Some of these organisms do not entirely relate to the subject of personal hygiene, as it may be that infection occurs as a result of some other problem, such as eating contaminated food, drinking contaminated water, through handling infected pets, or being bitten by a contaminated insect. The brief discussion illustrates how closely human beings live with potentially disease-causing organisms.

Fungal parasites

Fungal infections are caused by multicellular, mould-like organisms. Fungi are a simple form of vegetable life that group together to form filamentous colonies. They form a separate division in the plant kingdom and are unlike bacteria and viruses in that they are eukaryotic, meaning that each cell has a nucleus. However, they differ from other plants in that they are unable to photosynthesize. As such, they form parasitic and saprophytic relationships with other organisms. Diseases caused by fungus are known collectively as mycoses. Fungal disease is spread by spores and is highly communicable. These diseases are classified according to the site of infection (e.g. *tinea corporis*, or ringworm of the body). Infection of the skin, mouth, genital region and mucous membranes caused by this type of organism is quite common (see Case history 9.9); athlete's foot, thrush and ringworm are examples of this type of infection. Systemic disease is rarer, usually occurring when the immune system is compromised in some way.

Both males and females are susceptible to fungal infection and incidence is only partially age-related. That is to say, different age groups are prone to infection of different areas of the body:

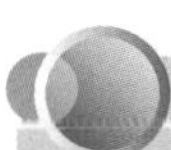

Case history 9.9

Caring for a patient with anogenital irritation

Mr Jones, is a 35-year-old type 2 diabetic, who is suffering from anogenital itching. Mark has been caring for Mr Jones and he is aware that a number of disorders can cause pruritus, including diabetes mellitus and HIV (human immunodeficiency virus) disease. The lowered immunity can cause furunculosis (fungal infection). Mark discusses this with his mentor who suggests he discusses with Mr Jones the possibility that he has non-specific pruritus or a fungal rash. Mark notes that Mr Jones is overweight and suspects that the problem may be non-specific dermatitis of the sort that occurs where there is skin-to-skin contact without much exposure to the air. In the latter case, it might clear up with washing 2–3 times per day with a mild soap then rinsing and drying well, and wearing loose-fitting clothing as much as possible. Another strategy is to make sure that his underpants are washed in a non-biological detergent, preferably one for delicate clothes, and that they are rinsed out thoroughly to make sure none of the detergent is left behind. Some detergents and incomplete rinsing can cause a localized pruritus. If the problem is not resolved by these strategies then Mr Jones might try one of the over-the-counter antifungal creams. If those measures don't help, then Mr Jones should see his doctor.

Mark documents his discussion with Mr Jones and records in his care notes that he consulted the nurse in charge of Mr Jones' care.

prepubescent children are more likely to contract *tinea capitis*, whereas adults tend towards *tinea pedis* or athlete's foot. Transmission is by both direct and indirect contact with the spores and occurs more frequently when environmental temperature and humidity are high. These organisms can be destroyed by the use of oral and topical fungicides (Watson & Walsh 2002, Walton et al 1994, Youngson 1994).

Protozoan parasites

There are over 65 000 species of protozoa. They are minute invertebrate creatures which have names that include a description of their shape, such as flagellates (lash-like), ciliates (hair-like), sporozoa (spot-like), amoebae and foraminifers. Many protozoa are amoebic; that is, a single-celled creature that moves by allowing its endoplasm to flow inside its ectoplasm to form a protrusion called a pseudopodium which is used to pull or push the organism through its environment (Roberts 1977). The commonest protozoan parasite of humans is *Entamoeba histolytica* and is the cause of amoebic dysentery. Malaria is caused by the amoebic parasites *Plasmodium vivax*, *Plasmodium malariae*, *Plasmodium falciparum* and *Plasmodium ovale* (Makins 1994, Youngson 1994).

Worm parasites

Worm parasites are referred to as helminths. They include roundworms (nematodes), flukes (trematodes) and tapeworms (cestodes). Roundworm larvae can enter the skin directly or be ingested with food or water or through biting the fingernails, once they have become infected with the parasite. This is a common route of infection in children, who scratch their itchy anus and chew their fingernails. The larvae can cause severe inflammatory reactions in the lungs. Some species invade muscle and other tissues, causing severe and sometimes fatal reactions. The tapeworm can develop in the human gut where it competes with its host for food, thus leading to weight loss accompanied by increased appetite, and possibly loss of blood. Its larvae can invade the muscles and brain causing permanent and harmful cysts. Other worm parasites invade the eye, lymphatic tissue, liver and bladder, producing various diseases according to their location (Youngson 1994). Treatment should be focused on the cause, such as preventing and stopping the cycle of infestation from fleas on pets.

Arthropod parasites

This group of parasites includes mites, ticks, lice, fleas and mosquitoes. At the very least these parasites can cause very distressing dermatitis, but they may also transmit diseases such as typhus, plague, impetigo typhoid and malaria (Youngson 1994).

Viruses

Viruses are microscopic infectious agents which, unlike bacteria, cannot perform any metabolic function without first entering the cell of another organism. They are not cells, but consist of deoxyribonucleic acid (DNA) or ribonucleic acid (RNA) surrounded by a protein coat called a capsid. Because of their inability to reproduce without another host cell, there has been some debate regarding the status of viruses as living organisms. The word 'virus' comes from a Latin word meaning a slimy, poisonous liquid or venom. In 1892, a Russian botanist named Dimitri Ivanovsky discovered that tobacco mosaic disease could be transmitted from plant to plant by the use of infected tobacco plant sap that had been strained through a filter, the pores of which were small enough to inhibit the passage of all known bacteria. At that point, the cause of the disease within the sap was unknown, but the sap was described as containing a filterable virus. During the 19th century the term virus continued to be vague, referring to any 'poison' produced by disease. As medical science progressed, it became apparent that the infectious agent causing tobacco mosaic disease and other diseases was indeed a micro-organism and it is these types of micro-organism that have come to be called viruses. They vary in size from about half the diameter of the smallest known bacterium down to the dimension of a large molecule. They also vary in shape because of the differing nature of the protein capsid. The genetic material of a DNA virus is in the double-helical form, whereas

RNA viruses have a single-strand genome that is often present in two, identical copies.

Viruses enter the body by a number of routes. They can be ingested with food or fluids or inhaled in airborne droplets. They can pass through minute skin abrasions or through mucous membranes of the eye, genital tract and rectum. They may be borne into the body in the bite of animals and insects or on contaminated hypodermic needles, medical equipment and products. As soon as viruses enter the body they invade local cells. They spread from cell to cell, increasing in number exponentially. As viruses enter the cell, some discard their capsid in order to expose their genetic material, while others pass through the host cell wall intact and only discard the capsid once inside. Inside the host cell, the virus can make use of the host cell's organelles to ensure its reproduction. The virus may even integrate itself within the host's genome and become established indefinitely. When virus genome is incorporated into host cell DNA without killing the host, then the changed DNA will be passed on with each generation of the host cell line. Cells that are changed in this way by viruses acquire new properties. These new properties may give rise to tumours in the host. However, more common conditions caused by viruses include the common cold, genital herpes, cold sores, glandular fever, influenza, warts, measles, mumps, hepatitis A, encephalitis, myocarditis and AIDS (acquired immune deficiency syndrome) (Watson & Walsh 2002, Youngson 1994).

Bacteria

Bacteria are micro-organisms. They are prokaryotic, meaning that they lack a cell nucleus, making them distinct from all other living cells. Bacteria exist everywhere. Most are not pathogenic. Those that do cause human disease are a small proportion of all bacteria and are specially adapted to life within the human body. It is believed that bacteria resemble the earliest forms of cellular life that evolved on the planet. Fossilized bacteria have been identified in rocks estimated to be at least 3 billion years old.

The classification of bacteria has proved problematic. The question is, are they animal or plant? Bacteria, like plants, have rigid cell walls but, in the main, do not photosynthesize. They also behave like animals, in that they may move about and assimilate organic matter for food. Early classifiers referred to bacteria as plants, but another system gives them their own, separate domain. They are classified in this latter system as prokaryotes or single-celled organisms that do not have a defined nucleus. Bacteria are measured in micrometres (sometimes called microns, the term we shall use here). A micron is one millionth of a metre. Most bacteria are between 0.1 and 4.0 microns wide and between 0.2 and 50 microns long. Some bacteria are spherical structures about 1.0 micron in diameter. Individually, bacteria are microscopic but colonies are visible to the naked eye.

Bacteria are very resistant to changes in their environment. Some can survive in temperatures close to boiling point, others can survive long periods of freezing. Bacteria exist at extremely high altitude where there is almost no air, and in the depths of the ocean where they are seemingly unaffected by the huge pressure at such depths. To survive such extremes, many bacteria enter a spore stage during which they are surrounded by a tough, protective capsule. The reproduction of bacteria is by binary fission (i.e. division into two). Under the appropriate conditions, one bacterium can give rise to more than a million cells in 6 hours. The destruction of most bacteria can be brought about by high temperatures. Most disease-causing bacteria can be destroyed at the temperature of boiling water. However, spore-bearing organisms require higher temperatures to be destroyed with, for example, compressed steam in the autoclaves used in operating departments to sterilize some surgical equipment.

Antiseptics and disinfectants chemically alter the structure of bacterial organisms or inhibit their reproduction. However, many antiseptics are harmful to human tissues and are therefore not appropriate for use to control infection in humans. Medical control of pathogenic, bacterial infection in humans is attained primarily by antibiotic medication. Generally, antibiotics are taken into the body orally. From the stomach, they are transported into the bloodstream, where they attach themselves to the bacterial cell membrane they are targeted to find. Antibiotics interfere with the metabolic functions of the bacterial cell thereby bringing about its destruction. Antibiotics may also be administered intravenously (Watson & Walsh 2002, Youngson 1994).

Hand hygiene and infection control of MRSA

Myatt & Langley (2003, p 675) described MRSA (methicillin-resistant *Staphylococcus aureus*) as:

> *An organism that is found in the normal skin flora. Colonization of the skin with the bacterium means that it is present on or in the body without causing any harm.*

However, MRSA is a bacterium that is resistant to many antibiotics, having emerged in the late 1950s after the introduction of semi-synthetic penicillin (Solberg 2000), and is responsible for outbreaks of infection in hospitals (Karchmer et al 2002, Nolan 2001). It is considered to be endemic (Myatt & Langley 2003), and preventing its spread is an important issue since it is one of the most common causes of infection and death of patients in hospitals in the UK. MRSA accounts for 5000 deaths per year in the UK, and the number of patients affected has increased by 600% in the last decade (Akid 2001, Reid 2004). It has been reported that the treatment and control measures associated with MRSA cost approximately £1 billion per year in the UK (Akid 2001, Reid 2004). MRSA infection is a major challenge worldwide because of the morbidity and mortality rates and associated costs related to infections (Lepelletier & Richet 2001). In Europe, the incidence of MRSA varies from 1% in the Scandinavian countries to more than 30% in Spain, Italy, France, Turkey and Greece (Kotilainen et al 2001, Tramier et al 2003). Exceptionally low rates can be found in the Netherlands (2%) (Aycliffe et al 1998) and Switzerland (1.8%) (Aycliffe et al 1998, Kotilainen et al 2003).

Research has shown that MRSA infections increase the cost of treatment per patient infected. Hospitals are attempting to address questions that have been raised about cost and ethical considerations regarding the protection of patients from infection and death (Herr et al 2003, Karchmer et al 2002, Solberg 2000). The way to address the problem of MRSA is the maintenance of effective personal and oral hygiene and to follow the British recommended guidelines (Aycliffe et al 1998), which involve wearing aprons and gloves during patient care, hand-washing prior to and following contact with each patient during nursing care, isolation of infected patients (Arnold et al 2002) and the use of protective clothing (barrier nursing: cap, gown and gloves, goggles and mask if sputum is positive).

MRSA definitions and terminology

To help understand the rationale for guidelines associated with the management of MRSA, you need to understand the current terminology that is used in relation to the various guidelines. A glossary of these terms is given in Box 9.10.

Prevention of cross-infection

Infection is seen as a clinically apparent, adverse reaction in response to contamination by microorganisms. Prevention of cross-infection is a crucial part of nursing care, and by understanding how cross-infection happens and by taking the appropriate actions you will be able to ensure that you do not contribute to the chain of events and so help to prevent cross-infection (Brooker & Nicol 2003, Nicol 2004). The two most critical elements in health care are good hand-washing technique and effective practice of universal precautions.

Universal precautions

Universal precautions are designed to protect both health care personnel and their patients from cross-infection from other patients or from other health care staff. Universal precautions are a set of standard procedures to be observed and practised at all times, thus reducing the risk of accidental contamination and transmission of infection (Horton & Parker 1997). Because nursing involves contact with blood and other body fluids during routine activities, such as dressing wounds (Figure

Box 9.10

Glossary of terms associated with guidelines for the management of MRSA

Airborne. Transmission of the bacteria through droplets containing micro-organisms that are suspended in the air may be carried long distances and may even become inhaled. Dust particles containing the infectious bacteria can be a form of airborne transmission (HICPAC 2004).

Carrier. A person who has MRSA organisms with no expression of clinical disease, but is a potential source of infection (Aycliffe et al 1998).

Colonization of the skin. Bacteria are present on or in the body without causing any harm, but have the potential to multiply (Aycliffe et al 1998).

Common vehicle. Transmission of the bacteria whereby the micro-organisms are transmitted/conveyed, for example, through contaminated medication or medical devices and equipment such as suction equipment, ventilators (HICPAC 2004).

Contact. Transmission of the bacteria occurs by direct contact with an infected wound, person or objects. Examples include: bathing someone with suppurating wounds or pustules; contact with wound dressings; having contaminated hands or gloves that are not changed between patients (HICPAC 2004).

Droplet. Transmission of the bacteria through droplets generated during coughing and sneezing, and procedures such as suctioning or bronchoscopy. 'Transmission occurs when droplets containing micro-organisms generated from the infected person are propelled a short distance through the air and deposited on the host's conjunctivae, nasal mucosa or mouth' (HICPAC 2004).

Infection. The entry and multiplication of the bacteria in the tissues of the host, where they can cause tissue damage (Aycliffe et al 1998). The Healthcare Infection Control Practices Advisory Committee (HICPAC) of the Centers for Disease Control and Health Prevention indicates that there are four main routes for the spread of the bacterium *Staphylococcus aureus*; these are contact, droplet, common vehicle and airborne (HICPAC 2004).

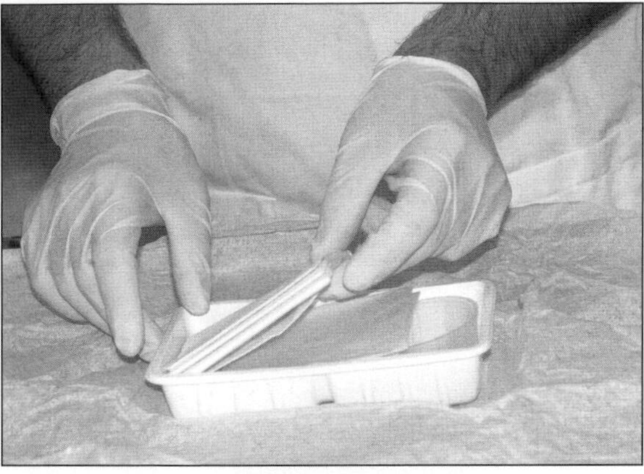

Figure 9.10 • Handling a sterile dressing.

9.10), care of infusions and assisting with toileting, nurses and other health care personnel need to wear protective clothing to prevent contamination (Nicol 2004).

People who are most at risk from introduced infections are people whose immune system is already under challenge, either due to trauma such as injury or surgery or if they are suffering from ill-health or malnutrition. You are likely to encounter such people in your everyday nursing practice and so it is vital that you learn how to practise safely for the benefit of your patients (Brooker & Nicol 2003). Another factor that you need to remember is that, when people are in enclosed spaces such as prisons, nursing homes or hospitals, they are exposed to a much wider range of infective organisms than if they were at home. The most efficient way for infective organisms to move from one vulnerable person to another is to hitch a lift, and the most effective transport agent is the staff of the hospital or the nursing home, as they work with a wide range of people every day. So the potential for cross-infection is great and nurses, health care support workers and doctors, as well as other health care staff, are at the front line for either promoting cross-infection or for breaking the chain of events and stopping it. To break this chain of actions it is important that you develop and maintain the necessary skills of effective hand hygiene, wearing of apron and gloves (Figure 9.11), disposal of clinical and domestic waste, and safe use and disposal of needles and other sharps (Nicol 2004).

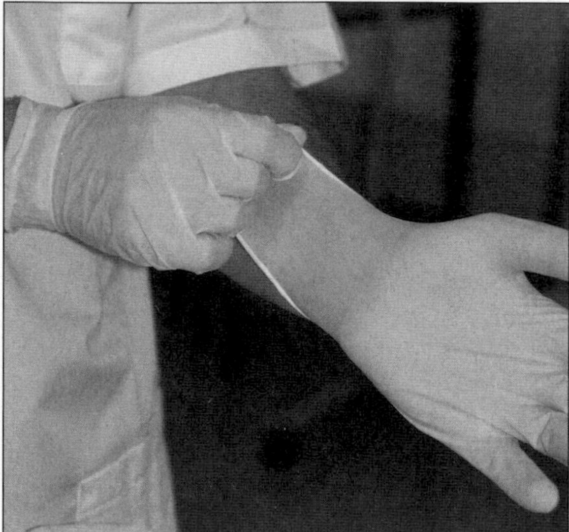

Figure 9.11 • Putting on sterile gloves.

You will find more information about infection control in Chapter 13.

Conclusion

Throughout this chapter we have discussed a range of factors that can influence your capability to provide effective hygiene care. The 'Essence of care' benchmarking toolkit for personal and oral hygiene developed by the Department of Health (2003) provides a useful framework. Understanding the structure and functions of the skin can alert you to any differences from normal and help you to identify people who need further help and assistance from other members of the health care team.

We have used the Department of Health (2003) definition of personal hygiene: 'The physical act of cleansing the body to ensure that the skin, hair and nails are maintained in an optimum condition'. They describe oral hygiene as the 'effective removal of plaque and debris to ensure the structures and tissues of the mouth are kept in a healthy condition', and that a healthy mouth is 'clean, functional, comfortable and free from infection'. We have also introduced you to some of the principles of cross-infection and the practice of universal precautions, particularly as they relate to MRSA (you can read more about this in Chapter 13).

The skill of providing effective care lies not only with the technical process but also with all the other activities that good nursing entails, including effective observational and interpersonal skills. Whatever care you provide, we urge you to consider your patient as a whole person with feelings and spiritual needs. Your care should always be provided as a result of careful assessment and documentation of your patients' needs and planned in collaboration with your patient or their carers and delivered using evidence from best practice. Whilst delivering personal hygiene care it is important that you think of it as an opportunity to get to know your patient better and to share some of yourself. This is essential even when your patient is unconscious or confused, as hearing is often the sense that is retained and can help your patient to maintain a sense of reality. Observing and monitoring your patient's condition is a more sophisticated skill, especially when you are able to correctly recognize changes that need further attention and documentation.

You may find it helpful to familiarize yourself with different nursing models and textual descriptions of personal care, as these describe some of the many different ways to care for patients (see Leddy et al 2005). If you are able to read widely and develop a profound understanding of nursing, medical disorders and the normal functioning of the body, you will be able use this knowledge to adapt your care to the individual needs of your patient and to monitor their condition effectively.

References

Akid M 2001 Now wash your hands. Nursing Times 97(49):11

Arnold MS, Dempsey JM, Fishman M et al 2002 The best hospital practices for controlling methicillin-resistant staphylococcus aureus: on the cutting edge. Infection Control and Hospital Epidemiology 23(2):69–75

Aycliffe G, Duckworth G, Cookson B et al R 1998 Working party report: Revised guidelines for the control of methicillin-resistant *Staphylococcus aureus* infection in hospitals. Journal of Hospital Infection 39(4):253–290

Aycliffe GAJ, Fraise AP, Eddes AM et al 2000 Control of hospital infection. A practical handbook. Arnold, London

Benbow M 2002 The skin. 1: Its structure and functions. Nursing Times 98(25):43–46

Botek AA, Lookingbill DP 2001 The structure and function of sebaceous glands. In: Freinkel R, Woodley T (eds) The biology of the skin. Parthenon, New York, p 87–100

Brooker C, Nicol M 2003 Nursing adults in the practice of caring. Edinburgh, Mosby, p 253–270

Byrne DJ, Phillip G, Napier A et al 1991 The effect of whole body disinfection on intra-operative wound contamination. Journal of Hospital Infection 1(2):45–48

Campbell A 1984 Moderated love. A theology of professional care. SPCK, London

D'Avanzo CE, Geissler EM (eds) 2003 Cultural health assessment, 3rd edn. Mosby, St Louis

Department of Health 2003 Essence of care. Department of Health, NHS Modernisation Agency, London

Dougherty L, Lister S (eds) 2004 The Royal Marsden Hospital manual of clinical nursing procedures, 6th edn. Blackwell, Oxford, p 570–586

Fullbrook S 2004 The human right to dignity v. physical integrity in manual handling. British Journal of Nursing 13(8):462–468

Greaves A (1985) We'll just freshen you up dear. Nursing Times 81(10):S3–8

Haake A, Scott G, Holbrook KA 2001 Structure and function of the skin: overview of the epidermis and dermis. In: Freinkel R, Woodley T (eds) The biology of the skin. Parthenon, New York, p 19–46

Healthcare Infection Control Practices Advisory Committee (HICPAC) 2004 Recommendations for isolation precautions in hospitals. Online. www.cdc.gov

Herlihy B, Maebius NK (2003) The human body in health and illness, 2nd edn. Saunders, Philadelphia

Herr C, Heckrodt T, Hofmann F et al 2003 Additional costs for preventing and spread of methicillin-resistant *Staphylococcus aureus* and a strategy for reducing these costs on a surgical ward. Infection Control and Hospital Epidemiology 24(9):673–678

Horton R, Parker L 1997 Informed infection control practice. Churchill Livingstone, Edinburgh

Hurley HJ 2001 The eccrine sweat glands: structure and function, In: Freinkel R, Woodley T (eds) The biology of the skin. Parthenon, New York, p 47–76

Karchmer TB, Durbin LJ, Simonton BM et al 2002 Cost-effectiveness of active surveillance cultures and contact/droplet precautions for control of methicillin-resistant *Staphylococcus aureus*. Journal of Hospital Infection 51(2):126–132

Kotilainen P, Routamaa M, Peltonen R et al 2003 Elimination of epidemic methicillin-resistant *Staphylococcus aureus* from a university hospital and district institutions in Finland. Emerging Infectious Diseases 9(2):169–174

Leddy S, Pepper J, Hood L 2005 Conceptual basis of professional nursing. Lippincott, Philadelphia

Lepelletier D, Richet H 2001 Surveillance and control of methicillin-resistant *Staphylococcus aureus* infections in French hospitals. Infection Control and Hospital Epidemiology 22(11):677–682

Makins M (ed) 1994 Collins English dictionary. Harper Collins, Glasgow

Marieb EN 2005 Human anatomy and physiology, 8th edn. Benjamin Cummings, California

Martini FH, Welch K 2005 A& P applications manual. London, Pearson

McCance KL, Huether SE 2002 Pathophysiology. The biologic basis for disease in adults and children, 4th edn. Mosby, St Louis

Myatt R, Langley S 2003 Changes in infection control practice to reduce MRSA infection. British Journal of Nursing 12(11):675–681

Nicol M 2004 Essential nursing skills. Mosby, London

NICE 2006 www.nice.org.uk.

Nolan JL 2001 A flexible approach to methicillin-resistant *Staphylococcus aureus* (MRSA). Nursing Times 97(46):57–58

Pellowe C, Loveday H, Harper P et al 2001 Preventing infections from short-term indwelling catheters. Nursing Times 97(14):34–35

Penzer R 2002 Nursing care of the skin. Butterworth-Heinemann, Oxford

Perry A, Potter P (eds) 2002 Clinical nursing skills and techniques, 5th edn. Mosby, St Louis, p 116–150

Quinless FW, Blauer RE (eds) 1992 Nursing procedures. Springhouse Corporation, Pennsylvania, p 79–95

Quinn AG 2000 Biology of the skin and dermatological disease. Medicine 28(11):1–3

Reid J 2004 MRSA in hospitals. Sky News, London (5 July 2004)

Richardson M 2003 Understanding the structure and function of the skin. Nursing Times 99(31):46–48

Roberts MBV 1977 Biology: a functional approach, 2nd edn. Thomas Nelson, Middlesex

Scanlon VC, Sanders T 1995 Essentials of anatomy and physiology, 2nd edn. FA Davies, Philadelphia

Smith P 1992 The emotional labour of nursing. Macmillan, London

Solberg C 2000 Spread of *Staphylococcus aureus* in hospitals: causes and prevention. Scandinavian Journal of Infectious Diseases 32(6):587–595

Tramier B, Schmit JL, Lescure F et al 2001 Evaluation of the contribution of isolation precautions in prevention and control of multi-resistant bacteria in a teaching hospital. Journal of Hospital Infection 47(2):116–124

Twigg J 2000 Bathing: the body and community care. Routledge, London, p 1–60

Walton J, Barondess AJ, Lock S (eds) 1994 Oxford medical companion. Oxford University Press, Oxford

Watson J, Walsh M 2002 Watson's clinical nursing and related sciences, 6th edn. Baillière Tindall, London, p 61–84

Woloski-Wruble A, DeKeyser F, Levi S et al 2000 Patients' attitudes towards use of gloves by healthcare staff. British Journal of Nursing 9(17):1146–1152

Young L 1991 The clean fight. Nursing Standard 5(35):54–55

Youngson RM 1994 The Guinness encyclopaedia of the human being. Guinness Publishing, Middlesex, p 122–123, 130–137

Section Three

Care management

Mike Cook

CHAPTERS

In this section of the book you will be exploring the nature of managing care as a foundation course nursing student. We will introduce the concepts of effective teamworking and the contributions other people make that enable effective care to be delivered, including the involvement of other carers. You will see how you play an important part in ensuring that high-quality care is delivered. As a novice learner in health care you will be faced with many different situations. You may find the numerous daily activities and demands on your time confusing, so we shall be exploring different ways in which you can learn how to manage your time in your placement setting and how to set priorities by assessing need. We shall also be discussing the importance of effective documentation to ensure information is effectively communicated.

Teamwork in nursing has been emphasized by many leading nurses and is reflected in several research reports. Chapter 10 introduces some important ideas for you to consider in terms of effective teamwork. Try to read this chapter in the context of your practice experiences in all your practice areas. You will encounter highly effective teams, and some not so effective teams. From your placement learning what sort of team player are you? What are your strengths and what areas do you need to improve? A part of the chapter provides a number of approaches as to how you can work effectively as a nursing student in a care team. Try to use the reflective practice models and questions to add to your learning log and portfolio.

Chapter 11 explores the important area of managing yourself in the placement setting as you move from being a nursing student to a qualified practitioner. Three elements of being a student are introduced. These include how to present yourself, how to manage your time and how to communicate in the placement setting. Each element examines these in the role of the developing practitioner, raising issues that arise through the process. Safeguards that promote ethical practice and prevent the misuse of power in the caring professions are discussed.

Chapter 12 introduces you to decision-making ideas that are useful for health care practitioners. This chapter is intended to stretch your thinking and introduces some complex issues. Health care is a complex working environment and the chapter is intended to provide a framework for you to use for your practice. We hope that you may find the information in this chapter helpful and that you will draw on the ideas and suggestions when you are giving care. You may even find the ideas helpful in other parts of your life and it might be worthwhile practising some of the activities at home and with your friends and monitoring which ones suit you best. It is also worth exploring how your colleagues arrive at their decisions. Do you see your mentors use a framework to make their decisions? Talk to your nursing mentors and supervisors in practice. What are their views? Ask other members of the health care team. Can they explain the range of decisions that are made?

The final chapter (Chapter 13) in this section and in this book is introduced by a quote from a very influential nurse, Florence Nightingale (1859) who stated that 'The very first requirement in a hospital is that it should do the sick no harm'. Given the learning you have undertaken so far, is this possible? Do you agree with this quote? What about health care delivered in the community or in people's homes? How does it apply to the particular area of nursing you most enjoy and what are the dangers that can cause harm to people you meet as part of your nursing practice?

Chapter Ten

10

Working in a team

Scott Reeves

Key topics

- The nature of teams and their characteristics
- Teamwork and the delivery of health care
- Factors leading to poor and good teamwork
- Case histories of different health care teams in different settings
- Working effectively as a nursing student in a practice placement team

Introduction

Teamwork is an essential feature of modern life. Teams can be found in every type of work, from the airline industry to the catering industry. As a nursing student, you will be required to work in a number of teams during your pre-qualifying programme. As well as working in student teams while in your higher education institution, when on practice placement you will also work as a member of a nursing team, with a number of qualified nurses and health care assistants. It is also likely that you will be a member of a larger multidisciplinary team made up from other health and social care professionals such as doctors, occupational therapists, physiotherapists and social workers.

Working in an effective manner within your student, nursing or multidisciplinary team requires an understanding of how teams operate and an awareness of why teams function well and why they sometimes function poorly. This chapter explores a variety of issues related to teamwork to provide an understanding of how care teams are organized, why they are needed, and why they sometimes encounter problems.

This chapter has three aims:

To provide an insight into the issues related to working in a team made up of students and/or qualified professionals from nursing or from a range of other health and social care professions.

To help prepare you for your future work in a range of different care teams.

To further enhance your understanding of becoming a nurse and entering the nursing 'community of practice'.

Teamwork: the basics

This part of the chapter outlines and discusses the key characteristics of teams and teamwork. It also offers an explanation of why teams are crucial to the delivery of health and social care, before providing an insight into the issues that underpin successful teamwork as well as issues related to the challenges that can occur while working in a care team.

Teams and teamwork: underpinning ideas

Across different work settings, teams are formed when groups of people come together to complete a task that one person would have difficulty in achieving on their own. In this context, the terms 'group' and 'team' are employed interchangeably. This use of terminology follows the work of authors such as Douglas (1983) and Adair (1986), who regard the interactions that occur within groups and teams as similar. For example, Douglas (1983, p 1) states:

> *Teams are cooperative groups in that they are called into being to perform a task, a task that cannot be performed by an individual.*

Sundstrom et al (1990) emphasize three other elements that help characterize a team. First, they point out that individuals should hold a *shared identity* of themselves as 'team members'. Second, they argue that each team member should have their own *individual role* to ensure that members do not duplicate work. Finally, they note that teams should share a *collective agreement* around how they work together. Pritchard (1995) goes on to outline four distinctive features that help define a team:

- Members should share a *common purpose* for their work.
- Members should have an understanding of all team members' *role and function.*
- Teams need to *pool their skills and knowledge* if they are to work together.
- Teams need to be able to work by themselves in an *independent* fashion.

Working in health and social care teams

Although health and social care teams share several of the above characteristics, they also have attributes that are specific to their role in the delivery of care. For example, the main goal of care teams is that members work together in a collaborative and cooperative manner to deliver care to patients or clients (Henneman et al 1995, Williams & Laungani 1999). Also, as noted above, a care team can be made up from a number of people from the same professions, or it can be made up from people in different professions such as nurses, doctors, physiotherapists and social workers. This diversity of care teams led Meerabeau & Page (1999, p 31) to note that:

> *Teams come in many shapes and forms within health delivery, from . . . the multidisciplinary team, the pain control team or the cardiac arrest team.*

Working as a member of a care team can involve a number of activities, from 'hands on' work with patients to handovers and case conferences where professionals review, discuss and plan patient care. This type of work can also be undertaken on a 'real-time' basis, as, for example, when you and other colleagues are delivering nursing care together. In addition, teamwork can be undertaken on a time-delayed basis (e.g. delivering care following a decision taken in a multidisciplinary case conference).

Increasingly patients/clients are becoming involved in team meetings where decisions are taken about their care. As the Nursing and Midwifery Council state in the 'NMC Code of professional conduct' patients and clients are equal partners in their care and therefore have the right to be involved in the health care team's decisions.

Therefore, as well as containing members of the caring professions, one needs to be aware that care teams can sometimes include patients/clients and also their carers.

Types of teams

To develop a comprehensive understanding of teams and teamwork, a number of authors have outlined the different types of care team that can exist. For example, Bruce (1980) devised a model of teamwork that contained three types of teams:

- *Committed teams*, in which all members share a common goal, roles and responsibilities between team members are well understood and there is good communication and regular interaction between members.
- *Convenient teams*, in which a few members share a common goal, there is some understanding of members' roles and responsibilities, but there is only limited interaction and communication between members.
- *Nominal teams*, in which members do not share a common goal, members have little idea of each other's roles, communication is poor and there is generally little interaction between members.

Katzenback & Smith (1993) developed a model that contained five different types of team:

- *High-performance teams*, in which members hold a clear understanding of their roles, share common team goals and encourage members' personal development.
- *Real teams*, in which members share common goals, hold collective team goals and share some accountability.
- *Potential teams*, in which members are beginning to work in a collaborative manner as they have a few of the factors needed for effective teamwork, such as sharing common team goals.
- *Pseudo-teams*, in which members are labelled as a 'team' but in reality there is little shared responsibility or coordination of their teamwork.
- *Working groups*, in which members hold some shared information and undertake some team activities, but there is no joint responsibility or clear team roles.

Such models are helpful to think about when you are working in a team, as they can help to pinpoint what type of team you are in. They might also be used to help individuals who are in poorly performing teams work towards achieving a more collaborative approach to their work.

Teams as families and tribes

An interest in the emotional dimension of teams has led some authors to compare team relations to those of *family members* (Woodhouse & Pengelly 1991). For example, it has been noted that interpersonal rivalry that can develop between team members has a similarity to sibling (brother or sister) tensions that emerge when one family member is competing to gain advantage over another for the attention of a parent (or a team leader).

Firth-Cozens (1998, p 4) draws on this idea when she notes that such emotions can have a problematic affect on teams and the way they work together:

> *Like families, a team's emotional life can at times be fraught . . . causing distress and stopping the team from functioning well.*

Similarly, interprofessional teams (consisting of two or more different care professions) have also been compared to different *tribes* (Beattie 1995, Pirrie 1999). It is argued that professions, like tribes, are protective of their individual identities, cultures and beliefs. Consequently, interaction between tribes (or professions) can be strained and, on occasions, can lead to friction. The challenges related to working in an interprofessional team are discussed in more depth later in the chapter.

Teams over time

It is important to recognize that teams develop and change over time. Tuckman & Jensen (1977) devised a model of group development to help understand the different stages groups and teams pass through as they work together. They identified five different stages:

Stage 1: 'forming'. This stage is characterized by ambiguity and confusion as members struggle to begin working together.
Stage 2: 'storming'. Friction is generated between members as they begin to adopt roles and negotiate how they can work together.
Stage 3: 'norming'. Members begin to find some agreement around how they work together and which roles different members might adopt within the group.
Stage 4: 'performing'. Members reach agreement around how they can work together; they understand one another and collaborate in a well-coordinated fashion.
Stage 5: 'adjourning'. In this final stage, members disband following completion of their collective goals and tasks.

Although Tuckman & Jensen considered that most groups would progress directly from stage 1 to stage 5, they did acknowledge that in problematic situations, for example in groups who experience a high degree of membership change, some of the stages would be repeated. Recent research into the nature of teamwork has revealed that Tuckman & Jensen's model can usefully track the different stages of team development (Farrell et al 2001, Janicik & Bartel 2003).

Why work in teams?

It is often argued that effective teamwork is an essential ingredient for delivering safe, high-quality care (Gregson et al 1991, Shaw 1970, Zwarenstein & Reeves 2002). Writing in 1974, Eichhorn offers an early example of why teams are needed in the delivery of care (Eichhorn in Larson & LaFasto 1989, p 17):

> *Because health problems have become defined in complex and multifaceted terms, health organizations have discovered it is necessary to have the information and skills of many disciplines in order to develop valid solutions and deliver comprehensive care to individuals and families.*

This early view has been echoed more recently by Firth-Cozens (1998, p 3), who argues:

> *Teamworking is seen as a way to tackle the potential fragmentation of care; a means to widen skills; an essential part of the need to consider the complexity of modern care; and a way to generally improve quality for the patient.*

Similar arguments have been regularly emphasized in national policies (Department of Health 1988, 1997, 2000a,b, Department of Health and Social Security 1974) and international policies (World Health Organization 1976, 1988) related to the delivery of health and social care. Indeed, research has indicated that effective teamwork can make a number of improvements for students, staff and patients/clients. It can:

- Create a more satisfying work environment (Iles & Sunderland 2001, McGrath 1991).
- Improve communication and coordination between professions (e.g. Borrill et al 2001).
- Reduce clinical error (Sexton et al 2000).
- Enhance the quality of care delivered to patients/clients (Litaker et al 2003, Schmitt 2001).

The need for effective teamwork has also led the organizations that regulate health and social care to stress the need for their practitioners to collaborate effectively within care teams. For example, the Nursing and Midwifery Council (NMC) states in the 'NMC Code of professional conduct' that qualified nurses and midwives are expected to work co-operatively within teams and to respect the skills, expertise and contributions of colleagues.

Similar statements can be found in the professional regulatory bodies for other health and social

care professions, such as doctors (General Medical Council 2001) and occupational therapists (College of Occupational Therapists 2000).

A number of 'benchmark statements' have also been developed to ensure that students develop the appropriate knowledge attitudes and skills of teamwork during their pre-qualifying programmes (Quality Assurance Agency for Higher Education 2000, 2001, 2002, 2004). Consequently, many higher education institutions are offering opportunities for students to learn together on an interprofessional basis to develop the range of attributes needed to become effective team players. For example, Ponzer et al (2004) describe an interprofessional ward experience where nursing, medical, occupational therapy and physiotherapy students worked together in teams to deliver care to orthopaedic patients.

The role of interprofessional team training is discussed in more depth later in the chapter.

Box 10.1

Essential criteria for effective teamwork

- Clear team objectives
- Clear and meaningful roles for each team member
- A high level of interaction by team members
- Low turnover of members entering and leaving the team
- Commitment to quality
- Equality among team members
- Trust
- Regular feedback on team goals and tasks
- Flexible decision-making processes
- Open communication systems
- Facilitative leadership
- Support for introducing new ideas
- Support from senior management

Making the team work

A large number of research studies has now been undertaken on how members of care teams work together (e.g. Borrill et al 2001, Øvertveit 1993, 1997, West & Slater 1996). As a result, there is a good deal of evidence on what constitutes effective teamwork. Box 10.1 outlines some of the issues identified by this research.

As Box 10.1 indicates, effective teamwork requires attention to a variety of factors. The remainder of this section draws together these factors in four separate subsections ('team preparation', 'leadership issues', 'team reflection' and 'external supports') to discuss their impact upon how teams work together.

Team preparation

Øvertveit (1997) argues that teams need to spend time undertaking preparatory work to achieve clarity around team roles, responsibilities and goals. Such preparation can provide a team with opportunities to agree how to coordinate their collaborative work in an efficient and mutually satisfying manner.

An important outcome of this preparation work is that teams develop a 'team policy', which explicitly records the collective aims, roles and responsibilities of the team. It also helps to ensure that a team has a formal document that provides members with 'defining details of how they operate' (Øvertveit 1997, p 272). Øvertveit saw that each team policy should contain a number of key elements:

- An outline of the overall purpose of the team.
- Information on team membership.
- Clarification of individuals' roles within the team.
- Details on the processes of teamwork.
- Shared targets/milestones.

For Øvertveit, on-going discussion between team members is required to ensure that their team policy is regularly updated and amended if, for example, a new member joins and there is a need to modify a previously agreed policy. Research has revealed that where team members spend time undertaking this form of preparatory work, they can be more effective in their collaborative work (Larson & LaFasto 1989, Meerabeau & Page 1999).

Leadership issues

Team leaders play a central role in ensuring that teams work together in an effective manner. Cook (2003, p 84), for example, provides a helpful definition of a care team leader as:

> *An expert involved in providing or supporting direct care services who influences others to improve the care they provide.*

Based on his research into the nature of leaders in care teams, Cook identifies a number of personal attributes required for such leaders. These include the ability to motivate staff, take effective decisions, encourage innovation and release the talents of the team members.

As well as requiring a variety of personal attributes, Adair (1983) found that an effective leader needs to attend to three central functions in relation to their team:

- *Individual team members' needs*: this ensures that individuals feel their contributions to the team are worthwhile and valued.
- *The team's tasks*: to ensure that the team is completing its agreed collective work.
- *The team's collective needs*: this ensures that team members can work in a collaborative and well-coordinated fashion.

It has also been argued that an individual's style of leadership can have a significant impact on how a team works together. Bass (1997), for example, identified two main types of leadership style: 'transactional' and 'transformational'. For Bass, a transactional leader adopts an authoritative approach to their work with team members. They also tend to work in isolation from the team and will take decisions without including other team members. In contrast, a transformational leader adopts a democratic approach to their work. In doing so, they work flexibly with the members of their team and they promote creative problem-solving among members.

Team reflection

For West (1996), a team that can spend time together reflecting upon their collaborative work can develop a 'reflexive' (e.g. integrated and well coordinated) way of working together. As West (1996, p 13) stated:

> *Reflexivity involves the members of the team standing back and critically examining themselves, their processes and their performance to communicate about these issues and to make appropriate changes.*

West identified that the development of a reflexive team approach can help ensure that members are able to adapt and respond effectively to any changes they encounter. This is an important quality to have for teams working in the NHS, as change is an ongoing factor that needs to be managed by students and staff.

A key aspect to achieving a reflexive approach is the creation of an environment where members value one another's contributions, feel safe to share their ideas openly and trust one another to acknowledge their shortfalls and mistakes. While West noted that the development of a reflexive approach to teamwork will take team members both time and effort, the benefit gained from this input is worthwhile.

Research into effects of incorporating shared reflection time has revealed that this activity can help produce a more effective team effort. For example, in her study of a care team, Opie (1997, p 275) found that when team members engage in shared reflection they are more likely to 'fuse together' their different knowledge bases and perspectives and achieve a more integrated way of working together.

External supports

As well as attention to the roles and processes that occur within a team, one also needs to be aware that effective teamwork requires support from outside (external) sources. In particular, it is vital that teams have the support of senior management (Onyett 2003). Such support ensures that the team has the resources (i.e. time and money) to

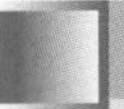

work together in focusing on the needs of patients/clients. The failure to obtain support of senior management can result in a team that cannot action its decisions on delivering care.

Another form of external support that teams can access is information technology. Reeves & Freeth (2003) argue that the use of information technologies is beginning to offer health and social care teams an additional means of supporting their collaborative work. They note that, whereas traditional forms of teamwork depend on members sharing the same physical space (i.e. a ward or a team room) to collaborate, the demands of managing patient caseloads in different locations often restrict time for this type of collaboration. The use of information technologies can help overcome such problems. They can provide an 'electronic bridge' (Reeves & Freeth 2003, p 81) to support teamwork, especially when there is little time for interaction or a need to rapidly access remote forms of information. Examples of technologies that can be used for this purpose include e-mail, e-conferencing and e-databases (e.g. electronic patient notes).

Box 10.2

Main challenges faced by team members

- Role overlap/blurred roles
- Geographical separation
- Heavy workloads
- Large teams
- Lack of trust between team members
- Different management lines between different professionals
- Steep team hierarchies
- Power and status differences
- Lack of knowledge/skills for effective teamwork
- Little critical thought about teamwork
- Belonging to multiple teams

Team challenges

Although, as discussed above, there is a good deal of evidence as to what constitutes an effective team, research has also revealed that teams often encounter a number of challenges while working together (e.g. Engel 1994, Miller & Freeman 2003, Reeves et al 2003). Box 10.2 outlines the key challenges identified by this research.

Box 10.2 reveals that teams and their members can encounter a range of different challenges while working together. This section goes on to draw together the difficulties identified in Box 10.2 in six separate subsections ('professional issues', 'time and space', 'roles and membership', 'team size and hierarchy', 'conflict' and 'team training') to provide a better understanding of how they can undermine team function.

Professional issues

Professions such as medicine and more recently nursing have undergone a process called 'professionalization'. For Friedson (1970), this process is undertaken in order to secure ownership of areas of knowledge and expertise. In obtaining this ownership, Friedson argued that professions secure a right to practise in an independent fashion, which in turn leads to financial reward and status enhancement. To protect the gains obtained from professionalization, Friedson claimed that professions guard the areas of knowledge and expertise they have claimed as their own primarily through the regulation of entry and the maintenance of professional standards. Tension and friction can therefore arise if a member of one profession perceives that a member from another is infringing their area of expertise.

A useful illustration of the difficulties that can arise in relation to professionalization is provided by Connolly (1995) in her evaluation of an interprofessional placement for nursing, social work, occupational therapy, nutrition and recreational therapy students. Connolly found that some students occasionally felt their professional boundaries were encroached when working together on the placement. These perceived professional boundary infringements were reported to cause friction, as students attempted to protect their own boundaries. In many senses, the discussion of teams as tribes mentioned above links into the issues of professionalization and the protection of professional boundaries.

Another difficulty that is encountered in multidisciplinary teams is the inequalities in terms of power and status that exist between the health and social care professions (Turner 1995). As doctors have the legal responsibility for the care of most patients/clients, they tend to have more influence (power) than nurses, therapists and social workers in the multidisciplinary team. As a consequence of this influence, they occupy a higher social status than their professional colleagues. As discussed above, given the need for equality within teams, such differences can cause interprofessional friction and tension, as a number of studies have revealed (e.g. Skjørshammer 2001, Walby et al 1994). However, as the section on teamwork in action indicates (see below), team members can often work together successfully despite such differences.

Time and space

Finding sufficient amounts of time to come together to meet as a team can be difficult given the heavy workloads professionals need to manage. For example, research by Annandale et al (1999) indicated that teamwork between nursing and medical staff based in an accident and emergency unit was restricted because of the heavy workloads each profession had to deal with. Similarly, Atwal (2002) found that nurses and other multidisciplinary team members such as occupational therapists and physiotherapists regularly encountered difficulties in attending discharge meetings due to heavy workloads.

Such time pressures led Engeström et al (1999) to question whether the traditional ideas of teamwork (discussed above) fit the realities of working in a care team. These authors argued that in most care settings, especially in acute care settings, many interprofessional relationships are short-lived and continually shifting between individuals. Teamworking could therefore be seen more as a process of 'knotworking', in which individuals tie, untie and re-tie separate threads of activity during their brief interactions.

Similarly, as discussed above, an important aspect of teamwork is the need for members to interact together regularly, in the same physical space (e.g. a ward or a meeting room). Research has indicated, however, that health and social care professionals find it difficult to do so. For example, Handy (1999) found that a single flight of stairs separating a team reduced their interactions by 30%. In relation to care teams, Allen (2002) found that teams of doctors and nurses often found problems meeting as their clinical work resulted in them being located in different parts of a hospital and at different times of the day. Opportunities for face-to-face interaction were therefore limited.

Roles and membership

As noted above, the need for team members to have clear roles and responsibilities within the team is essential for successful teamwork. However, a growing trend in health and social care teams is to attempt to work in a more 'generic' fashion in which different team members share roles. Unsurprisingly, it has been found that where generic working occurs, it usually results in the generation of friction between team members as they are often unclear as to what they should be doing within their team (e.g. Brown et al 2000, Stark et al 2002).

As discussed above, as a nursing student you will usually belong to a number of different student, nursing and multidisciplinary teams. For Zagier Roberts (1994), membership of a team normally carries an emotional attachment. Often people are more attached to one of the teams they work within, normally because they have a commitment to a particular team's aims or enjoy interaction with certain team members. Because of the number of years it takes for students to become qualified practitioners and the socialization (in which students adopt the beliefs and behaviours of their chosen profession) that occurs during this time, health and social care professionals normally identify most strongly with their own professional team. Consequently, they may prioritize that team's work at the expense of their multidisciplinary team.

Team size and hierarchy

It has been found that teams with large numbers of members (usually over 13 people) encounter more difficulties working together than do smaller teams (Øvertveit 1993, Williams & Laungani 1999). For large teams, it can be difficult to meet together at the same time. Consequently, members tend to have fewer interactions than do the members of smaller teams.

Handy (1999, p 155) argues that large teams do have some advantages in terms of a greater amount of 'talent, skills and knowledge'. However, Handy also argues that, in large teams, there is usually more absenteeism and lower morale as members tend to meet less often.

It has also been noted that small 'subgroups' can emerge within large teams (Douglas 2000). Subgroups occur when a small number of members who hold interests and ideas that diverge from those held by the majority of members work together in an exclusionary fashion. Although the emergence of subgroups can help a team to function well and complete its tasks, it has been found that they can sometimes cause tension between members (Reeves 2005).

As noted above, one of the requirements for effective teamwork is the need for equality between members. Therefore teams need to organize themselves into a 'flat' structure, without members occupying distinctly higher and lower levels of a hierarchy. Greenwell (1995) argues that one of the main difficulties for teams is that, although they require flat or horizontal structures, they are formed from health and social care professionals who are organized in steep hierarchies. For example, hospital-based nursing is based around a hierarchy that incorporates junior staff nurses, senior staff nurses, junior sisters/charge nurses, senior sisters/charge nurses, ward managers and lead nurses.

Although hierarchies are helpful in ensuring that more experienced staff take responsibility for junior staff so that they are well supported in their clinical practice, such structures can have an inhibiting effect on teamwork in some teams. For example, team hierarchies can disempower students and junior staff from making potentially valuable suggestions to the more senior staff for improvements in the delivery of care. The issue of hierarchy is explored in more depth in the next part of the chapter.

Conflict

As previously outlined, in general, conflict between team members, whether it is produced from professional frictions or a lack of clear team roles, is a problematic feature of teamwork and something that should be avoided. However, team conflict can also have a positive effect in terms of producing creative and effective teamwork among members. As West (1994, p 71) stated:

> *Conflict is . . . desirable in teams. Team conflict can be a source of excellence, quality and creativity.*

Nevertheless, West did note that conflict needs to be well handled within a team; if not, it can become damaging to the interpersonal relationships of team members.

It has also been found that an absence of conflict or friction within a team can develop a problem called 'groupthink'. Groupthink was devised by Janis (1982) from his analysis of how management teams dealt with highly stressful situations. Janis found that a lack of disagreement, debate and friction between members undermined their decision-making abilities. In such teams, rather than seeking opposing views and opinions during their discussions, members preferred to focus upon reaching agreement. Consequently, these teams failed to consider a range of possibilities around how they could solve a problem. Research into the nature of decision-making in teams continues to reveal that a lack of critical analysis in their discussions, in favour of an emphasis on consensus and agreement, is more likely to generate groupthink (e.g. Hart et al 1996, Reeves 2005).

Team training

As outlined above, working as an effective member of a health or social care team is a complicated task and it is surprising to discover that most professionals have traditionally received no formal training in how to become skilled team players.

Given this 'gap' in the knowledge and skills needed for teamwork, a growing number of initiatives have been implemented across care settings to begin developing the skills and knowledge for effective team working. For example, Zwarenstein et al (2003) described the introduction of an interprofessional training programme that aimed to improve collaboration between nurses and doctors based in an acute hospital. As well as reorganizing staff into small interprofessional teams, Zwarenstein et al described how staff were offered a series of team-building sessions focused on highlighting shared goals and clarifying each profession's contribution to care. It was found that the nurses and doctors communicated more frequently and in a more effective manner following their interprofessional training.

There has also been an increase in interprofessional education for pre-qualification students to better prepare them for their future professional practice. For example, Ker et al (2003) described the use of a simulated ward environment for medical and nursing students. After a briefing about the patients, students were allocated into interprofessional teams and were asked to take responsibility for the ward for a shift. At the end of their shift, the students prepared a joint report, which was presented to their tutors in the form of a ward handover. Student teams then received feedback on their performance by the tutors. It was found that students enjoyed working together in the simulated ward. It was felt that the ward provided a sufficiently realistic environment to help them learn about the demands related to interprofessional teamwork when attempting to organize and deliver care to patients.

Teamwork in action

The first part of this chapter provided background information on the ideas and issues related to working in a team. This part offers eight examples, presented as individual cases drawn from acute and community settings, of teams in action. This should provide you with an understanding of the range of issues related to working in a care team.

Teams working in acute care settings

Four different cases from teams working in acute care settings are presented here. As well as a description of each case, key messages are drawn from the case.

Case 1: Hierarchy and teamwork

Cott's (1998) study revealed how a team member's position in the hierarchy of the team has an important influence on their perceptions of teamwork. She examined the meanings and structures of teamwork of nurses, doctors and therapists who worked in a hospital-based long-term older-adult care unit. Interviews with team members revealed the existence of two distinctive subgroups within the multidisciplinary team:

- A subgroup of doctors, therapists and social workers who occupied a high position in the team hierarchy.
- A subgroup of junior qualified and unqualified nursing staff who occupied lower positions in the hierarchy.

Cott's study also revealed that team members in both subgroups held varying perceptions of teamwork, and these views were largely dependent upon their location in the team hierarchy. As Cott (1998, p 849) stated:

> *Staff in different structural positions held different perceptions of meanings of teamwork because they were engaged in different kinds of teamwork.*

It was found that the subgroup consisting of doctors, therapists and social workers collaborated as equals in the team, discussing and agreeing aspects of patient care. When they needed to ask one of the nurses to undertake a task, they generally spoke to the senior nurses, who in turn would talk to one of their juniors or one of the unqualified staff. In addition, for the subgroup of doctors, social workers and therapists, teamwork was essentially viewed as vital for improving quality of care they delivered to the patient. In contrast, the subgroup consisting of junior qualified and unqualified nursing staff viewed teamwork in less-positive terms, as it involved being told what to do by their senior colleagues.

Cott goes on to conclude that teamwork for the doctors, therapists and social workers was regarded as a rewarding activity as they occupied a high position in the team hierarchy and could influence the work of the junior nurses and the unqualified staff. Indeed, for the junior nurses and the qualified staff, who had little influence on patient care, teamwork was regarded in a different light.

This study provides a rare insight into how hierarchy affects members' views of teamwork. Importantly, it revealed that not all members share the same view of their collaborative work. Differences exist. It is therefore important that team members explore these differences to understand their possible effect on how they work together.

Case 2: Formal and informal teamwork

In a study by Reeves & Lewin (2004), difficulties in communication between team members who worked across a number of hospital wards meant that staff had to develop a number of informal mechanisms to support their teamwork. The authors examined the nature of teamwork in multidisciplinary teams consisting of nurses, doctors, therapists, pharmacists and social workers based in six wards within a general and emergency medical directorate of an inner city hospital.

Interviews and observations revealed that patients assigned to a particular doctor could be located in any one of the six wards in the directorate. This meant that while doctors were supposed to be based in a 'home' ward with their team, they regularly had to work across a number of wards to care for their patients. Consequently, doctors had only limited formal opportunities for teamwork with the nurses, therapists, pharmacists and social workers based on their home ward. Typically, interactions with their team were restricted to weekly multidisciplinary team meetings. However, heavy workloads meant that nurses and doctors failed to attend many of the weekly meetings. Teamwork therefore tended to be brief and irregular in nature.

To help overcome this lack of interaction, staff initiated a number of informal mechanisms to exchange information. These included:

- Talking to colleagues in the corridors while walking between wards.
- Asking the nurses to be an interprofessional 'go-between' to pass information between staff.
- Using patients' notes as a tool to communicate with one another.

Reeves & Lewin (2004) went on to conclude that the use of informal methods of communication are crucial in teams that have difficulty finding sufficient amounts of time to meet on a formal basis.

This study was helpful in describing a dimension of teamwork that is often overlooked: informal teamwork. Therefore one needs to be aware that both formal and informal types of collaboration can exist. Indeed, as this study revealed, staff were creative in finding alternative routes of communication to overcome their formal communication problems.

Case 3: A team in name only

A study by Meerabeau & Page (1999) provides an interesting insight into the difficulties nurses and doctors can encounter when working in cardiopulmonary resuscitation (CPR) team. Meerabeau & Page examined how CPR teams worked together. They noted that CPR teams usually differ from teams that work in accident and emergency departments or intensive care units. CPR team members tend not to know one another, as this type of team is formed from a variety of different staff trained in resuscitation techniques. Thus the same members are not always present in a CPR team.

Audio recordings from de-briefing sessions of team members who had recently attended a cardiac resuscitation were collected to provide an understanding of the nature of CPR teamwork. It was found that there was often an absence of leadership within a CPR team, especially when only junior and inexperienced staff arrived to give resuscitation. In addition, it was found that a number of members had only a poor idea of their role and input within the team during resuscitation. These two factors, combined with the stress of a resuscitation situation, often resulted in a lack of smoothly coordinated teamwork.

Meerabeau & Page argued that while CPR teams have a common shared purpose, their roles are generally unclear and there is often a lack of effective leadership. Furthermore, as CPR team members have 'no opportunities for teambuilding' (Meerabeau & Page 1999, p 38), their ability to function in an effective manner is limited. Consequently, the authors argued that in many ways a CPR team is not a team, rather they are a loosely connected work group.

This study indicated that simply coming together to work does not necessarily mean a team is really a team. If key attributes are missing (e.g. clear roles/functions and the input of an effective leader), teams display the characteristics of 'working groups' (Katzenback & Smith 1993), as mentioned at the beginning of the chapter.

Case 4: Flexible forms of teamwork

A study undertaken by Gair & Hartery (2001) examined the interprofessional relationships between two teams who worked in a hospital-based older-adult assessment unit. They observed the weekly case conference meetings of two teams who worked with older people to understand the nature of the relationships. Both teams were made up of nurses, doctors, occupational therapists, physiotherapists, health visitors, social workers and speech therapists.

Findings from this study revealed that a doctor always chaired (and also led) the meetings. However, as Gair & Hartery noted, given that doctors hold legal accountability for patients, their leading role in discussion and decision-making was accepted by the other members of the team. Nevertheless, in terms of the contribution made by the various professionals during their discussions, Gair & Hartery found broadly similar patterns for doctors (who contributed to 30% of discussions) and nurses (who contributed to 26% of discussions). Physiotherapists contributed to 20% of the discussions and occupational therapists contributed to 17%. In contrast, social workers only contributed to 4% of discussions, speech therapists to 2% and health visitors to 1%. These findings suggest that there was a core group of four professions who collectively dominated the meetings and decisions taken.

Consequently, while medical staff in general took the lead role in the teams, their decisions on patient management and discharge required input from a core of nursing, and, to a slightly lesser extent, physiotherapy and occupational therapy team members. The input of health visitors, social workers and speech therapists was much more limited.

This study indicated that, in meeting the needs of older adults, some team members had more input than others. Given the medical and nursing needs of most patients/clients, it is likely that these professions will work closely together, with additional input from physiotherapists, occupational therapists, social workers, speech therapists and other professionals when required.

Teams working in community settings

This section presents four different cases from teams working in community or primary care settings. Again, key messages are drawn out from each case.

Case 5: Success and challenges in mental health

Norman & Peck (1999) examined the experiences of community mental health team (CMHT) members to understand the key issues related to how they work together. They ran a number of workshops in which CMHT members (nurses, occupational therapists, social workers, doctors) were asked to generate accounts of their own role and identity as CMHT members. Data gathered from the workshops revealed a range of successes and challenges associated with working in a CMHT.

A number of areas were identified in which team members felt they were working well together. These included:

- A strong commitment for teamwork.
- A shared understanding of each other's roles and professional cultures.
- Regular contact between team members.
- Clear systems for referring clients between members and across different care agencies.
- Senior management support for teamwork.

In addition, the authors identified a range of factors that challenged CMHTs to work effectively. Most were linked to an underpinning uniprofessional culture that impeded the development of collaborative work. Evidence of this culture was identified as:

- Ambiguous professional responsibilities between team members.
- A lack of agreement around how team members work together in a cooperative fashion.
- Differences in professional power and status between members.
- Conflicting caseload priorities between team members.
- The use of different models of care, which generated different objectives and working methods between members.

This study revealed that, while teams can function in an effective manner, their collaborative work can also contain a number of challenges, all of which need to be managed if the team can successfully work together.

Case 6: Developing a new care team

Bateman et al (2003) collected observational data to understand the processes associated with the development of a new primary care team. The team comprised two doctors, two nurse practitioners, a child and family nurse, a pharmacist, a practice manager and four administrative staff. At the formation of the team, members met to agree a shared approach to their work. Based on these early discussions, it was agreed that their collective work should be grounded on a number of principles, which included:

- The adoption of a 'flat' management style to encourage team equality.
- That all members should use their skills and expertise to enhance patient care.
- To develop relationships with patients so they could play a part in the evolution of the team.

Despite laying these foundations, a number of difficulties were encountered in the months that followed the team's formation. Specifically, it was found that team members were uncertain about their own professional role, contribution and worth within the team. In addition, it was found that imbalances in workloads inhibited members' time to develop good relationships with their colleagues.

The team subsequently met to begin resolving these initial problems. It was found that ongoing discussions helped clarify the roles and responsibilities, and that a re-distribution of caseloads achieved more balance between members' workloads.

This study provides an insight into an innovative project that attempted to create an effective interprofessional team. The use of initial agreements over the key principles of good teamwork helped ensure that members worked together. Despite these efforts, a number of difficulties were still encountered. This study therefore indicates that such team arrangements need to be monitored to ensure that they are functioning. Clearly, where problems do arise, further team discussion will be needed to revise previously agreed approaches.

Case 7: Humour and teamwork

A study by Griffiths (1998) revealed that humour was an important mechanism for improving the quality of interprofessional relationships. She explored the role and influence of humour within two CMHTs. Both teams consisted of doctors, nurses, social workers and occupational therapists. Audiotape recordings of team meetings were gathered over a 12-month period to develop an in-depth understanding of how each team used humour in their collaborative work.

Findings from the study revealed that humour in both teams was used as a way of 'letting off steam' (Griffiths 1998, p 892) in relation to the general stresses and strains of working together.

Humour was also regarded as a mechanism that helped team members support one another in their difficult work with patients who had serious mental health problems. In addition it was seen as useful in helping to maintain cooperative relationships between the team leader and the other team members.

Griffiths found that humour could be employed by team members to question their team leader's approach to, or opinion on, issues related to the delivery of care. Specifically, the study revealed that team members used humorous comments to 'signal their unease about certain referrals' (Griffiths 1998, p 884) to their team leader, or question their leader's preferred course of action on a patient. Often, team members' use of humour resulted in a changed course of action by the team leader.

This study provides a rare account into the in-depth functions of a team. Importantly, it revealed that humour can make changes to a way a team works together. It can support/help a team's collaborative work and allow team members to raise sensitive questions about their work.

Case 8: Improving the delivery of care

A study undertaken by Lowe & O'Hara (2000) examined the impact of introducing an interprofessional team approach into a primary care clinic where staff had previously worked in isolation from one another. Lowe & O'Hara's study included nurses, occupational therapists, physiotherapists and speech and language therapists who worked in a primary care clinic. Traditionally, these professionals tended to work in isolation with clients. Consequently, staff had little regular communication or interaction, and they also lacked any shared clinical standards for the delivery of client care.

To improve the way staff worked together, it was agreed that they would introduce an interprofessional approach. They therefore undertook regular team meetings, initiated collaborative decision-making and undertook shared objective-setting and goal-planning. In addition, they attended a series of interprofessional training sessions to develop their teamwork skills.

An evaluation of this initiative revealed that all team members felt that they had a clear understanding of one another's roles and that there was an improved rapport between members. Staff also felt that the service they delivered to clients had improved, as there was more efficient use of time and less duplication of effort.

This study indicates that a careful and well-considered move towards team-based care can produce a number of positive outcomes for team members in terms of their satisfaction and an improved coordination of client care.

Starting work in a team

This final section of the chapter draws together the issues examined in the preceding sections in order to offer some ideas around how you can work effectively in a care team, especially when you are on a practice placement. Initially, it considers the issues related to when you start on a placement and how a mentor can support you. It then goes on to present some ideas designed to support your work as a student nurse in a care team.

Practice placements and mentorship

It is useful to remember that students starting on a practice placement often have difficulty adjusting to the demands of the new environment. Students can initially struggle to establish working relationships with qualified nursing staff and to collaborate with practitioners from other professional groups; they also encounter difficulties in being able to cope with delivering care to patients with unfamiliar clinical conditions. These difficulties are often compounded because most nursing students arrive on placements with a classroom-based knowledge of nursing care and only a limited experience of clinical nursing. As a result, many students find their initial entry to a new placement is stressful. The support and guidance of a mentor can therefore help alleviate many of these difficulties.

Mentors are experienced nurses who can offer you support and guidance during your placement. It has been found that mentors have four key roles: student supervision; assessment and feedback; teaching while engaged in clinical practice; and emotional support (Dewar & Walker 1999, Spouse 1996). Mentors therefore provide an excellent resource for nursing students. As well as supporting and guiding you through your early experiences in a new clinical environment, mentors can help you reflect upon your clinical learning and plan future learning activities to extend clinical knowledge. In addition, as experienced clinical practitioners, mentors should be able to provide advice on issues related to nursing-specific and interprofessional teamwork.

Given the importance of mentorship, if you do feel overwhelmed during your time on a placement do not be afraid to ask your mentor for support and guidance; they are there to help. Indeed, Spouse (2003) found that effective support from mentors significantly increased nursing students' ability to adjust to clinical settings, as they helped students integrate into the clinical nursing activities and therefore made them feel a part of the community of practice.

Ideas for teamwork

This section considers three separate approaches that might be useful in supporting your early experiences as a student nurse in a care team.

Stages of team learning

Hilton et al (1995) outlined three stages of development that students need to pass through before they have the attitudes, knowledge and skills to be an effective team worker:

- *Stage 1 (first year)*. Students need to develop an awareness of teamwork by exploring the professional goals of various team members. They also need to understand what other professionals know and do in a care setting. In addition, students need to appreciate the function of a care team, as well as be able to communicate with other students and qualified staff.
- *Stage 2 (second year)*. Students need to identify the areas that are unique to each member of the care team. They also need to participate actively in cooperative goal-making in relation to patient/client care. In addition, students should value the opinions of colleagues and be willing to give, receive and share information.
- *Stage 3 (third year)*. At this stage students should have the attributes (attitudes, knowledge and skills) gained from stages 1 and 2 to be able to work collaboratively as a valued member of a care team.

In essence, this model provides some idea of the attributes students need to develop during the 3 years of their pre-qualifying education. It might therefore be a useful tool to use in discussion with your mentor to help structure a range of different team-oriented learning activities that would be useful to your professional development.

Team roles

Belbin's (1981) model of team member roles provides another useful approach for students who are starting work within a team. Belbin identified eight different roles (see Box 10.3).

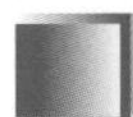

Box 10.3

An overview of Belbin's team members' roles

The chairman: a person who coordinates the team; they are focused and delegate tasks to other members.

The shaper: an enthusiastic person who will take over from chairman if absent; this person is usually keen to complete tasks.

The plant: an imaginative and creative person with good problem-solving skills.

The monitor-evaluator: an analytical person who offers careful examination of the team's ideas.

The resource-investigator: a sociable and popular person who can act as a diplomat if required.

The company worker: a person who likes to work along the team's agreed lines; someone who can turn ideas into manageable tasks.

The team worker: a supportive and uncompetitive person, who usually has a harmonizing effect on the team.

The finisher: a person who likes to check information and helps to ensure that the team complete its tasks.

Belbin went on to note that, if one type of role dominated, a team would encounter difficulties in their collaborative work. He also noted that teams containing too few roles may not be able to complete all its tasks. However, Belbin pointed out that, in small teams, it was normal for one person to undertake a number of different roles.

This model may be useful to you when you start to work in a team. It could provide you with some idea of the type of team members who you are working with, as well as identifying their roles, some of which you may want to discuss with your mentor. In addition, Belbin's model may help to identify the potential strengths and weaknesses that exist within a team. Further information on this model and how to use it can be found at http://www.belbin.com/.

Teamwork tasks

Zwarenstein & Reeves (2002) have outlined four key tasks to help ensure smooth and well coordinated teamwork between members:

- *Task 1*: agree on a shared definition of patient/client well-being which incorporates ideas from the different perspectives of team members.
- *Task 2*: identify the information to be shared in order to allow other professionals to work, and agree how this is to be shared; define the work each profession does alone and does together.
- *Task 3*: understand the differing demands and pressures each profession faces in delivering care; this can help lead to mutual support between team members.
- *Task 4*: acknowledge that delivering care is difficult, not always successful and can cause anxiety.

This model offers a set of practice guidelines, in the form of four team tasks, to encourage an interprofessional team to work in a more effective manner. If your care team is experiencing problems working together during one of your practice placements, this model could be helpful to incorporate when discussing such issues with your mentor. Indeed, it might also be employed to initiate a discussion with staff around how they might enhance their approach to teamwork.

Concluding comments

As discussed in the chapter, working in a team requires attention to a variety of factors. Importantly, the chapter outlines and discusses the key criteria that ensure team members can work together in an effective manner, for example, the sharing of common team goals, clear roles and responsibilities and regular interaction. In addition, the chapter presents a range of challenges team members need to be mindful of when working together in a team, such as unclear or blurred roles, geographical separation, steep hierarchies, professional power and status differences and a lack of skills required for teamwork. The chapter also presents a number of different case studies of teams in action to help develop an in-depth understanding of the issues related to teamwork. Finally, some ideas that could support you when you start to work in a clinical environment are outlined.

In collating the literature on teamwork and applying it to a nursing student context, it is hoped that the chapter will provide you with a useful source of information to support your work in the variety of care teams during your entry into nursing's community of practice.

References

Adair J 1983 Effective leadership. Gower, London

Adair J 1986 Effective teamworking. Pan, London

Allen D 2002 Time and space on the hospital ward: shaping the scope of nursing practice. In: Allen D, Hughes D (eds) Nursing and the division of labour in healthcare. Palgrave, Basingstoke

Annandale E, Clark J, Allen E 1999 Interprofessional working: an ethnographic case study of emergency health care. Journal of Interprofessional Care 13:139–150

Atwal A 2002 Nurses' perceptions of discharge planning in acute health care. Journal of Advanced Nursing 39:450–458

Bass B 1997 Transformational leadership. Lawrence Earlbaum Associates, Boston

Bateman H, Bailey P, McLellan H 2003 Of rocks and safe channels: learning to navigate as an interprofessional team. Journal of Interprofessional Care 17:141–150

Beattie A 1995 War and peace among the health tribes. In: Soothill K, Mackay L, Webb C (eds) Interprofessional relations in health care. Edward Arnold, London

Belbin M 1981 Management teams: why they succeed or fail. Butterworth-Heinemann, Oxford

Borrill C, Carletta J, Carter A et al 2001 The effectiveness of health care teams in the National Health Service. Aston University, Birmingham

Brown B, Crawford P, Darongkamas J 2000 Blurred roles and permeable boundaries: the experience of multidisciplinary working in community mental health. Health and Social Care in the Community 8:425–435

Bruce N 1980 Teamwork for preventive care. Wiley, Chichester

College of Occupational Therapists 2000 Code of ethics and professional conduct for occupational therapists. College of Occupational Therapists, London

Connolly P 1995 Transdisciplinary collaboration of academia and practice in the area of serious mental illness. Australian and New Zealand Journal of Mental Health Nursing 4:168–180

Cook M 2003 Interprofessional post-qualifying education: team leadership. In: Glen S, Leiba T (eds) Interprofessional post-qualifying education for nurses. Palgrave, Basingstoke

Cott C 1998 Structure and meaning in multidisciplinary teamwork. Sociology of Health and Illness 20:848–873

Department of Health 1988 Working together: a guide to inter-agency cooperation for the protection of children from abuse. HMSO, London

Department of Health 1997 The new NHS: modern, dependable. HMSO, London

Department of Health 2000a The NHS plan: a plan for investment, a plan for reform. Department of Health, London

Department of Health 2000b A quality strategy for social care. Department of Health, London

Department of Health and Social Security 1974 The Joseph report. HMSO, London

Dewar B, Walker E 1999 Experiential learning: issues for supervision. Journal of Advanced Nursing 30:1459–1567

Douglas T 1983 Groups: understanding people gathered together. Tavistock, London

Douglas T 2000 Basic groupwork. Routledge, London

Engel C 1994 A functional anatomy of teamwork. In: Leathard A (ed) Going interprofessional: working together for health and welfare. Routledge, London

Engeström Y, Engeström R, Vahaaho T 1999 When the center does not hold: the importance of knotworking. In: Chaklin S, Hedegaard M, Jensen U (eds) Activity theory and social practice. Aarhus University Press, Aarhus

Farrell M, Schmitt M, Heinemann G 2001 Informal roles and the stages of team development. Journal of Interprofessional Care 15:281–295

Firth-Cozens J 1998 Celebrating teamwork. Quality in Health Care 7(suppl):3–7

Friedson E 1970 Profession of medicine: a study of the sociology of applied knowledge. Harper and Row, New York

Gair G, Hartery T 2001 Medical dominance in multidisciplinary teamwork: a case study of discharge decision-making in a geriatric assessment unit. Journal of Nursing Management 9:3–11

General Medical Council 2001 Good medical practice. General Medical Council, London

Greenwell J 1995 Patients and professionals. In: Soothill K, Mackay L, Webb C (eds) Interprofessional relations in health care. Edward Arnold, London

Gregson B, Cartlidge A, Bond J 1991 Interprofessional collaboration in primary health care organisations. Royal College of General Practitioners, London

Griffiths L 1998 Humour as resistance to professional dominance in community mental health teams. Sociology of Health and Illness 20:874–895

Handy C 1999 Understanding organizations, 4th edn. Penguin, London

Hart P, Sterns E, Sundelius B et al 1996 Beyond groupthink: political group dynamics and foreign policy-making. American Political Science Review 93:766–767

Henneman E, Lee J, Cohen J 1995 Collaboration: a concept analysis. Journal of Advanced Nursing 21:103–109

Hilton R, Morris D, Wright A 1995 Learning to work in the heath care team. Journal of Interprofessional Care 9:167–174

Iles V, Sunderland K 2001 Organisational change. a review for health care managers, professionals and researchers. London School of Hygiene and Tropical Medicine, London

Janicik G, Bartel C 2003 Talking about time: effects of temporal planning and time awareness norms on group co-ordination and performance. Group Dynamics 7:122–134

Janis I 1982 Groupthink: a study of foreign policy decisions and fiascos, 2nd edn. Houghton Mifflin, Boston

Katzenbach J, Smith D 1993 The wisdom of teams: creating the high performance organization. Harvard Business School Press, Boston

Ker J, Mole L, Bradley P 2003 Early introduction to interprofessional learning: a stimulated ward environment. Medical Education 37:248–255

Larson C, LaFasto F 1989 Teamwork: what must go right, what can go wrong. Sage, Newbury Park

Litaker D, Mion L, Planavsky L et al 2003 Physician–nurse practitioner teams in chronic disease management: the impact on costs, clinical effectiveness and patients' perception of care. Journal of Interprofessional Care 17:223–238

Lowe F, O'Hara S 2000 Multi-disciplinary team working in practice: managing the transaction. Journal of Interprofessional Care 14:269–279

McGrath M 1991 Multidisciplinary teamwork. Avebury, Aldershot

Meerabeau L, Page S 1999 I'm sorry if I panicked you: nurses' accounts of teamwork in cardiopulmonary resuscitation. Journal of Interprofessional Care 13:29–40

Miller C, Freeman M 2003 Clinical teamwork: the impact of policy on collaborative practice. In: Leathard A (ed) Interprofessional collaboration: from policy to practice in health and social care. Brunner-Routledge, London

Norman I, Peck E 1999 Working together in adult community mental health services: an interprofessional dialogue. Journal of Mental Health 8:217–230

Nursing and Midwifery Council 2008 Code of professional conduct. Nursing and Midwifery Council, London

Onyett S 2003 Teamworking in mental health. Palgrave, Basingstoke

Opie A 1997 Thinking teams thinking clients: issues of discourse and representation in the work of health care teams. Sociology of Health and Illness 19:259–280

Øvertveit J 1993 Co-ordinating community care: multidisciplinary teams and care management. Open University Press, Milton Keynes

Øvertveit J 1997 Planning and managing teams. Health and Social Care in the Community 5:269–276

Pirrie A 1999 Rocky mountains and tired Indians: on territories and tribes. Reflections on multidisciplinary education in the health professions. British Education Research Journal 25:113–126

Ponzer S, Hylin U, Kusoffsky A et al 2004 Interprofessional training in the context of clinical practice: goals and students' perceptions on clinical education wards. Medical Education 38:727–736

Pritchard P 1995 Learning to work effectively in teams. In: Owens P, Carrier J, Horder J (eds) Interprofessional issues in community and primary health care. Macmillan, Basingstoke

Quality Assurance Agency for Higher Education 2000 Social policy and administration and social work: subject benchmarking statements. Quality Assurance Agency for Higher Education, Gloucester

Quality Assurance Agency for Higher Education 2001 Nursing: subject benchmark statements. Quality Assurance Agency for Higher Education, Gloucester

Quality Assurance Agency for Higher Education 2002 Medicine: subject benchmark statements. Quality Assurance Agency for Higher Education, Gloucester

Quality Assurance Agency for Higher Education 2004 A draft statement of common purpose for subject benchmarks for the health and social care professions: consultation. Quality Assurance Agency for Higher Education, Gloucester

Reeves S 2005 Developing and delivering practice-based interprofessional education: successes and challenges. Unpublished PhD thesis, City University, London

Reeves S, Freeth D 2003 New forms of information technology, new forms of collaboration? In: Leathard A (ed) Interprofessional collaboration: from policy to practice in health and social care. Routledge, London

Reeves S, Lewin S 2004 Hospital-based interprofessional collaboration: strategies and meanings. Journal of Health Services Research & Policy 9:218–225

Reeves S, Lewin S, Meyer J et al 2003 The introduction of a ward-based medical team system. City University, London. Online. Available: http://www.city.ac.uk/sonm/dps/research/research_reports/reeves_s/gem.pdf 19 Jan 2006

Schmitt M 2001 Collaboration improves the quality of care: methodological challenges and evidence from US health care research. Journal of Interprofessional Care 15:47–66

Sexton J, Thomas E, Helmreich L 2000 Error, stress and teamwork in medicine and aviation: cross sectional surveys. BMJ 320:745–749

Shaw M 1970 Communication processes. Penguin, London

Skjørshammer M 2001 Co-operation and conflict in a hospital: interprofessional differences in perception and management of conflicts. Journal of Interprofessional Care 15:7–18

Spouse J 1996 The effective mentor: a model for learner centred learning in clinical practice. Nursing Times Research 1:120–133

Spouse J 2003 Professional learning in nursing. Blackwell, Oxford

Stark S, Stronach I, Warne T 2002 Teamwork in mental health: rhetoric and reality. Journal of Psychiatric and Mental Health Nursing 9:411–418

Sundstrom E, de Meuse K, Futrell D 1990 Work teams: applications and effectiveness. American Psychologist 45:120–133

Tuckman B, Jenson M 1977 Stages of small group development re-visited. Group and Organisational Studies 2:419–427

Turner B 1995 Medical power and social knowledge, 2nd edn. Sage, London

Walby S, Greenwell J, Mackay L et al 1994 Medicine and nursing: professions in a changing health service. Sage, London

West M 1994 Effective teamwork. British Psychology Society Books, Leicester

West M 1996 Handbook of work group psychology. Wiley, Chichester

West M, Slater J 1996 Teamworking in primary health care: a review of its effectiveness. Health Education Authority, London

Williams G, Laungani P 1999 Analysis of teamwork in an NHS community trust: an empirical study. Journal of Interprofessional Care 13: 19–28

Woodhouse D, Pengelly P 1991 Anxiety and the dynamics of collaboration. Aberdeen University Press, Aberdeen

World Health Organization 1976 Continuing education of health personnel. Regional Office for Europe, Copenhagen

World Health Organization 1988 Learning together to work together. World Health Organization, Geneva

Zagier Roberts V 1994 Conflict and collaboration: managing intergroup relations. In: Obholzer A, Zagier Roberts V (eds) The unconscious at work: individual and organisational stress in the human services. Routledge, London

Zwarenstein M, Reeves S 2002 Working together but apart: barriers and routes to nurse–physician collaboration. The Joint Commission Journal on Quality Improvement 28:242–247

Zwarenstein M, Bryant W, Reeves S 2003 In-service interprofessional education improves inpatient care and satisfaction. Journal of Interprofessional Care 17:427–428

Chapter Eleven

11

Managing self and setting priorities in placements

Ann Jackson Fowler, Jane Akister, Mike Cook

Key topics

- Introduction
- Why are placements so important?
- What is a placement and who will support me?
- What can I do before I commence a placement?
- What is the role of the student/practitioner in a placement setting?
- Learning to prioritize
- Effective communication in the practice setting
- Maintaining confidentiality in the placement setting
- Promoting 'good practice'
- Looking after yourself and staying safe
- Asking for help
- Giving feedback

Introduction

> *Thirty years ago we were seen as 'angels'. We were revered and supported. It's not the same now.*
>
> (*Nurse*)

In this chapter you will look at some of the processes that you need to consider when working as a member of the clinical team whilst learning in your practice placements. A number of writers have remarked on the complexity of nursing and the demands made on nurses (Glouberman 2002, Revill 2005). Many recognize how the pressures of an increasingly technical age and government demands for greater efficiency – which is measured with through-puts rather than quality – makes compassionate caring more difficult to achieve (Shorr 2000). What is indisputable is the extent to which good nursing makes a difference to each patient's experience of care. Many practitioners strive to implement their vision of high-quality care that is patient-centred, but are often frustrated by the pressures under which they are working. As a nursing student learning in and from practice you will inevitably be exposed to the same pressures. This chapter will help you to think about managing your time and yourself in relation to other staff and in relation to patients or other service users whilst learning and working in your practice placement. We shall be exploring the following:

- Presenting yourself in the practice environment.
- Setting priorities and managing your work and patient care.
- Communication skills and documentation.
- Confidentiality.
- Looking after yourself.

Each of these aspects will examine elements in your role as a developing practitioner, raising issues that you might experience throughout the process. We will also be reconsidering some of the safeguards to promote ethical practice and prevent the misuse of power in the caring professions.

In Chapter 10 you explored some of the issues that arise when working in health and social care teams. The main goals of these health care team members are to collaborate to deliver care to patients or users and the nature of interprofessional working (Williams & Laungani, 1999). Chapter 10 also identified the challenges and barriers to becoming an effective team, which include power and status differences, heavy workloads and belonging to multiple teams (see Box 10.2). As a nursing student you will experience this in different ways, depending on the team setting in which you work. The hierarchy and demands on you in an acute care setting will be very different from those in a long-term care setting (Cott 1998). Strategies to prioritize the demands on you and to manage the competing claims of your role as student and as practitioner will help you to succeed in the practice placement setting and to complete your studies successfully.

Why are placements so important?

Under statutory regulations, all nursing students in the UK have to complete 4600 hours of learning, of which half (2300 hours) must be carried out in a practice placement undertaking direct patient care before they can become a registered nurse. This requirement is one of the reasons for ensuring that you keep an accurate record of all your placements. It is also important to ensure that you keep your own records up-to-date. All nursing students in the UK have to meet these requirements and all universities and partner placement providers will have a strategy in place to help you achieve this requirement. It is highly probable that you will undertake a range of placements to meet the curriculum requirements of your foundation programme and then your specialist branch requirements. Managing these placements for such a wide range of students and very frequently across large geographical areas is a highly complex activity. Changes to the delivery of patient care and policies that increase the range and number of people who receive health care in their own homes rather than in hospitals means that your learning in practice also needs to take place in such settings. Inevitably this means that you will have to travel to a placement, and this may be personally expensive and time-consuming. You need to consider how you are going to manage your time, your personal responsibilities (e.g. child care arrangements) to ensure that you arrive in your placements at the agreed times. You also need to be thoughtful about your arrangements for travelling home at unsocial hours. You should be aware of how you can claim your travel expenses and ensure that you follow local procedures. This will help ensure that your travel claim can be dealt with as quickly as possible.

In terms of the location of your placements, all universities have carefully developed policies and agreements with their partner placement providers about the numbers of students they can accommodate and ways of allocating students to particular patterns of placement. The intention is to ensure you receive the best possible learning opportunities across a range of placements according to professional and statutory requirements that have been laid down by the European Union and the Nursing and Midwifery Council. Some placements may not necessarily be convenient for all students. Some universities may allow students to change their allocated placement in exceptional circumstances. A more strategic approach is to negotiate your placement before it is planned, which is often

12 weeks before the placement is due to commence. This reduces the amount of work and disruption that last-minute placement changes incur not only for allocations staff but also for practice placement staff and your peers. Take time to find out your own university procedures so that, should you feel a particular placement would be very difficult for you, you know who you can talk to about this. It is critical that you arrange to meet with the relevant person before the change list is published (often 6 weeks before). Changing placements after this time, if it can be done, is generally very difficult and is very expensive to undertake as well as delaying other allocations lists.

What is a placement and who will support me?

A useful definition of a placement is provided by the Royal College of Nursing (2002, p 2):

> *A practice placement is where learning opportunities are available for you to undertake practice under supervision.*

In reality, this could be a wide range of different learning environments and will depend on the particular learning needs that you require at any specific time. You may spend time in different wards and departments in hospitals, community areas such as nursing homes, self-care homes, nurseries, working with specialist practitioners, visiting patients in their own homes or meeting them in clinics to name a few. Some programmes also provide opportunities for students to spend time in a range of non-health care work environments such as factories, offices or schools. These placements are designed to help you understand the dimensions of public health and ill-health and the factors that contribute to ill-health. They are also designed to introduce you to the core elements of nursing practice rather than to be an expert in all aspects of your chosen area of nursing practice.

In contemporary nursing education, a high percentage of nursing students are embarking on their second or third career and may be entering higher education for the first time. Many students now enter nursing with previous health care experience. It is therefore inevitable that you will be allocated to spend time in a practice setting that may be similar to an area that you have already experienced. In this situation, it is critical that you spend time before the placement reviewing your learning to date, reading your placement objectives carefully and deciding how you will use the experience to learn more. Try to use the opportunity to learn new skills and to develop knowledge that may previously either have not been relevant to your role or not available to you. Whatever practice placement you are allocated to, learning how to use your practical experience to increase your professional knowledge is a critical factor in your success. Chapter 6 provides some ideas about how to learn in and from practice.

Who will support me in practice?

Several different staff will be available to support you in your placement learning. Their job titles will vary slightly from placement to placement and across different settings and universities. However, the main person that will support you will normally be referred to as a mentor or supervisor or coach. Throughout this text we have used the term mentor. Your mentor is normally a member of the health care team and a registered nurse. Nurses providing mentorship receive special preparation for their role, but do not receive any remuneration either in the form of financial reward or relief from their normal caseload. Your mentor will facilitate and assess your learning, supporting you to achieve your required learning outcomes and competencies. In addition to the mentor role, many placements have a lecturer from the university who supports the practice placement staff and in some cases works with students in groups or as individuals. It is also common for partner placement providers to employ staff who work specifically to improve and develop the learning environment for students. These may be referred to as practice educators, practice education facilitators or clinical educational facilitators. In some cases, these staff will work exclusively to support nursing students and are qualified nurses. It is becoming more common, however, to appoint staff with other professional backgrounds to support all health care students. Find out in advance of the placement the names and contact points for the staff who will be available to support you.

What can I do before I commence a placement?

So that you can make the best use of learning from your placements, you can do quite a lot of preparation work prior to commencing. The Royal College of Nursing (RCN) has produced clear guidelines for students and mentors (RCN 2002, 2005). Key points from the guidelines have been extracted below with additional notes that others have found useful. Thus, before a placement, you have a responsibility for the following:

- *Know your own programme*. Read and understand your own programme/course handbooks. These handbooks contain a great deal of very useful material and have been devised to help you. Quite often students have problems because they failed to read their own programme course handbook or practice placement guidelines.
- *Know the policies relating to the practice placement*. Familiarize yourself with any policies and procedures concerned with your practice placement. These are likely to relate to your specific programme of study (these are correlated to practice placements).
- *Know your assessment*. Your programme course book will include information about your practice placement assessments and the pass/fail criteria. Quite often one practice placement may host students from several different programmes and from several different universities. So it is important that you accept responsibility for knowing the details of your own programme and your assessments, as it may mean that you are more aware of your specific needs than your mentor. All mentors will fully understand the importance of providing an effective learning environment for you.
- *Why this placement?* Understand the purpose of the placement experience and the learning outcomes you need to meet and ensure that your mentor is clear about these expectations. As you will read later in this chapter, it is important that you understand the priorities that mentors have to deal with in terms of supervising your learning and providing client care. Always ensure that you are working under the supervision of a registered nurse or midwife.
- *Be proactive about your placement*. Many placements have websites that you can visit or provide a welcome pack for students; these often contain useful information about the nature of care and relevant theoretical knowledge that you need in order to make the most of the placement. Use this information to ensure that you have some theoretical knowledge relating to the placement. No-one will expect you to be an expert in any particular area of care. You should, however, have learnt some of the key concepts. You can often find out about the type of client that uses the placement that you have been allocated to.
- *Know your strengths and weaknesses*. It is important that you prepare for your placement by identifying your own strengths and the areas of your practice that you want to improve. Arriving in your placement with this knowledge helps your mentor to understand your learning needs and to help you make a plan that will assist you.
- *Brush up your technical skills*. Before you start your practice placement it is a good idea to spend some time in the skills laboratory improving your technical skills. If, for instance, you are going to be working in the community, you may have the opportunity to give injections and deliver wound care, so it is a good idea to improve your techniques and confidence in these areas. If you are going to work in a mental health setting, you may want to think about how you present yourself and how you might respond to someone who is physically or verbally aggressive.

- *While you are on placement*. It is critical that you do not participate in procedures for which you have not been fully prepared or in which you are not adequately supervised. If in any doubt always ask a qualified member of staff. It is better that your patient waits until a qualified member of staff can deal with their needs properly, than you trying to undertake an activity that you are not prepared for.

The RCN guidelines suggest that you contact the placement and mentor prior to starting a placement. Although this is generally useful advice, it may not always be the preferred approach for some placements. You may find that you will be invited to a special induction day designed to introduce you to the key staff, the relevant policies and procedures and to your placement. You will probably be told which is the preferred approach, but it is a good idea to find out in advance of the placement start date and it is essential that you attend.

When you first meet your mentor it is worth being as open and honest as you can, and discuss with them any specific or special support that you need. This is important, as they may need to discuss your needs with other members of the placement team and possibly with relevant university staff.

First days in your practice placement

First impressions

As an ambassador for your university and for the profession it is critical that you always act professionally with regard to punctuality, attitude and image, and dress according to uniform policy. Wearing your uniform with pride is important as it communicates a great deal to the public and can either instil confidence or distrust. Your uniform should always be clean and smartly worn without the use of make-up, jewellery or flashy accessories! With the complexity of society in the UK and the wide range of values and beliefs, modesty is an important attribute to cultivate in the way you dress: short skirts, low necklines and tight-fitting clothes do not communicate a professional approach. Such an attire can cause deep offence to many patients and could also put you at risk of sexual abuse due to misunderstanding by some patients.

Punctuality

Practice placement staff are very busy people and can not wait for students who are poor timekeepers. So it is essential that you do not underestimate the importance of attending at the agreed times. In most nursing areas the handover is an important learning opportunity. If staff have to repeat information because you are late, this will detract from the care that they should be providing and may mean that patients miss out on essential care. You will miss out on learning opportunities and you are unlikely to achieve the required professional competencies. Naturally anyone can be late on very rare occasions for a variety of reasons. If you suspect you are going to be late, it is important that you leave a clear message including your anticipated arrival time. The same principal applies if you are unwell and not able to attend. It is essential that you develop and maintain effective communication with patients, mentors and link personnel from both the placement and university. We shall explore this point further on in other parts of this chapter.

Confidentiality

It is critical that you maintain confidentiality with respect to the patients that are using the services in your placement environment in accordance with the 'NMC Code of professional conduct'. Ensure that you respect the wishes of patients at all times and make sure that, at the first opportunity, your patients understand that you are a nursing student.

What is the role of the student in a practice placement setting?

Are you an extra pair of hands (i.e. supernumerary) or are you seen as part of the team with workload expectations? This is quite critical to the

scope for individualizing your practice experience to your particular learning needs. Being supernumerary means that you are not part of the staffing and skills mix of the practice placement.

As a nursing student you will be supernumerary, participating in the delivery of care under the supervision of a qualified professional. Usually your supervisor's background will be nursing, but not in all cases. It is important to clarify the team's expectations of you at the beginning of the experience. For example, you need to clarify whether or not you will be able to have study time as part of your shifts. In this context, study time would be time to complete requirements for your programme such as reflective learning logs or journals. This may sound like a small point but it may be crucial to your work/life balance as a student.

Box 11.1

Identifying staff in placements

Spend some time in your first placement identifying the wide range of staff that work in the environment.

- How do people dress?
- If staff wear a uniform is it obvious what experience people have?
- Can you tell from the clothes that they wear?
- If uniforms are not worn is the dress code smart or casual?

Talk to a visitor and a patient and find out how people who are using the services feel.

- Do you believe they can tell who is who?
- What are the implications of your learning for those that use the services?
- Is there a notice board with the photographs of staff and their names available for visitors to see?

How shall I present myself?

It can be difficult to present yourself as a nursing student in a situation where the patient is probably anxious about their condition or treatment and anticipating that an experienced practitioner will be caring for them. In some settings uniforms and badges immediately identify your status to others that are familiar with uniforms and badges. In other situations (e.g. some community settings such as in homes for people with learning disabilities or in mental health environments) it is difficult for patients to identify what role you might play, or your level of experience. Wearing your identification badge is essential for your protection as well as that of your patients. No matter where the practice setting is, you have to think about how to present yourself to people, not just those that you will be caring for but their carers and also to all members of the team. Box 11.1 provides some questions to follow up when you are next in a placement.

In terms of presenting yourself, you can see that it is important that you introduce yourself and explain your part in the team when you first start working with a patient. It is important that you explain that you are a nursing student and you are learning the necessary skills. Mentors and other supervisors working with you should explain your role to people when they are working with you. At times, however, it will be entirely appropriate that you are delegated a task to perform with minimal supervision. Introducing yourself and your role at the first opportunity is not only a good example of courtesy but can really help people understand, such as why you are perhaps taking more time than others to perform the task or need to seek additional help.

Starting a placement is an exciting time. Now is when the theory you have studied moves into the practical world of nursing. You will be anxious about your performance and keen to be competent and successful in the placement. At this stage some students find themselves trying to take on too much as a result of their enthusiasm and desire to learn and also in order to impress those others more experienced in the team. This may be particularly the case if you have worked in health care before starting your programme. Others feel paralysed by the new environment and are reluctant to take on responsibilities. This initial stage sets the scene for your whole placement experience and careful setting up of what is expected from you helps optimize the learning potential. Box 11.2 will help you organize your thoughts about this

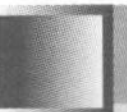

Box 11.2

Preparing for work in practice

The setting. What do I need to know about it?

Learning outcomes. I will be assessed during my time at the placement. Do I understand what I will be assessed on?

The team. Who will I be working with? Will there be other students from different health care professions there (i.e. will it be interprofessional)?

Presentation. Consider what is appropriate dress, language, behaviour, respect.

Recording. What will the requirements be?

Time-keeping. What are the expectations?

Confidentiality. Read the relevant code of practice.

Supervision. Think about the supervisory relationship. My mentor will be assessing my overall competence and performance.

process, and you should spend some time making sure that you can answer all the questions raised.

Once you are clear about what you need to achieve during the placement, and about the constraints of the setting, you need to move on and plan how to achieve this and to work out where any pitfalls may be.

How can I manage my time?

In Chapter 2 you will have learned about personal time management to help you balance your studies, social activities and other responsibilities. This chapter focuses more on achieving effective time management in your practice placements. Some of the same principles apply; for example, knowing how you spend your time and learning to allocate time to important tasks. But a critical learning element for providing effective care is knowing how to prioritize your time in placements when several competing demands are evident. For instance, in a children's setting, how would you deal with the situation described in Case history 11.1? On the surface this probably appears to be a simple example of conflicting demands. No doubt you can determine how you would prioritize

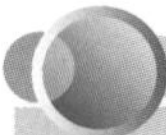

Case history 11.1

Responding to requests

Sofia is on placement in a nursing home for young adolescents with severe physical disabilities. She is comforting a teenager who is very distressed, when a visitor tells her that another resident in the side-room wants to use the toilet. At the same time, a physiotherapist comes up to ask Sofia to ensure that another resident that has fluid-balance difficulties needs to be assisted to have a drink.

these demands. You will encounter this scenario again later in this chapter. Other scenarios that you encounter will be more challenging.

Effective time management is an important lifelong learning activity. As life changes then so do the priorities that have to be dealt with. A significant number of books and websites exist that deal with effective time management. You may have noticed that most of the current NHS targets in all four UK countries are time-related. An example is the 4-hour waiting time for accident and emergency departments, which is a high-profile target frequently cited in the press and other media (Johnston 2005). This means that staff have to work quickly and still provide high-quality care. Knowing how to set priorities by selecting the right things to do at the right time is vital to make sure that patients' needs are met. Observing experienced staff working in placements can be stimulating, but as a person learning to undertake the same skills it can be a challenging prospect.

For a number of nursing students and qualified staff ineffective time management is a common reason for complaints to arise. When you are next in a placement listen out for any member of the team who says to a person that they will be with them in a minute, and then try to keep a watch out for how long this minute really is. Try to listen to yourself in placement settings. Do you ever say that you will be with someone in a short period of time and then forget to go back to them? Scheduling and managing time wisely is important. Omitting activities of care can lead to serious problems, resulting in distress, anxiety, frustration and guilt for carers and service users.

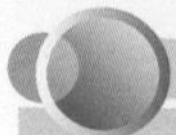

Case history 11.2

Consequences of delays

Jerome is working in a mental health ward where some patients have been admitted following an incident of self-harm. Jerome has been working alongside his mentor assisting her with her caseload. She has gone to discuss a matter with one of the doctors and, during her absence, Jerome notices that Mat is not in the day room or in the ward. Jerome wonders whether it is important and whether he should tell another staff member, or if he should go to find Mat.

Jerome decides that he will try to find Mat and, after searching around the ward, wonders if he has gone into the garden, which is where he finds him. Fortunately all is well with Mat.

Case history 11.2 provides an illustration of what often happens:

- What might have happened to Mat, if he was at risk of self-harm? What should have been Jerome's priorities? Should he have told a staff member what he was planning to do?
- What actions could Jerome have taken if he discovered Mat in the process of self-harming?
- How much time might have been saved if he had notified staff of his concerns and they had accompanied him to find Mat and prevent him from self-harming?

The dilemma Jerome faced was not knowing what had happened to Mat and whether he was 'making an unnecessary fuss' by raising the alarm. However, if Mat had been intent on self-harming, by raising the alarm and getting help Jerome might have saved everybody a great deal of time as well as saving Mat from self-harming.

Knowing your role in your practice placement is an essential aspect of learning how to use your time appropriately. The dilemma for foundation course nursing students is that it is hard to anticipate questions or situations when everything is so unfamiliar.

Other situations can be easier to manage, such as having a series of tasks to complete or having a small caseload of patients that provide you with your planned learning opportunities.

Knowing how you currently use your time and how to set priorities can be an important first step in learning how to prioritize your activities in this area of care.

Managing your time

To begin managing your time you first need a clearer idea of how you currently use your time. To get a reasonably accurate estimate, you might like to keep track of how you spend your time in your everyday life. Analyse how you set priorities and think about the principles you use. Now try the same exercise during a typical period in a your practice placement setting. This will help highlight areas where you are time-efficient and possibly help you identify areas where you might be able to improve. To be worthwhile, this exercise requires you to be very honest. Do not forget that, as a learner, some of the tasks that you are allocated will take you longer than more experienced staff will take. Ensure that you take time to complete any task safely. If in doubt, ask a more experienced practitioner for advice.

Learning what must be done: handover and note-keeping

Critical to any nursing system is providing care in a way that ensures all people that require care are receiving the care they need in the most effective manner. For those working in hospital-orientated care environments, one of the most important points for learning about the care to be delivered is obtained during the 'handover'. This is the time when staff share the care requirements at the start of the working period. You will note different approaches to achieving this handover. In some areas, staff will meet in an office or the nurses' station. In community nursing, handover could be in the car or in a car park.

Some staff will talk with the people they are caring for and exchange views about the requirements for the next period of care. Some staff use tape-recorded notes that you listen to. You will be exposed to a wide variety of approaches, but the critical thing is to learn as much as you can at the handover periods. If you hear terms that you are unfamiliar with, note these down and plan time to ask about them. It is not always convenient for staff to answer all your questions as you think of them. You can ask these later when a more opportune moment arises. It is also worth being aware of when and where you ask questions. You can unintentionally ask a question that compromises a person's confidentiality. So you need to ensure that you think about the environment and circumstance in which you are asking questions.

You will note that different staff use different methods of keeping track of the care that they are to provide during the care period. Some use a small notebook to note down key activities. Some may use a personal digital assistant (PDA), which might be connected to an electronic patient record system. Others use their patients' care plans and do not use any additional aid. In different settings you will find approaches that suit you and the setting in which you are learning. It is valuable, however, to keep short notes of questions and thoughts that arise during your placement. Some of these questions will be related to finding out more about a particular condition, treatment or care approach. It is better not to personalize your questions by referring to actual patient names or placement area details. This could result in a breach of confidentiality if you were to misplace your notes.

It is good practice to link your practice learning with your lecture notes, and vice versa, as soon as possible, or to formulate new questions to ask in class or through any group learning that you are doing. Doing this will help you remember things more effectively as you will be able to link actual care settings to the theoretical aspects of your course.

Learning to prioritize

In many of your practice settings, despite working under supervision, you will be having to think about more than one 'task' to complete at the same time period. Prioritizing these activities is very important as this helps to ensure that the more important items are dealt with first and the other items are dealt with later. However, learning to prioritize is not easy in the placement setting, when there are many interruptions and distractions.

You might find it useful to spend some time observing the staff in your first few placement visits to understand their normal routines. From this you can notice who seems to work most effectively and what it is that they do that makes things run smoothly. Try to keep a record of your observations and an action plan for yourself for when you work under the more distant supervision of your mentor. For instance, once handover is completed, what types of activities do staff get involved in? Make a short list of these, and in particular the ones that you will be undertaking or involved with. During your time in the placement, identify other tasks that you are involved with and identify if possible the amount of time that these activities take.

Your foundation programme will give you the opportunity to spend time in different care settings. You might want to compare the different approaches the nurses use to plan and organize their working time. Are they able to plan ahead? If so, is this for longer or shorter periods of time? In some acute adult hospital settings you might find that staff have very little time for proactive planning. The requirements of people can change rapidly and care plans are often organized over quite short periods of hours or days. In other areas, such as longer-term care, care plans are organized over weeks, months or even years. Take time to compare the care plans in the different areas. Think about the implications that these will have for the working time of nurses and other care staff.

When in the placement areas try to concentrate on results, not on being busy. Many people spend their days in a frenzy of activity, but achieve very little because they are not concentrating on the right things. This is summarized in the Pareto Principle, or the '80 : 20 rule'. This argues that typically 80% of unfocused effort generates only 20% of results. The remaining 80% of results are achieved with only 20% of the effort. Although the ratio is not always 80 : 20, this broad pattern of a small proportion of activity generating large returns recurs so frequently as to be the norm in many areas.

Another important consideration is exploring how you can work efficiently. This means planning your activities ahead of implementing the plan. For example, if you are going to help a patient mobilize, it is a good idea to assess their needs by discussing your plan with your patient first. Patients can often give you tips about how to work effectively as they are cared for by a range of nurses and they probably have views about the methods used.

Read Case history 11.3 about how Netta managed her patients' care. From this case history you can see that Netta had learned more than she had initially realized from her mentor and was able to use the knowledge in practising her care skills. She had learnt how to assess her patients' needs and to prioritize her workload such that it saved her from disruptions and she was thus able to work more efficiently.

Let us 'wind the clock back' and briefly consider what might have happened if Netta had not been so efficient with her time (Case history 11.4).

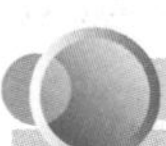

Case history 11.3

Netta's priorities

Netta is on placement in a medical ward and has three patients to care for this morning. All three of her patients are bed-bound following orthopaedic surgery; two of them are able to manage quite a lot of their care, but the third is still quite drowsy from her anaesthetic. Netta had noticed that her mentor always did a nursing round of her patients before starting any care delivery. This nursing round entailed going to greet each patient, telling them that she was going to be working with them and asking them if they had any worries or needs (such as pain relief or toilet needs). Netta used her mentor's approach and discovered that all the ladies desperately needed to use a bedpan and the postoperative care lady had some pain.

Netta alerted her mentor of her postoperative patient's need for analgesia and then gave each of the patients their bedpan. After washing her hands, she assisted her mentor in giving the analgesia and told the lady that she would come back in an hour, once the analgesia had worked, to help her wash. Netta then removed the bedpans and helped the other two ladies to get started with their morning wash. By the time they had finished this, the physiotherapist had arrived and so Netta was free to go and look after her postoperative patient.

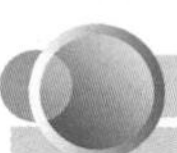

Case history 11.4

Netta and her patients' bad morning

Netta has been assigned three patients to care for this morning. Mrs Ondatije and Mrs Singh had their surgery 2 days ago and can get out of bed after they have had a wash. Mrs Brown had her surgery yesterday. Netta notices that Mrs Brown seems to be asleep so she decides to leave her until last.

Netta decides to give Mrs Singh her washbowl and then leave her to wash while she gives a washbowl to Mrs Ondatije. She sets Mrs Singh up with all her wash things and prepares to help Mrs Ondatije. She draws the water into the bowl and takes it the bedside, but, as she begins to prepare her things, the call-bell goes and it is Mrs Brown who is very upset as she is in pain and needs to use a bedpan. Netta leaves the washbowl (outside Mrs Ondatije's reach) and goes to find a bedpan for Mrs Brown. As she does this, Mrs Ondatije says she would also like one, so Netta returns to the sluice to get another bedpan. After making sure both patients are safe, she goes to find her mentor to provide Mrs Brown with some analgesia, but her mentor is busy with an emergency and cannot come immediately, but promises to do so as soon as she is free. Helping Mrs Brown off her bedpan is clearly a very painful activity for her as her hip is very sore and Mrs Brown is whimpering as she moves. By now, Mrs Ondatije has finished with her bedpan and her bowl of hot water is now cold, so Netta has to replace it and set Mrs Ondatije up for her wash. However, just as she is about to do so, the physiotherapist arrives and insists she gives Mrs Ondatije her treatment, so the washbowl has to go back to the sluice.

By now Mrs Singh has been waiting to have her back and legs washed for 20 minutes and is feeling cold; she also needs to have a bedpan. Mrs Brown still has not had her pain relief, and Netta knows that the physiotherapist will want to give her some treatment when she has finished treating Mrs Singh in about 20 minutes' time.

It is now 11 o'clock and Netta has hardly started her morning's work and she has a patient who is in a lot of pain.

Consider these two approaches to prioritizing care on what seemed to be quite a light workload. In Case history 11.4, by poor planning, Netta spent a lot of time running around but not achieving her aims for the morning. To make matters worse, all her patients were inconvenienced by her lack of planning. One of them (Mrs Brown) suffered considerably as a result. The moral of the story is to assess your patients' needs before you do anything else, and then decide on your priorities and action them. Netta's plan to give Mrs Brown analgesia before she did anything else meant she could leave her in comfort knowing that by the time she was ready to give her a wash the analgesia would be working at its maximum potential and Mrs Brown would therefore be able to do quite a lot for herself. Another advantage is that Mrs Brown would be able to benefit from the physiotherapist's treatment, which may mean she can get out of bed sooner and be discharged home quickly. By giving the other ladies a bedpan at the beginning of the morning shift, Netta is remembering the normal rhythm of the body and that often after meals the gastrocolic reflex causes peristalsis and the call to defaecate; moreover, as a result of the diurnal rhythm of the kidneys and after fluids at breakfast, the bladder will be getting full. Taking note of these normal bodily rhythms, Netta was able to care for her patients in a way that met their needs without causing anxiety to them, and saved her from being interrupted while she was going about her work.

By learning to use your knowledge and to develop your organizational skills in this way you can optimize your efforts to ensure that you concentrate as much of your time and energy as possible on the important few activities rather than the trivial many. This ensures that you achieve the greatest benefit possible for your patients as well as for yourself, within the limited amount of time available to you.

Your learning versus their treatment

Is there a conflict between your need to learn and your patients' and agencies' needs for 'best practice' in their treatment? Having clarified what the placement expectations are of you, there is a need to think about your learning needs in relation to your patients' needs. As you are supernumerary, there should be capacity in the team to cover the patients' needs and scope to shape your experience around your learning needs. As you progress through your programme, you become more involved and start to work as an integral member of the team. You are likely to have core tasks to perform and a tension may arise between the patients' needs and your needs as a student practitioner. It is helpful to identify how you would cope with this. What support strategies are available to you? First, from your initial meeting with your mentor there should be a clear learning agreement in place so that you and the placement setting are clear about the expectations of you. Second, you will have a mentor in the workplace and a link lecturer overseeing you from the university perspective. If you experience any difficulties, make sure that both the university and the placement setting are aware of these. Your handbook will contain details about how to get help and what you can expect; it is highly likely that staff in the university will have spent time discussing some of the issues with you before your placements. But no matter how often you are told about these aspects of the programme, you have to experience them for yourself to truly understand.

Becoming a thoughtful practitioner student

An important consideration is how you can manage your time effectively to complete the tasks required of you as a practitioner and as a student. As a practitioner, there will be recording requirements relating to the direct work with your patients or their carers. As a student you will have some combinations of practice reports, learning and journals and assignments to complete. A 'last-minute.com' approach will not work. It is all about 'getting organized'.

At times it is hard to balance all these competing demands. Although the demands of practice are compelling, your academic work is also important. An effective, qualified practitioner is someone who is able to integrate theory into their practice and to learn how to learn from practice. If you are finding it difficult to balance your practice requirements and academic workload, it is vital that you seek help, as soon as possible (Duffy 2004).

However, even if you are well organized, it is useful to think about the strategies that can be used to collect material to meet your programme requirements. Some students keep a daily journal to record their experiences, then reflecting on them and noting where they might provide evidence for their placement competencies. Other students keep a box file and put relevant materials in it, including articles they may want to refer to in assignments. Others write their own placement reports as they progress through the placement, adding material either on a daily basis or relating to specific learning in the form of practice learning summaries. Whichever method you use, the more you write about your practice experiences and try to analyse them the more you will learn, and you will become more successful and happy in your programme.

What system is going to suit your personal learning style and enable you to meet your course and placement requirements? Quite a lot of research has been done into personal learning styles to try and help students maximize their learning potential. Knowledge of your learning style not only helps you, but can also guide practice supervisors to providing you with appropriate learning opportunities (Cartney 2004).

Table 11.1 identifies some learning styles (Honey & Mumford 1986). You will see that the table contains some '*?'s. Spend a little time working on this, so wherever a '*?' occurs try to think of other points under each of the headings. Once you have spent some time thinking about how to complete the queries, you should be able to identify what you think your own learning style, or combination of styles, might be. This will help you to develop an awareness of your strengths and to identify those areas where you need to improve as a learner.

Whatever your learning style, reflective journals are a good way of building up material through the placement. 'Getting started' on reflection and the advantages and disadvantages of the reflective process are discussed in Chapter 2. Here, we look at how reflective practice can help you collect and organize material to meet your placement competencies.

Reflective practice can be thought of as a cycle such that your reflections alter how you practice

Table 11.1 Learning styles (based on Honey & Mumford 1986)

Style	Characteristics	Good points	Areas of concern
The activist	Jumps in at the deep end Gets immersed in the placement Enjoys hands-on practical experience	Likes a challenge Quick to take action *?	May make mistakes May become bored *?
The reflector	Keeps a low profile and listens Takes into account a wide range of perspectives	Thoughtful Looks at the past and the present *?	Too cautious May progress too slowly *?
The theorist	Puts observations into theories and models Thinks through situation in an organized way	Rational and objective Can work out a structure based on a wide range of facts *?	May not be flexible and intuitive May not be able to deal with an unstructured organization *?
The pragmatist	Puts theory into practice Has a practical problem-solving approach	Practical Shows understanding of the theory practice link *?	Task-orientated 'let's get on with it' Acts quickly *?

See text for explanation of *?.

(Schon 1983) (see Figure 11.1). From Figure 11.1 you can see that reflective practice is concerned with thinking about the actions you take, your responses to a situation and your analysis of your response in the way that you did. Here you need to use your reading and theoretical models to help you understand the consequences of your actions. In this way, the reflective process enables you to analyse the strengths and weaknesses in your practice and think of ways to improve this in the future. Box 11.3 gives two possible formats for your learning journal.

You may decide to collect your evidence using practice learning summaries rather than a reflective diary. To help you with this, the template in Figure 11.2 can be used or adapted for this purpose.

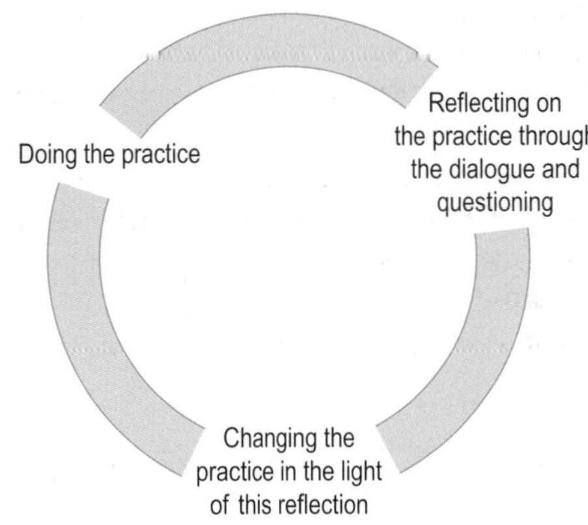

Figure 11.1 • The reflective cycle.

Box 11.3

Reflective learning journal: two possible formats

Format 1: a diary with headings for each placement day

Description of practice

- What I did.
- What was the outcome?
- Could I have done anything differently?
- Should I have involved anyone else?
- What learning from my classroom learning did I use?

Reflections on my learning

- Can I use this as evidence in my assessment?
- What theories are relevant?

Format 2: a diary with entries focused on each learning objective

- What was the event?
- What happened?
- What was my part in the event?
- Why did I behave in this way?
- What was the outcome?
- How does this relate to this particular learning objective?
- Reflections on my learning?
- Can I use this as evidence in my assessment?
- What theories are relevant?

Practice learning summaries

Date:
Type of activity (please state):
(you may want to adopt a specific nursing model to guide you)

1. Reason for patient episode:
2. Description of activities/and or interaction with patients, carers, staff group and other professionals:
3. Reflection on process and main learning points:
4. Discussion about what learning the activity evidences and how:
5. Discussion about how this activity reflects values and ethics and the 'NMC Code of professional conduct:
6. Discussion about how this activity demonstrates the needs of different people, including cultural aspects:

Figure 11.2 • Template for practice learning summaries.

Once you have decided on the best way to collect your evidence of learning in your practice placement, there is still the issue of preparing assignments for your university. You are likely to experience assignments as a competing demand on your time. There are ways that you can use your assignments to help with your learning; after all, they are designed for you to show off how much you have learned! A good strategy is to build up assignments in a stepwise fashion by developing the core components throughout your placement. The 'patchwork text' approach (Winter et al 1999) involves writing small pieces of work (patches) relating to components of the assignment you are doing. Ideally, these are then shared in your student learning group where you can further develop your understanding and ideas (learning), before you put all the pieces of the patchwork together into an integrated text with reflective comments (Akister 2003). Another approach is to develop a grid in which you can record your placement learning, any relevant articles and book chapter notes that you have read and note their contents and where they may help you in your writing (appendix 4 in Hart 1998).

Becoming an effective communicator in practice

Developing effective communication skills requires significant effort. This is mainly because by adulthood we have developed a range of virtually automatic communication responses to a range of situations. Learning to 'unlearn' these behaviours requires different approaches. In the clinical setting, you will be faced with a wide range of circumstances, many of them new. These situations will require you to respond in different ways. You will no doubt spend time learning a range of communication skills with staff that are teaching you. These are critical skills in becoming an effective health care worker.

Verbal communication

Appropriate language in the placement setting is important (see Box 11.4). You are likely to find yourself working with a wide range of patients who may represent a wide ethnic mix and span the age range. Similarly, you will need to communicate with other professionals. This can be quite daunting at first. However, good preparation can really help you.

Remember that communication in your placement is about professional relationships. These relationships differ from 'friendships'; thus communications in a professional setting such as a hospital ward, general practice surgery or community setting should be structured as demonstrated in Box 11.4. Non-verbal communication, such as expression, posture and gaze, are also important; they too impact on your relationship with the patient. Try Activity 11.1 and see how different types of communication might take place in a professional setting. Reflecting on your own experiences both as a patient/user and as a practitioner will help you to improve and develop your professional communications (see Figure 11.1).

A common experience for patients, who are usually anxious about their condition, is that they

Box 11.4

Elements of professional communications (Jack 2001)

Purposive. Communication with a patient or other professional will have a purpose. You will be undertaking a particular task that is part of the function of the placement setting.

Time-limited. In most cases work with patients will have a beginning, middle and end, unlike friendships which could literally last a lifetime.

Accountable. You are accountable for your actions to patients, your professional body and to your mentor/assessor.

Altruistic. Communication is concerned with servicing the patients' needs.

Statutory. In some cases the relationship with the patient may be the result of legal action (e.g. patients held under sections of the Mental Health Act).

Guided. Communication in a professional relationship should be guided by the knowledge, skills, ethics and values of the profession.

Activity 11.1

You might like to reflect on your own experiences of talking to a 'professional': perhaps a visit to a general practitioner, your dentist or being a blood donor. Try and identify one positive and one 'not so positive' experience. Write down your experiences using the following headings:

- Verbal (tone, use of language including jargon, attitude).
- Non-verbal (including eye contact, expression, attitude).
- Symbolic (including comfort in the environmental setting).

Once you have done this, reflect on whether or not it was a positive experience. How could the professional have related to you to improve the experience?

do not retain the information they are given. For example, if someone is awaiting test results, the relief at hearing the results are 'normal' often means that the patient fails to ask the questions that they need to, such as what other explanation is there for their symptoms. Conversely, the acute anxiety of an 'abnormal' result may mean that they do not retain other information given at the time.

When reflecting on your experience in the placement, try to identify a situation where the effectiveness of verbal communication was restricted by the patient's circumstances. Think about ways that you could improve things for service users.

Written communication

Patients need and want written information as well as verbal information to reinforce the communication. There is evidence that giving written information increases overall satisfaction with the care given by health care professionals (Semple & McGowan 2002). Written material can be factual, as in information sheets, or therapeutic. An example of a therapeutic written communication is where letters composed by clinicians to the family between clinical sessions have been used as extensions of clinical work with families. The influences of therapeutic letters are connected to the meanings which the recipient attaches to them (Moules 2002). Moules suggests that these meanings are products of the intersection between the intended meaning of the nurses and the received or interpreted meanings of the families (messages received not necessarily being the same as the message the sender intended.)

The need for effective written communication is therefore clear, whether this is recording medicines that have been dispensed (to avoid over- or under-medicating), or whether it is recording a therapeutic conversation in a mental health setting. All agencies will have guidelines about what to record and how this should be done. There will also be handovers when shifts change involving written and verbal communications to promote continuity of patient care.

While the guidelines you receive for recording written communication will probably seem quite straightforward, there are two questions to consider as you approach the recording task. First, the question of whether the information you want to record is 'fact' or 'opinion'. Second, what are you going to include, and what are you excluding? It is never possible to record every part of an interaction and your judgement as a practitioner will determine what you record. Try to consider what the record actually is, what it does and what it means in terms of the communication process between the user, worker and agency. All report writing involves deciding what to include and what to omit to achieve the desired communication.

Your opinions based on hunches, hypotheses and guesses and rooted in theoretical frameworks are valuable, but it should be clearly stated that they are opinions and these should only be noted where necessary (e.g. to justify actions). An example from social work is described in Box 11.5. The 'opinion' about the adequacy of mothering is not helpful recording because it does not give the reader any of the facts that informed the opinion.

How you complete reports will very much depend on the purpose for which you are writing. A 'handover' report between shifts will include different material from a daily log or from a report for other agencies. Even apparently simple 'handover' reports require a complex process to select the material you decide is relevant to pass on. The process of synthesizing material into a concise report involves your professional judgement as to

Box 11.5

Distinguishing fact from fiction: an example from health visiting

Instead of: 'Mrs J is an inadequate mother. (*Opinion*)

Record: 'Mrs J quickly comforted C when she fell down. In other respects, I felt concern about her care of C who was very dirty, wore few clothes despite the cold and had nothing to play with.' (*Fact*)

Plan for next contact: Check with Mrs J.

- Is she depressed?
- Is she satisfied with her mothering of C? (*Analysis*)

This format:

- Doesn't cause offence.
- Records evidence.
- If shared with Mrs J, would reassure her that the health visitor was thinking about her.

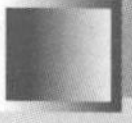

Box 11.6

Example of different communications and their interpretation

Scenario: Patient presents in accident and emergency with a burn.

Report 1: This patient was aggressive and uncooperative. (*Opinion*)

Report 2: This patient was clearly in pain. They seemed to find the waiting room situation stressful and became verbally abusive to the receptionist. In the consultation they remained agitated. (*Fact*)

Questions to clarify: Why are they responding like this? Is it symptomatic of drugs or alcohol consumption, mental health problems or other functional issues (e.g. brain tumour)? Will their responses affect this treatment episode? Do they need referral to another service?

what is relevant to pass on and also involves an interpretation of the patient's position. The situation described in Box 11.6 illustrates how different conclusions can be drawn from the same observations. It may help you to be aware of this to think that, for everything you include in a written report, there is something you decided not to put in. This helps maintain your awareness that there are very few situations in which there is only one interpretation. It helps you to stay alert to continually observing the status of your patient and to identify the relevant theoretical frameworks.

Given that you have to do a report for a specific purpose, be clear about the following:

- What information do you need?
- How are you going to get the information?
- That for everything included, something is excluded.

It is important to remember that your written records are likely to be a major source of information about a person. These records can be used for various purposes over different lengths of time. Initially they are for immediate use by other nurses and a range of other health care workers.

Your written records can help promote a safe environment and good clinical experience. For example, an accurate record of a reaction to a particular clinical intervention will help decide a course of action. Recording preferences will help promote comfort.

Over time, the written record can be used as part of an investigation into a complaint. Some complaints lead to further independent investigation, and in many cases a lack of effective record-keeping and ineffective communication channels are found to be a significant cause of the complaint. For relevant examples it is worth visiting the following websites: http://www.ombudsman.org.uk/; http://www.scottishombudsman.org.uk/; http://www.ni-ombudsman.org.uk/pubslist.htm.

Maintaining confidentiality in the placement setting

As a nursing student, and subsequently as a practitioner, you will have privileged access to a wide

range of confidential information. Ethical practice demands patient confidentiality. What does this mean in practice? As you read this you may begin by thinking that this is really quite straightforward. If a patient asks you 'not to tell anyone' what they have told you, you must respect their request. In your professional nursing role there will be times when you cannot respect their request as you have a responsibility to safeguard the welfare of the patient themselves and also other patients in your care. Sometimes the appropriate response will be more obvious (e.g. when a patient threatens suicide). At other times, there will be an ethical dilemma between the patient's rights to confidentiality versus your responsibilities for their welfare and possibly the rights of other patients. So who can you talk to about which aspects of patient care? How do you respond to ethical dilemmas? Ideas about what is ethical practice change over time.

> *Every generation (of practitioners) will be faced with certain abstract questions of morality, fairness and justice that will only find answers within the actual practice of therapy.*
>
> (Rivett & Street 2003, p 162)

If you read Chapter 4, and joined the virtual ethics class, you will remember one of the members discussed a situation in which an assurance of confidentiality was a difficult promise to give. Practice in all the caring professions is guided by professional codes of conduct (e.g. General Social Care Council 2002, NMC 2008). Your code of professional conduct will help to guide your practice. However, no code of practice provides the answer to every situation and ethical dilemmas in relation to confidentiality and your responsibilities as a professional will still arise. This is where safeguards, such as supervision are necessary to ensure ethical and safe practice (see the section on safeguards to promote good practice, below).

What is an ethical dilemma?

An ethical dilemma presents in a situation where there are two or more good reasons to make two or more reasonable decisions (Burkemper 2002). This captures the core of the dilemma; that is, that there is more than one reasonable decision that could be made and, therefore, there has to be some ethical basis on which to make a decision. There are different types of reasoning that can be used to help make decisions in practice. The concepts of 'care reasoning' and 'justice reasoning' can be used to appraise the dilemma in its simplest form (see Box 11.7).

Two ethical dilemmas are described in Box 11.8. As you read these, try to pause and decide what decisions you would make about keeping this information confidential. Before progressing, also consider whether you have based your decision on either predominantly care reasoning or predominantly justice reasoning.

A research study presented these dilemmas to individual and family therapists. The findings were quite astonishing. The results showed that both the individual and the family therapists had adopted a model of decision-making that focused on values identified with an ethic of care.

> *When the outcome of this study is viewed with an understanding that the ethical codes of professional organizations emphasize a justice ethic, it clarifies the concerns professionals express about their professional ethical codes.*
>
> (Newfield et al 2000, p 182)

Box 11.7

Care reasoning and justice reasoning: what are they?

Essentially, care reasoning and justice reasoning propose a value base which can underpin ethical decisions. The care perspective considers the actual consequences of a decision for the involved parties, how the decision would affect the relationship, the context, the need to avoid hurt, and the issues of altruism. Justice reasoning highlights issues of fairness, rights and obligation. Clearly, a decision based on justice reasoning may also take care reasoning into account. The point of separating these two concepts is to try to understand which type of reasoning is dominant in different situations and whether professionals agree about this.

Most professional codes of practice emphasize justice reasoning.

Box 11.8

Two ethical dilemmas

(Newfield 2000)

Dilemma 1: Individual – hypothetical

A patient informs you that he has tested positive for AIDS (acquired immune deficiency syndrome). When you discuss this with him, he demonstrates an understanding of the disease process and mode of transmission. Although he has been aware of this condition for several months, he has continued to engage in sexual relationships, and also indicates an unwillingness to discontinue sexual activity or to discuss this information with past and present sexual partners.

Dilemma 2: Family – hypothetical

A family referred itself to a Child and Adolescent Mental Health Team for help with communication problems. The family consisted of five persons at home: mother, father, two daughters and a son. After several sessions, it was disclosed that father had sexually abused the oldest daughter. The father had stopped the abuse several months ago, and the family indicated that the primary reason for seeking therapy was to address issues related to the abuse. The family members had kept this a secret, and only confided in you with the request that you not appraise or involve others because they felt the problem was being resolved. To date, this family has worked hard in therapy, and all family members, including the father and daughter, seem highly motivated to continue the therapy. The father has agreed to a contract with your mentor regarding the issues of abuse.

This all goes to emphasize that there is nothing simple about 'confidentiality' in the caring professions. This is why we need 'safeguards', to promote good practice and protect both staff and patients or service users.

When in practice settings, it is likely that you will come across situations which you might be concerned about in terms of confidentiality. Do not hesitate to share these concerns with your mentor. As an experienced nurse they will be able to use their enhanced knowledge to provide guidance and reassurance.

Confidentiality in student assignments

On a different note, what about 'confidentiality' in your assignments? Anonymizing material that could identify patients, users or colleagues is essential when preparing your assignments or portfolios. You may also need to take steps to anonymize the placement setting if it is easily identified. This is because your assignment lies outside the workplace with its safeguards designed to protect sensitive material, and could even be left on a bus to be read by passers-by. Your work is also likely to be on computer, memory disk or other electronic storage medium, which again can fall into the wrong hands. Password-protecting documents is relatively easy to do and helps to provide a reasonable level of security. If you submit work electronically remember to advise the assessor of the password or disable it before submitting.

Safeguards to promote 'good practice'

With your professional role, even as a nursing student practitioner, comes power. Power in how you exercise your judgement. Power in how observant you are. The unobservant practitioner in the caring professions misuses their power to care and protect. The practitioner who perceives themselves as 'just following instructions' fails to engage their professional abilities and may collude in poor practice. (Hugman 1991). So with power comes responsibility for ethical practice. It is not easy in a busy workplace to always get this right. For this reason, the safeguards, such as supervision and evaluating practice, are crucial for the safety of both the person being cared for and you, the practitioner (see Box 11.9).

Looking after yourself and staying safe

Looking after yourself and staying safe is key to a long and successful career in nursing. It is some-

Box 11.9

Safeguards to promote good practice (Mantle & Akister 2001)

Supervision. As well as providing opportunities for learning and development, supervision can act as a vital check on the use/misuse of power. Supervision is a two-way process, not just the supervisor's responsibility. Therefore you should prepare for it by thinking about the issues you need to discuss with your supervisor.

Policy and procedures. Rules, procedures and other 'red tape' sometimes seem to get in the way of day-to-day practice. Procedures are also an important safeguard, and policy gives us the mandate to practice.

Evaluation. This offers an opportunity to research evidence-based practice and to identify good practice.

User/patient perspective. Feedback from users and patients helps form our procedures and improve practice.

Complaints procedures. These offer an opportunity for poor practice to be identified.

times helpful to think about the different aspects of looking after yourself; we have divided these into physical, psychological, social, technical and financial. We start with physical, as staying safe physically is critical because many nurses and other caring professionals experience physical threat or actual assault at some time in their career. All the other aspects are important too and the psychological impact of your experiences should not be underestimated.

Physical safety

In a survey of 6300 nurses in Minnesota, USA, 13.2 assaults a year per 100 nurses were recorded. The incidence increased with additional hours of shift duration and decreased when the nurses carried personal alarms or mobile phones (Gerberich et al 2005). In UK accident and emergency departments, violence and aggression continues to be a significant problem and studies are examining the characteristics of individuals who assault the staff (Ferns et al 2005).

Unfortunately, violence and aggression towards nurses do occur and you will need to think about your physical safety in a number of ways. First, as a student nurse, when working unsocial hours do not take any risks in your journey to and from work, such as taking shortcuts across parks late at night. Second, how should you handle aggressive patients? This is a huge subject, but make sure you are aware of and have discussed safety procedures with your mentor and take any opportunities that present themselves in the way of training for handling aggressive patients. Third, avoid working alone. If you are in a situation where this is required, prepare carefully and listen to your own responses. If you feel afraid you must take action to change the situation. Do not wait until it is too late (Mantle & Akister 2001).

Psychological well-being

A UK study examined occupational stress in four areas of high-dependency nursing: theatres, liver/renal, haematology/oncology and elective surgery (Tyler & Ellison 1994). It was found that the amount of stress experienced was similar across all four departments, but its sources varied. Theatre nurses experienced less stress than other nurses, through patients' death and dying. They also found that social support was beneficial to psychological well-being.

The emotional demands of caring for and treating patients are great. Some situations, such as a child dying, are clearly distressing and the treatment team usually finds ways to help each other deal with this distress. At other times, it can be hard to know when you need to look after your psychological or emotional well-being. You don't feel quite right, but you don't know why. This is why regular supervision giving you an opportunity to review your work experiences and your reactions to these is critical to safe and effective practice in all the caring professions.

Social well-being

Here we are thinking about the personal and professional boundaries in your relationships with patients. There are many examples in literature, where the patient falls in love with the nurse who helps them back to health despite extreme injuries or illness (as, for example, in 'The English patient' by Ondaatje, 1993). Neither is it uncommon for nurses to believe they are in love with their patient. Often when people are in a position of vulnerability and dependency they project earlier similar feelings onto the care giver, the kinds of feelings they may have had towards their primary carer, their mother or their father. This can be quite confusing for a novice nursing student.

What is the appropriate way to conduct yourself in relation to your patients, especially if you find yourself attracted to a patient or if a patient is attracted to you? Your code of professional conduct will give some guidance on this and it is helpful to reflect on this possibility and how you should handle such an event before you start your placement.

Technical safety

This is a rather different, but equally important, aspect of staying safe. Your phone number and your e-mail address give direct access to you personally. Who should you give these to? Definitely do not give these to patients. Also, what about Internet 'chat rooms'? These can be useful for a number of purposes, but again you need to think about what kind of information it is safe for you to post there.

Another aspect of safety is to rely on others to behave with the same integrity that you might. It is not good practice to e-mail your university assignments to any of your friends for instance. If they decide to copy and paste some of your assignment into theirs you may find yourself involved in a case of plagiarism!

Financial safety

Although as a student nurse you will probably have limited funds, you may find yourself under pressure or even wanting to lend patients money. If you find yourself in this situation seek advice and guidance. It is probably a good indicator that you are becoming overinvolved with the patient and their difficulties. How to deal with patients' financial needs should be a decision made by the treatment team not by any individual.

Asking for help

Throughout your nursing career, but particularly as a student, there will be situations in which you do not know what to do. Learning to identify the boundaries to your professional competence and seek help is fundamental for all professionals. This can occur when the situation is outside the limits of your experience and knowledge and you need to extend your knowledge base. It can also occur in situations where the expertise of other professionals is needed. Within your profession you must be able to identify sources of expertise and guidance. As a student nurse this will often be your mentor. Once you have qualified you will also need to identify appropriate sources for advice and consultation.

In an increasingly interprofessional environment you will also need to seek expertise beyond your own profession. Interprofessional training and multidisciplinary teams will help you develop an understanding of the role, function and expertise of the different professions. If you do not seek help you may leave patients and/or other professionals at risk. This applies not only while you are a student but throughout your professional life. You should therefore familiarize yourself with policies concerned with safe practice. If you are in any doubt about this area you should seek guidance from your mentor.

As a student you can help contribute to improving care standards. In some placement areas you are likely to find very high standards of care. It is worth highlighting these in any feedback sessions that you have. This can help to raise the profile of the placement or the mentor and contribute to quality improvement. It is also possible that you will experience care that does not meet the expected quality standards. It is important that you raise these issues with your mentor in the first place and if necessary the link lecturer or your personal tutor. Most universities have policies and procedures that need to be followed if you raise any matter of concern. Be reassured that you will be taken seriously and you will be supported.

What if my mentor and I are not getting on well?

On rare occasions, a small number of students and mentors for a variety of reasons are not able to work well together. If you feel that this is happening to you, you need to seek advice and help quickly. The sooner that a resolution can be found, the sooner you can focus on your learning again. Your handbook is likely to contain some useful advice in this regard and you should follow the relevant advice. A good option to start with is to let your mentor know that you are experiencing difficulties. This is a difficult thing to do, but unless they know that you believe that there is a problem they cannot help to improve the situation with you. If you do not feel right in talking directly to your mentor, then you can talk the situation through with a link tutor, the practice education facilitator or a more senior member of staff in the area. It is important that you do this quickly. It may be that your relationship with your mentor could jeopardize your achievement of your competencies in the placement.

Giving feedback

Just as you will benefit from and appreciate the feedback that your mentor will give to you as you learn, mentors appreciate feedback from you. Take some time during your mentor interviews to let them know what you find helpful. It is likely that other students will benefit from this praise as they are more likely to repeat this behaviour. If you find areas that they can improve then you have a responsibility to let them know this as well. Do recognize the constraints that many mentors are working under in terms of having to prioritize giving care and supporting your learning. You will also have some form of evaluation sheet to complete, or discussion to share your views of the placement. Do take time to participate in these activities.

Concluding comments

This chapter has reflected on the opportunities and challenges your placement will present. It has identified preparations you can usefully make prior to beginning the placement (see Box 11.2). It has also invited you to think carefully about how to use your time on placement to optimize your learning and meet your learning objectives.

In the placement there will be written and verbal communications. You will have the opportunity to develop your skills in professional communication (Box 11.6) and in report-writing and handover skills. As your skills in practice develop you are likely to come across more complex presentations which will challenge your assessment skills and may present ethical dilemmas in terms of confidentiality.

As you progress through your nurse education try and find time to revisit this chapter to remind yourself of some of the structures that can help your learning experience. These include ways to collect material for your assignments (e.g. reflective journals) and the need, in all placements, for clear contracts.

References

Akister J 2003 Designing and using a patchwork text to assess social work students undertaking a module in family therapy. Innovations in Education and Training International 40(2):202–208

Burkemper EM 2002 Family therapists' ethical decision-making processes in two duty-to-warn situations. Journal of Marital & Family Therapy 28(2):203–212

Cartney P 2004 How academic knowledge can support practice learning: a case study of learning styles. Journal of Practice Teaching 5(2):39–50

Cott C 1998 Structure and meaning in multidisciplinary teamwork. Sociology of Health & Illness 20:848–873

Duffy K 2004 PhD studies 'failing to fail'. Nursing and Midwifery Council, London

Ferns T, Cork A, Rew M 2005 Personal safety in the accident and emergency department. British Journal of Nursing 14(13):725–730

General Social Care Council 2002 Code of practice for social care workers and employers. GSCC, London

Gerberich SG, Church TR, McGovern PM et al 2005 Risk factors for work-related assaults on nurses. Epidemiology 16(5):704–709

Glouberman S 2002 Structures, power and respect: the nurse's dilemma. Online. Available: www.healthandeverything.org/pubs/Nursing_Paper

Hart C 1998 Doing a literature review. Sage, London

Honey P, Mumford A 1986 The manual of learning styles. Ardingley House, Maidenhead

Hugman R 1991 Power in the caring professions. Macmillan, Basingstoke

Jack R 2001 Communication and interviewing skills in social work. Open Learning Foundation, London

Johnston I 2005 Hospitals under pressure over four-hour A&E waits. The Scotsman 26 August 2005. Online. Available: http://news.scotsman.com/health.cfm?id=1843652005 3 Jan 2006

Mantle G, Akister J 2001 Social work power & responsibility. Open Learning Foundation, London

Moules NJ 2002 Nursing on paper: therapeutic letters in nursing practice. Nursing Inquiry 9(2):104–113

Newfield SA, Newfield NA, Sperry JA et al 2000 Ethical decision making among family therapists and individual therapists. Family Process 39(2):177–188

Nursing and Midwifery Council (NMC) 2008 The NMC Code of Conduct. NMC, London

Nursing Standard 2004 Editorial. Online. Available: www.nursing-standard.co.uk/students/worklife.asp

Ondaatje M 1993 The English patient. Picador, London

Revill J 2005 Why angels must spread their wings. The Observer 24 April

Rivett M, Street E 2003 Family therapy in focus. Sage, London

Royal College of Nursing 2002 Helping students get the best from their practice placements: a RCN toolkit. RCN, London. Online. Available: www.rcn.org.uk

Royal College of Nursing 2005 Guidance for mentors and student nurses and midwives: an RCN toolkit. RCN, London. Online. Available: www.rcn.org.uk

Schon D 1983 The reflective practitioner. Basic Books, New York

Semple CJ, McGowan B 2002 Need for appropriate written information for patients, with particular reference to head and neck cancer. Journal of Clinical Nursing 11(5):585–593

Shorr A 2000 Has nursing lost its professional focus? Nursing Administration Quarterly 25:89–94

Tyler PA, Ellison RN 1994 Sources of stress and psychological well-being in high-dependency nursing. Journal of Advanced Nursing 19(3):469–476

Williams G, Laungani P 1999 Analysis of teamwork in an NHS community trust: an empirical study. Journal of Interprofessional Care 13:19–28

Winter R, Buck A, Sobiechowska P 1999 Professional experience and the investigative imagination. Routledge, London

Chapter Twelve

12

Decision-making in practice

Verina Waights

Key topics

- **Evidence-based practice**
- **Decision-making**
- **The nursing process**
- **Using models of assessment**
- **Using frameworks**
- **Making decisions on-your-feet**
- **Documentation and record-keeping**

Introduction

This chapter is about making decisions in practice, which is an integral part of care delivery. Indeed, as Thompson (2003) states:

> *It is clinical decisions that commit scarce resources to patients, determine the clinical outcomes associated with care, and, in part, shape the health care experience for patients and professionals alike.*

This chapter focuses on making clinical decisions associated with care, as opposed to making financial or staffing decisions, as these are the first type of decisions that you will become involved with as a student nurse. Nurses are responsible for their decisions at a professional level; the Nursing and Midwifery Council make this clear in the 'NMC Code of professional conduct' (NMC 2008).

Every day of their working lives, health care practitioners make clinical decisions about patients' health and well-being. These decisions may be taken at several different points in a patient's care. Some decisions are made during initial assessment of a patient, and others are made in response to changes in their condition, which may occur over time or may occur very quickly. Indeed, research has shown that nurses on an Australian intensive care unit make one decision every 30 seconds! (Bucknall 2000). Having to make such decisions may seem quite threatening, yet you are actually quite experienced in making decisions, you may just not have thought about it before.

In your personal life, you are making decisions all the time. Some of these decisions you take on your own and others you make after consulting one or more people, but all require some background information about the issue in question. For example, if you are deciding whether to catch a bus or to walk to work, you need to know the bus routes, timetable and fares. You also require information based on your experience, such as how long it will take you to walk that distance, and you need information based on the current situation, such as 'it is raining at the moment'. You need to be able to think about all the relevant pieces of information and draw them together to make your decision. This is also true of making clinical decisions. To make effective decisions about patients' care you need to acquire sound background knowledge and develop good decision-making skills. These are sophisticated skills and you will need practice to enable you to become an experienced and confident decision-maker.

Evidence-based practice

The emphasis in health care today is on evidence-based practice. In 1998, clinical governance was initiated in the UK Government's white paper 'A first class service: quality in the new NHS (Department of Health 1998). This initiative aimed to put clinical quality at the heart of Trusts' agendas, and included expectations of continuing quality improvement focused on clinical services and effective use of evidenced-based practice. UK Trusts are audited by the Healthcare Commission from which reports for each Trust that has been audited can be obtained (www.healthcarecommission.org.uk).

So what is evidence-based practice? Muir Gray (1997) stated that evidence-based practice is:

> *An approach to decision-making in which the clinician uses the best evidence available, in consultation with the patient, to decide upon the option which suits the patient best.*

This means that decisions taken by health care practitioners for each individual patient are supported by the best evidence currently available, not just on experience or their own personal feelings. Indeed, McKibbon (1998) suggests that evidence-based practice is the formalization of the care process that the best clinicians have practised for generations. However, you will be aware of the so-called 'postcode lottery' in the UK, in which the type of treatment available for a particular condition varies depending on where you live. Evidence-based practice should reduce this effect, as everyone should be using the same evidence to support their care. It should also ensure that the latest research evidence about a topic is incorporated into the treatment of the patient. This is problematic though, as we cannot just accept a research paper at face value. You need to be able to evaluate research findings in order to determine the degree of confidence you have in the results of the research and the conclusions drawn by the researchers. Your training will include learning how to evaluate research evidence, and you can keep up-to-date with research relevant to your practice in a variety of ways. Sources of evidence-based information are given in Box 12.1.

One source of relevant information is the Cochrane Library of Systematic Reviews. Each review evaluates research related to a particular topic and gives a recommendation as to the reliability and usefulness of the data. This means that the evaluation is carried out by experts so you don't have to evaluate the data for yourself. For example, should colloid solutions (which contain particles that remain in the bloodstream) or crystalloid solutions (which readily cross cell membranes) be given to reduce the risk of death due to blood loss in healthy adults? Roberts et al (2004) reviewed the research in this area and concluded there was no evidence to support one solution being superior to the other, so which solution to use is still a matter for debate.

Box 12.1

Sources of evidence for use in nursing practice (all accessed July 2006)

Bandolier (journal), evidence-based thinking about health care: www.jr2.ox.ac.uk

Centre for Evidence Based Nursing: www.york.ac.uk

The Cochrane Library: www.cochrane.co.uk

Database of Abstracts of Reviews of Effectiveness (DARE), The NHS Centre for Reviews and Dissemination, UK: www.york.ac.uk

Evidence-based Healthcare & Public Health (journal): www.harcourt-international.com

Journal of Evidence-based Medicine: www.bmjjournals.com

Journal of Evidence-based Nursing: www.bmjjournals.com

National Institute for Health and Clinical Excellence (NICE): www.nice.org.uk

RCN Clinical Guidelines: www.rcn.org.uk

Scottish Intercollegiate Guidelines Network (SIGN): www.sign.ac.uk

Wales Centre for Evidence Based Care: A Collaborating Centre of the Joanna Briggs Institute (JBI): www.cardiff.ac.uk

Much research can be accessed through databases such as MEDLINE, CINAHL and TRIP, which should be available through your practice Internet service provider. The NICE (National Institute for Health and Clinical Excellence) frameworks are also evidence-based and we will be looking at one of these in more detail later. You can also find out about new developments through articles in professional magazines.

If you find some interesting research that you think may help your patients you must *never, ever* act on it by yourself. Discuss the article with your mentor or senior nurse. If they think it is useful they will discuss it with everyone at a team meeting and decide what action, if any, they will take. As mentioned before, your training will include learning how to evaluate evidence but it will be a long while before you can implement research findings yourself.

Decision-making

Bucknall (2003) observed that nurses feel more comfortable and look more confident making clinical decisions when they make decisions regularly and are able to compare situations either mentally or with colleagues. So what does decision-making involve? It has been described as:

> *A process by which a person, or group of people . . . identifies a choice or judgement to be made, gathers and evaluates information about alternatives and selects from among the alternatives.*
>
> *(Carroll & Johnson 1990)*

Matterson & Hawkins (1990) further suggest that a decision 'ends doubt and debate and occurs when the solution to a problem is uncertain'. This latter issue is very important. If a particular problem has a specific solution, there is no need for anyone to make a decision about the action to be taken. So how do you think in a structured way about making a decision? Carroll & Johnson (1990) suggested a model of decision-making that comprises seven stages. These stages do not need to be followed one after another, but each stage can be returned to as long as the stage is helpful in assisting the practitioner to make a decision. The seven stages are:

- Recognizing the situation.
- Forming an explanation.
- Forming alternative explanations.
- Searching for information/evidence to clarify each explanation.
- Making a choice between possible explanations, i.e. making a decision.
- Acting on the decision.
- Obtaining feedback to check the effectiveness of the decision.

We will look at these stages in more depth later in the chapter.

The nursing process

Making decisions may be easier if you have a framework or guidelines for making them.

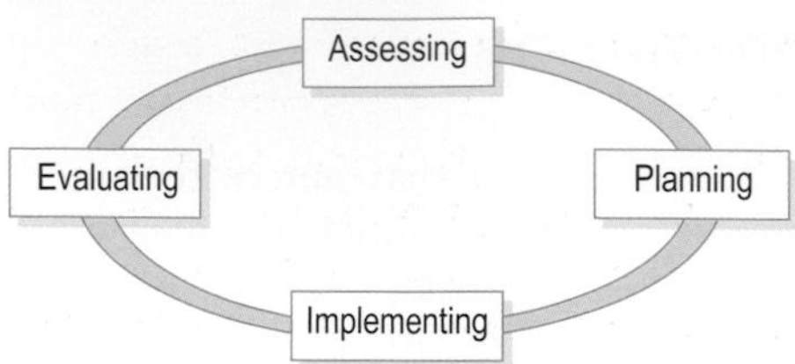

Figure 12.1 • The nursing process.

Frameworks and guidelines also ensure that each patient is treated similarly and important aspects of their care are not overlooked. These frameworks and guidelines are not used in isolation, however, but are commonly used within a cyclical problem-solving procedure described as the 'nursing process' (see Figure 12.1). This process was developed in the 1970s and was quickly adopted by nurses worldwide (Habermann & Uys 2005). Briefly, the cycle is as follows.

Assessing

This describes the way you consider all of a patient's individual needs. This holistic assessment should identify the patient's physical, psychological, emotional, social and spiritual needs. This is the stage when you can use a model of assessment to collect relevant information, enabling you to make appropriate decisions about the patient's plan of care (using models of assessment is discussed later in the chapter).

Planning

This is the stage of the process when you, in conjunction with the patient and, if appropriate, their carers, set realistic goals and plan how they can best be achieved. In common with goal-setting in other professions and situations, the goals set should be SMART (i.e. **S**pecific, **M**easurable, **A**chievable, **R**ealistic and **T**ime-limited).

- *Specific*. The goals may be short term (e.g. nothing by mouth prior to a patient having surgery) or long term (e.g. enable a client with a learning disability to prepare and cook their own food).
- *Measurable*. Goals need to be measurable, otherwise you will not be able to evaluate whether the goals have been met or how effective the interventions have been towards achieving the goals.
- *Achievable and realistic*. It is vital that you recognize the patient's individual needs and set goals that are achievable and realistic, so as to avoid disappointment if a goal is not achieved. You should encourage patients to participate in setting their own goals as everyone views their condition differently. A newly diagnosed diabetic, for example, might want to take immediate control of their care, whereas others might need a little time to take on this new role.
- *Time-limited*. It is important to determine a time period within which the goals should be achieved so that the patient's progress can be evaluated.

Once the goals for the patient have been identified, you need to determine what activities need to be done, when they should be carried out, and who will be doing them to enable the patient to achieve these goals. You write this information into a care plan, which aids communication between all members of the multidisciplinary team concerned with the patient's care. But it is important to remember that primarily you are writing the plan for the patient and their carers and they are entitled to read them (discussed later in the chapter, under Record-keeping). So you need to write the care plan in a clear and explicit way that the patient can understand. It should give the patient a clear picture of the stages of the care, which may encourage them to participate in the plan. The plan must give very clear instructions as to who is to do what and when. Here are a few examples:

- The mother will feed the baby, using prepared bottles of milk, every 3 hours.
- The client will get up each morning at 7.30 a.m., wash and dress themselves before breakfast at 8.30 a.m.
- The health care assistant will help with personal hygiene needs until the patient is able to do it unaided.

Integrated care pathways

Many clinical areas use integrated care pathways (ICPs). Each ICP is based on evidence and best practice and describes the plan of care that should be given to a patient with a specific condition (e.g. those who have chronic heart failure, or schizophrenia, or are undergoing knee replacement surgery). ICPs are followed by all members of the multidisciplinary team and so reduce the complications of different parts of the care being recorded on discrete notes that are kept separately. It also enhances greater understanding within the multidisciplinary team, enabling them to deliver an agreed plan of care for the patient as everyone is aware of what other professionals are doing. The patient also benefits from this by having a total picture of their care.

However, if you are using an ICP, you need to be aware that all patients are individuals and may have particular needs in addition to the needs identified through the ICP for their main condition. You need to record these individual needs and the associated goals in the ICP to make sure these additional needs are not overlooked. ICPs are explored in more detail in Chapter 13.

Implementing

This is the stage where you, the patient, their carers and other members of the multidisciplinary team, as appropriate, follow the care plan or ICP. You must ensure relevant interventions are carried out to enable the patient to achieve their goals.

Evaluating

This is the most important step of the process as it informs the patient, their carer(s) and the multidisciplinary team whether goals have been achieved or are being achieved. Your evaluation should determine future action. You may be noting success and stating that no further action is required or reassessing the situation and planning new goals, which takes you back to the beginning of the process. It is thus important that you set achievable goals so that the patient will be encouraged rather than discouraged. For example, it is possible to set short positive goals to note progress rather than regression; for example, a terminally ill patient in pain may have a goal of being pain-free for 1 hour, whereas a patient with chronic arthritis may have a goal of being pain-free for 6 hours. Setting measurable goals in the initial care plan helps you to evaluate your patient's progress more effectively.

Using models of assessment

Many of your practice settings will be using a model of assessment. However, this may not be immediately recognizable as the team may have taken one of the known models and adapted it to be more appropriate for patients with conditions that they typically nurse. Your responsibility in each practice setting is to identify whether a model is being used, and, if so, to determine which one and to learn about it to enable you to deliver care in the same way as the rest of the team. This section does not describe all the nursing models available but highlights five that are representative of different ways to approach the decision-making process.

Biomedical model of care

This is the traditional model of practice, which has influenced nursing and medicine for a long period. There is a great deal of evidence to suggest that many nurses and doctors base their practice on this model, and many medical schools use the concepts within the model in the preparation of doctors (Pearson et al 2005). Hence, it is important that you have an insight into this model of care.

Nursing models are based on the following three components, which makes it easier to compare them:

- Beliefs and values.
- Goals of care.
- Knowledge required to achieve the outcomes.

The beliefs and values of the biomedical model are that humans are made up of biological components. Specialized cells make up tissues that comprise organs, such as the heart, liver and lungs. Groups of organs are linked together as systems, such as the digestive system, and all the systems interact together to achieve a balance, termed 'homeostasis'. An imbalance is regarded as 'disease' with little or no consideration being given to psychosocial issues. Yet it is known that these issues can have significant effects on patients' well-being; for example, stress can lead to an increase in colds and flu, irritable bowel syndrome, circulatory disorders, anxiety and depression. The goals of the biomedical model of care are to cure or treat the imbalance to restore homeostasis. Decisions regarding care are based on knowledge from biological subjects, such as anatomy and physiology, biochemistry, microbiology, pathology and pharmacology.

This type of model works well with traditional physical care and has a long history of success, but it makes no allowances for the individuality of the person. Indeed, critics of this model dislike the fact that it reduces a person to a set of parts that can be repaired or replaced, much like a machine. Recently, this model has been extended into the biocultural model of care (Morris 2000), which is based on scientific knowledge of human biology but also encompasses culture, thus recognizing that each patient's beliefs, values and experiences influence their health and well-being. Prior to this biocultural model being proposed, some nurses, who recognized that their patients were all different, developed models to encompass the individual needs of their patients, including their psychological, social, behavioural and spiritual needs. Four of these models are described further.

Roper, Logan and Tierney model

This is probably the model most commonly used in the UK, particularly in adult nursing. It is based on a concept of nursing proposed by Henderson (1966):

> *The unique function of the nurse is to assist the individual, sick or well, in the performance of those activities contributing to health or its recovery (or to a peaceful death) that he would perform unaided if he had the necessary strength, will or knowledge, and to do this in such a way as to help him to gain independence as rapidly as possible.*

Henderson suggested 14 'activities of daily living' and, from these, Roper et al (1980) developed the 12 activities which 'people engage in to live'. Since its inception, these authors have continued to refine the model, the most recent version being published in 2000 (Roper et al 1996, 2000). The activities are listed in Box 12.2.

These activities of living are then set against a lifespan continuum where conception through childhood and adulthood to death is aligned to a continuum from total dependency to independence and possibly to some level of dependency. When you assess a patient's needs, the activities of living can be plotted on the continuum, enabling you to identify the stage of the continuum to which they are trying to return. For example, if a patient who eliminates independently has a temporary colostomy formed to aid recovery from major bowel surgery, they will be dependent for care of the colostomy until taught how to care for it themselves. In the long term, they will be fully independent again when the colostomy is reversed to enable normal bowel actions to resume.

The goals of the model are to enable patients to have maximum independence for the 12 activities of living, using medically prescribed treatments to overcome illness or its symptoms. In addition to the lifespan continuum, each activity of living

Box 12.2

The 12 activities which 'people engage in to live'

- Maintaining a safe environment
- Communicating
- Breathing
- Eating and drinking
- Eliminating
- Personal cleansing and dressing
- Controlling body temperature
- Mobilizing
- Working and playing
- Expressing sexuality
- Sleeping
- Dying

may be influenced by biological, psychological, sociocultural, environmental and politicoeconomic factors. A patient's health, therefore, will be influenced by a unique set of factors, which will be reflected in their living patterns. To help a patient to achieve the goals of the model, you need to know about their living patterns and the role each of these influencing factors plays in their lives.

Case history 12.1 shows an assessment of a patient using the 'activities of living model'.

Once you have used the model to identify a patient's needs, you need to decide on a plan of care that will address those needs and write it up as described previously (see the section on planning, above). However, one of the criticisms of this model is that, although it is a more holistic approach to assessment than the biomedical model, it may still concentrate on the physical aspects of care rather than on other areas. Murphy et al (2000) carried out a small research study in Ireland and found the model was unsuitable for psychiatric nursing. It was as a result of this type of criticism that a plethora of other models were developed.

Roy's adaptation model of nursing

This model of nursing was described by Roy in the 1960s and has been used widely in the field of psychiatric nursing (Roy 1976, Andrews & Roy 1997). Roy suggests this model embraces client-centred nursing and requires professional accountability. The framework suggests that each person responds or adapts to changes, termed 'stimuli', within their body or in the surrounding environment. Everyone is an individual and the way each person reacts to the environment is central to this model. Rambo (1984) described these assumptions as follows:

- Each person, as an integrated whole, comprises biological, psychological and social parts, and interacts with the environment.
- People adapt to change from within their body or in the environment in order to maintain homeostasis.
- The stimuli to which people respond are of three types:

Focal. These are direct causes of the problem and may be either within their body or affecting the person at the time (e.g. a leg wound or bereavement).

Contextual. These are indirect causes within the body or in the environment that might result in a poor response to the focal stimulus; for example, malnutrition may prevent healing of a leg wound, poor social circumstances may make it more difficult for a person to cope with bereavement.

Residual. These are the person's beliefs, attitudes and past learning that may influence their current response. For example, one woman might tolerate pain during childbirth because she accepts that it is part of the process, whereas another might believe labour in the 21st century should be pain-free and therefore will expect to be given analgesia.

Everyone is an individual and will therefore adapt to situations differently. Providing stimuli are within the coping adaptations of that person, the responses to the stimuli will be adaptive or positive and homeostasis will be maintained. If, however, the stimuli are too large, the responses made will not be adequate to maintain balance; this is known as maladaptive or negative. For example, following the loss of a job, one person might think of it as another opportunity in life, enabling them to adapt positively and cope well. Another person might find losing their job is beyond their coping capacity, and respond negatively with anger, sleeplessness and poor appetite.

Roy suggests that there are four adaptive modes used to respond to stimuli to maintain balance:

- *Physiological*. As the name suggests, this is associated with the structure and function of the body and in particular the standards and ranges that are regarded as normal with respect to oxygen and circulation, fluids and electrolytes, elimination, nutrition, exercise and rest, regulation of temperature, senses and endocrine activities.
- *Self-concept*. This focuses on the way a person perceives themselves. Self-concept can be

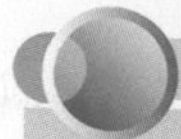

Case history 12.1

Mrs Bartlet

Mrs Bartlet, aged 77 years, lives in a 'granny annexe' at her daughter's home. She is admitted to the ward via the accident and emergency unit following a fall that morning. She is diagnosed with a fracture of the neck of her left femur.

Assessment using the 12 activities of living (Roper et al 1980) was as follows:

- *Maintaining a safe environment*. Mrs Bartlet fell on the stairs and will need a handrail fitted before discharge. Has lived alone safely since her husband died 4 years ago.
- *Communication*. Mrs Bartlet is able to explain how she fell. She wears glasses for reading and watching the television but not when moving around the house. She has no problems with hearing. Her body language shows that she is in discomfort from her injury. Mrs Bartlet is aware of the name of the ward to which she has been admitted.
- *Breathing*. Mrs Bartlet has no problems with her breathing. Her respiration rate is 20.
- *Eating and drinking*. Mrs Bartlet prepares her own breakfast and snack at lunchtime. She has her main meal with her daughter and her family at 6 p.m. She has a cup of tea with her breakfast, coffee at mid-morning and after lunch. A small cold drink is taken with her evening meal. At present she is nil by mouth in preparation for her operation.
- *Eliminating*. Mrs Bartlet normally has her bowels open once a day. She needs to get out of bed at least once during the night to pass urine but has no incontinence. At present she is unable to get out of bed and so will need to use a bedpan.
- *Personal cleansing and dressing*. Prior to her accident, Mrs Bartlet was self-caring. She has a shower every morning but admits that she preferred it when she could get into a bath. She will need assistance with this at present.
- *Controlling body temperature*. Mrs Bartlet says that she enjoys the central heating in her home and was appropriately dressed for the time of year. Temperature 36°C.
- *Mobilizing*. Mrs Bartlet is now immobile. Prior to this accident she says that, although a little slow, she is able to get around her home and, when her daughter takes her there, is able to walk around the shops. She uses no aids. Waterlow assessment will be undertaken to assess her risk of pressure sores.
- *Working and playing*. Mrs Bartlet has not worked since having her two children (55 and 53 years old). Her husband was an accountant. She has many hobbies including reading, television, attending church and spending time with her grandchildren.
- *Expressing sexuality*. Mrs Bartlet enjoys shopping for clothes. A local hairdresser comes to her house every 2 weeks to wash and dry her hair and cut it when necessary.
- *Sleeping*. Her normal pattern of sleep is 10.30 p.m. until 6 a.m. and she says she often has a little nap after lunch.
- *Dying*. Mrs Bartlet was able to discuss the risks of a general anaesthetic at her age, but said 'I have had a good life'.

This example highlights how an elderly person can become dependent on carers following an accident but, despite her age, following successful surgery, she could return home and continue living almost independently. You may also notice that, although the activities of living cover a broad spectrum, other assessments and measurements will need to be undertaken (e.g. Waterlow risk assessment, temperature and respiration rate). From the assessment, the following actual problems can be identified:

- Pain
- Immobility
- Personal hygiene: needs help at present
- Elimination: needs help at present
- Eating and drinking: nil by mouth prior to surgery.

The potential problems for this lady are:

- Pressure sores from immobility
- Thrombosis from immobility
- Dehydration from surgery preparation.

Hence, from using a model, the nurse can obtain a clear picture of the patient and the patient's needs and plan the appropriate care.

divided into two parts: the physical self, and the personal self. The physical self is concerned with how people perceive themselves either physically or mentally; for example, does the person perceive themselves to be ugly because their surgery resulted in a large scar, or frightened because they have to have another operation? The personal self is concerned with maintaining personal standards, behaviours and morals; for example, does the person feel anxious because they cannot maintain their personal standards when confined to bed-rest?

- *Role function*. The focus here is on social integrity and the roles each person plays within society. These roles can be described at three levels (Rambo 1984): primary and predetermined (e.g. gender, age, race); secondary, mainly permanent and chosen (e.g. parent, carpenter, Member of Parliament); and tertiary, fairly minor and chosen (e.g. union representative or choral singer). Illness can impact on one or more of these roles, and often it is the impact on secondary roles that leads to maladaptation. For example, illness might cause a person to be anxious that they are having time off work or unable to care for their child.
- *Interdependence*. This focuses on social integrity and the ability to maintain a balance between independence and dependency on others. For example, an older person living alone may be independent in cooking meals for themselves but dependent on others for shopping and providing the food to be cooked.

A person must make positive adaptations to stimuli to remain healthy and this is dependent on having the ability and energy to do this. Illness occurs when the adaptations needed are too great for the individual to make a positive response. The goals for nursing in this model must therefore be to support the patient's adaptation to these stimuli. This can be achieved by :

- Assessing behaviour in relation to the four adaptive modes: physiological, self-concept, role function and interdependence.
- Identifying focal, contextual and residual stimuli influencing responses.
- Drawing up a care plan that:
  Identifies problems.
  Sets achievable goals.
  Selects appropriate interventions.
- Evaluating care.

Roy's adaptation model is a useful framework to use for patients as it considers them as individuals within the larger environmental setting. Case history 12.2 illustrates an assessment using Roy's adaptation model within the mental health branch of nursing.

Orem's self-care model

Orem first described her model of nursing in 1971; more recent updates were published in 1985 and 1991 (Orem 1971, 1985, 1991). It is based on the philosophy that all individuals wish to have control over their lives. Bennett (1980) drew our attention to this issue, saying:

> *When nurses discuss self-care, they need to remember that individuals, healthy and ill, are demanding increased control of their health care. They want to be active in the decision-making process; that is, they want to be able to identify their self-care needs, to establish their learning goals and to evaluate their self-care behaviour . . . [they] want to assume responsibility for their own care.*

This understanding links well to theories of health education and promotion and has been developed by the Expert Patient Programme (Department of Health 2001), in which patients with a good knowledge and understanding of their condition help other patients with a similar condition to care for themselves. You will find this model particularly useful in the fields of rehabilitation and community care. Its concepts fit well with recent UK Government initiatives to develop the role of nursing in the community, such as the establishment of community matrons (Department of Health 2004a, 2005) and the publication 'Supporting people with long term conditions to self

Case history 12.2

Tom's story

Tom is 35 years old, unmarried and lives in a housing association flat. He has been in contact with the mental health services since the age of 22, when he was diagnosed with schizophrenia. The community psychiatric nurse who administers injections of antipsychotic drugs every 3 weeks maintains his condition. Tom will not admit that he is ill but agrees to the medication.

Tom's sleep is disturbed at times and he is regularly heard talking to himself. He is self-caring but a heavy smoker. He is unemployed, with few social contacts except for the friends he meets at the day centre. He has little contact with his parents.

	Behaviour	Focal	Contextual	Residual
Physiological				
Oxygen/circulation	Tom smokes 30 cigarettes a day and is often breathless when walking	Smoking is an irritant	Poor social conditions	His social contacts smoke
Fluids/electrolytes	Tom enjoys making and drinking tea			
Elimination	No problems with micturition and elimination			
Nutrition	Tom eats instant/ready-prepared meals; he does not enjoy shopping for food	Poor nutritional status	Can buy burgers and chips readily from nearby shop	Tom thinks cooking is a woman's job
Rest/activity	Tom is unemployed and has little interest in doing anything; he attends the day centre 3 days a week	Unemployment causes financial restraints	Few opportunities for employment	Other social contacts are unemployed
Regulation	Respirations are a little rapid	Smoking affects Tom's breathing	Temperature and pulse within normal limits	
Self-concept				
Physical self	Tom is not interested in how he dresses or looks	Tom thinks he is appropriately dressed	Little money available for clothes	Dresses similarly to friends
Personal self	Tom does not accept that he is ill	Tom accepts his medication to help the voices he hears	He has always talked to the voices in his head	
Role function				
Primary	Single male	Tom is happy by himself	Difficult to find a partner	His friends are single too
Secondary	Unemployed	Does not want to go to work	Very little money to spend	Other friends are unemployed

(*Cont'd*)

Case history 12.2

Tom's story *(Continued)*

Behaviour	Focal	Contextual	Residual	
Role function				
Tertiary	Son	Tom has little contact with his parents	Parents could not accept/understand Tom's behaviour	Tom does not see his brother either
Independence				
	Lives alone in housing association flat	Tom likes his independence	Tom found communal living difficult	Poor social conditions but an improvement from institutional care
	Needs medication	Dependent on community psychiatric nurse	Nurse encourages Tom with social skills	

care' (Department of Health 2006). However, it is important to remember that not all patients wish to take responsibility for their own care; some wish to be cared for by expert professionals and to leave all the decisions regarding their care to them. Some critics of this approach believe that self-care is a way to cut NHS costs, although practitioners in favour of self-care believe it is actually just as costly, but that money is spent in primary care rather than in acute care (Pearson et al 2005).

Also, some people are not able to care for themselves. For example, it is impossible for a baby to be self-caring, and so the self-care is actually carried out by their parent or guardian. They gradually teach the child to be self-caring within the developmental stages of life. Indeed, if you have a placement with a health visitor, you will see that one of their roles is to ensure that these developmental stages are being reached, by checking each child at specific milestones. If these stages are not being reached, the health visitor may decide to refer the child to other agencies for specific help, such as speech therapists or paediatricians. This continuum of life is also a key element of the Roper et al (1996) model of nursing.

In the same way, you may become the self-care agent for a person who becomes ill and is unable to care for themselves. The goal of this model is to return the patient to being self-caring. If, however, this is impossible (e.g. in the case of a client with severe learning difficulties and mental illness), then a self-care agent will undertake the activities that the client is unable to achieve. Such activities are known as self-care deficits. These deficits can be compensated for in three ways:

- *Total compensation*. Here, you or their carer totally undertakes all activities for a patient to meet their self-care needs. For example, a terminally ill patient or an unconscious patient will be totally dependent on others.
- *Partial compensation*. Here, you or their carer works with a patient to meet their self-care needs. In this way the patient is able to feel in control of their care but has support for the activities that they cannot manage by themselves. For example, a patient discharged home from hospital following surgery for a hip replacement may require help with shopping and personal hygiene but be otherwise independent.

- *Educative/supportive compensation*. In this case, you are required to teach patients or carers how to deliver care themselves. For example, a patient with newly diagnosed diabetes who requires insulin injections has the potential to be self-caring but needs to be taught how to undertake this new care. Similarly, in the case of a child with diabetes, the parents or guardians might need to be taught how to inject insulin to partially compensate for the child until the child is ready to do it for themselves.

When you assess a patient, you will need to decide whether they need total or partial compensation or some education to meet their self-care needs. Orem's model (1985) describes the basic human needs, or 'self-care requisites', that she considers are common to all people for effective living. They are:

- *Air*: able to breathe sufficient air } to maintain life.
- *Water*: able to drink sufficient water } to maintain life.
- *Food*: able to eat enough food } to maintain life.
- *Elimination*: in control of elimination and excretion processes.
- *Activity/rest*: in control of the balance in their life between activity and rest.
- *Solitude/social activities*: able to seek solitude or to participate in social activities as they desire.
- *Hazards*: able to prevent hazards to themselves.
- *Normality*: able to interact in society and with chosen groups of friends.

Orem's model (1985) also includes two more categories of self-care requisites, which you need to consider during your assessment:

- *Developmental requisites*. A patient may have additional needs due to the developmental stage of life at which they are, such as childhood, or to changes in their life such as loss of a job or poor living conditions.
- *Health deviation requisites*. These occur when a patient requires a change in self-care due to illness (e.g. a patient needing dialysis for kidney failure).

Thus, the care plan you draw up after assessing the patient's needs and implementation of this care would need to be compensatory for self-care deficits in any of these requisites.

Case history 12.3 shows an assessment of Ben, a patient with Down's syndrome, using Orem's model of care.

The plan of care for Ben would need to be detailed (e.g. helping Ben with dressing). This would need to be broken down into many stages; here are a few examples of the stages:

- Ben chooses what clothes he will wear. Carer dresses Ben.
- Ben puts on his underwear unaided. Carer does the rest.
- Ben puts on his underwear and trousers. Carer does the rest.
- Ben does up the zip and buttons on his trousers after putting them on. Carer does the rest.

The series would be continued for as long as Ben was able to progress. For Ben, this partial compensation is a long process in comparison to the partial compensation required for a patient postoperatively or to the total compensation for an unconscious patient who regains consciousness following an anaesthetic. When working with patients with learning difficulties, you will need to enquire if a model of assessment is used and how it has been developed to adapt to patients' long-term requirements.

Casey's partnership model

When nursing children, it is vital to remember that they are not 'mini-adults' but have differing physiological, psychological, social and emotional needs to adults. It has been recognized for some time that children, whether at home or in hospital, benefit most if care is given by their family in partnership with health care practitioners. This approach has been emphasized in many reports, including the UK Children Act (Department of Health 1989), and has led to the recent 'National

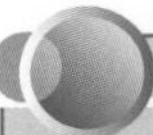

Case history 12.3

Ben

Ben Smith, aged 42, has Down's syndrome and has recently been moved from a large institution to a 17-bed nursing home for people with severe learning disabilities.

Ben was assessed on admission to the home and a care plan written for him. Ben's care plan will be very different from those you may have experienced in a hospital ward or the community. His care will be for the rest of his life as he has no living relatives and needs constant care. The plan will be amended as he reaches his goals but it may take several months/years for him to achieve a goal. Hence, each goal will need to be broken down into small achievable targets for Ben.

	Self-care	Total compensation	Partial compensation	Educative/supportive compensation
Air	Ben has no problems with breathing			
Water	Ben is able to drink unaided	Drinks need to be supplied for Ben to drink with meals		To encourage Ben to get his own drinks when needed
Food	Ben is able to feed himself	Ben needs his food supplied	Ben likes to choose what he eats	To teach Ben to prepare some of his food. To encourage Ben to accompany a carer to do the shopping for food
Elimination	Ben is self-caring			
Activity/rest	Ben attends a day centre for activities. He is taken in the mini-bus			To encourage Ben to make choices
Solitude/social	Ben enjoys watching television and is able to switch this on and off	Ben does not like mixing with people he does not know	Carers to accompany Ben on social outings that he has requested	To teach/support Ben in socializing
Prevention of hazards	Ben is unaware of any dangers such as traffic			To try to make Ben aware of danger
Promotion of normality	Ben mixes well within the home	Ben needs help with socializing outside the home	Carers need to take him out to socialize	To teach/support Ben in socializing in unfamiliar situations
	Ben will wash himself if taken to the bathroom and given all the toiletries	Ben needs help with personal hygiene		To encourage Ben to wash and dress himself appropriately

service framework for children, young people and maternity services: change for children – every child matters' (Department of Health 2004b). As the report says:

> *At the heart of the Children's National Service Framework is a fundamental change in thinking about health and social care services. It is intended to lead to a cultural shift, resulting in services which are designed and delivered around the needs of children and families using those services, not around the needs of organisations.*

The report highlights the need to 'treat children, young people and parents as partners in care' (Department of Health 2004b, p 13). Here we are using 'parents' as a generic term to represent those with everyday responsibility for a child, be it their parents, grandparents, or carers. In particular, this means recognizing that:

- Parents are usually the experts on their child.
- Their presence is a positive factor in aiding a child's recovery.
- Their practical contribution to care is often essential.
- They may have other children to care for, and will have to balance their needs with the needs of the ill child.

Consequently, if you are involved in the care of a child or young person, you will need to develop a care plan in conjunction with both the child and their parents. The extent of involvement of the child is dependent on their age, but even very young children may have an opinion, and their wishes must be taken into account if possible. The plan of care must clearly identify the roles of the child, their parents and health care professionals to ensure that all parties understand and accept their responsibilities.

A framework for delivering this care is required, and the one most commonly adopted is Casey's (1988) model. Lee (1998) does not consider this to be a true model, according to Fawcett's analysis of conceptual models (Fawcett 1989). However, irrespective of whether or not it is a model in the strict sense of the term, it was the first to focus on caring for children and families. This was acknowledged during 2002, when Anne Casey was made a Fellow of the Royal College of Nursing in recognition that the development and implementation of the partnership model is one of her most significant contributions to nursing. Casey defends the model as being based on concepts of the person, health, the environment and nursing. The 'person' concept is split into two parts: the family and the child. The child's needs are protection, sustenance, stimulation and love.

Casey (1988) describes a continuum, starting at conception through to maturity. At the start of the continuum, the child is dependent on carers for all its needs, but by maturity it is independent and self-caring. The process of functioning, growing and developing is based on the following aspects:

- Physical.
- Emotional.
- Intellectual.
- Social.
- Spiritual.

When carrying out an assessment, you need to explore the structure of the family, with great sensitivity, to establish who normally undertakes the caring role. With more women in full-time employment, some grandparents are assuming the role of main carer and, in families with only one parent, older siblings might take on this role. Also, with a rise in divorce and remarriage the family structure is getting more complicated. It is essential you have an understanding of the family structure to enable effective communication in planning the child's care.

The process of assessment and subsequent care for the child will be negotiated between the child, the family carer, yourself and other members of the multidisciplinary team as appropriate. Casey (1988) does not suggest a list of needs to be considered but takes a broad approach. Hence your assessment should be based on the following areas:

- What family care the child routinely receives.
- The child's present condition, both physical and psychological.

- What nursing care the child needs.
- The ability and willingness of the child and/or family to participate.

Case history 12.4 illustrates the use of the Casey model with a child with asthma.

This simple framework can also be followed if you are working in a hospital setting. Most parents like to continue caring for their child, but you need to plan this care with them. It is vital they fully understand what is expected of them and are happy to participate. You will find some parents just wish to continue to help with personal care while others have the confidence to be actively involved in administering oxygen or managing the care of their child's tracheotomy. You need to support the family as they adjust to this new role. For example, you may need to teach them to give the care required or, once taught, encourage them to continue.

Choosing the most suitable care model

As you will have become aware, the nursing models discussed above are just a few of the models available. The most important point to consider is, which model helps you to make decisions on behalf of a particular patient. For example, would Orem's model or the Roper, Logan, Tierney model be most helpful in enabling you to make decisions for care of a patient recovering from major surgery in the intensive therapy unit or for a child with mobility difficulties. Discussing with your mentor the models in use in your practice setting will

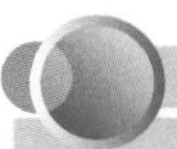

Case history 12.4

Emma

Emma is nearly 5 years old and was diagnosed with asthma at the age of 3 when her mother brought her to see her general practitioner as she was waking at night with a cough. Since then she has been reviewed every 6 months by the practice nurse who is a specialist in the care of asthma. On this visit, Emma is being reviewed prior to commencing school full time.

The care plan that was being reviewed was as follows:

Emma

- To use metered inhaler with spacer device.
- To do a peak flow measurement every morning and evening and watch mother record in book.
- To tell an adult when she is short of breath or has a cough so she can use her inhaler.

Family

- To keep a symptom diary stating when Emma becomes short of breath (e.g. when playing, sleeping or running).
- To record Emma's peak flow measurements.
- To encourage Emma to use her inhaler.
- To encourage Emma to participate in exercise (e.g. swimming).
- To provide Emma with a balanced diet.
- To visit school and talk with teachers and school nurse about medication.

Nurse

- To review Emma's peak flow recordings and symptom diary.
- To check Emma's inhaler technique.
- To weigh and measure Emma.
- To educate family and child about asthma and in particular about use of different inhalers.
- To encourage Emma to participate in all school activities.

This plan enabled all those involved to have clear guidelines as to what was expected of them and to make evaluation easier by reviewing each step. You can see how the partnership between the child, family and nurse was established. Once at school, there will be a need to include the teachers within the plan so they understand which inhaler Emma should use. They will also need to discuss with the family the safe-keeping of the inhaler while she is at school. Other children in the class might also be included in the care as they can help by telling the teacher if they notice Emma is coughing but unable to ask for help herself. Other children with asthma might also be introduced to Emma.

Activity 12.1

Take the assessment and care plan for a patient in your care, and rewrite them based on each of the models described above.

- Do you have sufficient information from the original notes to enable you to complete an assessment based on each model?
- What additional information would you seek?
- What changes, if any, would you make to the patient's care when you take into account the perspectives of each model?

give you insights into why particular models were chosen (for some insight, try Activity 12.1). You may find that your practice setting has developed a single assessment model that incorporates features of several recognized models, as none of these are considered adequate to meet the needs of the particular patients in their care.

Using frameworks and guidelines

There are many frameworks available for assessing patient's needs, such as the Glasgow Coma Scale, pain assessment charts and wound-healing guidelines. These guidelines help to ensure that patients receive care based on the best evidence available. One set of frameworks available to assist health care practitioners in their decision-making is the NICE clinical guidelines, which have been developed by the UK National Institute for Health and Clinical Excellence (NICE). The role of NICE was set out in the white paper 'Choosing health: making healthier choices easier' (Department of Health 2004c).

NICE produces guidance in three areas of health (NICE 2005):

- *Public health*: guidance on the promotion of good health and the prevention of ill health, for those working in the NHS, local authorities and the wider public and voluntary sector.
- *Health technologies*: guidance on the use of new and existing medicines, treatments and procedures within the NHS.
- *Clinical practice*: guidance on the appropriate treatment and care of people with specific diseases and conditions within the NHS.

Similar guidance has been developed by NHS Quality Improvement Scotland (technology appraisals) and the Scottish Intercollegiate Guidelines Network (SIGN).

Once NICE publishes guidance for a particular condition, health professionals and the organizations that employ them are expected to take it fully into account when deciding what treatments to give patients with that condition. However, NICE guidance does not replace the knowledge and skills of individual health professionals who treat patients; it is still up to them to make decisions about a particular patient in consultation with the patient and/or their guardian or carer when appropriate.

Since January 2002, NHS organizations in England and Wales have been required to provide funding for medicines and treatments recommended by NICE in its technology appraisal guidance. The NHS normally has 3 months from the date of publication of each technology appraisal guidance to provide funding and resources. However, this time limit can be extended if the technology cannot be acquired in time or if insufficient staff are available to deliver the treatment.

When NICE publishes clinical guidelines, local health organizations should review their management of clinical conditions against the NICE guidelines. This review should consider the resources required to implement the guidelines, the people and processes involved, and how long it will take to do so. It is in the interests of patients that the NICE recommendations are acted on as quickly as possible.

NICE frameworks often take the form of an algorithm. An algorithm is a type of flow-chart that describes a course of action in a particular situation. For example, NICE has published guidance for chronic heart failure (NICE 2000), which includes an algorithm for the pharmacological treatment of systemic heart failure. This algorithm describes the progression of treatment that is followed for patients with heart failure until their

Activity 12.2

First, read the following case history:

My name is Vila and I am 74 years old. I had a heart attack a couple of years ago, which left me feeling tired all the time and I couldn't work up the enthusiasm to do anything much at all. My consultant put me on beta-blockers and furosemide, and for a time I was able to do virtually everything that I did before. But, recently, my breathing has been getting worse; just going up the stairs is a real effort. My consultant is now talking about adding spironolactone and possibly digoxin to my medication. I don't want to take more medicines but I think I may have to as I am finding it increasingly difficult to join in things with my husband and the rest of my family.

Then find the NICE guideline for chronic heart failure on the NICE website (www.nice.org.uk). Begin by finding the box at the top of the algorithm (labelled new diagnosis) and follow the boxes one-by-one until you have included all of the medication that Vila is taking. Now identify where on the algorithm Vila's treatment currently lies. Note that running alongside the boxes, on the left-hand side, are recommendations concerning the use of diuretics and digoxin. Both of these pathways need to be included in your assessment.

You will note that Vila's treatment is just about to move on to another level with the addition of digoxin and spironolactone, so her condition has clearly been deteriorating of late.

condition is stabilized. Activity 12.2 is based around this particular NICE guidance.

Making decisions on-your-feet

Clinical decision-making is one aspect of being able to reflect-in-practice or, as Schön (1988) described it, 'reflect-in-action' and think on your feet. Being able to reflect-in-practice is a vital skill to develop. Unless you can 'think on your feet' with confidence, you may find it difficult to make sound clinical judgements in response to the changing needs of your patients, thereby compromising the care that you are able to deliver.

Earlier in this chapter we looked briefly at Carroll & Johnson's stages of decision-making. It is in the arena of reflecting-in-practice that these stages are invaluable:

- *Recognizing the situation*. This stage is vital. As Schön (1988, p 65–66) highlights: 'In real world practice, problems do not present themselves to the practitioner as givens. They must be constructed from the materials of problematic situations which are puzzling, troubling and uncertain.' You need, therefore, to be able to recognize that a problem is developing so that you can take steps to avert it or address it.
- *Forming an explanation*. Here you draw on your knowledge of the patient, your knowledge and understanding of the condition(s) and your previous experience to form the most likely explanation for the problem.
- *Forming alternative explanations*. It is important to also think about other possible explanations for the particular problem in question; otherwise you may miss important cues regarding the situation. Research has shown that expert decision-makers can be distinguished from students by their ability to use their knowledge to generate more possible explanations (or hypotheses) and to perceive the important aspects of a problem more quickly (Botti & Reeve 2003).
- *Searching for information/evidence to clarify each explanation*. Is there any evidence in the patient's notes to support an alternative explanation, or would asking more questions or carrying out further assessment yield additional information? Depending on the circumstances, this may have to be carried out very quickly.
- *Making a choice between possible explanations (i.e. making a decision)*. Here you weigh up the explanations for the problem that is occurring and decide which one is the most likely. You may make this decision on your own or in consultation with other colleagues depending on the severity of the problem. Remember that to be a safe practitioner you must always recognize your limitations and seek help whenever necessary.

- *Acting on the decision.* Once you have identified the most likely cause of the problem, you need to act to overcome the problem. If the action is unequivocal, you will simply carry out that action. For example, if a patient's vital signs are giving cause for concern you must consult a senior nurse immediately. However, if there are several possible options to resolve the problem, you must go through the decision-process again to determine the action you will take.
- *Obtaining feedback to check the effectiveness of the decision.* Finally, you need to obtain feedback from your patient, or from other members of the team, to check that your decision had the desired effect. This is a vital stage in the process, but one that can be easily overlooked.

We are now going to look at some of the skills that you need to make decisions about your patient's well-being when you are carrying out care.

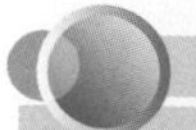

Case history 12.5

The importance of looking at your patients

Mrs James is recovering from the abdominal surgery she had yesterday. She seems comfortable, and all routine 4-hourly observations of blood pressure and pulse suggest she is stable. The ward is very busy and the nurses are well occupied with other patients. As the student nurse walks into Mrs James's bay, she notices that Mrs James is slightly restless, a little sweaty and rather pale. This patient is not inclined to make a fuss or say much at any time so she does not complain. The nurse asks her if she is OK and Mrs James admits that she does feel a bit light-headed but presumed it was normal to feel like this so soon after the operation.

The student reports her findings to the staff nurse, who quickly comes and checks Mrs James's blood pressure. She discovers that it is very low. She calls for the doctor and it soon transpires that Mrs James is suffering from postoperative reactionary internal haemorrhage. A regimen of care is put into place immediately to restore Mrs James's blood pressure and she eventually goes to theatre for the cause of the bleeding to be found and repaired.

The importance of nursing observations

One of the most important skills that you need to develop is 'how to see'. Using your eyes and understanding what you are looking at is perhaps one of the most sophisticated skills you will use in your nursing. Health care is provided with an impressive array of devices designed to monitor organ function; however, none of them is as effective as a knowledgeable practitioner who is able to recognize and interpret accurately the signs and symptoms of organ dysfunction and patient unease. So learning how to observe your patients is one of the most significant nursing activities. With increasing professional knowledge you become skilled at noticing even very small changes in your patients' condition, and these observations can be life-saving.

Case history 12.5 illustrates how a nurse noticed something a little unusual which turned out to be a very important observation.

It is essential you observe closely any particularly vulnerable patients such as: infants, whose condition can deteriorate very suddenly and quickly; people with learning disability; the mentally ill; frail older people; and people who cannot tell you how they feel. There may also be special reasons for observing patterns of behaviour of people with mental health problems or those with learning disability because changes may be signals that intervention is required.

Routine clinical nursing observations and tests

An essential aspect of observing your patients is to conduct routine monitoring observations and tests. These can tell a lot about how the body is responding to disease and treatments. The main observations to carry out are the following.

Temperature, pulse and respiration

These are always checked when a person is admitted to an acute care setting – as an emergency or for planned care – to ascertain baseline levels and any deviation from the normal range. Thereafter, frequency of checking will be according to the patient's condition and care plan. Sudden changes in pulse and respiration may indicate cardiovascular problems, shock, respiratory obstruction. Increased temperature may indicate infection, allergic reactions to drugs, or a reaction to a blood transfusion. Temperature recording is very significant in infants with fever and in anyone with hypothermia. A range of temperature monitors are used, because of the risks of mercury in glass thermometers, and you need to know how to use all of these.

Blood pressure

Accurate taking and recording of blood pressure is vital as it provides a good measure of how the body is functioning. This is always checked on admission to acute health care and thereafter, if required and according to the care pathway. As a clinical measurement of cardiovascular function, blood pressure changes denote critical changes or potential changes in a patient's condition. Postoperatively, it is important to check and record at regular and frequent intervals patients' blood pressure for hypotension (caused by fluid loss and shock), particularly for trauma patients, also for patients who have hypertension, cardiac failure, myocardial infarction or renal failure. Patients in long-stay care, mental health community care or learning disability care do not normally need to have their blood pressure taken unless it is part of a general physical assessment or they become acutely physically ill.

Peak flow measurement

This assesses the rate of flow of exhaled breath in patients where there is, or might be, an obstructive airways disorder which reduces the effectiveness of breathing and gaseous exchange at the alveoli. This observation is commonly required for patients with long-term respiratory diseases such as asthma, chronic bronchitis and emphysema. The frequency of recordings will vary. It is often used to check the effectiveness of treatment with nebulizers or other inhalers by carrying out before and after peak flow tests.

Pulse oximetry

This is a sophisticated test to check the patient's blood oxygen level by placing a sensor on the finger or ear. Patients with obstructive airways disease or cardiovascular disease will usually have this test carried out to check the efficiency of the lungs in absorbing oxygen in exchange for carbon dioxide, and thus the severity of their condition.

Neuro-observations

These are measured and recorded when any patient is at risk of brain damage. Common situations are when a patient has suffered a head injury, had a cerebrovascular accident, taken poisons, or is admitted unconscious for any reason, or when it appears that their general condition and alertness are deteriorating. The observations include checking the person's mental orientation (if possible), the responses of their pupils to light, responses to touch or stronger stimuli on the limbs, hands and feet if the person is unconscious. Temperature, pulse and blood pressure and respirations (vital signs) are another important part of this set of observations. A conscious patient will also be checked for the level of strength in arms and legs, to see if there is any weakness and whether or not it is equal on both sides of their body. Alterations from the normal range of function are indicators of brain damage, and recordings will be taken regularly to ascertain major deterioration or recovery. Most hospitals will use a special recording chart, such as the Glasgow Coma Scale chart. This measurement is carried out frequently within accident and emergency departments and in neurology units and, less often, in general acute adult and children's wards.

Skin colour and texture

Looking at a patient's skin, its colour, skin tension and tenderness can tell the skilled practitioner a great deal. Pallor may indicate anaemia or shock, although this may be difficult to detect in patients with darker skin. A yellowing of the conjunctiva and the skin indicates different diseases. Swelling and pain may occur in a range of abnormalities from heart and renal failure to infection.

Reddening may be an early indicator of pressure damage. Intolerance of being touched may indicate poisoning or neurological damage. Bruising may be a very significant finding if injury or non-accidental injury is suspected. Severe dehydration affects skin texture and suppleness. The skin extremities on any splinted limb must be observed for abnormal swelling and checked for normal sensation. The need to observe and the frequency of skin observation will vary from patient to patient, but this simple detection is one of the most important in nursing.

Urine testing

Routine testing of urine is carried out to assess the volume of a range of normal waste products of body metabolism, as well as the abnormal presence of substances such as protein, blood, ketones, bilirubin and glucose. The urine pH, specific gravity and colour are also checked for hydration levels. Testing urine provides an easy and non-invasive way of assessing the patient's condition and to identify abnormalities such as diagnosis of diabetes or infection. Urine is often collected for different tests, including collecting an uncontaminated sample from a urinary catheter or catheter bag specimens, or collecting only the mid-stream sample for culture if infection is suspected; 24-hour collections of urine are used to check renal function.

Monitoring and maintaining adequate hydration

Monitoring and maintaining a patient's fluid intake is a significant aspect of your role to prevent deterioration of your patient. This is particularly true for older people in mental health settings, because, although it is known that they can be at risk of dehydration, this may be overlooked (Brown & Marland 2002). Even minor changes in the body's fluid balance at cellular level can have major consequences for health. When a person is identified as being at risk of dehydration, or may have some other ailment that requires the fluid intake to be carefully maintained, your role is critical in ensuring that fluid balance is checked and recorded. You may need to work very closely with people to encourage them to drink by checking them frequently and providing the most acceptable beverages or alternatives (e.g. ice lollies). Although they may not be receiving complicated treatments, older people, children, people with learning disabilities and some people with mental illness can easily become seriously dehydrated if they are not encouraged to drink. In extreme cases of dehydration or where the person is unable to tolerate oral fluids (e.g. following major surgery), intravenous fluids may be given.

One important aspect of care of the person with dehydration is mouth care. Enabling these patients to keep a moist and fresh mouth adds greatly to their feeling of well-being and may enable them to take oral fluids more easily. It also protects them from developing painful infections of their salivary glands.

Fluid-balance charts

Whenever there is any concern about a patient's level of hydration, either dehydration or even overhydration, accurate records of the patient's fluid intake and output (fluid-balance chart) are essential. Most people undergoing surgery have their fluid balance monitored while they recover from the anaesthetic, to monitor the amount of fluid lost from wound drains, or as a result of intestinal dysfunction. This is continued until the patient can maintain their hydration independently. Medical patients whose hydration balance is compromised because of their condition, such as major organ failure (e.g. heart, kidney or liver), must have a careful record of their total intake and output of fluids recorded on a fluid-balance chart. These records tell the physician how effectively the treatment is working and indicate the extent of the organ failure.

You will probably find that different health care providers use slightly different documents to chart the information, although the types of fluid monitored are the same. If possible, you should engage your patient's cooperation in monitoring their fluid balance. By explaining the reasons for recording intake and output and how they can help (e.g. measuring their own urine), the likelihood of accuracy is increased. Fluid-balance charts need to be monitored regularly and frequently (every hour at a minimum). Accurate recording of both intake and output is vital to be able to calculate the fluid balance, which is totalled at the end of each 24-hour period. Often records are supplemented by accurate weighing of the patient every day, as increased fluid retention increases weight and vice versa.

Pain assessment

This important observation can often be overlooked in the busy world of health care, unless you are working in a specialist palliative care setting. However, it is vital in all areas of care, not just when working with cancer patients or the terminally ill. Postoperative patients, burns patients and patients with arthritis are among those who can suffer extreme pain and for whom accurate assessment of their pain and the effectiveness of analgesia is important.

Prevention of the complications of immobility

One of your key functions is to protect your patients from harm. People who are having difficulty moving or changing their position are at risk of suffering complications that can be prevented with good-quality care. Deep-vein thrombosis and pressure sores are the two main complications of immobility, both of which are painful and unpleasant for the patient, costly for the Trust concerned, and can be life-threatening. The existence of pressure sores for patients in NHS care is taken extremely seriously.

Monitoring cardiac function

Recognizing that someone is suffering from sudden cardiac failure is difficult. Sometimes it looks like a fit; at other times you will notice that they are not breathing normally and their colour has changed. The first action is to use the emergency bell, or call out to get help. Second, check the carotid or femoral artery for a pulse and, if it is absent, begin resuscitation. Of course, a walking person may suddenly collapse and fall to the ground, but the immediate process of care is just the same.

Recording the findings

All the various observational activities you undertake are very important to aid decision-making, but they are of no value unless you keep accurate records. The charts or the relevant section in the care plan/pathway form part of the legal record of the patient's care and may sometimes be used in cases of investigation or review of care in relation to complaints or police matters. Not only is it important to record, but it is also important to record accurately. If you find any result from your observation that is abnormal, unusual or differs from previous recordings, it is important that you tell the nurse in charge of the patient immediately and make a record of doing so in the patient's notes. We will be looking at record-keeping in more detail later in the chapter.

Frequency of nursing observations

The frequency with which the above observations are made depends on the patient's health. A patient in the intensive therapy unit, or undergoing surgery, will need to be observed more frequently than a patient waiting in accident and emergency for a small cut to their finger to be treated. When observing your patient, it is essential that information from all of these observations are considered together to ensure that any deterioration in their condition is identified quickly and appropriate action is taken. The link between early observation of patients' deterioration and access to prompt expert treatment was raised in the government report 'Comprehensive critical care' (Department of Health 2000). This report proposed setting up critical care outreach services to link intensive care units with other patient areas within hospitals to ensure that expert treatment is available when necessary.

Guidelines for the establishment of such critical care outreach services emphasized the importance of ward staff systematically observing patients' vital signs for deterioration (Intensive Care Society 2002). The Intensive Care Society noted that a systematic approach did not take place on all general wards. Indeed, some patients admitted to intensive care units from wards had deteriorated further than patients admitted straight from accident and emergency or theatres (Goldhill & Sumner 1998). To prevent this deterioration, which has serious implications for the prognosis of the patient, various types of early warning scores (EWSs), including the modified early warning score (MEWS), have been developed in several hospitals (Rees 2003). These systems are based on measurements of five physiological signs (temperature, pulse rate, systolic blood pressure, respiratory rate and mental response) and usually also include an assessment of the patient's urinary output.

The chart shown in Figure 12.2 is used for patients considered to be at high risk of developing a critical illness, such as emergency admissions, unstable patients, postoperative patients, patients whose condition is causing concern, patients who have stepped down from a higher level of care, patients with a chronic health problem or who are failing to progress. The readings for each observation are recorded and given a score against the readings on the chart. The total score for the patient is determined and used to decide the next course of action. As you can see, if the score reaches 3, the nurse taking the observations is expected to alert the senior nurse, who, depending on the current frequency of observations may decide that they need to be monitored more regularly. Usually a score of 4 or more triggers the ward staff to call for a special team to give advanced care (see Figure 12.3).

Thus, as you can see, an important part of responding to patients' needs and making decisions about the care required is recording the subsequent care delivered and the underpinning rationale.

The importance of effective documentation

However effectively you have been making decisions for your patients and delivering appropriate care, this is not sufficient. Good care includes documenting it in a timely, clear and full manner. Written records demonstrate that nursing care has been performed (Abraham 2003), enable it to be evaluated (Department of Health 2003) and researched, and may provide evidence in a legal inquiry (NMC 2002). Most importantly, these records can be accessed widely, ensuring continuity of care and enabling subsequent practitioners to make informed decisions that improve the quality of care patients receive. Indeed, Martin et al (1999) suggest that documentation of nursing care is the foremost source of reference and communication between nurses and other health care providers.

In addition to recording interventions carried out and actions taken, these records should include evidence of meeting patients' psychological, spiritual and cultural needs, thereby demonstrating a holistic approach to care. Korst et al (2003) have shown that nurses on a day shift spend nearly 20% of their time documenting care, which is not surprising when you consider the influence documentation has on the quality of patient care.

Despite this, there is evidence that the quality of nursing care documentation needs to be improved (Idvall & Ehrenberg 2002). A study by Taylor (2003) showed that a number of factors contribute to poor documentation, ranging from lack of time to devote to record-keeping and undervaluing time spent writing, to nurses writing minimal records or only recording positive outcomes in order not to compromise themselves legally, ethically or professionally, or because they lack, or think they lack, adequate literacy skills. In addition, records may be inadequate because patients' needs identified during assessment are not reflected in their care plans (Abraham 2003, Idvall & Ehrenberg 2002), or information is misplaced and therefore unavailable (Martin et al 1999).

The NHS is moving to a single patient record and to using electronic patient record systems, although, at the time of writing, the majority of NHS trusts are still working towards achieving this and have separate medical and nursing notes.

Routine biographical documentation is made for any patient or client seeking care (i.e. name, address, age, date of birth) (see Box 12.3). This information forms part of the nursing assessment, and gives you the opportunity to meet your patient/client and practise your communication skills. This is also an ideal time to use your observa-

EARLY WARNING SCORE

For all emergency and compromised post ITU patients

This should be assessed on all emergency admissions, major surgery, all patients returning from ITU/HDU and any patient that you are concerned about. *If outside this range call cardiac arrest team.

Date of admission	Affix patient label here
Consultant	
Ward	

Date															
Time															
HR 30–180*															
BP <60*															
Resp. rate 8–40*															
Central Nervous System															
Temp.															
Urine															
Score															
Doctor Y / N															
Grade if called															

Score	3	2	1	0	1	2	3
HR per minute		<40	41–50	51–100	101–110	111–129	>130
BP systolic	<70	71–80	81–100	101-199		>200	
Resp. per minute		<8		9–14	15–20	21–29	>30
Central Nervous System				Alert	Drowsy/ rousable to voice or newly confused	To pain	Unresponsive
Temperature		<35		35.1–37.5	>37.5		
Urine output	Nil	<20 ml/2 hrs or has not voided within 4 hrs of admission	20–50 ml/2 hrs or has not voided within 4 hrs of admission	>50 ml/2 hrs			

If the patient has a score of 3 or more, follow the flowchart in Figure 12.3

Figure 12.2 • Early warning score (EWS) chart. (Adapted from Table 1 in Rees 2003.)

tion skills in assessing the patient's physiological and psychological status. Note also that you must ensure confidentiality regarding any knowledge you may acquire of a patient/client; this is both a legal and a professional requirement.

Although it is the custom in Western countries to use the family name as the main means of identification, this may not be so in all cultures, so it is important to record the 'correct' family name. The use of first names is now more frequent for

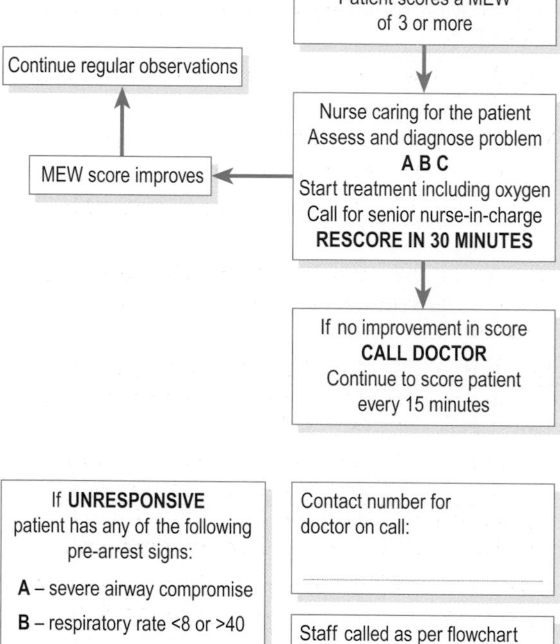

Figure 12.3 • Responding to early warning score (or modified early warning score). (Adapted from Figure 1 in Rees 2003.)

both patients and staff. However, care should be taken, and it is preferable to ask all patients how they wish to be addressed, rather than taking it for granted that they are happy with the one you have chosen for them! Not all patients like the name they were given and may prefer that you use a different name.

You need to always keep in mind the purpose of anything you record and the audience for whom it is intended. Many records are used by multidisciplinary teams, and patients are now allowed access to their records. You must record facts, not opinions, and these should be stated precisely, clearly and accurately. It is also important to avoid bias and misinterpretation. Similarly, abbreviations should not be used as these can lead to misunderstanding, unless they are in common usage and well known to all those using the records. Further guidance on good record-keeping can be found in the Nursing and Midwifery Council 'Guidelines for records and record keeping' (NMC 2002).

Nursing observations have been discussed earlier; these should be recorded, accurately and

Box 12.3

Typical biographical details required from a patient on admission to an acute setting

- Full name
- Preferred name (the name by which the patient likes to be addressed)
- Address
- Telephone number
- Date of birth and age
- Preferred language
- Ethnicity
- Religion
- Mobility and visual aids
- Diet requirements
- Allergies (this question is normally placed in a prominent position on the first page of the notes to alert carers to it)
- Next of kin or contact
- Address and telephone number of next of kin or contact
- Second contact name
- Address and telephone number of second contact person
- General practitioner's name, address and telephone number
- Occupation
- Social circumstances (this is important information for discharge planning and may be included in the model assessment or in the biographical details. Does the patient live in a house or a bungalow? Does the patient live alone? Where is the bathroom? Are there steps in the house?)
- Past medical history

clearly, on the relevant charts, as soon as they are taken. Never make these up; a patient's treatment and even life may depend on what has been recorded. If you have been unable to complete any observations, you must report this to the person in charge of the ward immediately.

Concluding remarks

In this chapter we have discussed making decisions in practice from several perspectives, from using models of assessment and clinical frameworks to monitoring your patient and thinking-on-your-feet whilst carrying out care. We have also considered the importance of recording the outcome of your decisions; that is, the care that you subsequently gave.

In conclusion, it is important to remember that:

> *If we are to have dialogue with other professionals and with clients [it is not sufficient to make decisions on our patients' behalf] . . . , we need to be able to articulate the basis for our judgements.*
>
> *(Taylor & White 2000, p 193)*

References

Abraham A 2003 Inadequate nursing care and the failure to keep adequate records. Professional Nursing 18:347–349

Andrews HA, Roy C 1997 The Roy adaptation model. Appleton and Lange, Norwalk

Bennett JG 1980 Foreword to the symposium on the self-care concept of nursing. Nursing Clinics of North America 15:1

Botti M, Reeve R 2003 Role of knowledge and ability in student nurses' clinical decision-making. Nursing and Health Sciences 5:39–49

Brown J, Marland G 2002 Hydration in older people with mental health problems. Nursing Times 98:38–39

Bucknall T 2000 Critical care nurses' decision-making activities in the natural setting. Journal of Clinical Nursing 9(1):25–36

Bucknall T 2003 The clinical landscape of critical care: nurses' decision-making. Journal of Advanced Nursing 43:310–319

Casey A 1988 A partnership with child and family. Senior Nurse 8:8–9

Carroll J, Johnson E 1990 Decision research: a field guide. Sage, California

Department of Health 1998 A first class service: quality in the new NHS. HMSO, London

Department of Health 1989 Children Act. HMSO, London

Department of Health 2000 Comprehensive critical care: a review of adult critical care services. HMSO, London

Department of Health 2001 The expert patient: a new approach to chronic disease management for the 21st century. HMSO, London

Department of Health 2003 The essence of care: patient focused benchmarking for health care practitioners. Department of Health, London. Online. Available: www.dh.gov.uk April 2006

Department of Health 2004a NHS improvement plan putting people at the heart of public services. HMSO, London

Department of Health 2004b National service framework for children, young people and maternity services: change for children – every child matters. HMSO, London

Department of Health 2004c Choosing health: making healthier choices easier. HMSO, London

Department of Health 2005 Case management competences framework for the care of people with long term conditions. HMSO, London

Department of Health 2006 Supporting people with long term conditions to self care: a guide to developing local strategies and good practice. HMSO, London

Fawcett J 1989 Analysis and evaluation of conceptual models of nursing, 2nd edn. Davis, Philadelphia

Goldhill DR, Sumner A 1998 Outcome of intensive care patients in a group of British intensive care units. Critical Care Medicine 26:1337–1345

Habermann M, Uys L 2005 The nursing process: a global concept. Churchill Livingstone, Edinburgh

Henderson V 1966 The nature of nursing. Macmillan, London

Idvall E, Ehrenberg A 2002 Nursing documentation of post pain management. Journal of Clinical Nursing 11:734–742

Intensive Care Society 2002 Guidelines for the introduction of outreach services: standards and guidelines. The Intensive Care Society, London

Lee P 1998 An analysis and evaluation of Casey's conceptual model. International Journal of Nursing Studies 35:204–209

Korst LM, Chamorro T, Eusebio-Angeja AC et al 2003 Nursing documentation time during implementation of an electronic medical record journal. Nursing Administration 33:24–30

Martin A, Hinds C, Felix M 1999 Documentation practices of nurses in long-term care. Journal of Clinical Nursing 8:345–352

Matterson P, Hawkins J 1990 Concept analysis of decision making. Nursing Forum 25(2):4–10

McKibbon KA 1998 Evidence based practice. Bulletin of the Medical Library Association 86:396–401

Morris DB 2000 How to speak postmodern medicine, illness and cultural change. Hastings Centre Report 30:7–16

Muir Gray JA 1997 Evidence-based healthcare: how to make health policy and management decisions. Churchill Livingstone, London

Murphy M, Cooney A, Casey D et al 2000 The Roper, Logan and Tierney model: perceptions and operationalization of the model in psychiatric nursing within a health board in Ireland. Journal of Advanced Nursing 31:1333–1341

National Institute for Clinical Excellence 2000 NICE guideline. Chronic heart failure. Management of chronic heart failure in adults in primary and secondary care. Online. Available: www.nice.org.uk April 2006

National Institute for Clinical Excellence 2005 Online. Available: www.nice.org.uk July 2006

Nursing and Midwifery Council 2002 Guidelines for records and record keeping. NMC, London

Nursing and Midwifery Council 2008 Code of professional conduct. London, NMC

Orem D 1971 Nursing concepts of practice. McGraw-Hill, New York

Orem D 1985 Nursing concepts of practice, 3rd edn. McGraw-Hill, New York

Orem D 1991 Nursing concepts of practice, 4th edn. McGraw-Hill, New York

Pearson A, Vaughan B, FitzGerald 2005 Nursing models for practice, 3rd edn. Butterworth-Heinemann, Oxford

Rambo BJ 1984 Adaptation nursing: assessment and intervention. WB Saunders, Philadelphia

Rees J 2003 Early warning scores. World Anaesthesia 17, article 10. Online. Available: www.nda.ox.ac.uk July 2006

Roberts I, Alderson P, Bunn F et al 2004 Colloids versus crystalloids for fluid resuscitation in critically ill patients. Cochrane Database of Systematic Reviews Series 4, CD000567. Wiley, Chichester

Roper N, Logan W, Tierney A 1980 The elements of nursing: a model for nursing based on a model of living. Churchill Livingstone, London

Roper N, Logan W, Tierney A 1996 The elements of nursing: a model for nursing based on a model of living, 4th edn. Churchill Livingstone, London

Roper N, Logan W, Tierney A 2000 The Roper Logan Tierney model of nursing. Churchill Livingstone, London

Roy C 1976 Introduction to nursing: an adaptive model. Prentice Hall, New Jersey

Schön D 1988 Educating the reflective practitioner. San Francisco, Jossey-Bass

Taylor H 2003 An exploration of the factors that affect nurses' recordkeeping. British Journal of Nursing 12:751–758

Taylor C, White S 2000 Practising reflexivity in health and welfare: making knowledge. Open University Press, Buckingham

Thompson C 2003 Clinical experience as evidence in evidence-based practice. Journal of Advanced Nursing 43:230–237

Chapter Thirteen

13

Promoting safe practice

Anne Harriss, Mike Cook

Key topics

- An introduction to clinical governance
- Essential principles of safe practice:
- Adopting a questioning approach
- Informing your practice with up-to-date knowledge and evidence
- Knowing your limitations
- Being aware of hazards in the environment
- Remembering that prevention is the key
- Taking prompt action in the event of an emergency
- Communicating effectively
- Reporting concerns

Introduction

> *The very first requirement in a hospital is that it should do the sick no harm.*
>
> *(Florence Nightingale 1859, 2001)*

In this chapter you will explore what fundamental practice skills you need to learn during your foundation year and beyond so as to provide safe, high-quality practice that will enhance the health of the people that you care for and 'do your patients no harm'.

Florence Nightingale's remark about the environment in which health care is delivered continues to be relevant more than a century later. Furthermore, it is a sentiment that applies equally well to all sectors of health care and to all branches of nursing. Reports in the public press indicate that, despite the best endeavours of many health care workers, we cannot take for granted the fact that health care practice causes 'no harm'. Sadly, within health care, harm is still being caused to patients. The reasons for this are not straightforward, and in some situations, such as pioneering surgery or testing out new drug regimens, risks are taken to achieve clinical outcomes. But in many cases practitioners could have avoided errors. In this chapter you will learn that you have an important part to play in maintaining safety for the people you care for and other staff.

The scope of the problem

The NHS Litigation Authority (NHSLA) is a special health authority (part of the NHS) that is responsible for handling negligence claims made against NHS bodies in England. As well as dealing with claims they also have an active risk-management programme to help raise standards of care in the NHS and hence reduce the number of incidents leading to claims. The NHSLA was established in 1995. Some of the following figures indicate the nature of the situation within England in terms of claims for clinical negligence. It can be seen that the NHS has to spend increasing amounts of money in cases of clinical negligence.

In 2004–2005, 5609 claims of clinical negligence and 3766 claims of non-clinical negligence against NHS bodies were received by the NHSLA. This compares with 6251 claims of clinical negligence and 3819 claims of non-clinical negligence in 2003–2004.

In 2004–2005, £502.9 million was paid out in connection with clinical negligence claims; this figure includes both damages paid to patients and the legal costs borne by the NHS. In 2003–2004, the comparable figure was £422.5 million (NHSLA 2006).

The costs of treating hospital-acquired infection, including extended length of stay, are difficult to measure with certainty, but a report in 2005 (House of Commons Committee of Public Accounts 2005) estimated that each year in England there are at least 300 000 cases of hospital-acquired infection, causing around 5000 deaths and costing the NHS as much as £1 billion. The report states that critical to managing this situation is a shift towards prevention at all levels of the NHS. This would require commitment from everyone involved and a philosophy that prevention is everybody's business, not just the specialists'.

Not all hospital-acquired infection is preventable, since the very old, the very young, those undergoing invasive procedures and those with suppressed immune systems are particularly susceptible. However, in 1995 the Hospital Infection Working Group of the Department of Health and Public Health Laboratory Service believed that about 30% of hospital-acquired infections could be avoided by better application of existing knowledge and realistic infection-control practices. One of the most important strategies for reducing hospital-acquired infection is effective hand-washing; this is covered later in this chapter. It is probable that specific sessions will be provided by your university or placement area on hand-washing. It is vital that you attend these sessions to ensure that you are familiar with local policies and protocols.

During the 1990s, a number of prominent service failures in areas such as bone tumour diagnosis, paediatric cardiac surgery, cervical screening and wrong injection routes for powerful drugs have undoubtedly caused the public to revise their perception of the health care system and the people who work within it (Nicholls et al 2000). Although these examples may have made headline news, daily practice events remind us that we must constantly question our assumptions that health care is automatically safe practice. For example, hospital-acquired pressure sores (decubitus ulcers), methicillin-resistant *Staphylococcus aureus* (MRSA) and preoperative anxiety are all conditions that can have immensely detrimental physical, psychological and social consequences for people who require care and their carers. As the news about health service investigations change quite rapidly, it is worth looking at the local press for details about incidents in your area. When reading any press articles try to be critical in your reading (see Activity 13.1).

Activity 13.1

Be critical in your reading:

- How is the news reported?
- Which side of the story is being reported?
- What is the tone of the language in the report?
- Are other points of view not represented?
- Why might the news story be reported in this way?

During this activity try to draw on your own learning about providing care.

Websites for exploring more information about NHS services and investigations can be found for all countries of the UK. In England and Wales it is the Healthcare Commission. In Scotland this role is undertaken by NHS Quality Improvement Scotland. In Northern Ireland the role is undertaken by the Committee for Health, Social Services and Public Safety. All these bodies have statutory duties to assess the performance of health care organizations.

In the 21st century, given the complexity and pace of change within health care, we need to be clear and explicit in our attempts to assure both ourselves and the general public that our practices are safe and effective. Indeed, along with all the other regulatory bodies of health care practitioners, the Nursing and Midwifery Council of the UK (NMC) has produced a code of practice to guide practitioners and protect the public. The 'NMC Code of professional conduct' states that practitioners are personally accountable for their practice. This means that, once qualified, you will be answerable for your acts and omissions, regardless of advice or directions from another professional and that you have a duty of care to your patients and clients, who are entitled to receive safe and competent care.

Exercising your duty of care

You will recall that the 'NMC Code of professional conduct' expects you:

- To protect and support the health of individual patients and clients.
- To act in such a way that justifies the trust and confidence that the public have in you.

In this chapter we describe activities related to prevention of illness or disability or which alert nurses to potential clinical problems. All of them are aspects of care which every foundation course nursing student will encounter; they include ensuring adequate nutrition and hydration of patients and clients, preventing the complications of immobility and carrying out clinical observations. All of these nursing duties may be seen as routine; indeed, they form part of the daily work of the nurse and experience of the patient, but they are far from routine and ordinary in their consequences if they are not fulfilled as required within the patient's care plan.

What is quality?

Everyone seems to have a general understanding of quality. It describes how individuals value particular aspects of a service or product that they either actually use or are considering using. One useful definition is:

> *. . . quality can . . . be defined as what the customer states it is . . .*
>
> *(Wiggans & Turner 1991, p 183)*

Quality in public service can be defined as:

> *. . . fully meeting customer requirements at the lowest cost . . .*
>
> *(Øvretveit 1992)*

Others define quality as features of the service, for example: accessibility, relevance to need equity, social acceptability, efficiency and effectiveness (Maxwell 1984). This definition makes an important point as it is not only important to produce satisfaction for those health care 'customers' who receive the service, but to ensure that all those that need the service can and do get it. It is important to include, alongside the patient's judgements of the service, a professional definition of need, and a professional judgement of the extent to which a service meets the patients' needs. However, even this reference to need becomes complex as patients may not know what they need, or may ask for treatments that are really inappropriate or harmful. Therefore, the provider must gain an understanding of the perceived needs of the person. It is also important to determine who these customers are. A wide definition of customer is required; this includes staff working in the organization, employers, patients, relatives, health authority purchasers, NHS executive bodies, and health service providers.

Clinical governance

Clinical governance was introduced into the British health care system by the Labour government in 1998. It has now become firmly established as an important framework for assuring and improving the quality of health care. It is described as: 'a framework through which NHS organisations are accountable for continuously improving the quality of their services and safeguarding high standards of care by creating an environment in which excellence in clinical care will flourish' (Department of Health 1998). It is important to note that this definition refers to the organizations in which individual practitioners work as well as the accountability that practitioners adhere to as part of their codes of conduct.

Clinical governance encourages safer practice and places accountability for this practice and for improving quality directly and personally with the chief executive officer of the health care institution. This means that chief executives have to focus on achieving financial balance and assuring clinical quality. Since the 1980s, quality has been high on the health care agenda. Concepts such as audit, clinical effectiveness, evidence-based practice and risk management are important elements of clinical governance.

Clinical governance is intended to foster learning from situations that go wrong. The emphasis is on learning rather than on punishment. It is designed to help practitioners, managers and all other members of the health care team to be open and honest so that risks can be identified and errors can be prevented and acted upon quickly when they do occur.

The importance of patient/client and public involvement at all levels of service development is recognized as being a critical factor in clinical governance. This has led to patient advisory councils being formed in each health care trust to provide communication channels between service providers and service users.

The National Institute for Health and Clinical Excellence (known as NICE) identifies good practice through the development of national service frameworks and clinical guidelines.

Adopting a questioning approach

The first principle of delivering safe and effective care is to adopt a questioning approach to your own practice and that of others. This involves not only being able to account for your actions, explaining why you are undertaking a particular activity and ensuring that you have the necessary knowledge and skill, but also reflecting on past situations and events to ensure that you maximize the learning available to you. You will recall that some of the techniques for using reflection in practice were introduced in Section One of this book.

Inform your practice with up-to-date knowledge and evidence

The use of the best available evidence to support practice is intended to enhance care, and lead to consistency in practice and a better-informed public. It is hoped that this in turn will contribute to an increase in the public's confidence in the health care system. From the nurse's perspective it is anticipated that the use of evidence to inform decision-making will assist us to account for our practice, and that the generation of such evidence will contribute to our body of knowledge as nurses. From an organization's perspective, the use of the very best evidence to inform practice should contribute to a reduction in risk (and associated litigation), the best use of resources and an enhanced reputation.

There are many tools that provide a summary of the available evidence and help to deliver safe and effective practice (see Activity 13.2 to help identify guides to safe practice).

Activity 13.2

- Try to identify any tools in your placement area that health care professionals use to guide this practice.
- Make a list of these and then compare with the examples in the rest of this chapter.

Policies, protocols and care pathways

The best available evidence is often translated locally into guidelines, protocols, principles of practice and policies which are defined as follows:

- *Policies*. Statements that guide decision-making and require employees of an organization to work within certain parameters.
- *Guidelines*. Systematically developed statements to assist practitioner and patient decisions about appropriate health care for specific clinical circumstances (NHSME 1996; further information can be found on the NHSME website).
- *Protocols*. A term often used to refer to a way of prescribing exactly what must be done in often high-risk situations.
- *Principles of practice*. A statement which explains how things should be done.

It is important for you, as a student nurse, to ensure that you become familiar with the evidence sources that are used locally. You will need to know the existence of policies and procedures in your practice placements, even if you are not expected to use them immediately. Such policies will include things such as care of drugs, patient or client control and restraint, care of patients' property, speaking out policy, patient resuscitation, fire procedures, Mental Health Act implications for patients' leave, child protection. There are many more, some examples of which are described later in this chapter or elsewhere in the book.

Care pathways

Integrated care pathways were introduced in Chapter 12. This approach is described in a little more detail here, together with a specific exercise to undertake. The use of care pathways has become increasingly important within health care today. A care pathway is an outline of anticipated clinical practice for a particular group of patients/clients with a particular diagnosis or set of symptoms. Successful care pathways are normally constructed by interdisciplinary care teams and are derived from evidence-based practice.

Kitchiner & Bundred (1998) comment that an integrated care pathway determines locally agreed multidisciplinary standards based on evidence, where available, for a specific patient group. Documentation associated with care pathways is an important part of clinical records as this identifies the planned clinical care.

For examples of care pathways and more information, please refer to http://libraries.nelh.nhs.uk/pathways.

It is impossible in the space available here to give examples for all programme branches. Integrated care pathways are complex and result in the creation of large documents which constitute the patient's live record of care. The use of care pathways is still being developed in the NHS but you are most likely to see those that are for patients with conditions most often encountered. Care pathways generally identify the total care regimen, including emergency admission to perhaps an accident and emergency department, through to a specialist unit such as a coronary care unit and via a general ward to discharge into the care of a rehabilitation team such as a cardiac rehabilitation nurse. All aspects of the care are based on evidence-based 'best practice' for both medicine and nursing. At this stage, you will not necessarily know about all the medical treatments and drugs used, but the pathway does show the integration of all aspects of a person's care.

Important features of successful pathways include the following:

- They are agreed by all members of the multidisciplinary team or agencies involved in the patient's episode of care.
- Their focus is the patient/client rather than any one professional group.
- The care contained within the pathway is based upon the very best evidence available.

Try reflecting on care pathways as suggested in Activity 13.3. Some of your reflective ideas might have included the potential of care pathways to improve communication, not only between those delivering care but also between health professionals

Activity 13.3

- Reflect on the description of care pathways using any of the reflective models identified in Section One of the book.
- Try to identify any advantages or limitations of care pathways.

and the patient or client. This is an important benefit. Expectations are clearly mapped out in advance. Care pathway development necessitates the review of existing practice and continually monitoring the evidence. They can also help to promote evidence-based practice and reduce unwanted variations in care delivery. You may also have identified that some of your lecturers and mentors use care pathways as teaching tools for you and other new team members. In short, care pathways promote many of the activities required to ensure the delivery of safe and effective care.

However, care pathways are not without their critics. For example, there is a thought that they will reduce clinical judgement or be used unthinkingly, resulting in poorer, rather than enhanced, care. Clearly this depends on how they are introduced. Whether care pathways are in place or not, nurses and other health care professionals are still accountable for their actions, and decisions still need to be made about the appropriateness of standard actions for individual patients/clients. Professional judgement and patient preference cannot be suspended if practice is to be safe and effective rather than routine.

Audit

Care pathways are not the only method of ensuring that practice is evidence-based. Audit is another important strategy and widely used in all areas of health and social care today. Audit of practice is usually integrated within a care pathway, but it can be undertaken independently in conjunction with guidelines and standards. Audit involves reviewing practice and ensuring that it is in accordance with that defined as 'the best', and that action is taken to rectify the situation when shortfalls occur.

Care bundles

A newly emerging term within hospital-based acute settings is 'care bundles'. This idea emphasizes the importance of clinical teams delivering the best evidence-based care to patients. The technique of 'care bundles' measures how often therapies that should be given are actually given in practice. If a therapy is administered as proposed under best practice guidelines, then compliance is achieved. Measuring compliance in this way gives a good focus for teams to improve the care given to patients.

An example of this type of measurement is used within the critical care area when monitoring blood glucose levels. Current research (e.g. van den Berghe et al 2003) suggests that carefully controlling blood glucose can reduce mortality. Many critical care units will have protocols related to glucose control, and these may be adhered to, but they do not record how good at actually controlling blood glucose, within the target range, the units are. In other words, the measurement of blood glucose may be taken, but appropriate measures to control a person's blood glucose levels might not be implemented. Care bundles use agreed measurement frequencies to match best evidence against actual practice.

A very useful article that relates this concept to reducing health care associated infections has been written by Storr et al (2005). The article identifies the few critical activities that health care practitioners can undertake to help reduce healthcare-acquired hospital infections. More practical information can be found in the Department of Health document 'Saving lives' (Department of Health 2005). This is discussed later in this chapter.

Delivering safe and effective care based on the very best evidence requires active efforts to keep up-to-date with new knowledge, and national and international strategies are in place to facilitate this process. Evidence of continuing professional development (which involves keeping up-to-date with the latest knowledge and evidence) is a requirement to remain on the professional register as a nurse and is vital if we are to be accountable practitioners, able to reason for our actions. Section

One of this book provides details of the continuing professional education requirements for nurses today; this chapter reinforces the importance of this for practice.

Know your limitations

When you consider the expectations placed on nurses in practice today, it is little wonder that they are sometimes faced with new and complex situations beyond their existing knowledge and experience. For a student of nursing this is clearly to be expected, yet given the dynamic and changing face of health care it is a situation that you can expect to face well beyond registration. Progress means that as nurses we are expected continually to learn and develop our practice, for example through reflection, further academic study and supervised practice.

As discussed in Section One, nurses are accountable for their practice; that is, they must be able to explain the reasoning behind their decisions and actions. The accountability of nurses and other health care professionals is primarily to the patients/clients in their care, but nurses are also accountable to the employing organization, to other members of the profession and to the professional body, the Nursing and Midwifery Council (NMC).

Accountability means not only knowing how to carry out a particular aspect of care, but also being clear about the limitations of your knowledge and experience. Although as nursing students your accountability is limited, the principles still apply as listed in the 'NMC Code of professional conduct'. In order to be safe in practice, it is vital that you are aware of your limitations as well as your strengths, and that you know when to seek advice and support. This may not always be easy, especially in the early stages of your programme.

Activity 13.4 ask you to explore why it might be difficult to seek help. Your response to the question might have included some, or perhaps all, of the following:

- You may have feared looking foolish.
- You may have already asked once before but were unable to remember or did not grasp the response.

Activity 13.4

Although it is an important part of providing safe and effective practice that we do not undertake tasks for which we do not feel prepared and for which we are not competent, it can sometimes be very difficult to say 'no' or to seek help. Why might this be the case?

Activity 13.5

Think of a situation in which you felt unprepared to undertake the task asked of you. Use one of the frameworks described in Chapter 2 to reflect upon this incident.

- What was your response?
- Did you undertake the task or ask for help?
- Why did you behave in this way?
- What factors influenced your judgement?
- Would you deal with the situation in the same way next time, or would you do things differently?

- The nurses may have looked busy and you did not wish to interrupt them.
- You may have asked questions in the past and received a curt response.

It is important to understand the concept of accountability and to know how to handle situations for which you feel ill prepared. Activity 13.5 asks you to reflect on a difficult situation. Then Case history 13.1 describes a situation in which a student nurse is reflecting on facing up to her limitations and how she would act differently in future, to ensure safe and effective care.

Professional self-regulation

Self-regulation, the type of regulation that has been granted to nurses and midwives, is a privilege granted by parliament. It is not a right. It has to be earned continually to sustain public trust and confidence in the profession. Integral to self-regulation is the onus placed on each and every member of a profession, including the nursing profession, to ensure that their practice is safe and effective. Section One covers this in some detail.

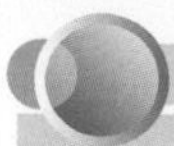

Case history 13.1

Knowing my limitations

It was during my first placement on an orthopaedic ward that the incident took place. My mentor had arranged for me to attend fracture clinic, something I was looking forward to. When I got there it was suggested that I join the doctor and nurse covering clinic 'A'. I spent the first hour watching patients being booked in, called through, seen by the doctor and departing. It was interesting and a lot busier than I'd expected. I was then sent to fetch some medical notes that had been left in reception. On my return, the staff nurse was nowhere to be seen and the buzzer for the next patient was sounding. I didn't know what to do, I looked around, and all staff appeared to have vanished. The doctor came out. I explained that I was unsure where the staff nurse had gone. He said 'Not to worry, you can do it. Call in the next patient or we will be running late'. I had watched the staff nurse, so I did as I thought she had done. I soon realized how difficult it was. I was unfamiliar with the abbreviations used, I had never heard of half of the words used and found it quite impossible to spell them. When I was asked for the simplest thing it took me ages to find it and I just got more and more flustered.

I felt really distressed by the time the nurse returned. She apologized immediately and told me that I should have fetched someone else. I went home and worried . . . what if I had heard the doctor's instructions incorrectly or if what I had managed to write down did not make sense? Would the patient get the 'wrong' care? I began to feel angry for being put in the situation. I was angry with both the doctor and the staff nurse, it was their fault!

On reflection the nurse was right; I should have persisted in my attempt to get some assistance, but I panicked and did not want to look foolish. The fact that I didn't know the staff seemed to make getting help harder. I wasn't sure how they would respond as they were clearly busy. Would they be angry? I did not want to be a nuisance.

I learned a great deal about myself from this incident. I like to be seen as competent and helpful and I find it very difficult to say 'no' when asked to do something.

However, I now recognize that I was putting my need to look good before the safe and effective care of the patients. Perhaps the staff nurse should not have left me, but this will happen occasionally. Although I recognize that as a student I do not carry full professional accountability in situations such as this, it is my responsibility to make the limitations of my knowledge and experience known. Next time, if faced with a situation I feel ill-prepared for, I will speak out. This will not only reduce my anxiety about being left in similar situations, but will be in the interests of safe patient care.

Health and safety for patients and staff

Environmental awareness begins shortly after birth and continues throughout life and, ideally, people make choices in the nature and style of their personal environment. This is true for all people, whether they are well or ill or have some form of disability, who devote much energy towards accomplishing tasks to fulfil their wish of being master of their personal environment. The quality of the health and safety of our environment is greatly affected by the environment itself, and never more so than in the health care setting, where patients and clients may be more vulnerable than when in their own homes. Florence Nightingale suggested that patients in health care settings may be harmed just by being there. As previously discussed in this chapter hospital acquired infection in the UK highlights the need for health care professionals to be vigilant about this and other potential hazards to patients. So, a major task for all is to promote and maintain a safe environment. Of course, the health and safety of staff is also important and the Health and Safety at Work etc. Act (Great Britain Parliament 1974) places a general duty on all employers to ensure the health and safety of their employees.

Promoting a safe environment is one of the many functions of the nurse. As you read at the beginning of this chapter, the Nursing and Midwifery Council (NMC) makes this explicit by requiring nurses to ensure that no action they

undertake is detrimental to the safety and well-being of patients, and to ensure that they report any unsafe practice or environmental danger that might affect the safety of either patients or staff. Within this section of the chapter only four specific nursing activities are covered; these are infection control, food hygiene, moving and handling, and the safe administration of medicines. All foundation students will experience elements of these. The important issue of the prevention of pressure sores is covered later.

Infection control and the role of the nurse

Chapter 9 identified some important elements of infection and you will have noted that disposable items such as dressings, gloves, aprons, eye protection and other equipment are the norm in hospitals and in the community. To be effective, these disposable items have to be used correctly and the principles of infection need to be understood.

The document 'Saving lives: a delivery programme to reduce healthcare associated infection (HCAI) including MRSA' (Department of Health 2005) highlights five high-impact interventions that have been developed for the clinical practice related to infection control, each with distinct evidence-based elements of the clinical process. They are:

- Preventing the risk of microbial contamination.
- Central venous catheter care.
- Preventing surgical site infection.
- Care of ventilated patients (or tracheostomy where appropriate).
- Urinary catheter care.

This chapter focuses on the first of these high-impact changes as this is the one that is most likely to involve you as a foundation student. You will learn about the other four high-impact changes as you progress through your programme. High-impact change 1, preventing the risk of microbial contamination, is based on best evidence and highlights the key points listed in Box 13.1.

Box 13.1

High-impact change 1: preventing the risk of microbial contamination

Hand hygiene

- Decontaminate hands before and after each patient contact
- Use correct hand hygiene procedure.

Personal protective equipment

- Wear examination gloves if risk of exposure to body fluids
- Gloves are single-use items
- Gowns, aprons, eye/face protection may be indicated if there is a risk of being splashed with blood or body fluids.

Aseptic technique

- Gown, gloves and drapes as indicated should be used when invasive devices are being inserted.

Safe disposal of sharps

- Sharps container available at point of use
- No disassembling of needle and syringe
- Not passed from hand to hand
- Container should not be overfilled.

Nurses play an important role in managing aspects of these high-impact interventions. As you progress through the foundation programme into your specific branch, you will learn more about aspects of these specific procedures that are relevant to your area of practice.

What is infection?

An infection is caused when the body is invaded by pathogenic (disease-producing) organisms: either bacteria or viruses. Infection is usually accompanied by a high temperature (pyrexia) and sweating and sometimes even causes a rigor. If the infection is associated with a wound then this will be red, hot and inflamed and the patient will complain of pain around the inflamed area. All these signs and symptoms are the body's response to the presence of a pathogen.

Box 13.2 shows how cross-infection can occur from person to person, or from implements or the atmosphere.

Hospital infection

> *Whatever the setting, everyone who works in health care establishments is responsible for maintaining a safe environment.*
>
> *(Parker 1999)*

Despite a great increase in the legislation governing working practice in hospitals aimed at reducing cross-infection, the situation appears to be getting worse rather than better. Parker's statement is therefore very relevant and demonstrates that such an important issue cannot be considered to be the sole responsibility of the microbiology department or the infection control nurse. One of the simplest measures to prevent cross-infection, and probably the single most important contribution to its prevention, is hand-washing (Figure 13.1), which nurses and all clinical staff are taught as a matter of priority and yet is sometimes rushed or neglected altogether.

Disposable gloves may protect you, but they do not protect your patients unless you wash your hands and change your gloves between each procedure or patient. Reducing the spread of infection in all health care areas is a major priority. Charge nurses are being urged and supported to insist that all medical and other staff wash their hands between every patient on every round and in every clinic. Knowing how to wash your hands is important (Box 13.3) (see also Figure 13.2).

The operating theatre 'scrubbing up' area is a good area to see hand-washing performed at its best. This would be a good learning opportunity if you could arrange to visit this area.

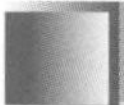

Box 13.2

Routes of cross-infection

- Ingestion through the mouth (e.g. ingestion of contaminated food or water).
- Inhalation through the nose (e.g. breathing in micro-organisms from the atmosphere, particularly bacteria and viruses) causing sore throats, coughs and colds, leading to chest infections. The respiratory system may also succumb to more contagious aerobic bacteria such as *Mycobacterium tuberculosis*, which causes tuberculosis. Patients on artificial breathing machines are especially at risk.
- Via the skin, through abrasions, wounds (including open pressure sores) and 'compound' fractures (i.e. the bone has broken through the skin). Burns, particularly those covering large areas of the body, are so prone to infection that these patients have to be nursed in specially designed units aimed at reducing infection to the minimum. An incision made in order to undertake an operation may be sutured afterwards, but still provides a portal of entry for infection. There is the potential for infection to occur when the skin is broken.
- Injections of any kind, intravenous fluids, central venous pressure lines, and transfusing blood and blood products including contaminated blood.
- Invasive procedures such as catheterization, bladder washouts, chest drainage, wound drainage.
- Changing of dressings.

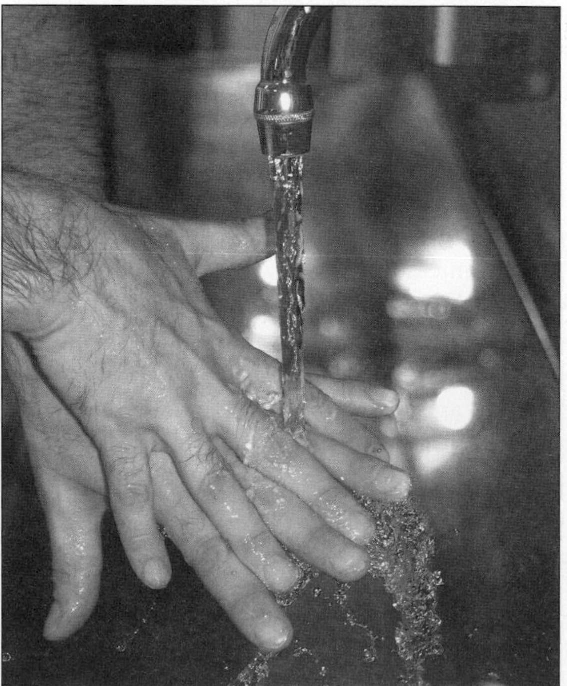

Figure 13.1 • Hand-washing.

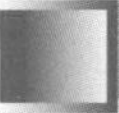

Box 13.3

Hand-washing

- The hands should be washed before and after all patient contact.
- To prevent cross-infection, jewellery should not be worn; a plain wedding ring only is permissible, and it is preferable not to wear a watch on the wrist.
- A waterproof, occlusive dressing should cover any cuts or abrasions.
- A sink with elbow- or foot-operated mixer taps is best; the temperature of the water should be adjusted so that it is comfortable and the flow steady so that it avoids splashing the surrounding area.
- Liquid soap or antiseptic detergent hand-washing solution should be used, applying sufficient to create a good lather; scrubbing the skin with a nailbrush is *not* recommended as this causes abrasions, but the fingernails may be scrubbed.
- Wash hands thoroughly under running water and then rinse them, making sure that all traces of soap/detergent are removed.
- Turn off the taps using elbows or feet, but keeping your hands pointing upwards, to avoid water from the wrist area and above which has not been washed coming into contact with the washed area.
- Dry hands well to minimize growth of micro-organisms and to prevent the hands from becoming sore.
- Dispose of used towels in a foot-operated waste bin.

Disposable aprons and gloves

Disposable aprons and gloves do more harm than good if they are not used and disposed of correctly. A habit of abiding by some simple principles will give greater protection to your patient against cross-infection.

Aprons

Sometimes plastic aprons are supplied in different colours for different tasks (e.g. for serving meals or doing dressings). Aprons should be worn:

- For all situations in which there is direct contact with the patient.

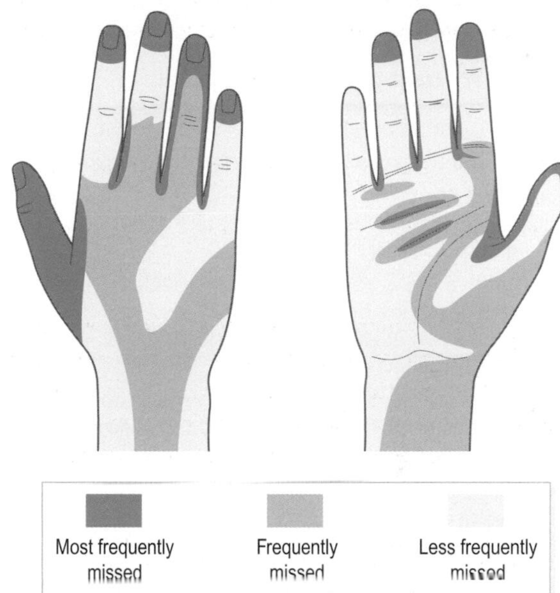

Figure 13.2 • The areas of the hand most often missed during hand-washing (Nicol et al 2000).

- Where there is contact with body fluids.
- When handling bed linen, excreta or clinical waste.
- When handling items that have been in contact with infectious disease, including clothes and books.

Box 13.4 details the procedure for the use of aprons.

Disposable gloves (non-sterile)

The use of gloves does not reduce the need to wash the hands before and after the gloves have been worn. This is because the hands sweat and create a warm, moist environment that will encourage micro-organisms to thrive. Another reason for this is that the gloves may not completely protect the hands as they have been shown to develop tiny puncture holes that go undetected, but allow micro-organisms to enter. Seamless, single-use latex or vinyl gloves are recommended. These come in three sizes and fit either hand.

Gloves should be worn whenever patient care involves dealing with blood or other body fluids, depending on the procedure, when providing care

Box 13.4

How to use an apron

- Wash and dry hands before putting on the apron.
- Pull the apron over your head, trying to avoid touching the hair or uniform.
- Tie the apron loosely at the back so that any liquid will quickly run off.
- Remove the apron by pulling the neckband and the sides, thus breaking the ties, and fold the apron in on itself to prevent the spread of micro-organisms.
- Do not allow your hands to touch your uniform, and discard the used apron into the yellow clinical waste bag.
- Wash and dry your hands thoroughly.

Box 13.5

Use of gloves

- Wash and dry hands thoroughly.
- Take the correct size of glove from the appropriate area.
- To remove the gloves, do not touch your wrists or hands with the dirty gloves. Using a gloved hand, pinch up the cuff of the other hand and pull the glove off inside out. Using the ungloved hand, insert it behind the cuff, and pull the other glove off, turning it inside out (Figure 13.3).
- Gloves that have been used for clinical procedures should be discarded immediately into the yellow clinical waste bag.

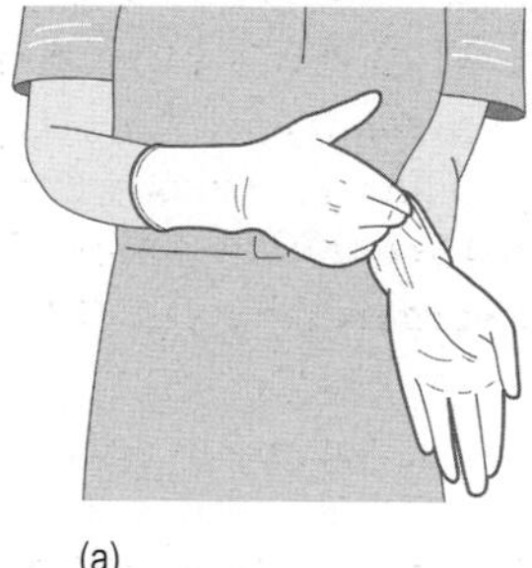
(a)

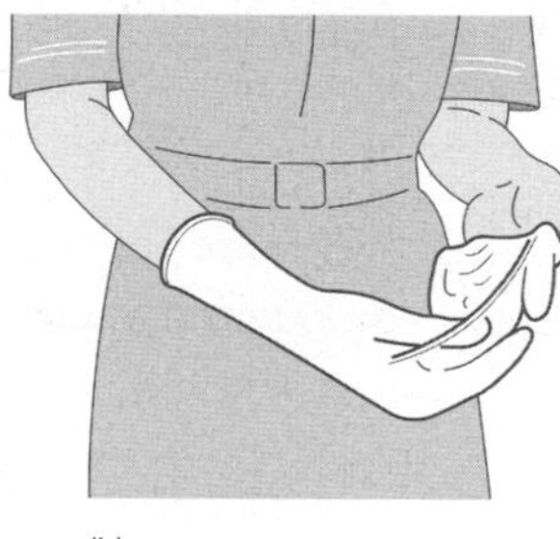
(b)

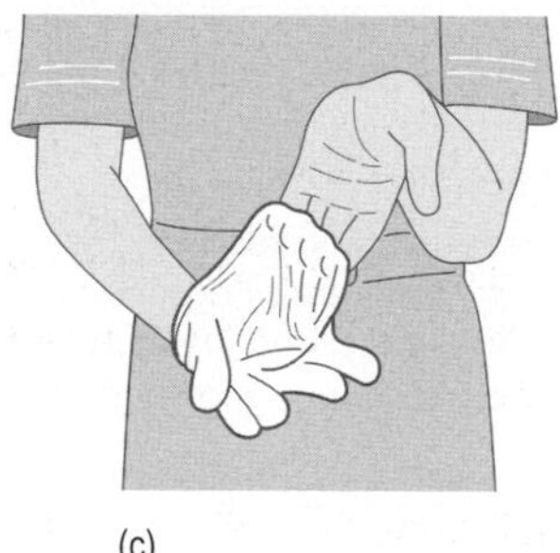
(c)

Figure 13.3a–c • Safe removal of gloves (Nicol et al 2000).

for a patient who has an infection (e.g. hepatitis, HIV, MRSA or TB) and when giving certain intramuscular drugs (e.g. antibiotics).

Choosing the correct size of glove is important as gloves that are too large or too small could impair dexterity. If gloves are required for a clean procedure these should be taken from the clean area rather than those stored in the sluice.

Box 13.5 details the procedure for the use of gloves.

Eye protection

Many clinical areas provide suitable eye protection which should be used when situations determine this. Local guidelines will exist, and they are likely to include times when you may be exposed to splashes from blood or other bodily fluids.

When selecting eye protection the following should be considered:

- Eye and face protection should be selected with the particular risk in mind.
- Is the protection comfortable and does it fit properly? It should not hinder movement or visibility. Fit is important as you do not want to be adjusting eye protection with potentially contaminated gloved hands.
- The working environment; for example, spectacles or visors may be preferable in humid or hot conditions as goggles may steam up.

> **Activity 13.6**
> - Find out who your infection control nurse is, and how they can be contacted.
> - Locate your infection control manual and identify the key nursing elements.

The infection control nurse and infection control policies

Every hospital trust will have an infection control team which will include a specialist infection control nurse. Infection control nurses are qualified experienced nurses, who have usually taken a further course on infection control. They are there to advise staff on how to prevent cross-infection and care for patients with infectious diseases, and to assist in the interpretation of hospital policies and procedures dealing with infection control (try Activity 13.6). They are very much involved in finding and implementing the latest research on infection control, advising on new products and updating nursing procedures. They work closely with the microbiology department and the health and safety officer.

Policies and procedures in relation to infection control

Much can be achieved by reducing the level of pathogenic organisms in the environment by routine cleaning. With the amount of movement of personnel, visitors and the high turnover of patients, any environment where patients or clients are nursed or are resident can quickly become contaminated with dust, soil and debris, along with organic matter and potentially infectious organisms. A safe environment can be achieved by following simple guidelines on the disposal of contaminants and by introducing routine and effective cleaning. Hospitals in particular are introducing clean-up campaigns as part of the drive to reduce hospital-acquired infections.

Chadwick & Oppenheim (1996) stated that cleaning the hospital environment is a cost-effective method of controlling infection. Routine cleaning with household detergents and hot water is considered sufficient to maintain the appearance of the building and reduce the number of microbes in the environment (Collins 1988). A clean environment inspires confidence in patients, relatives and staff. It is also well known that certain organisms responsible for hospital-acquired infections such as *Staphylococcus aureus* and *Escherichia coli* survive for long periods in most environments. If the environment is not cleaned regularly there will be a build-up of dust and debris that will support the growth of these and other micro-organisms. The report from the Standing Medical Advisory Committee (SMAC) subgroup on antimicrobial resistance states that the role of hospital cleaning staff is fundamental to controlling the spread of multi-resistant micro-organisms (SMAC 1998). At the same time, the House of Lords Select Committee on Science and Technology (1998) wants infection control and basic hygiene to be placed 'at the heart of good hospital management and practice'.

All hospitals have to produce an infection control policy and you should be introduced to the key elements that will effect you and your practice by your mentor. The topics that should be included in any infection control policy are listed in Box 13.6.

Medical devices and safety

As a result of European legislation, the Medicines and Healthcare Products Regulatory Agency (MHRA) is the government agency that is responsible for ensuring that medicines and medical devices work and are acceptably safe. The MHRA has been given full responsibility to carry out the directives as required under UK legislation. The definition of medical devices is any instrument, apparatus, appliance or material or other article, whether used alone or in combination (including software) on human beings for the purpose of diagnosis, prevention, treatment, investigation, replacement or modification of the anatomy, control of conception, and certain pharmacological products.

The Department of Health has issued guidance on all medical devices that need to be inspected, serviced, repaired or transported, and the requirement of a declaration of contamination status (Medical Devices Agency 1996). Staff should

Box 13.6

Topics that should be included in an infection control policy

- Contact telephone numbers of appropriate personnel such as the infection control nurse, and key personnel in the microbiology department who will give advice and guidance.
- Admissions, transfers and discharges (patients with known or suspected infection).
- Cleaning, disinfection and decontamination, if necessary, of medical equipment.
- How to handle outbreaks of diarrhoea, hepatitis, meningitis and other notifiable infectious diseases.
- Specific guidance on handling patients with MRSA and HIV infection.
- Handling laundry.
- Food handling.
- Waste disposal.
- Disposal of 'sharps' (i.e. syringes and needles), including dealing with injuries.
- Collection of specimens.
- Control of pests (e.g. cockroaches, fleas).
- Control of hazardous substances and spillages.

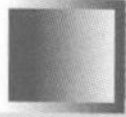

Box 13.7

Some definitions

(Medical Devices Agency 1996)

- *Cleaning*. A process which physically removes contamination but does not necessarily destroy micro-organisms. The reduction of microbial contamination is dependent upon many factors, including the efficiency of the cleaning process and the initial amount of microbial contamination. Cleaning removes micro-organisms and the organic material on which they thrive. It is a necessary prerequisite of effective disinfection and sterilization.
- *Disinfection*. A process used to reduce the number of viable micro-organisms but which may not necessarily inactivate some microbial agents, such as certain viruses and bacterial spores. Disinfection may not achieve the same reduction in microbial contamination level as sterilization.
- *Sterilization*. A process used to render an object free from viable micro-organisms, including viruses and spores.

refuse to handle such equipment if it is not accompanied by documentation indicating that it has been decontaminated.

Devices are designated for single or multiple use (Medical Devices Agency 1996), and this should be adhered to. Recycling items such as opened packs of wound care products, unused swabs and dressings from packs, or sharing topical creams between patients, re-using nebulizers, oxygen masks, failing to change sheets, pillowcases, blankets or duvets between patients, all increase the risk of cross-contamination.

Disposing of waste and equipment

As student nurses you will need to be aware of the exact procedures in your practice placements. If in doubt regarding the disposal of waste or equipment, ask! There is always someone to help. The procedure will be explained either in the local infection control manual or in the health and safety manual. Ask your mentor or, if you really cannot find any other local help, call the infection control nurse. It is important to understand what is meant by the terminology 'cleaning', 'disinfection' and 'sterilization' (see Box 13.7).

Clinical waste

Any waste generated in the health care setting that has been in contact with blood or other body fluids is classified as clinical waste and must be *incinerated*. Examples are soiled dressings, swabs, wound drainage tubes and bags, catheters, urine drainage bags, sputum pots, incontinence pads, used gloves and aprons.

All clinical waste should be disposed of in *yellow plastic bags*, which are then incinerated.

Needles and other 'sharps'

Many clinical procedures require the use of a needle, scalpel or lancet which is capable of puncturing the skin. Consequently, these 'sharps' become contaminated and could pose a danger to health care workers if they are not used and disposed of in a responsible manner. All sharps must be discarded into a special *yellow sharps bin*, which complies with BS 7320 (see Figure 13.4). These containers are rigid, puncture-resistant and leak-proof. They will have a special opening that is designed to allow sharps to be dropped in, but will not allow them to be taken out or spill out should the container topple over. Sharps bins should not be used once they are three-quarters full; they should then be sealed so that they cannot be re-opened.

The safe disposal of needles and sharps is the responsibility of the user, and they should not be left for someone else to clear away. Used needles should not be re-sheathed and should not be separated from the syringe. They should be disposed of as soon as possible in a sharps bin. Always make sure you know where the sharps bin is before you use any sharp implement or need to move any sharp implements after any procedures.

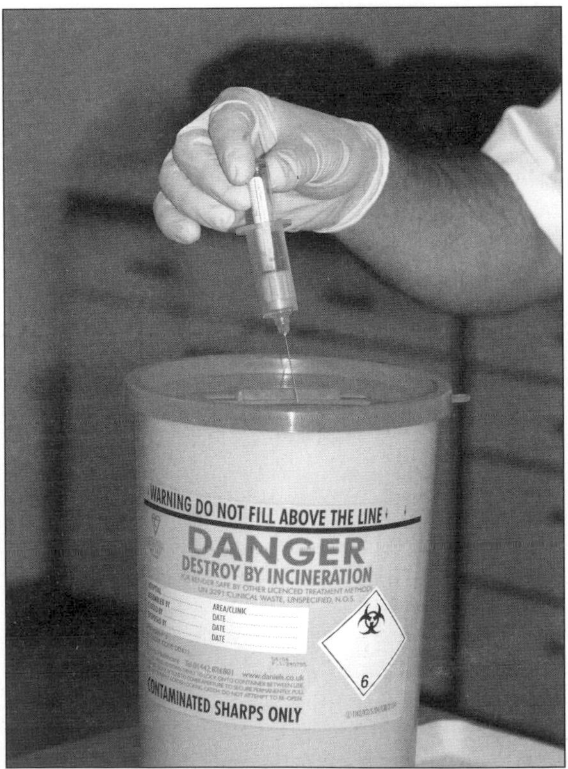

Figure 13.4 • Disposal of sharps.

Non-clinical waste

Non-clinical waste includes general waste that poses no risk to the public (e.g. packaging, dead flowers and paper hand-towels). Non-clinical waste should not be disposed of with clinical waste; rather, it is disposed of as general non-hazardous waste and placed in a black plastic bag. This is important, as clinical waste is disposed of via incineration which has significantly higher costs than those associated with the disposal of general household waste. Clinical waste disposal costs are approximately ten times higher than that of household waste; inappropriate disposal of household waste is therefore a waste of valuable financial resources.

Dealing with used and soiled laundry and general equipment

Used linen refers to the majority of laundry that has been used but is not soiled (e.g. sheets, towels, clothing). To prevent contact with your uniform a plastic apron should be used when making beds or handling used linen. Used laundry should be placed immediately into a polythene or fabric linen bag.

Soiled or *fouled* laundry refers to fabric materials, such as bed sheets and towels that have been contaminated with blood or other body fluids or excreta. To prevent contamination of other articles through leakage, this laundry should be placed in a plastic bag indicated for this purpose (you need to check the policy for disposal of soiled laundry in the trust where you are on placement) and then placed in the bag for used laundry. It will then be handled separately in the laundry.

Infected linen refers to laundry from patients with infectious conditions such as MRSA, salmonella, hepatitis, pulmonary tuberculosis or HIV. This linen is placed in a specific plastic bag identified for this purpose and then in another linen bag (often red or with red markings, but check your local policy). The linen is not handled by anyone as the plastic bag has special water-soluble seams which dissolve when they come into contact with the high temperature wash at 95°C.

General equipment such as washbowls, commodes, mattresses and beds must be washed with hot water and detergent and dried thoroughly between each patient to avoid cross-infection. Washbowls in particular can be a source of infection if not cleaned correctly. Abrasives, such as scouring pads or cream cleansers, should not be used as this roughens the surface, giving a good surface for micro-organisms to adhere to and multiply. Once washed and dried, it is preferable to store bowls upside down in a pyramid to allow air to circulate rather than stacking them one inside the other.

Methicillin-resistant *Staphylococcus aureus* (MRSA)

As mentioned above, most hospitals have a specific policy regarding patients with MRSA. Because of the concern over the rising number of cases of MRSA it is worth considering the management of such cases. MRSA infection was first reported in the UK in 1961 and has been responsible for many outbreaks of infection. As we have seen, *Staphylococcus aureus* is a common bacterium that may be carried naturally in the nose of healthy people and not cause problems. Alternatively, it may cause wound or skin infections, but these respond to antibiotics. It is only when the bacterium becomes resistant to certain antibiotics that it is referred to as MRSA.

MRSA has become more prevalent both in the UK and worldwide as a result of the increased use of antibiotics. Patients sometimes bring MRSA into hospital without their or our knowledge, from other hospitals at home or abroad. For this reason, it is important to screen such patients. There is no evidence that MRSA poses a risk to health care workers or their families. Similarly, there is no justification for discriminating against people who have MRSA by treating them with prejudice or refusing them admission.

How to prevent the spread of MRSA (also applicable to HIV infections and TB)

Basic infection control principles are adequate to prevent spread and protect staff from MRSA. These are as follows:

- *Hand-washing* is essential and should be carried out as described in Box 13.3. This should occur after any contact with the patient/client and before contact with another patient.
- *All cuts and grazes* should be covered with waterproof plaster. Staff with skin problems such as eczema or psoriasis must not attend patients with MRSA.
- *Wear gloves and apron* for all patient contact and discard immediately on leaving the patient.
- *Any equipment* that comes into contact with the patient should be thoroughly cleaned with soap/detergent and water before use by anyone else.
- *Laundry* should be bagged separately and identified as infected linen (usually a red bag).
- *Cutlery and crockery* should be washed as usual.

Food hygiene

Food regulations

In 1984 there was a devastating outbreak of salmonella food poisoning at the Stanley Royde Hospital in Wakefield (DHSS 1986) when 19 patients died. Since then, recorded incidents from hospitals have been less frequent and less severe, probably due to improved safety routines.

In 2004, investigators in a North-East hospital were unable to track down the source of a food poisoning incident. The inquiry into the salmonella outbreak at the University Hospital of North Durham in November 2004 concluded that it was highly likely that the outbreak was linked with eating food from the hospital restaurant. The team concluded that the outbreak revealed a failure of routine hazard-control systems within the kitchen. Ten people were affected by the outbreak; two people were admitted to hospital. The investigators advised that the management structure and supervision within the hospital's kitchen should be strengthened to prevent the opportunity for future errors that could cause food-borne illness.

In 2001, the 'Better hospital food' programme (Department of Health 2001) was implemented which aimed to ensure the consistent delivery of high-quality food and food services to people in care. Hospital food is an essential part of care. Good food can encourage patients to eat well, aiding their recovery from surgery or illness. The 'Better hospital food' programme aims to ensure the consistent delivery of food to patients that is safe, of good quality, nutritious, well presented and served at a time convenient to them. Activity 13.7 explores how the people that you care for are being served.

Several pieces of legislation have been passed regarding the preparation and serving of food, although major outbreaks of food poisoning continue to occur, especially in the domestic situation. This indicates that people are not abiding by this legislation and that even greater care needs to be take when preparing and serving food. The Food Safety (General Food Hygiene) Regulations 1995 (Great Britain Parliament 1995) forms the basis of good practice in any catering establishment, and this includes hospitals. The regulations cover the training of food handlers and details the processes required in order to provide food that is fit for consumption and avoid food poisoning. Nurses are closely involved with food preparation, food handling and assisting patients with their meals, and you should observe the safety points listed in Box 13.8.

Although the preparation of food is usually the responsibility of the kitchen staff and catering manager, it is useful for nurses to be aware of the commonest reasons for the outbreak of food poisoning (Barrie 1996):

- Preparing food too far in advance of the event.
- Storing food at room temperature.
- Cooling food too slowly before putting in the refrigerator.
- Not reheating food to a temperature that would kill food-poisoning bacteria.
- Using food that is already contaminated, especially poultry.
- Undercooking meat, meat products and poultry.
- Inadequate thawing of frozen foods.
- Cross-contamination between raw and cooked food.
- Keeping hot food below 63°C.
- Infected food handlers.

Does your own domestic approach to food storage, serving and handling comply with the above points? If not, what do you need to improve?

Nurses have a responsibility to see that all patients are appropriately fed. In part this means

Activity 13.7

Look critically look at the diet that is being served to people you care for:

- Does the food look appealing?
- Is the food served at the correct temperature?
- Is the food served at a convenient time?
- Do the portions appear appropriate?
- Are people encouraged and assisted to eat?
- What could you do to improve this aspect of care?

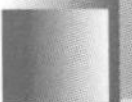

Box 13.8

Safety issues that nurses should observe when handling food

(Department of Health 1990)

- Wash hands before touching or preparing food.
- Wash hands after dealing with patient's needs.
- Wash hands after using the toilet or seeing to a patient's toiletry needs.
- Cover cuts and sores with blue-coloured waterproof plaster so that it can be easily identified if it falls into food; that food is then disposed of.
- Do not cough or sneeze over food.
- Do not pick your nose, touch your hair, lips or mouth when serving food.
- Keep equipment and utensils clean.
- Keep food clean and covered, and handle it as little as possible.
- Keep lids on waste sacks and dustbins.

keeping hot food hot (above 63°C) and cold food cold (below 5°C). Meals should be served immediately they arrive; if there is any delay, a fresh meal should be requested. Meals should not be reheated in the microwave in a placement area, unless it can be confirmed that the food reaches a temperature of 75°C and has been heated uniformly. All placement areas will issue guidelines regarding the handling of food, and failure to follow these may result in prosecution under legislation such as the Food Safety (General Food Hygiene) Regulations 1995.

Moving and handling

Learning how to move and handle patients and any heavy items within the workplace is an enormous topic that can not be addressed adequately within a textbook alone. But in this section we will discuss some of the important factors that you should consider to ensure the safety of your patients, your colleagues and yourself. Injury to the spine and back through unsafe moving and handling results is one of the commonest causes of nurses taking time off from work. In 1992, the Manual Handling Operations Regulations (Health and Safety Executive 1998) gave specific duties to employers for the manual handling of patients. The Management of Health and Safety at Work Regulations (MHSWR 1992, reg: 6:34) stated that employers must have access to competent help in applying health and safety law. Despite the introduction of the legislation, research in 1996 suggested that every year an estimated 80 000 nurses were still damaging their backs and that approximately 5% had to leave the profession as a result of back damage. From a patient's viewpoint, being moved and handled with care and safety is critically important if you are immobile, disabled, critically ill or in pain (or any combination of these). Most patients suffering from a period of immobility will need help with moving if they are to recover without complications or delay.

Learning how to move a patient safely is an essential part of learning to nurse. This is for your own health and well-being as well as that of those you care for. It is one of the earliest practical skills that you will learn and before you are allowed to enter the practice setting you have to demonstrate that you can do this safely and that you have completed the relevant part of your course as part of health and safety legislation. For the safety of the people you care for and yourself you should ensure that you attend these sessions.

Manual handling and the law

The implementation of a number of European directives in 1992 led to important changes in health and safety legislation in the UK (Great Britain Parliament 1992), particularly with regards to regulations covering the manual handling and moving of loads. These regulations stipulate that employers have a duty to ensure the safety of all employees involved in manual handling and moving tasks (including the moving of patients). Employers have a responsibility to make a thorough assessment and implement measures to avoid risk or minimize it to the greatest possible degree (Health and Safety Executive 1998). Employees also have a responsibility to follow appropriate policies and procedures put in place by their employer in relation to moving and handling and to act with reasonable care and skill. Employers have a responsibility to provide a sufficient number of suitable lifting aids, and appropriate training (and updating) in moving and handling. Employees have a duty to use the aids and attend all available training.

Many health care organizations are working towards safer handling or no-lifting policies. The provision of, and training in the use of, no-lifting equipment, such as hoists, transfer aids (used when transferring a patient from trolley to bed, bed to bed, etc.) has extended considerably during the last 10 years. Not only does this help to prevent injury for the nurse, but it also ensures that people are not damaged by poor lifting and moving, which can result in shearing force on the skin of back, buttocks and heels or dislocation of shoulders by being heaved up the bed with an underarm lift. Description of the techniques involved is not possible in this book, and safe moving and lifting can only be learned in practice with a skilled instructor. But the main principles to be applied to any handling situation are provided in Box 13.9.

Box 13.9

Principles of safe handling

- From your first day in practice, never put yourself at risk, never lift alone, and find out where all the lifting aids are.
- Assess the situation for moving the patient.
- Communicate clearly with your partner(s) so that all know what to expect and do.
- Avoid tensing your muscles.
- Adopt a stable stance; this usually means having your feet about a hip-width apart.
- Keep your knees 'soft' or bent.
- Keep the load as close to your body as possible and avoid stretching.
- Avoid twisting or bending sideways.

Moving and handling patients within an acute hospital setting, with the availability of other colleagues and lifting aids, is more easily achieved safely than trying to move a patient in their own home, in a low bed, perhaps with little space to move and without the support of staff and mechanical aids. Community nurses are able to obtain lifting aids and will always take a colleague to assist with lifting. The principles of safe moving and handling must still be applied.

Using visual display equipment safely

An increasingly important aspect that can help you maintain your own healthy back is in relation to using computers and visual display equipment. It is probable that you will spend time working with computers as part of your course and in the practice area. It is surprising how many regular computer users are unfamiliar with the correct use of work stations, leading to back, visual and repetitive strain injuries. To help prevent these problems you need to consider posture and your working environment carefully. This means making sure that your chair, desk, display screen, mouse and keyboard are in the correct position and used correctly at all times. Even though you may be very used to working with computers and display screen equipment it is easy to get into bad habits. It is useful to check your own set-up from time to time. Also, in practice settings, many staff use machines and adjust the working environment to suit their own needs. So get used to checking your work space before getting engrossed in the work that you are doing. Take regular breaks to stretch to prevent back problems and change your focal point by looking away from the screen to help reduce headaches. Several websites provide useful guidance and it is likely that your university will also provide guidance that you should consult. The following web links are very useful, but be aware that websites change frequently: http://www.vduhealthandsafety.org/, http://www.learninglink.ac.uk/site.htm.

Pasting the term 'VDU' or 'computer workstation safety' into a computer search engine will reveal useful sources of practical advice.

Trips, slips and falls

Slips and trips resulting in falls are the most common cause of major injuries in all workplaces in Great Britain and the second biggest cause of over-3-day injuries.

Within health care settings the Health and Safety Executive estimates that over 2000 injuries to employees in health care, attributed to slips and trips, are reported each year. Many patients and visitors also receive injuries, but figures are not as easy to collate for this area. Simple slip injuries (broken bones, etc.) often lead to complications in older people, such as thromboses or embolisms, which may be fatal. A National Audit Office report (National Audit Office 2003) highlighted slips and trips as a main type of accident to workers and patients. The report includes recommendations that NHS trusts should review their health and safety risk-management policies and improve accident-reporting systems. Nurses have an important preventative role to play in this regard. Areas that you undertake placements in are likely to have local policies and you should ensure you are aware of your role in implementing these.

The four main causes of slips-and-trips accidents in health care settings are:

- Slippery/wet surfaces caused by water and other fluids.
- Slippery surfaces caused by dry or dusty floor contamination (e.g. plastic, lint or talcum powder).
- Obstructions, both temporary and permanent.
- Uneven surfaces and changes of level, such as unmarked ramps.

Human factors include:

- Employees rushing.
- Running or carrying heavy/cumbersome items.
- The wearing of unsuitable footwear.
- The use of improper cleaning regimes.

Prevention

Advice on preventing falls is applicable to everyone.

General advice

Small changes in and around the home and health care settings can make a big difference in reducing accidents:

- Mop up spills promptly, or ensure that they are cordoned off and a member of staff is alerted to deal with the spill.
- If you identify clutter, trailing wires or frayed carpets, make sure that you report these to your mentor or other supervisors.
- Ensure that handrails in bathrooms and other areas are available to use.
- If you find any non-slip mats and or rugs then ensure that these are reported and removed if safe to do so.
- Ensure that suitable lighting is always used so that you and those that you care for can see. This can be difficult at night when you do not disturb others, but using a torch can really help.
- If you are in the community setting look to see how the home is organized. You might suggest that things are rearranged so that the need for the person to climb, stretch and bend for items is kept to a minimum, and they are not as likely to bump into things.

Advice for older people

Box 13.10 gives advice for older people (taken from the NHS Direct website) and provides useful reminders that you can pass on.

Box 13.10

Advice for older people to help prevent falls

- Have regular eye tests. Separate types of glasses are better than bifocals or varifocals.
- Take exercise, keep physically active, and keep muscles as strong as possible.
- Take fewer risks in your routine, slow down, take things gradually.
- Look after your feet, and wear well-fitting sensible shoes with thin soles, high sides and good grip.
- Don't walk on slippery floors in socks or tights.
- Avoid wearing loose-fitting trailing clothes which might trip you up.
- Get a flu jab; being unwell can make people more prone to fall.
- Don't mix alcohol with medication; this may cause dizziness and loss of balance.
- Let your GP know if you feel dizzy; review your medication with your GP regularly.
- If you feel unwell, let your family, friend, or neighbour know.
- Jerky movements may make you feel dizzy, particularly if you have arthritis.
- Keep your home warm, cold muscles lead to accidents.
- Have enough calcium and vitamin D in your diet to keep bones strong and reduce the risk of fracture. Calcium is found in dairy products (choose lower-fat ones). Vitamin D is found in oily fish and meat, but is added to cereals; it can be formed by exposure to sunlight. Or use a vitamin supplement.
- Hip protectors, worn under clothes, reduce the risk of hip fracture by at least 50%.
- Get help to do things you can't do safely yourself.
- Consider using a personal fall-alarm system.

Risks

There are countless causes of slips, trips and falls, but the most common are:

- Unsafe ladders. Be careful if you need to use steps or ladders to locate any equipment that you might need.
- Unsafe stairs, steepness of stairs, or slopes. Be vigilant when working in unfamiliar areas, especially if working in the community.
- Slippery surfaces.
- Obstructions, things to trip over.
- Poor footwear.
- Untidy areas.
- Running.
- Low lighting.
- Hurried or careless movements.
- Distractions.
- Poor manual handling, carrying large objects badly, or with no hands free to break a fall.

In summary, by being vigilant and by thinking ahead you can do a lot to keep yourself and others safe.

Safe administration of medicines

As with other important practical skills, we are not able to provide you with all the knowledge needed for you to administer medicines. You have a responsibility to become familiar with the local policies regarding administration of medicines and the guidance provided by your lecturers and your mentors. Administration of medicines is an important responsibility for all nurses. The most important aspect of administering medicines is to ensure that you do this safely, and while you are a nursing student only under the direct supervision of a professionally qualified practitioner. The Nursing and Midwifery Council stresses the importance of administration of medicines in professional practice. It makes it clear in the 'NMC Code of professional conduct' (NMC 2008) that all practitioners, including student nurses, are responsible and accountable for the safe administration of medicines. In the 'Guidelines for the administration of medicines' (NMC 2000) the NMC recommends that all medicines should be administered by a first-level nurse or midwife.

The importance of pharmacology

With the wide range of medicines that is increasing almost daily, you have the difficult responsibility to ensure that you have a sound understanding of your responsibilities as well as a good knowledge of the medicines that you encounter in your daily placement experiences. You need to understand the reason for the drug being prescribed, the way in which the drug acts on the body, the side-effects the drug can have and how you can recognize them, the patient's needs and the environment in which the drug should be given. Unfortunately, prescribing or administering the wrong drug or the wrong dose can happen. Another hazard is theft of controlled drugs from the health care setting. This can present a potential hazard to patients and other people.

Management of drugs and their administration is, therefore, a strictly controlled process and one which you need to learn in the early stages of your programme. One major problem for health care provision is the number of patients who do not take their prescribed drug therapy. This results in millions of pounds worth of wasted resources, and patients not making the recovery or having the level of health they could have had if they followed the correct prescription. Educating patients about their drug regimens is an important teaching activity for the nurse.

In your foundation year, you will almost certainly be involved in assisting with the administration of drugs. In some settings, drugs are administered from each patient's own stock of medications. If they are hospitalized, the drugs are stored by their bedside; if they are at home, they are stored in a safe place, out of reach of children. The aim is to protect patients from misadministration of drugs. In other settings, drugs and medicines are administered from a drug or medicine trolley that is taken around the patients' beds and administered at the bedside. Whenever medicines and drugs are being administered it is a serious and responsible activity governed by strictly enforced principles of storage, administration and record-keeping. Quite often the hospital or local pharmacist is involved in monitoring patients' prescriptions and ensuring that the prescribed drugs are compatible. So nurses are key members in a team of practitioners working to ensure the safe administration of drugs. As a result, it is essential that you work at developing your knowledge of pharmacology. You may find it helpful to keep a pocket notebook of all the different medicines and drugs that you encounter and write notes about their purpose, normal dosage, side-effects and actions to any side-effects.

Calculating correct amounts of drugs to administer is critical, and many mistakes still occur as a result of poor skills amongst many nurses. The reasons for these are varied. According to some researchers, the mathematical skills are not good enough; others identify that performing drug calculations in the classroom and in practice are very different skills. A summary of research in this area has been documented by Wright (2005). It is critical that you are aware of your own skills and can undertake the range of calculations that will be expected of you in practice. Some tools to help you learn are available on the web. One such example has been devised by Lanarkshire NHS in Scotland (see www.lanpdc.scot.nhs.uk/calculations/dc.asp).

Delivery routes

Patients will be prescribed medicines for therapeutic, diagnostic or preventative purposes. 'Medicines' or 'drugs' can be delivered in a range of forms and modes such as: oral tablets, pills, capsules; drugs given rectally through suppositories or enemas; drugs given subcutaneously, intravenously and intramuscularly, as well as through inhalation (e.g. anaesthetics or pain killers); topically to the skin through medicated dressings or corticoid creams. The young and old are particularly vulnerable to drugs and great care is taken to ensure the dose is correct for their body to metabolize and excrete.

Administering drugs safely

The safe administration of medicines involves five main principles:

- Safe storage.
- Safe prescribing.
- Safe administration.
- Receipt from the pharmacy.
- Accurate recording.

Storage and the law

The law of the UK requires that all medicines and drugs are safely stored, and provides strict guidelines for the storage of different types of drugs. It is part of the nurse's role to see that the law is respected according to local policy. Some drugs that are likely to cause addiction, or are particularly toxic, are governed by the Controlled Drugs Act. The main principles are listed in Box 13.11.

Prescribing medications and the nurse

In health care settings, a doctor or other professional with specific prescribing qualifications prescribes all medicines and drugs before they can be administered. This means that on no account can a nurse prescribe and administer any form of drug or medicine (e.g. paracetamol) without the prescription having been made by the patient's doctor, nurse or other professional with extended skills training.

Whenever a medication is going to be administered, the nurse must ensure that the prescription meets the criteria listed in Box 13.12.

Administering medications

Medicines can only be administered by a registered nurse. In principle, this means that a registered nurse 'takes charge' of the task and oversees all aspects of it. It will be reasonable to expect a student nurse to participate in the giving of medications under the supervision of a registered nurse. Student nurses can expect to give oral, intramuscular, subcutaneous and topical medicines according to the correct procedure and when trained to do so, under the direct supervision of the registered nurse.

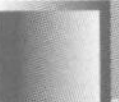

Box 13.11

Principles for the safe storage of drugs

- All medicines, lotions and reagents (except intravenous fluids and drugs used in emergency situations) must be stored in a locked cupboard. Drugs for emergency use have to be readily available and are therefore allowed to be stored in a sealed container that is replenished and re-sealed after use.
- All medicines should be stored at the correct temperature recommended by the manufacturers, particularly intravenous fluids and drugs that require refrigeration. The fridge should be one designated for this purpose and not one that is also used for food.
- Medicine cupboards and drug trolleys should be kept locked at all times when not in use. Drug trolleys should be secured to the wall.
- All stock should be rotated so that it is used before the expiry date.
- Labels on medicine containers must not be altered or added to. Any damaged or obliterated labels or ones that require changing in any way must be returned to the pharmacy department.
- Medicines must not be transferred from one bottle to another.
- Borrowing from other wards or departments should be discouraged except in an emergency, when it should be documented and the pharmacy department notified.
- Medicines held in wards, units and departments must only be used for the patients for whom they have been prescribed and not be issued to hospital personnel or visitors.
- Controlled drugs should be kept in a separate cupboard with the key kept separate from the other drug keys. A controlled drug register must be kept, and all controlled drugs given must have two signatories and be accounted for in the register. Local policies will dictate the ordering, receipt and checking procedures for controlled drugs.
- No unauthorized person must be allowed access to the drug cupboard keys.
- The security of the medicines is the responsibility of the qualified nurse in charge.

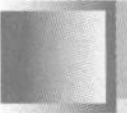

Box 13.12

Criteria for the safe prescription of medications

- It should be written legibly (or printed) in ink and dated. The approved generic name should be used. It should not be altered once written and should be written out again in full if it is necessary to change the dose or frequency. When a prescription is to be cancelled, it should be crossed out (indicating the start and finish of the line) and signed and dated by the qualified prescriber. The nurse should not administer the medicine if the prescription is illegible. She should not guess the name of the drug to be given.
- It should clearly and accurately identify the patient. In an acute care setting, it should match the name on the wrist band.
- It should specify the preparation to be given (e.g. tablets, capsules, suppositories, etc.).
- It should state the strength, the dose, the timing and the frequency. For certain drugs (e.g. antibiotics), the proposed duration for which the drug is to be given should be stated.
- It should state the route of administration.
- It should be signed and dated by the doctor or other registered prescriber.
- In an emergency a first-level nurse may take a telephone message for the administration of medicines. The prescription must be written and signed for by the nurse, stating that it was a verbal request, and giving the time, the date and the doctor's name. The doctor should countersign the prescription as soon as possible. No orders given over the telephone should be repeated.

The following principles apply to the administration of all medicines, whatever the route. Ensure that you have:

- The right medication.
- The right time.
- The right patient.
- The right amount.
- The right route.

Local policy may require that two nurses check certain medicines before administration. Two nurses are required to check and administer all controlled drugs. Box 13.13 gives the procedure for the safe administration of medicines.

Patients' self-administration

In some hospitals, and in many community care settings, patients often have responsibility for taking their own prescribed medication. When patients are at home they take responsibility for the safe storage and administration of their medications. In institutions such as hospitals, clinics and nursing homes, the organization has responsibility for safety and storage of medications. The organization must have an effective system of storage of medications according to the requirements of the law. This involves providing cupboards that can be locked and secured for individual storage of medications. Some criteria need to be agreed to ensure the safety of the patient when self-medicating. These include that: the medical condition of the patient is stable, so the drug regimen will not change frequently; the drugs can be dispensed individually by the pharmacy department; the patient is able to take the medications as prescribed. When patients take several different drugs at different times of the day (polypharmacy), it is easy to forget, so systems of indicating the day of the week and the time of the day have been developed to help correct administration. The nurse has an important role to liaise with the pharmacist and to ensure the patient understands and is able to adhere to the drug regimen.

Receiving medicines

This refers to the ordering and receiving of medicines from the pharmacy department, checking that they are correct and ensuring they are stored in the appropriate locked cupboard. Local policies will give guidance on this and on stocktaking.

Accurate recording

Stocktaking within hospitals and in residential settings must take place at appropriate intervals. This involves recording, checking stocks and disposing of unwanted medicines according to legislation and local policy. Any discrepancies in the stock

Box 13.13

Safe administration of medicines

- Check the location of the patient before dispensing medication.
- Do not leave the unlocked trolley unattended, or medicines out on a locker or a table to be administered later.
- Make sure the patient understands the reasons for the medication being given when possible, and check whether the patient has any drug allergies.
- Wash and dry hands thoroughly.
- Prepare the medicines to be administered (see Figure 13.5) and the appropriate equipment for the route of administration.
- Check the prescription chart has the patient's full name and hospital number.
- Check the prescription, bearing in mind the points outlined above.
- Check it is the correct time to administer the medicine and that the patient has not already received it. Check any special observations (e.g. blood pressure) or requirements (e.g. before, with or after food) relating to the medication.
- Check the medicine container against the prescription to identify that it is the correct medicine. Check the expiry date of the medicine.
- Calculate how much is required to achieve the dose prescribed.
- Check the patient's identity, using the patient's name band, with the prescription.
- Administer the medicine as prescribed.
- Ensure the patient is comfortable and understands any instructions related to the medication.
- Sign the prescription chart according to local policy. Document if the medication was not given. This is a most important aspect of the process and contributes to the legal record of care.
- Monitor the effects of the medication and report and record any abnormal side-effects (e.g. antibiotic rash).
- Wash and dry hands thoroughly.

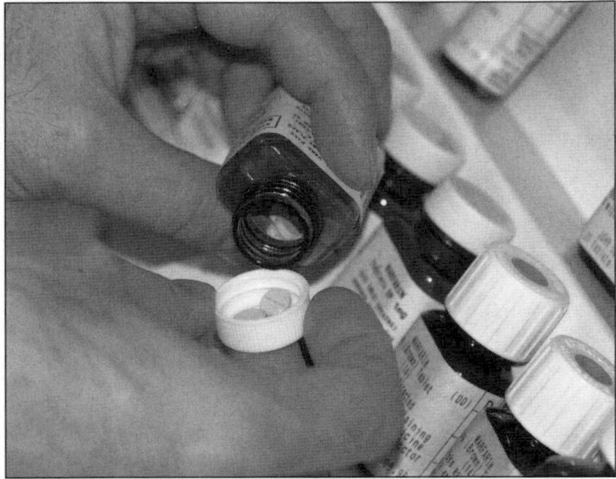

Figure 13.5 • Preparing medicine for administration.

must be reported immediately to the nurse in charge and investigated.

Practical skills of giving medication

As a foundation nursing student you will be expected to develop the skills of giving injections, applying topical lotions, inserting suppositories and overseeing intravenous infusions. There are several good texts that can help you understand the techniques, and the 'Further reading' list at the end of the chapter provides some recommendations. Advanced skills in relation to safe practice and medications are required for nurses working in chemotherapy units, transplant centres and possibly in community psychiatry. There is a great deal more to safe practice in dealing with medication than just handing out pills.

Prevention of the complications of immobility

People who are having difficulty moving or changing their position are at risk of suffering complications that can generally be prevented with good-quality care. Pressure sores and deep vein thrombosis (DVT) are the two main complications of immobility, both of which are painful and unpleasant for the patient, costly for the organization, and can be life-threatening.

Pressure sores

Pressure sores or decubitus ulcers are normally found over bony surfaces of the body such as the coccyx, the heels, elbows and shoulder blades. They are one of the most difficult nursing problems to address. They are extremely painful, prone to infection and can be life-threatening (for detailed information about the structure of the skin and the processes of healing, see Chapter 9). The incidence of pressure sores is complex and related to a number of factors associated with the general health of the patient as well as the environment the patient is in and the quality of care they receive. The existence of pressure sores in patients under NHS care is taken extremely seriously.

It is good practice to assess your patients when they are first admitted to your care for their vulnerability to developing a pressure sore. A number of different assessment tools are available and each area is likely to use the one most suitable for their type of patient. One in common use is the Waterlow scoring system (Table 13.1).

Whatever assessment tool is used in your placement area the tool in use will include most if not all of the factors listed in Box 13.14.

When making an assessment, each of the factors identified in Box 13.14 is scored in relation to its likely impact on the risk of developing a pressure sore. The total score for all the factors is then provided as the full-risk assessment. The risk score indicates to the care team the appropriate care programme required to prevent pressure sores developing in that patient. Different wards and departments will all have developed their 'plans of care to match score' based on their experience and best evidence. But all care pathways will have certain features in common, as described in Box 13.15.

Deep vein thrombosis

People who are immobile, undergoing surgery or who have predisposing factors such as dehydration or hypotension are at risk of developing deep vein thrombosis (DVT). High-profile airline-related legal cases means that people are becoming more aware of the risks of DVT. It is vital that you

Table 13.1 Waterlow pressure sore prevention/treatment policy. Ring scores in table, add total; several scores per category can be used

Build/weight for height	★
Average	0
Above average	1
Obese	2
Below average	3

Continence	★
Complete/ catheterised	0
Occasion. incont.	1
Cath./incontinent of faeces	2
Doubly incontinent	3

Skin type Visual risk areas	★
Healthy	0
Tissue paper	1
Dry	1
Oedematous	1
Clammy (temp. ↑)	1
Discoloured	2
Broken/spot	3

Mobility	★
Fully	0
Restless/fidgety	1
Apathetic	2
Restricted	3
Inert/traction	4
Chairbound	5

Sex Age	★
Male	1
Female	2
14–49	1
50–64	2
65–74	3
75–80	4
81+	5

Appetite	★
Average	0
Poor	1
N.G. tube/ fluids only	2
NBM/anorexic	3

Special risks	★
Tissue malnutrition	★
e.g. Terminal cachexia	8
Cardiac failure	5
Peripheral vascular disease	5
Anaemia	2
Smoking	1
Neurological deficit	★
e.g. Diabetes, M.S., CVA, motor/sensory paraplegia 4–6	
Major surgery/trauma	★
Orthopaedic: below waist, spinal	5
On table >2 hours	5
Medication	★
Cytotoxics, high dose steroids, anti-inflammatory	4

Score	**10+ at risk**	**15+ at risk**	**20+ very high risk**

Source: Waterlow 1991 (obtainable from Newtons, Curland, Taunton TA3 5SG).

monitor your patients for any signs or symptoms of the complication. You should check your patient's legs daily for signs of redness or tenderness in the calves, especially when they flex and extend their foot, which are the main signs of DVT.

Wherever possible, you need to encourage your patients to move their legs and feet, to transfer their weight off their coccyx and, if part of their care plan, to walk around as much as possible. Patients who have had surgery are particularly at risk and it is important to teach them how to reduce venous stasis in the legs and so reduce the risk of developing DVT. Physiotherapists and nurses teach patients how to do foot and leg exercises ensure they practise them postoperatively or during periods of immobility. If the patient is unable to do these exercises for themselves (e.g. if they are unconscious or are too confused to cooperate), the nurse can carry out gentle passive leg movements on the patient. Physiotherapists will usually assist with this and other aspects of patient activity to reduce DVT risk.

Blood flow to the legs is impeded when people cross their legs either when sitting in a chair or when in bed. It is therefore useful to discourage this posture, especially amongst those in whom problems might develop.

Box 13.14

Risk assessment for pressure sores

- *Weight, height, build*: an overweight or very thin person is at greater risk of pressure damage.
- *Level of mobility*: any immobility increases the risk of damage.
- *Nutritional state*: poor nutritional health, emaciation or eating difficulty can all increase the risk.
- *Skin condition*: oedematous, dry, thin, clammy skin is all more prone to pressure sores; any pre-existing sores or blisters should be noted.
- *Medical condition*: vascular disorders, some cancers, diabetes, pain and a period of time on an operating table can all predispose to the development of pressure sores.
- *Mental condition*: depression, apathy and lethargy can mean greater risk of development of pressure sores because these patients are less likely to want to move about, eat, etc.
- *Any special medication*: some drugs can cause sedation and increased immobility; steroids affect the property of the skin.

Box 13.15

Preventing pressure sores

- *Ensure that pressure on the body is relieved regularly*. For some patients, encouraging them to get out of bed, stand, walk and move about will be sufficient if done frequently enough. Postoperative patients should be encouraged to walk as soon as their condition will allow. If this is painful, following surgery or because of a painful condition such as arthritis, adequate pain relief must be administered. For the bedridden patient, the person's body must be moved at least every 2 hours, so that different parts of the body are in contact with the bed. It is now usual for every immobile patient to be nursed on a pressure-relieving mattress and the nurse must ensure that this happens. But these patients will still need turning frequently. The frequency of mobilizing and turning patients will vary according to the risk assessment score and care plan.
- *Ensure the patient is receiving adequate nutrition and hydration* to maintain healthy skin.
- *Keep the skin clean and dry at all times*. Episodes of incontinence should be dealt with promptly; talcum powder should be used sparingly because it can become clogged and lumpy on the skin.
- *Check buttocks and bony prominences frequently* for signs of reddening and soreness. It may be necessary to alter the care regime slightly or add further pressure-relieving aids to elbows and heels.
- *Avoid shearing forces and mechanical injury to the skin*. This is the result of unsafe lifting technique where a patient is dragged up the bed or chair, or sheets remain crinkled.

Another factor that helps reduce the incidence of DVT is deep breathing exercises, which speed up the venous return to the heart and thus reduces sluggishness in the venous circulation. Good hydration through regular intake of fluids reduces the viscosity of the venous blood and so again improves venous circulation. There are now special machines available which carry out the equivalent of these leg exercises on a patient and are often used for patients who have had major leg and knee surgery where movement and walking is initially very painful. Many patients undergoing surgery, and almost all patients undergoing hip and leg surgery, are encouraged to wear special anti-embolism stockings (such as the stockings recommended for long airline journeys), which should be worn for several days, possibly weeks, after their operation.

Responding to emergencies

Responding to emergency situations is probably the most daunting aspect of learning to become a nurse and the ones that are most feared are 'fire' and the 'crash call' (when a person is expected to require resuscitation and life support).

Learning how to respond when there is a fire alarm is an important part of mandatory training activities that all health care staff working in institutions must attend each year. So it is essential that you meet these requirements as a nursing student who will work in a clinical setting.

Another emergency situation is knowing how to respond when a patient stops breathing or has a cardiac arrest and cardiopulmonary resuscitation (CPR) is necessary. As a nursing student you will be taught this in the early part of your course. Before giving information about the process of resuscitation, it is important that on each placement you learn about the following during your first week:

- Where the resuscitation trolley is stored, what is on it and how the equipment works.
- How to make the crash call wherever you are working in practice.
- What action to take (prompt action is essential and can save life).

If you witness your patient's collapse shout for help/press the alarm and immediately begin the process of ensuring the person's safety. This involves ensuring that help is called for. Once help arrives ensure that you follow their instructions. As a foundation programme nursing student it is likely that you will only be expected to watch the proceedings rather than take a key role. You may be asked to support the remaining patients who will probably be distressed by events. Usually these events look chaotic to the outsider even though they are often well rehearsed by the emergency team and they are mindful of the health and safety of staff and others around the event so it is important to listen to and respond to instructions carefully.

The process of cardiopulmonary resuscitation

Recognizing that someone is suffering from sudden cardiac failure is difficult because sometimes it looks like a fit, other times you will notice that they are not breathing normally and their colour has changed. The first action is to use the emergency bell or call out to get help. Then check the person's airway for any obstruction and, after ensuring a patent airway, check the person's breathing by observing the chest for movement and remove any tight clothing if easy to do so. Check the person's circulation by checking the carotid or femoral pulse; if it is absent, begin resuscitation. Of course, a walking person may suddenly collapse and fall to the ground (see Box 13.16 for possible causes of collapse), but the immediate process of care is just the same.

First, it is important to assess the patient rapidly to determine the specific course of action required. Not all collapsed individuals need all aspects of cardiopulmonary resuscitation (CPR) and some do not need anything more than being placed in the recovery position. Case histories 13.2 and 13.3 describe two collapsed patients who required very different care.

The principles of CPR are well described in Figure 13.6 and in the case examples. In a hospital setting, the presence of trained nurses, doctors and the crash team ensures a streamlined, efficient and rapid programme of care. However, you will be trained to carry out CPR on your own in a non-clinical situation in case that is necessary. All nursing students, whatever specialist branch they choose, must know how to care in this particular emergency situation.

Informed consent

The 'NMC Code of professional conduct' stresses the importance of respect for the patient or client

Box 13.16

Possible causes of collapse

Possible causes include the following, although the list is not exhaustive:

- Simple faint
- Haemorrhage
- Choking
- Drugs that cause respiratory arrest
- Cardiac arrest
- Fitting
- Hypoglycaemia
- Febrile convulsions
- Cerebrovascular accident

In every case, the approach to the patient is the same as described in Figure 13.6, even though the subsequent care for each is very different.

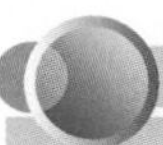

Case history 13.2

Mr P

Mr P was a 53-year-old man admitted to the medical assessment unit for further investigations into intermittent chest pains. On the morning following his admission he had been out to the bathroom for a wash and was sitting on his bed, looking in his locker for his book. He suddenly experienced an intense crushing pain in the centre of his chest, and cried out before slumping backwards onto the bed.

Assessment and action

A student nurse who had been walking towards the bed saw Mr P collapse and ran towards him. Checking that the area round the bed was safe, she approached the patient, and called his name out, shaking him by the shoulders at the same time. There was no response, and she then pulled the emergency call button to summon more help. She also pulled the curtains round the bed. By this time two staff nurses had arrived and together they laid Mr P flat on the bed, removing all pillows and the bed-head in order to gain better access for assessing him.

The staff nurses had brought with them the emergency trolley containing equipment and emergency drugs. One staff nurse lifted the patient's chin to open his airway, did a mouth sweep to check for obstruction, and checked for signs of respirations. Having established that the patient was not breathing, the staff nurse told the student nurse to run and telephone for the resuscitation team, using the emergency code number. She then gave Mr P two rescue breaths, establishing the rise and fall of his chest. The second staff nurse checked the carotid pulse to establish whether there was circulation. There was no pulse present, and she then began external cardiac compressions.

Meanwhile the first staff nurse had connected the Ambu (breathing) bag to a mask and oxygen tubing and attached it to the wall oxygen supply at 10 litres per minute and prepared a Guedel airway for insertion. After the two rescue breaths, the staff nurse inserted the airway upside-down into the mouth then turned it over into position over the back of the tongue, which ensured a clear airway. While the external cardiac compressions continued, the first staff nurse continued to give breaths, lifting the chin, holding the mask to the face, and compressing the Ambu bag. Thus cardiopulmonary resuscitation continued at a rate of 2 breaths to 15 compressions. The student nurse was, in the meantime, standing by the emergency trolley, and the first staff nurse explained what would be required next. First the patient was attached to the cardiac monitor so that any heart activity could be seen. Then some of the drugs normally used in a cardiac emergency were prepared (e.g. adrenaline, atropine).

By this time the medical team had arrived and assessed the situation and obtained a brief history of events from the staff nurse. The anaesthetist took control of the airway. Although the patient was still unresponsive, not breathing and without a pulse, the cardiac monitor indicated that his heart was fibrillating. The staff nurse prepared the defibrillator and pads, and the medical registrar administered two shocks, bringing the patient's heart back into sinus rhythm. A pulse was now present and the patient was beginning to breathe unaided, although he continued to receive oxygen via the Ambu bag until able to expel the Guedel airway.

Mr P was still seriously ill and would require several more hours of intensive treatment and observation. However, the prompt action of all the nurses in initiating cardiopulmonary resuscitation proved life-saving in this instance.

---

as an individual and obtaining consent before giving any treatment or care (NMC 2008).

Some hospitals issue leaflets to people receiving care, informing them that students in training will be based in their care area. The leaflet will ask for their cooperation and support in helping students to learn about their future roles, but also informing them of their rights. Examinations or treatments on patients/clients should not normally be carried out without their prior consent, which will have been obtained following an explanation of the procedures involved.

The purposes of gaining the patient's consent are:

- To ensure that the patient understands the nature of the treatment or examination, including alternatives and possible potential

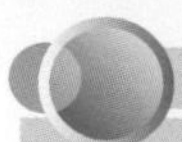

Case history 13.3

Mrs B

Mrs B was a 42-year-old woman who had come into the accident and emergency department with heavy p.v. (per vaginum) bleeding and cramping abdominal pain. She had been assessed by the staff nurse in triage and was waiting to be called through and be seen by the doctor. Approximately 20 minutes after being assessed, she walked out to the toilet. Another patient waiting to be seen witnessed Mrs B come out of the toilet and suddenly slump to the floor. He ran to call the staff nurse working in the triage area.

Assessment and action

The staff nurse could see that the patient was unresponsive and not moving. Checking the immediate area for safety, he then approached the patient, first calling out her name, and then gently shaking her shoulders. There was no response and the staff nurse asked the receptionist at the triage desk to telephone through to the main department and ask for immediate assistance. He then ensured the patient's airway was open by tilting the head and lifting the chin. He assessed whether she was breathing, looking for chest movements, listening for breath sounds, and feeling for air on his cheek. Having ascertained that she was breathing but was still unresponsive, he placed her into the recovery position. This he did by placing her on her side, with the uppermost hand under her cheek, and the uppermost knee bent to prevent her from rolling onto her stomach.

Having been reassured by the receptionist that help was coming, the staff nurse stayed with the patient, checking that she was continuing to breathe spontaneously. He also checked her carotid pulse, which indicated that she was tachycardic. By this time more help had arrived in the form of a doctor, staff nurse, porter and a trolley with an oxygen supply. The patient was carefully transferred to the trolley and kept in the recovery position, with the nurse continually observing her respirations and checking her pulse. Oxygen was administered at 4 litres per minute through a mask and she was taken to the resuscitation area of the accident and emergency department. While on her way to that area she began to move and make groaning noises and after a few more minutes had opened her eyes and was asking the staff nurse what had happened to her.

The staff nurse was able to reassure Mrs B that she had fainted in the waiting room while waiting to see the doctor, but that she was much better now, although she needed further observation and treatment from the medical team to ensure a full recovery.

complications or risks, thus allowing them to make an informed decision.

- To indicate that the patient's decision was made without pressure, and to protect the patient against unauthorized procedures.
- To protect the medical staff and the hospital against legal action by a patient who claims that an unauthorized procedure was performed.

The circumstances requiring written consent are any procedure that requires a general anaesthetic, any invasive procedure or those treatments carrying a side-effect or a substantial risk. Some drug therapy (e.g. cytotoxics) and therapy involving ionizing radiation also require written consent. If in doubt always ask a qualified member of the nursing staff or the doctor.

Before consent is requested for any examination or treatment and before the patient has any sedation, it is the nurse's responsibility to ensure that the patient is told about the options available in clear and simple terms by a doctor or health professional who should be experienced and knowledgeable. The nurse can help in explaining again anything that the patient was unsure about. Remember, anxiety often hinders concentration.

The information provided should include:

- Details of the diagnosis, prognosis and consequences if the condition is left untreated.
- Any uncertainties, including the need for further investigations.
- Options of treatments available, including the option not to treat.
- Description of the proposed treatment, any consequences, as well as substantive risks.
- Advice about whether the treatment is experimental or part of a research programme.
- How the patient's condition and treatment will be monitored or reassessed, the recovery period and the time involved.
- The name of the clinician who has overall responsibility for the treatment and, where appropriate, the names of the senior members of the team.
- Whether clinicians in training will be involved.

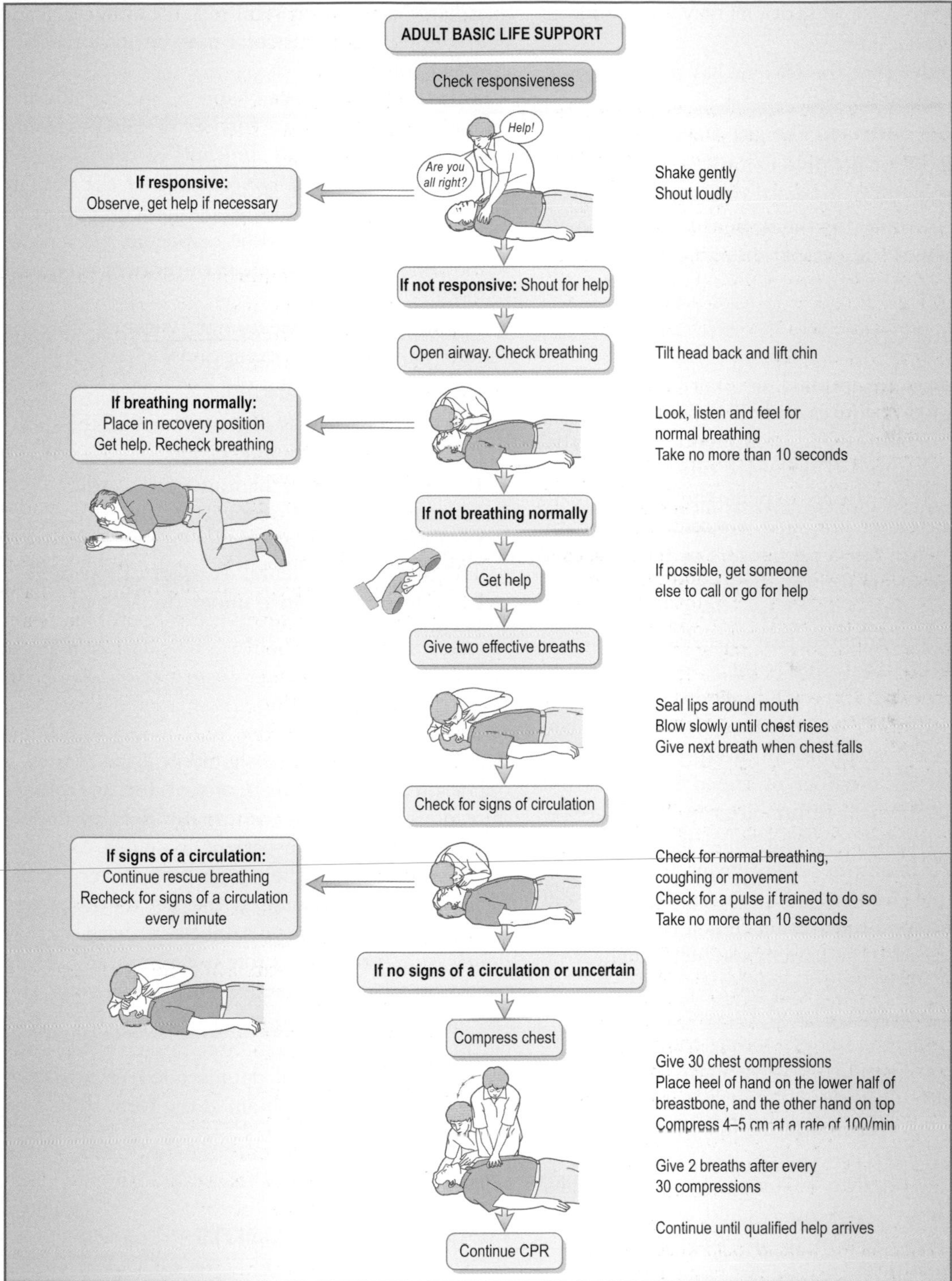

Figure 13.6 • Procedure for adult basic life support and CPR. (Reproduced with kind permission from the Resuscitation Council 2006.)

- A reminder that the patient may change his mind at any time.
- A reminder that the patient has the right to a second opinion.
- Details of costs and charges if applicable.
- A reminder of possible complications, disfigurement, or removal of parts.
- An opportunity for the patient to ask any questions of the person obtaining consent.

Obtaining consent

Consent may be implied or expressed. For the majority of procedures and treatments, including nursing procedures and treatments, only verbal consent is required. The golden rule before taking any action is to always explain the procedure to the patient/client. Implied consent may be by offering an arm for venepuncture or taking up the required position for the treatment, and this is taken that consent has been given. However, it should be remembered that this does not necessarily indicate that the patient has understood what is proposed. Expressed consent is that which is confirmed orally or in writing. If there are language difficulties, an official interpreter should be used. A family member or friend who does not understand medical terminology is not an appropriate interpreter. Certain religious beliefs may have an effect on the patient giving their consent, for example Jehovah's Witnesses, who do not agree with blood transfusions. Such issues need to be explored with the patient and help sought from one of their leaders if necessary.

A child between 13 and 16 years who is alone and has sufficient understanding may consent to an examination or to treatment by a doctor or other health professional, but not to a surgical procedure or anaesthetic. A full note should be made of the factors taken into account when assessing the child to be knowledgeable and their capacity to give consent. A child over the age of 16 years may consent to any surgical, dental or medical treatment.

For those patients who are unconscious or not considered to be 'responsible', a parent or guardian's signature is required. If neither is available, the duty administrator may be authorized to give the consent.

Refusal to consent can happen, and initially the patient should receive a further detailed explanation (preferably by the clinician) of the proposed treatment and why it is necessary. If the patient still refuses to agree and is deemed competent to do so, the refusal should be respected and a note, witnessed if possible, made in the patient's medical records.

Examination or treatment without consent should only occur in exceptional circumstances, for example:

- When the patient is unconscious and the procedure would be life-saving.
- In some cases when the minor is a ward of court and the court decides that the treatment would be in the child's best interests.
- Treatment for a mental disorder of a patient liable to be a detainee under the Mental Health Act 1983.

Consent form

A different consent form should be signed for each operation or procedure. Consent for one procedure does not give any automatic right to undertake any other. If the patient is unable to write, an 'X' to indicate their signature is acceptable if there are two signed witnesses to the mark. For those with learning disabilities or with sensory deprivation, the nurse's role is essential in helping the patient to understand what is happening. The use of visual aids and drawings can be effective in getting the message across. Standard consent forms should be used and all details filled in correctly. Once the signature is obtained the form should be filed in the patient's notes.

Reporting concerns

National and local mechanisms are in place in all health and social care organizations to ensure that practice is safe and limitations are recognized. In addition to promoting continuing professional development, recent policy developments have encouraged the use of competency frameworks and personal development plans for all NHS staff. Many other employers have similar procedures. These initiatives help both individuals and their employing organizations to judge the level of support a practitioner requires in order to practise safely, and to identify their learning needs and, by implication, their limitations.

'Speaking out' policies are now in place in many NHS trusts and other health and social care employing agencies. Supported through the implementation of clinical governance, individuals are encouraged to bring to the attention of the organization their concerns about practitioners who are underperforming or, frankly, performing dangerously or harmfully to patients or the organization. Together with clinical incident and 'near-miss' reporting, this initiative is designed to ensure that action is taken promptly to prevent unsafe practice. Associated with the success of these developments, is the presence of a 'no blame' culture, in which learning and improvement rather than reprisal is the focus, a culture which is also expected to make acknowledging our limitations a little easier.

NHS organizations are also required to have anti-fraud policies in place and to have a designated fraud officer in post. Part of reporting concerns includes reporting fraud or suspected fraud within the workplace. Although this will rarely affect the quality of patient care directly, unless patient property is the subject of the fraudulent act, it is important in relation to the honesty and integrity of the institution and the staff within it.

A particularly important area for reporting concern is when a nurse, or other professional, has noticed possible non-accidental injury of patients. While this is a particular issue in paediatric care (see Section One), it may also be seen in other client groups, particularly the elderly or mentally frail. Employers will have policies and procedures to follow when these things are suspected and student nurses should become familiar with them.

Concluding remarks

This chapter has introduced some important nursing activities which, if applied, will promote the safety of yourself, those you care for, their carers and other colleagues. Do not underestimate the importance of learning these key skills. Other nurses using these skills well, combined with a good underpinning knowledge, make a real difference to patient outcomes. Although you are not likely to be saving lives every day, you will be making a significant contribution to improving lives.

If in doubt about any area of your practice, ask; if you are worried, express your concerns. Learn to use all your senses. In this way, you will learn the skills that many of your mentors demonstrate with ease.

References

Alexander MF, Fawcett JN, Runciman PJ 2006 Nursing practice, 3rd edn. Churchill Livingstone, Edinburgh

Barrie D 1996 The provision of food and catering services in hospital. Journal of Hospital Infection 33:13–33

Chadwick C, Oppenheim BA 1996 Cleaning as a cost effective method of infection control. Lancet 347:1776

Collins BJ 1988 The hospital environment: how clean should it be? Journal of Hospital Infection 11(suppl A):53–56

Department of Health 1990 Food handler's guide. HMSO, London

Department of Health 2001 Better hospital food. HMSO, London. Online. Available: http://www.dh.gov.uk/PolicyAndGuidance/OrganisationPolicy/HealthcareEnvironment 3 Jan 2006

Department of Health 1998 A first class service: quality in the new NHS. Stationery Office, London

Department of Health 2005 Saving lives: a delivery programme to reduce healthcare associated infection (HCAI) including MRSA. Department of Health, London

Great Britain Parliament 1974 Health and safety at work etc. act 1974. HMSO, London

Great Britain Parliament 1992 The manual handling operations regulations statutory instrument 1992, no. 2793. HMSO, London

Great Britain Parliament 1995 Food safety (general food hygiene) regulations. Stationery Office, London

Health and Safety Executive 1998 Manual handling operations regulations 1992. Guidance on regulations, 2nd edn. HSE Books, Sudbury

House of Commons Committee of Public Accounts 2005 HC 554 incorporating HC 1044-i, session 2003–04. Stationery Office, London

House of Lords Select Committee on Science and Technology 1998 Resistance to antibiotics and other antimicrobial agents. Stationery Office, London

Kitchiner D, Bundred P 1998 Integrated care pathways increase use of guidelines. British Medical Journal 317:147

Maxwell RJ 1984 Quality assessment in health. British Medical Journal 288:470–471

Medical Devices Agency 1996 Sterilisation, disinfection and cleaning of medical devices and equipment. Guidance from Microbiology Advisory Committee to the Department of Health Medical Device Agency. Part 2: Protocols. HMSO, London

National Audit Office 2003 A safer place to work. Stationery Office, London

National Health Services Litigation Authority 2006 About the NHS Litigation Authority. Online. Available: http://www.nhsla.com/home.htm 3 Jan 2006

National Health Services Management Executive (NHSME) 1996 Clinical guidelines: using clinical guidelines to improve care within the NHS. Department of Health, Leeds

Nicholls S, Cullen R, O'Neill S et al 2000 Clinical governance: its origins and foundations. British Journal of Clinical Governance 5(3):172–178

Nicol M, Bavin C, Bedford-Turner S et al 2000 Essential nursing skills. Mosby, London

Nightingale F 1859 Notes on hospitals. Longman, London

Nightingale F 2001 http:chatna.com/author/nightingaleflorence.htm

Nursing and Midwifery Council 2000 Guidelines for the administration of medicines. NMC, London

Nursing and Midwifery Council 2008 Code of professional conduct. NMC, London

Øvretveit J 1992 Health service quality: an introduction to quality methods for health services. Blackwell Scientific, London

Parker LJ 1999 Managing and maintaining a safe environment in the hospital setting. British Journal of Nursing 8(16):1053–1066

Resuscitation Council (UK) 2005 Resuscitation guidelines 2005. Resuscitation Council (UK), London

Standing Medical Advisory Committee (SMAC) 1998 Sub-group on antimicrobial resistance: the path of least resistance. Department of Health, London

Storr J, Topley K, Privett S 2005 The ward nurse's role in infection control 19(41), 56–64

van den Berghe G, Wouters PJ, Bouillon R et al 2003 Outcome benefit of intensive insulin therapy in the critically ill: Insulin dose versus glycemic control. Critical Care Medicine 31:359–366

Waterlow J 1991 A policy that protects. The Waterlow pressure sore prevention/treatment policy. Professional Nurse 6(5):258, 260, 262–264

Wiggans T, Turner G 1991 Breaking down the walls. Total Quality Management 3(3):183–186

Wright K 2005 Unsupervised medication administration by nursing students. Nursing Standard 19(39):49–54

Further reading

Backcare 2003 Back care at work. Backcare, London

This publication is not written specifically for people working in health care but is aimed at anyone who lifts, moves or stores objects in order that they can do so without causing injury to themselves or others.

Backcare and Royal College of Nursing 1998 The guide to the handling of patients, 4th edn (revised). Backcare, London

Prepared with nurses for nurses and provides a definitive guide to safe lifting, moving and handling of patients to minimize the risk of injury to both patients and nurses.

Nicol M, Bavin C, Bedford-Turner S, Cronin, P, Rawlins-Anderson K, 2000 Essential nursing skills. Mosby, London

Written to help student nurses carry out clinical skills safely. It uses a step-by-step approach to over 100 essential skills of foundation nursing care. Its emphasis is on the care carried out in the general nursing setting but all common foundation students should find it helpful in the early stages of training.

Resuscitation Council (UK) 2005 Resuscitation guidelines 2005. Resuscitation Council (UK), London

This is a full procedure manual for basic life support care and covers the theory and practice in lively and accessible language. Used widely in accident and emergency departments, the ambulance services and all areas where life-saving procedures are carried out. Resuscitation guidelines are available online at the Resuscitation Council (UK) website: http://www.resus.org.uk

Royal College of Nursing 1996 Code of practice for patient handling. RCN, London

Guidelines and associated safety procedures for all aspects of patient handling. Written from a health and safety perspective for the prevention of back injury to nurses.

Skinner S 1996 Understanding clinical investigations. Baillière Tindall, London

Provides information about the rationale and procedure for all major observations carried out on patients.

Snowley G, Nicklin P, Birch J 1992 Objectives for care: specifying standards for clinical nursing, 2nd edn. Wolfe, London

Emphasizes the systematic approach to nursing care and embraces all care groups and care settings. Written to provide a link between theory and practice; links in with available research and accompanied by detailed bibliographies.

Appendix

NMC outcomes for entry to branch programme

Domain	Outcome
1. Professional & ethical practice	
1.1	Discuss in an informed manner, the implications of professional regulation for nursing practice: • demonstrate a basic knowledge of professional regulation and self regulation • recognise and acknowledge the limitations of one's own abilities • recognise situations which require referral to a registered practitioner.
1.2	Demonstrate an awareness of the NMC Code of professional conduct: • commit to the principle that the primary purpose of the registered nurse is to protect and serve society • accept responsibility for one's own actions and decisions.
1.3	Demonstrate an awareness of, and apply ethical principles to, nursing practice: • demonstrate respect for patient and client confidentiality • identify ethical issues in day to day practice.
1.4	Demonstrate an awareness of legislation relevant to nursing practice: • identify key issues in relevant legislation relating to mental health, children, data protection, manual handling, and health & safety etc.
1.5	Demonstrate the importance of promoting equity in patient/client care by contributing to nursing care in a fair and anti-discriminatory way: • demonstrate fairness and sensitivity when responding to patients, clients and groups from diverse circumstances • recognise the needs of patients and clients whose lives are affected by disability, however manifest.

(Cont'd)

Domain	Outcome
2. Care delivery	
2.1	Discuss methods of, barriers to and the boundaries of effective communication and interpersonal relationships: • recognise the effect of one's own values on interactions with patients and clients and their carers, families and friends • utilise appropriate communication skills with patients and clients • acknowledge the boundaries of a professional caring relationship.
2.2	Demonstrate sensitivity when interacting with and providing information to patients and clients.
2.3	Contribute to enhancing the health and social well-being of patients and clients by understanding how, under the supervision of a registered practitioner, to: • contribute to the assessment of health needs • identify opportunities for health promotion • identify networks of health and social care services.
2.4	Contribute to the development and documentation of nursing assessments by participating in comprehensive and systematic nursing assessment of the physical, psychological, social and spiritual needs of patients and clients: • be aware of assessment strategies to guide the collection of data for assessing patients and clients and use assessment tools under guidance • discuss the prioritisation of care needs • be aware of the need to reassess patients and clients as to their needs for nursing care.
2.5	Contribute to the planning of nursing care, involving patients and clients and, where possible, their carers, demonstrating an understanding of helping patients and clients to make informed decisions: • identify care needs based on the assessment of a patient or client • participate in the negotiation and agreement of the care plan with the patient or client and with their carer, family or friends, as appropriate, under the supervision of a registered nurse • inform patients and clients about intended nursing actions, respecting their right to participate in decisions about their care.
2.6	Contribute to the implementation of a programme of nursing care, designed and supervised by registered practitioners: • undertake activities which are consistent with the plan of care and within the limits of one's own abilities.
2.7	Demonstrate evidence of a developing knowledge base that underpins safe nursing practice: • access and discuss research and other evidence in nursing and related disciplines • identify examples of the use of evidence in planned nursing interventions.
2.8	Demonstrate a range of essential nursing skills, under the supervision of a registered nurse, to meet individuals' needs, which include: • maintaining dignity, privacy and confidentiality • effective observational and communication skills, include listening and taking physiological measurements • safety and health, including moving and handling and infection control; essential first aid and emergency procedures • administration of medicines • emotional, physical and personal care, including meeting the need for comfort, nutrition and personal hygiene.

(Cont'd)

Domain	Outcome
2.9	Contribute to the evaluation of the appropriateness of nursing care delivered: • demonstrate an awareness of the need to assess regularly a patient's or client's response to nursing interventions • provide for a supervising registered practitioner, evaluative commentary and information on nursing care based on personal observations and actions • contribute to the documentation of the outcomes of nursing interventions.
2.10	Recognise situations in which agreed plans of nursing care no longer appear appropriate and refer these to an appropriate accountable practitioner: • demonstrate the ability to discuss and accept care decisions • accurately record observations made and communicate these to the relevant members of the health and social care team.
3. Care management	
3.1	Contribute to the identification of actual and potential risks to patients, clients and their carers, to oneself and to others and participate in measures to promote and ensure health and safety: • understand and implement health and safety principles and policies • recognise and report situations which are potentially unsafe for patients, clients, oneself and others.
3.2	Demonstrate an understanding of the role of others by participating in interprofessional working practice: • identify the roles of the members of the health and social care team • work within the health and social care team to maintain and enhance integrated care.
3.3	Demonstrate literacy, numeracy and computer skills needed to record, enter, store, retrieve and organise data essential for care delivery.
4. Personal & professional development	
4.1	Demonstrate responsibility for one's own learning through the development of a portfolio of practice and recognise when further learning may be required: • identify specific learning needs and objectives • begin to engage with, and interpret, the evidence base which underpins nursing practice.
4.2	Acknowledge the importance of seeking supervision to develop safe nursing practice: • identify the roles of the members of the health and social care team • work within the health and social care team to maintain and enhance integrated care.

Index

C

D

E

H

M

O

P

Q

R

S

T

U

V

W

Z